Urologic Laparoscopy

SAKTI DAS, M.D.
Chief of Urology
Kaiser Permanente Medical Center
Walnut Creek, California

E. DAVID CRAWFORD, M.D.
Chairman, Department of Urology
University of Colorado
School of Medicine
Denver, Colorado

W.B. SAUNDERS COMPANY
A Division of Harcourt Brace & Company
Philadelphia ▲ London ▲ Toronto ▲ Montreal ▲ Sydney ▲ Tokyo

W.B. Saunders Company
A Division of Harcourt Brace & Company

The Curtis Center
Independence Square West
Philadelphia, Pennsylvania 19106

Library of Congress Cataloging-in-Publication Data

Urologic Laparoscopy / [edited by] Sakti Das, E. David Crawford.
p. cm.
ISBN 0-7216-3766-3
1. Genitourinary organs—Endoscopic surgery. 2. Laparoscopic surgery. I. Das, Sakti. II. Crawford, E. David.
[DNLM: 1. Urologic Diseases—surgery. 2. Urogenital Diseases—surgery. 3. Surgery, Laparoscopic—methods. 4. Laparoscopy—instrumentation. 5. Laparoscopy—methods. WJ 168 L2992 1994]
RD571.L3583 1994
617.4′6059—dc20
DNLM/DLC 93-47167

Urologic Laparoscopy ISBN 0-7216-3766-3

Printed in the United States of America.

Last digit is the print number: 9 8 7 6 5 4 3 2 1

Urologic

Laparoscopy

TO
Raja
and
Michael, Marc, and Ryan—
our pride and joy

Contributors

David M. Albala, M.D.
Assistant Professor of Urology, Loyola University Medical Center, Stritch School of Medicine, Maywood, Illinois; Staff Urologist, Hines Veterans Administration Hospital, Hines, Illinois
Laparoscopic Ureteral Surgery

Peter S. Albert, M.D., F.A.C.S.
Assistant Professor of Urology, SUNY Health Science Center at Brooklyn, Brooklyn, New York; Director, Urology, Staten Island University Hospital, Staten Island, New York
Extraperitoneal Endoscopic Surgery for Benign Renal Cysts; Extraperitoneal Endoscopic Gasless Pelvic Lymph Node Dissection

Ermanno Ancona, M.D.
Professor of Surgery, Medical School, University of Padova, Padova, Italy; Chairman, Institute of General Surgery II, University of Padova, Padova, Italy
Laparoscopic Treatment of Lymphoceles

Gopal H. Badlani, M.D., F.A.C.S.
Associate Professor in Urology, Albert Einstein College of Medicine, Bronx, New York; Associate Chairman, Department of Urology, Long Island Jewish Medical Center, New Hyde Park, New York
Laparoscopic Entry and Exit

David W. Bowyer, M.D.
Staff Urologist, Kaiser Permanente Medical Center, Vallejo, California
Laparoscopic Suturing: Principles and Techniques

Paramjit S. Chandhoke, M.D., Ph.D.
Assistant Professor of Surgery and Medicine and Chief, Endourology and Kidney Stone Disease, University of Colorado Health Sciences Center, Denver, Colorado
Laparoscopic Complications and Management

R. V. Clayman, M.D.
Professor of Urologic Surgery and Radiology, Washington University School of Medicine, St. Louis, Missouri; Attending Staff, Washington University School of Medicine at Barnes Affiliated Hospitals, St. Louis, Missouri
Laparoscopic Nephrectomy, Nephroureterectomy, and Partial Nephrectomy

E. David Crawford, M.D.
Chairman, Department of Urology, University of Colorado, School of Medicine, Denver, Colorado
Laparoscopic Retroperitoneal Lymph Node Dissection

Sakti Das, M.D.
Chief of Urology, Kaiser Permanente Medical Center, Walnut Creek, California
History of Laparoscopy; Laparoscopic Procedures in Pediatric Urology; Retroperitoneoscopy; Laparoscopic Extraperitoneal Pelvic Lymphadenectomy; Laparoscopic Reconstructive Surgery of the Urinary Bladder

Sandro Cassiano Esteves, M.D.
Resident Doctor, Division of Urology, University of Campinas Medical Center, Sao Paulo, Brazil
Laparoscopy in the Management of Intersex States

Ubirajara Ferreira, M.D.
Associate Professor, Division of Urology, University of Campinas Medical Center, Sao Paulo, Brazil
Laparoscopy in the Management of Intersex States

George Ferzli, M.D., F.A.C.S.
Associate Professor of Surgery, SUNY Health Science Center at Brooklyn, Brooklyn, New York; Director, Laparoendoscopic Surgery, Staten Island University Hospital, Staten Island, New York
Extraperitoneal Endoscopic Surgery for Benign Renal Cysts; Extraperitoneal Endoscopic Gasless Pelvic Lymph Node Dissection

Inderbir S. Gill, M.D., M.Ch.
Senior Resident, Division of Urology, Department of Surgery, University of Kentucky Chandler Medical Center, Lexington, Kentucky
Laparoscopic Reconstructive Surgery of the Urinary Bladder

Paul G. Hagood, M.D.
Chief Resident, Department of Surgery, Division of Urology, St. Louis University School of Medicine, St. Louis, Missouri; St. Louis University Medical Center, St. Louis, Missouri
Laparoscopic Varicocelectomy; Laparoscopic Cystectomy

Lawrence S. Hakim, M.D.
Chief Resident Urology, SUNY Health Science Center at Brooklyn, Brooklyn, New York
Extraperitoneal Endoscopic Surgery for Benign Renal Cysts; Extraperitoneal Endoscopic Gasless Pelvic Lymph Node Dissection

Diane M. Hartman, M.D.
Chief Resident, Genitourologic Surgery, University of Colorado Health Science Center, Denver, Colorado
Laparoscopic Complications and Management

Shinji Kageyama, M.D.
Fellow, Department of Urology, Hamamatsu University School of Medicine, Hamamatsu, Japan; Staff Urologist, University Hospital, Hamamatsu University School of Medicine, Hamamatsu, Japan
Laparoscopic Surgery for Adrenal Tumors

Louis R. Kavoussi, M.D.
Associate Professor of Urologic Surgery, The Johns Hopkins School of Medicine, Baltimore, Maryland; Chief of Urology, Johns Hopkins Bayview Hospital and Director of Endourology, Brady Urologic Institute, The Johns Hopkins Hospital, Baltimore, Maryland
Anatomic Perspectives During Laparoscopy; Laparoscopic Ureteral Surgery

Kazuki Kawabe, M.D.
Professor and Chairman, Department of Urology, Faculty of Medicine, The University of Tokyo, Tokyo, Japan; Urologist in Chief, University Hospital, Faculty of Medicine, The University of Tokyo, Tokyo, Japan
Laparoscopic Surgery for Adrenal Tumors

John J. Keizur, M.D.
Chief Resident in Urology, Oaknoll Naval Regional Hospital, Oakland, California
Retroperitoneoscopy

Mike Kozminski, M.D., F.A.C.S.
Private Practice, Phoenix Urology of St. Joseph, St. Joseph, Missouri
Laparoscopic Ureteroileocutaneous Urinary Diversion

Roger K. Low, M.D.
Chief Resident, Department of Urology, University of California at Davis, Sacramento, California
Laparoscopic Clipping and Stapling Techniques

Elspeth M. McDougall, M.D.
Assistant Professor of Urology, Division of Urologic Surgery, Washington University School of Medicine, St. Louis, Missouri; Attending Staff, Barnes Affiliate Hospitals, St. Louis, Missouri
Laparoscopic Nephrectomy, Nephroureterectomy, and Partial Nephrectomy; Laparoscopic Reconstructive Surgery of the Urinary Bladder

Terri G. Monk, M.D.
Assistant Professor, Department of Anesthesiology, Washington University School of Medicine, St. Louis, Missouri; Attending Staff, Barnes Hospital, St. Louis, Missouri
Anesthetic Considerations for Laparoscopic Urology

Michael E. Moran, M.D.
Clinical Assistant Professor of Urology, Albany Medical Center, Albany, New York; Attending Staff, Albany Medical Center and St. Peter's Hospital, Albany, New York
Laparoscopic Operating Room Setup, and Patient and Instrument Preparation; Laparoscopic Equipment and Instruments; Laparoscopic Clipping and Stapling Techniques; Future Perspectives in Laparoscopy

Nelson Rodrigues Netto, Jr., M.D.
Professor and Chairman, Division of Urology, University of Campinas Medical Center, Sao Paulo, Brazil
Laparoscopy in the Management of Intersex States

Raul C. Ordorica, M.D.
Assistant Professor, Division of Urology, Brown University, Providence, Rhode Island; Assistant Professor, Department of Urology, Rhode Island Hospital, Providence, Rhode Island
History of Laparoscopy; Laparoscopic Operating Room Setup, and Patient and Instrument Preparation; Laparoscopic Equipment and Instruments

Gary S. Oshinsky, M.D.
Chief Resident in Urology, Long Island Jewish Medical Center, New Hyde Park, New York
Laparoscopic Entry and Exit

Raul O. Parra, M.D., F.A.C.S.
Professor of Surgery and Chief, Division of Urology, St. Louis University School of Medicine, St. Louis, Missouri; Attending Staff, St. Louis University Medical Center, St. Louis, Missouri
Laparoscopic Varicocelectomy; Laparoscopic Cystectomy

Craig A. Peters, M.D.
Assistant Professor in Urologic Surgery, Harvard Medical School, Boston, Massachusetts; Staff Urologist, Boston Children's Hospital, and Consultant Urologist, Brigham and Women's Hospital, Boston, Massachusetts
Anatomic Perspectives During Laparoscopy

Adley Raboy, M.D.
Assistant Professor of Urology, SUNY Health Science Center at Brooklyn, Brooklyn, New York; Associate Director Urology, Staten Island University Hospital, Staten Island, New York
Extraperitoneal Endoscopic Surgery for Benign Renal Cysts; Extraperitoneal Endoscopic Gasless Pelvic Lymph Node Dissection

Paolo Rigotti, M.D.
Assistant Professor of Surgery, Medical School, University of Padova, Padova, Italy; Assistant Professor of Surgery, Institute of General Surgery II, University of Padova, Padova, Italy
Laparoscopic Treatment of Lymphoceles

Leslie A. Sharpe, M.D., F.A.C.O.G.
Clinical Associate Professor, Obstetrics and Gynecology, University of Minnesota, Minneapolis, Minnesota; Active Staff, Fairview Riverside Medical Center, Minneapolis, Minnesota; Courtesy Staff, Fairview Southdale Hospital, Minneapolis, Minnesota
Laparoscopic Intracorporeal and Extracorporeal Suturing

Irwin B. Simon, M.D., F.A.C.S.
Assistant Clinical Professor of Surgery, University of Nevada School of Medicine, Las Vegas, Nevada
Virtual Reality, Robotics, and Surgery in the Twenty-First Century

Arthur D. Smith, M.D., F.A.C.S.
Professor and Chairman, Long Island Campus for Albert Einstein College of Medicine, Bronx, New York; Chairman of Urology, Long Island Jewish Medical Center, New Hyde Park, New York
Laparoscopic Entry and Exit

Marshall L. Stoller, M.D.
Assistant Professor, Department of Urology, University of California School of Medicine, San Francisco, California; Attending Staff, Moffitt Hospital and San Francisco General Hospital, San Francisco, California
Physiologic Considerations in Laparoscopy

Kazuo Suzuki, M.D.
Associate Professor, Department of Urology, Hamamatsu University School of Medicine, Hamamatsu, Japan; Associate Chief of Urology, University Hospital, Hamamatsu University School of Medicine, Hamamatsu, Japan
Laparoscopic Surgery for Adrenal Tumors

Zoltan Szabo, Ph.D., F.I.C.S.
Director, Microsurgery and Operative Endoscopy Training (MOET) Institute, San Francisco, California; Associate Director, Videoscopic Surgery Training Center, Department of Surgery, University of California, School of Medicine, San Francisco, California
Laparoscopic Suturing: Principles and Techniques

Miles Tashima, M.D.
Staff Urologist, Department of Urology, Kaiser Permanente Medical Center, Walnut Creek, California
Laparoscopic Extraperitoneal Pelvic Lymphadenectomy

Raju Thomas, M.D., F.A.C.S.
Professor, Department of Urology, Tulane University School of Medicine, New Orleans, Louisiana; Attending Staff, Tulane University Medical Center, New Orleans, Louisiana
Laparoscopic Pelvic Lymphadenectomy

Daisuke Ueda, M.D.
Fellow, Department of Urology, Hamamatsu University School of Medicine, Hamamatsu, Japan; Staff Urologist, University Hospital, Hamamatsu University School of Medicine, Hamamatsu, Japan
Laparoscopic Surgery for Adrenal Tumors

Tomomi Ushiyama, M.D.
Assistant Professor, Department of Urology, Hamamatsu University School of Medicine, Hamamatsu, Japan; Attending Urologist, University Hospital, Hamamatsu University School of Medicine, Hamamatsu, Japan
Laparoscopic Surgery for Adrenal Tumors

Cliff Vestal, M.D.
Fellow, Division of Urology, University of Colorado, Denver, Colorado; Attending Staff, Phoenixville Hospital, Phoenixville, Pennsylvania; Valley Forge Urological Associates, Valley Forge, Pennsylvania
Laparoscopic Retroperitoneal Lymph Node Dissection

B. Craig Weldon, M.D.
Departments of Anesthesiology and Pediatrics, St. John's Mercy Medical Center, St. Louis, Missouri
Anesthetic Considerations for Laparoscopic Urology

J. Stuart Wolf, Jr., M.D.
Chief Resident in Urology, University of California School of Medicine, San Francisco, California
Physiologic Considerations in Laparoscopy

Preface

During the last decade there has been an explosion of minimally invasive techniques in urology. This has led to the rapid development of novel procedures that reduce iatrogenic trauma without compromising therapeutic outcomes. Percutaneous and transurethral endoscopic procedures in concert with technologic advances in use of imaging, laser, shock wave, ultrasonics, hyperthermia treatment, and the like are systematically eliminating open operation from surgical repertoire. Presently, the most revolutionary endeavor in this spiraling trend is laparoscopy. Pioneering works by Semm in gynecologic laparoscopy and by Dubois, Perissat, and Reddick in endoscopic cholecystectomy have paved the way for renascence of laparoscopy in urology.

The original development of laparoscopy at the beginning of this century necessitated the use of Nitze's urologic cystoscope. It is ironic that despite urologists' endoscopic heritage, our real interest in using laparoscopic techniques in urology was kindled only after the publicized excellence of the general surgeons in laparoscopic cholecystectomy. Thus initiated, the impetus for laparoscopic urology now continues to be fueled both by the publicity and by the demand from patients for this minimally invasive surgery. Starting from diagnostic laparoscopy for nonpalpable testes, laparoscopy has now encompassed all extirpative surgeries and most of the reparative and reconstructive surgeries in urology. There is no doubt that laparoscopic surgeries are exacting; they are also in a continuous state of evolution, aided by developments in video imaging and instrument technologies. New indications, procedures, and improvements are being reported nearly every day. But popular acceptance of laparoscopy in urologic practice can come only from the acquisition of skill and dexterity, the following of established principles and practices, and the continued upgrading of the available information in new developments.

In this text, we have culled internationally recognized stalwarts in laparoscopic urology to provide their practical and detailed insights into the various laparoscopic procedures, some of which are established while others are evolving. The book begins with homage to the historical beginnings of endoscopy in general and laparoscopy in particular. Practical and helpful chapters on laparoscopic instrumentation and setup are followed by narrative chapters on particular surgical procedures. Finally, the text culminates with two philosophic chapters on future perspectives and the potential shape of minimally invasive surgery in the coming century.

The ubiquitous impact of laparoscopy is very much perceptible in our urologic practice. Avoidance of disfigurement from large open incisions, reduction of postoperative morbidity and pain, and quicker recovery, allowing earlier resumption of productive vocations, are all significant benefits attributed to laparoscopy that are affecting the therapeutic decisions of our patients. Admittedly, laparoscopic surgery is difficult and time consuming and has a steep learning curve, but as the feasibility and benefits of these new procedures become established, it behooves us to provide our patients with those procedures that are minimally invasive as well as maximally effective. To that end, we hope that the contributions assembled in this text will help our interested colleagues in their journeys toward the challenging and rewarding therapeutic techniques of laparoscopy.

"Sometimes one should consider crossing the line of convention."

Robert Fulghum

SAKTI DAS
E. DAVID CRAWFORD

Contents

Color Plates

Plate 1

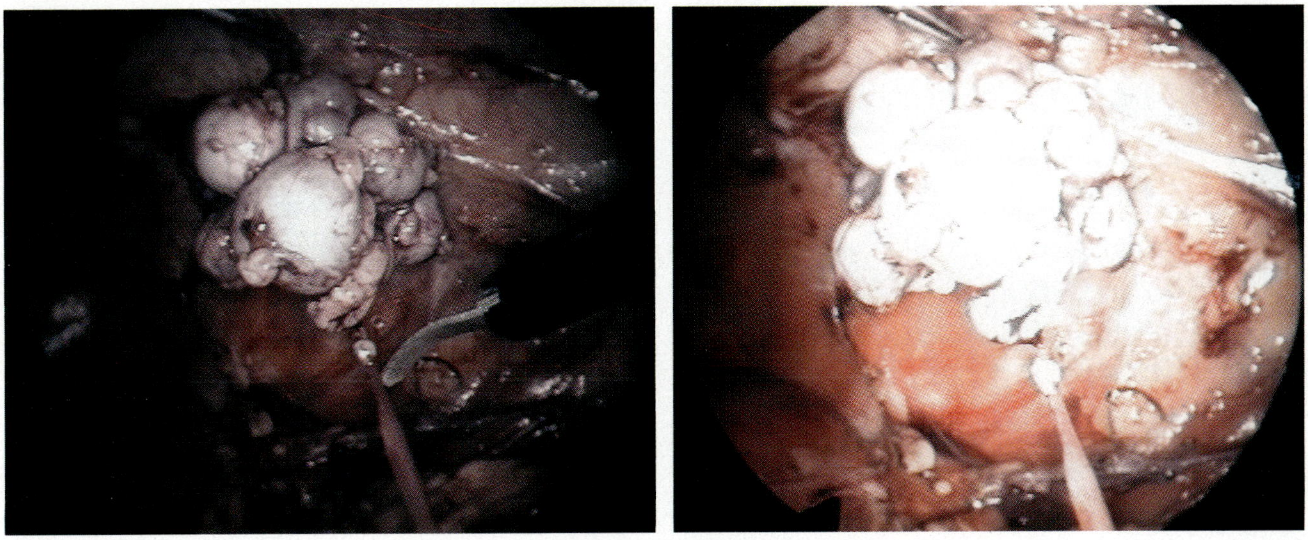

A B

Figure 3–3

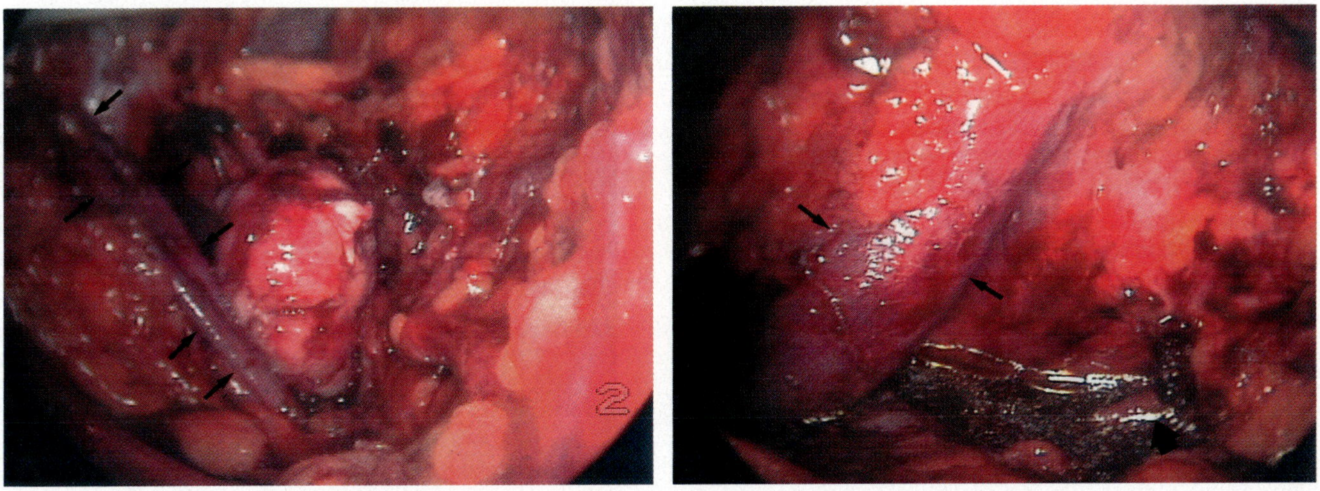

A B

Figure 3–5

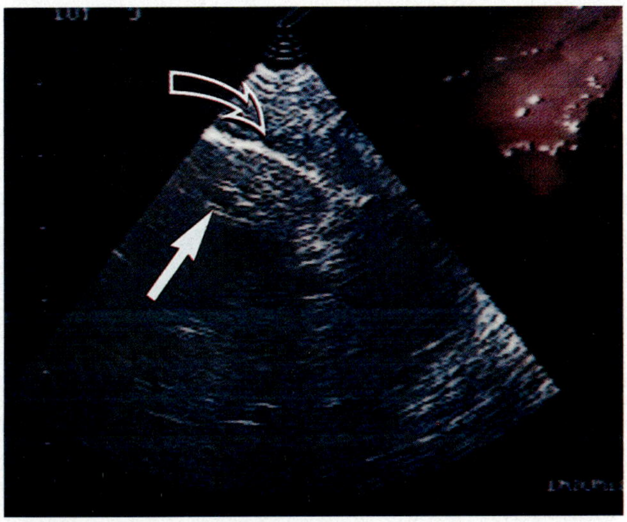

Figure 3–8

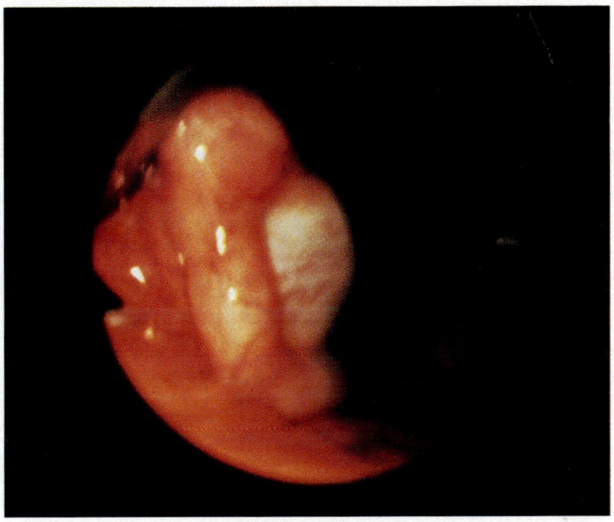

Figure 8–1

Plate 2

Figure 8–2

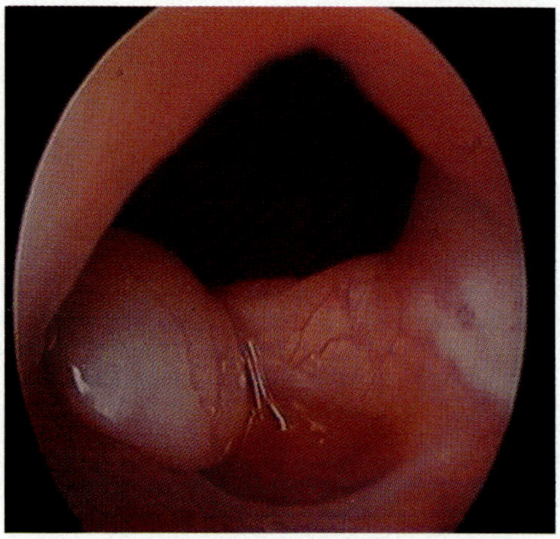

Figure 8–3

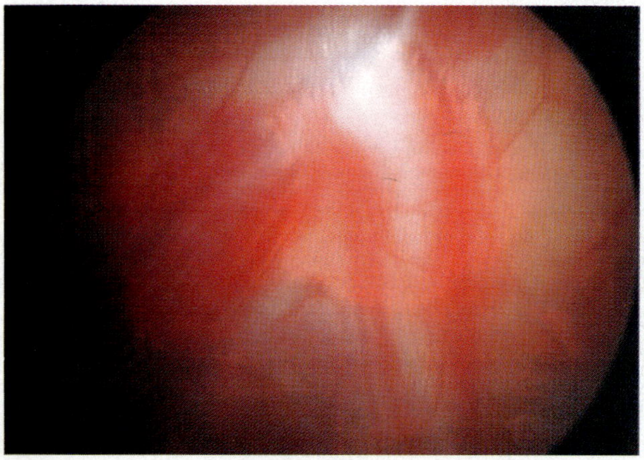

Figure 8–4

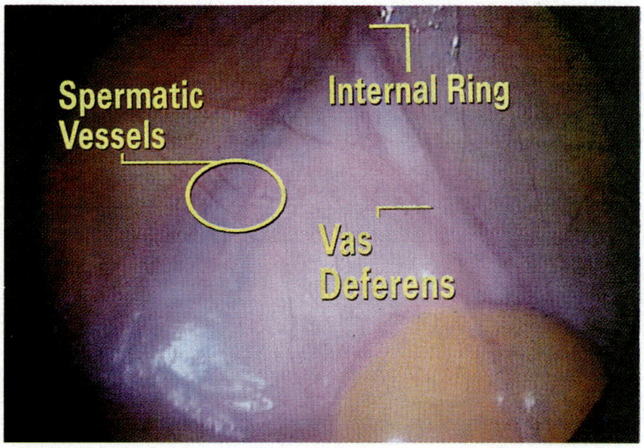

Figure 10–1

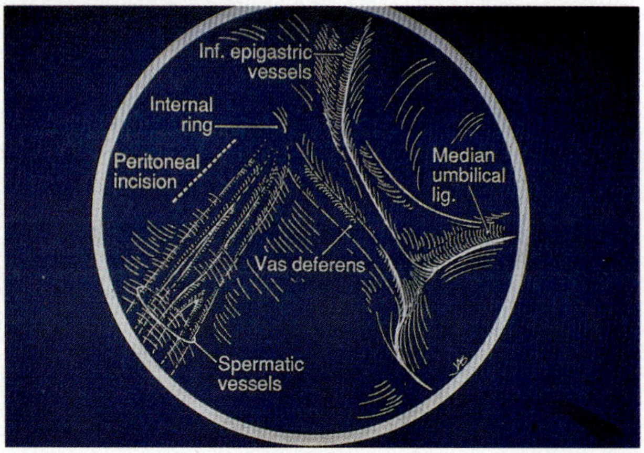

Figure 10–2

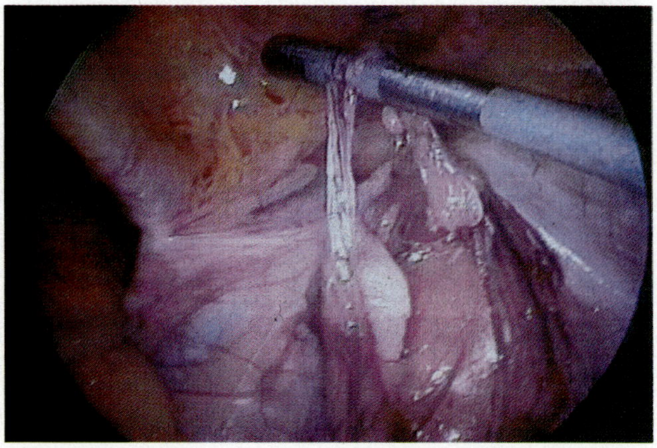

Figure 10–3

Plate 3

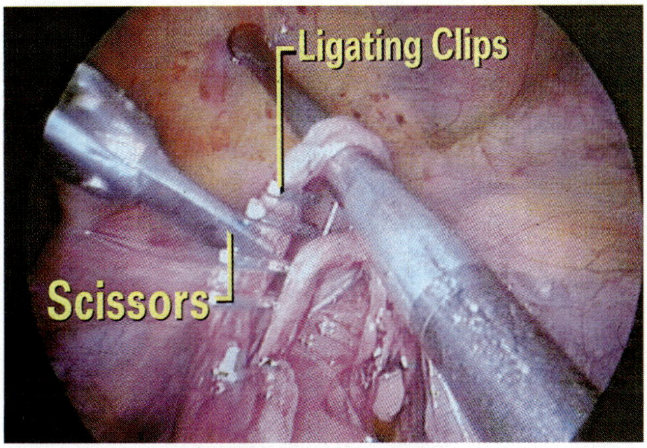

Figure 10–4

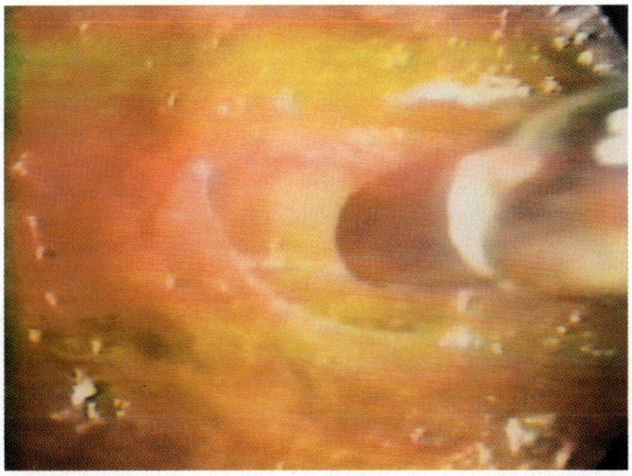

Figure 12–1

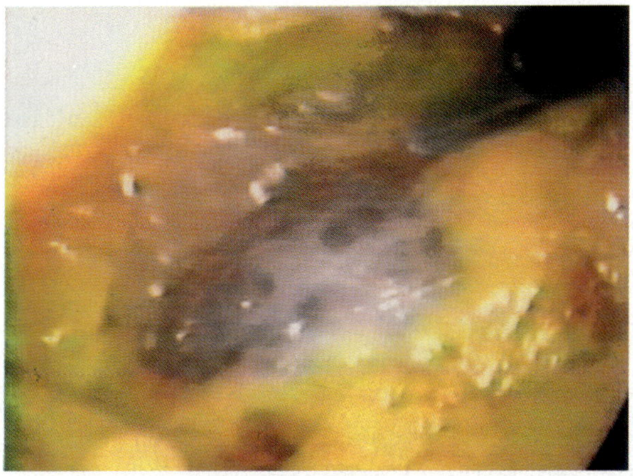

Figure 12–2

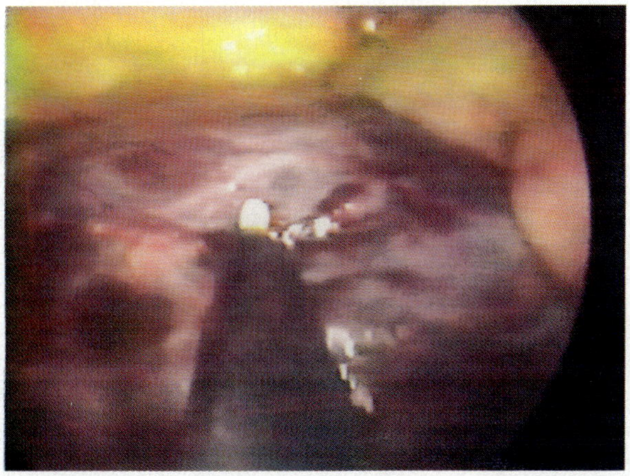

Figure 12–3

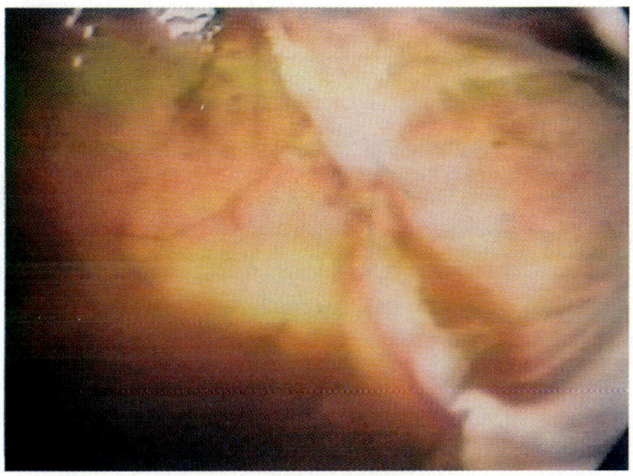

Figure 12–4

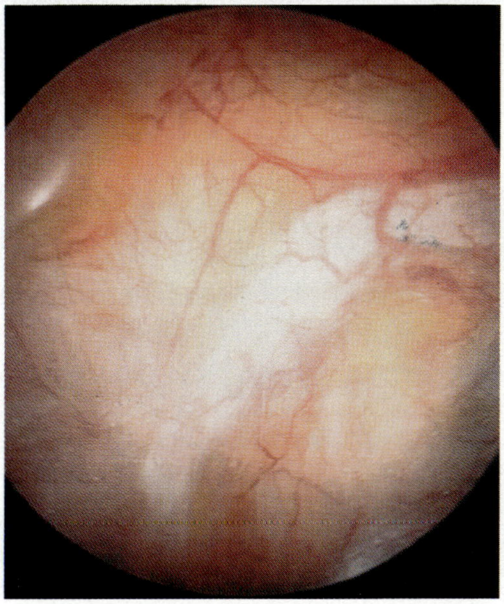

Figure 14–2

Plate 4

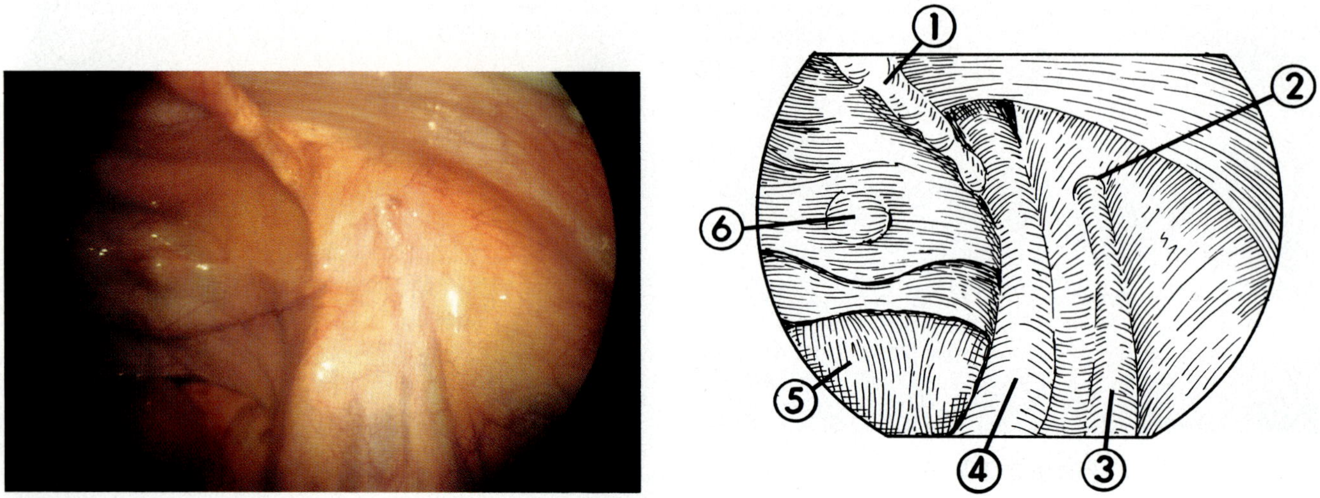

A B

Figure 15–2

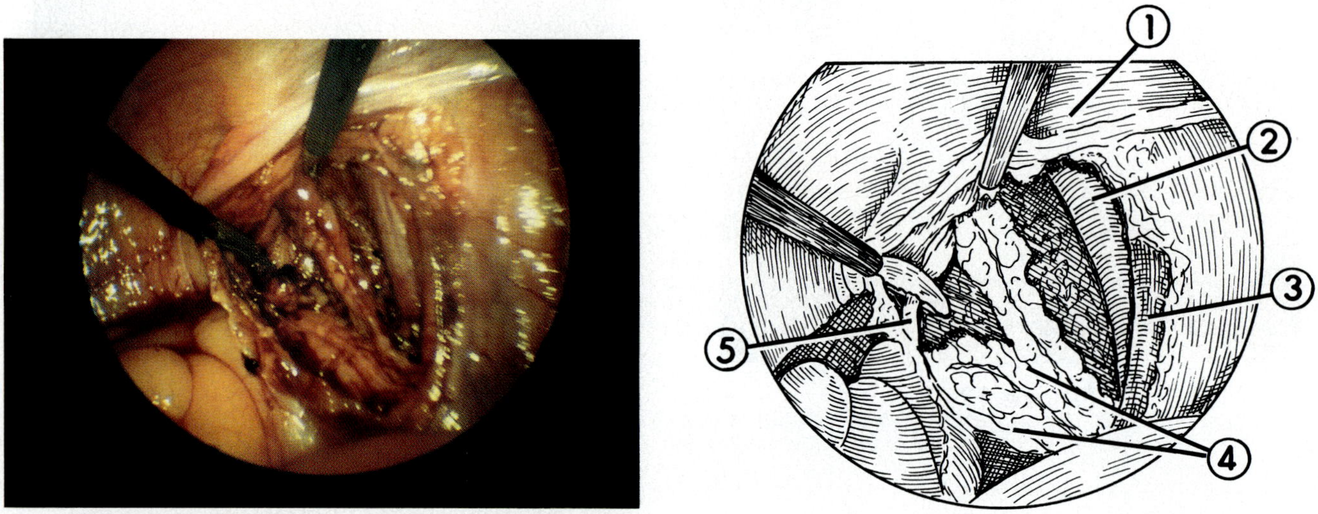

A B

Figure 15–3

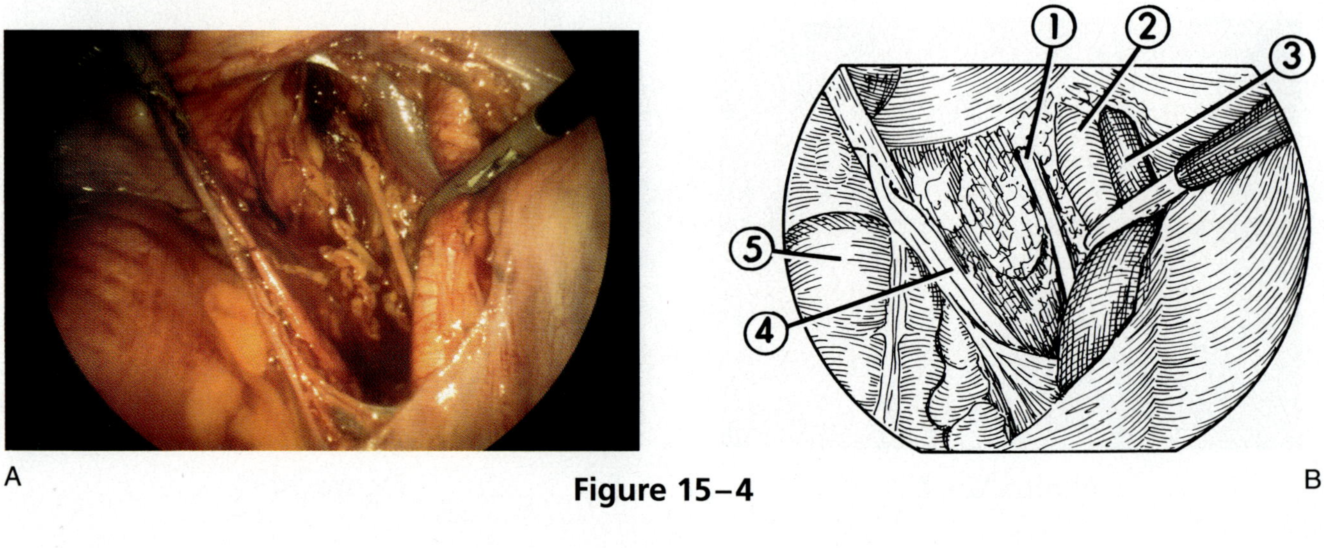

A B

Figure 15–4

Plate 5

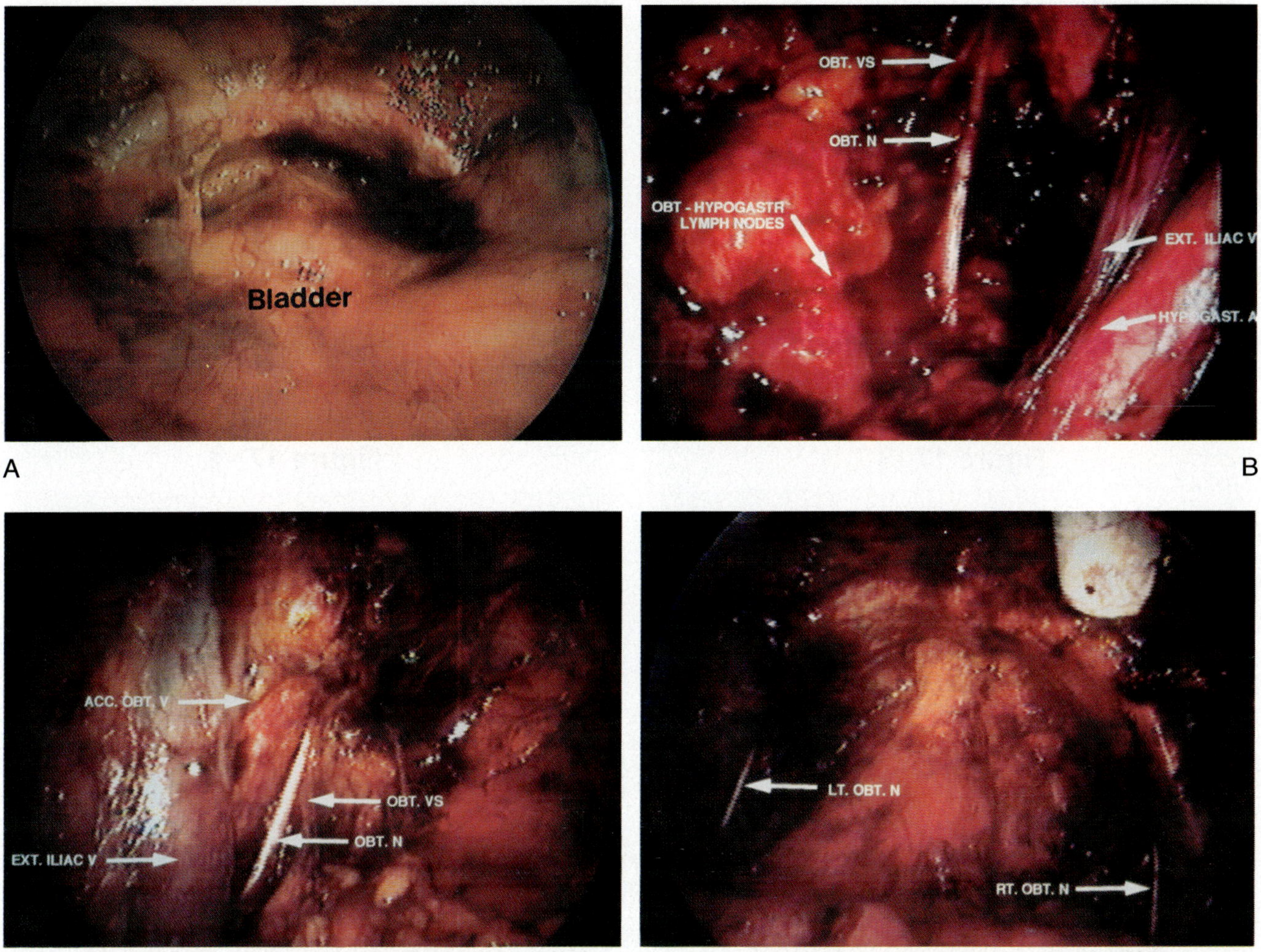

A B C D

Figure 16–2

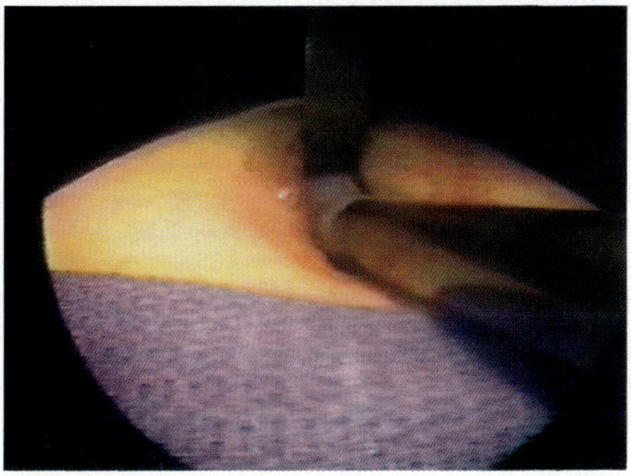

Figure 17–1

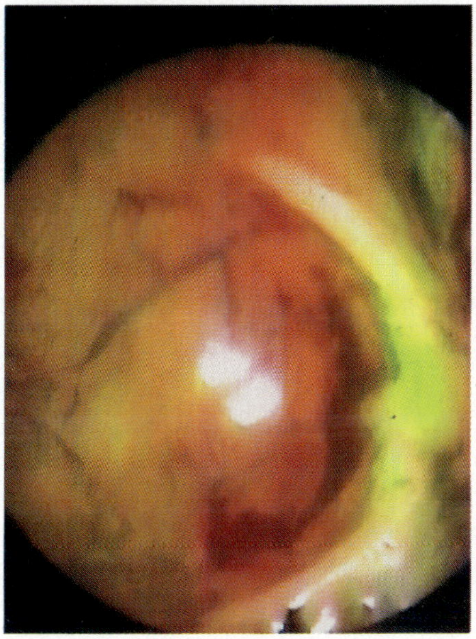

Figure 17–2

Plate 6

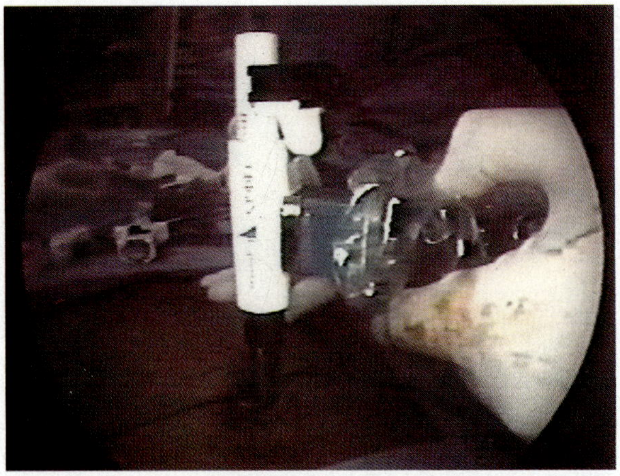

Figure 17–3

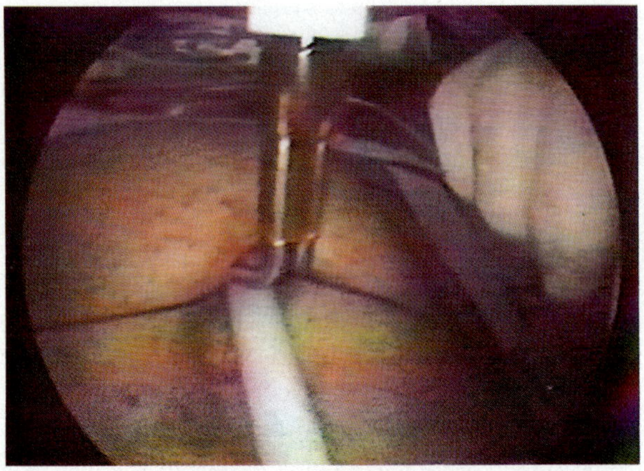

Figure 17–4

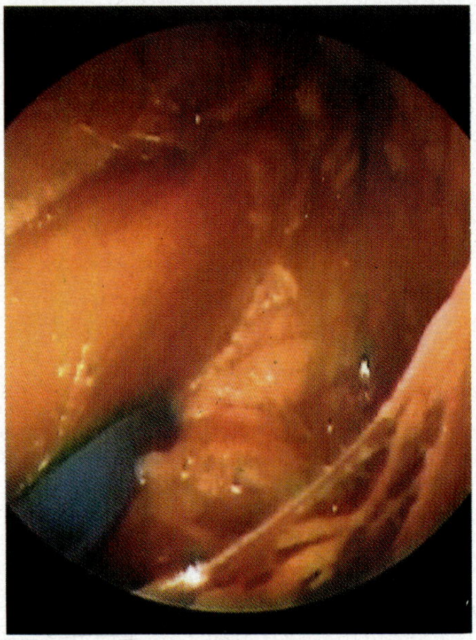

Figure 17–5

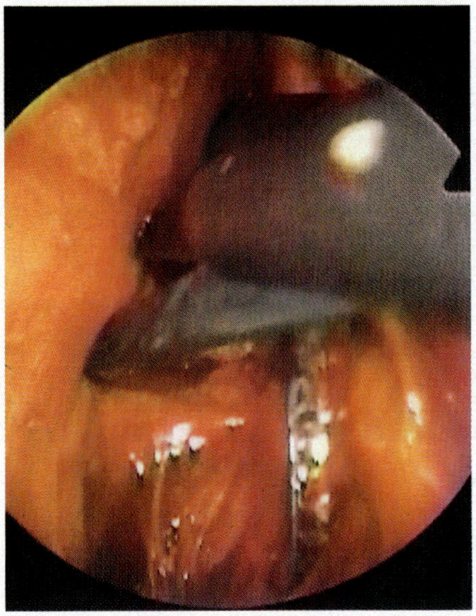

Figure 17–6

Plate 7

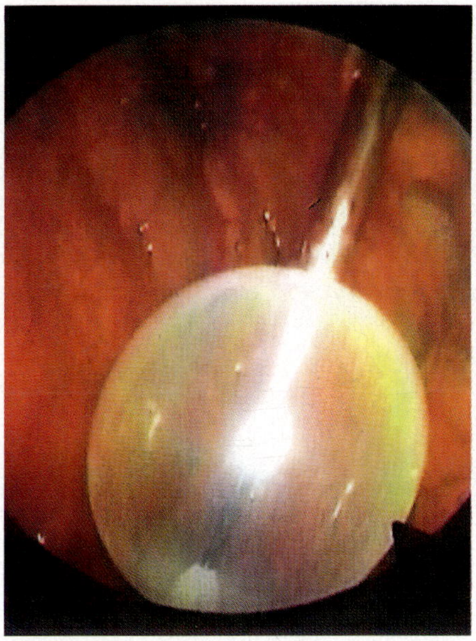

Figure 17–7

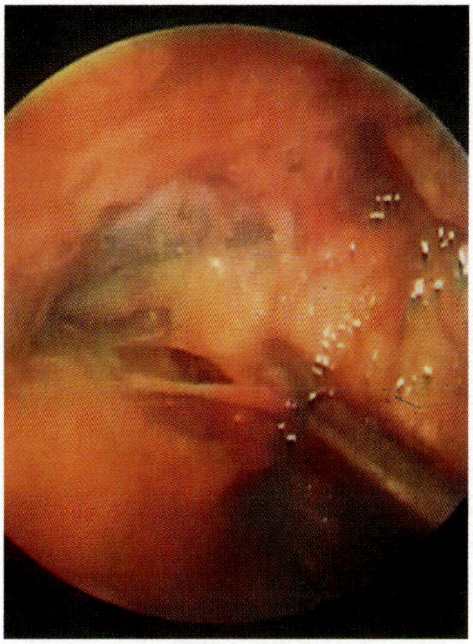

Figure 17–8

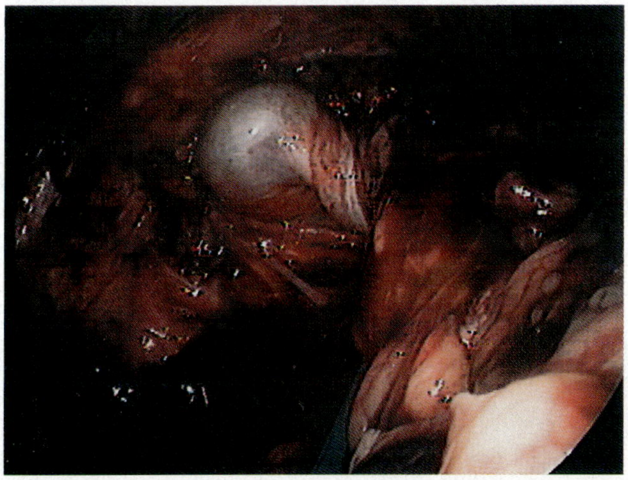

A

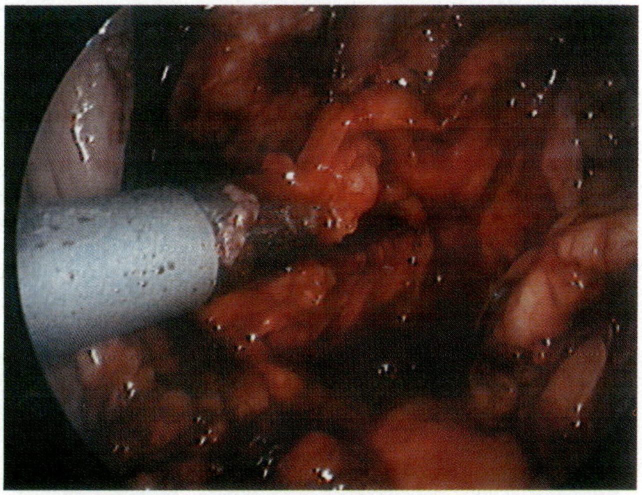

Figure 20–2

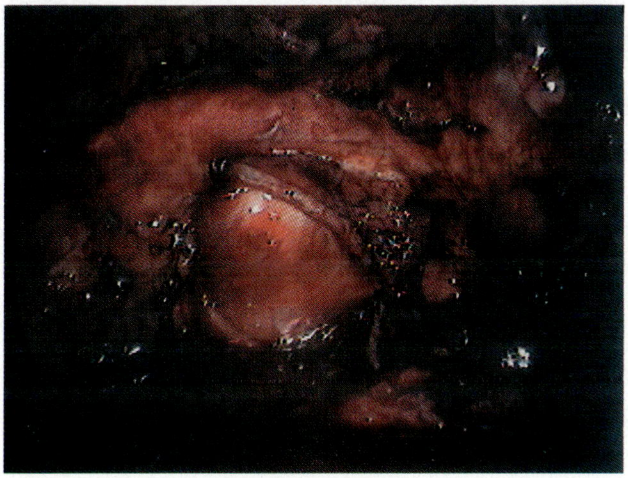

B

Figure 20–3

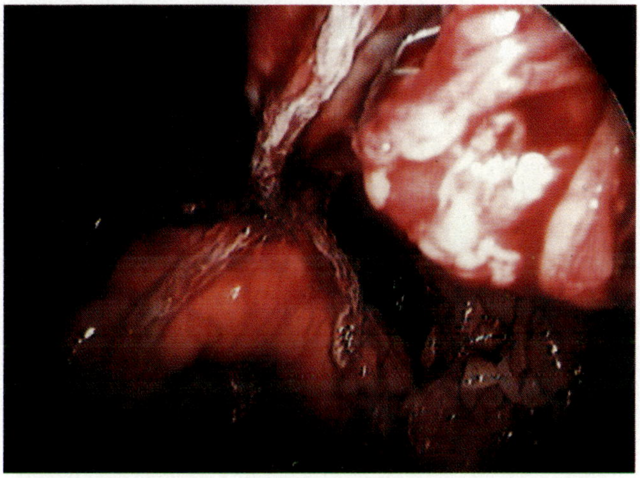

Figure 20–4

Plate 8

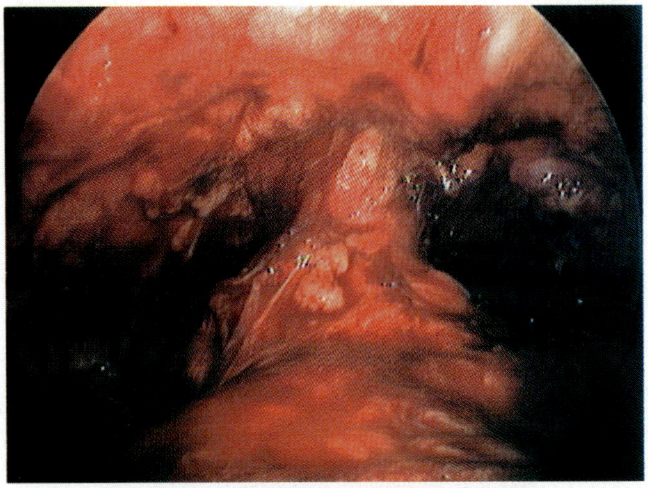

Figure 20-5

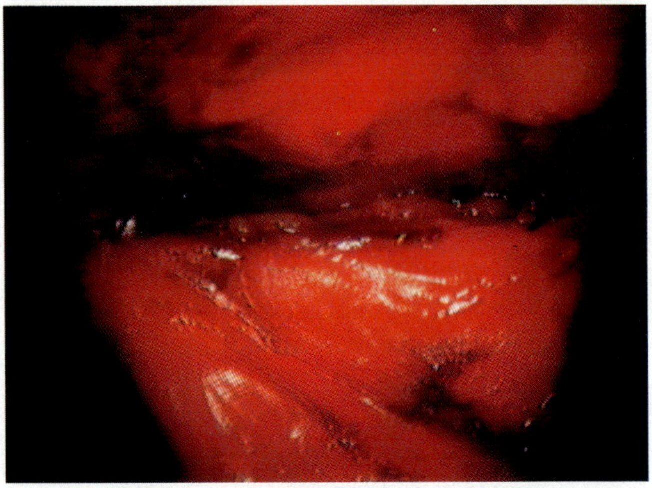

Figure 21-1

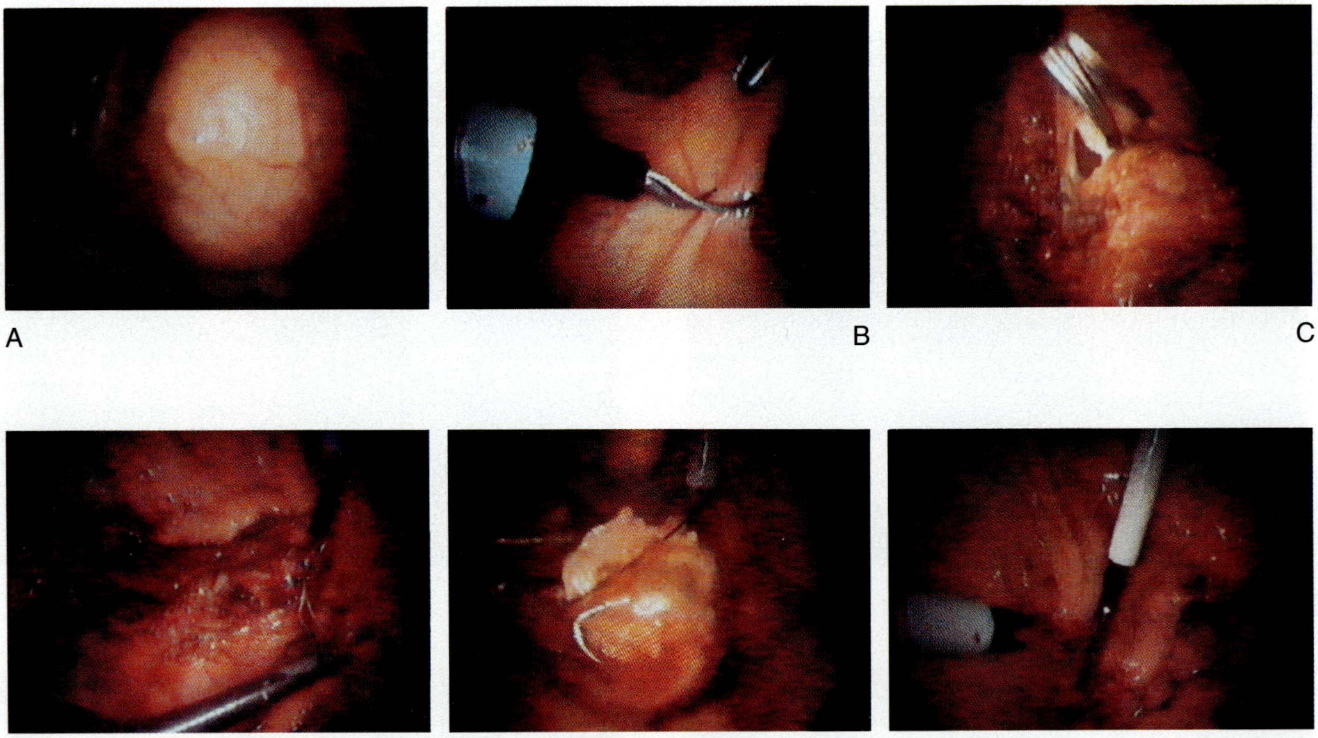

A B C D E F

Figure 21-3

SECTION I

HISTORICAL PERSPECTIVE

CHAPTER 1

History of Laparoscopy

Raul C. Ordorica, MD
Sakti Das, MD, FACS

"I have but one lamp by which my feet are guided, and that is the lamp of experience. I know of no way of judging of the future but by the past."

PATRICK HENRY
Speech in Virginia Convention,
Richmond, March 23, 1775.

Of late there has been a tremendous upsurge in the utilization of laparoscopy in general surgery and urology. Those unfamiliar with the craft may dismiss this intense interest as a passing phenomenon. However, by reviewing the historical development of laparoscopy we may better understand the current enthusiasm toward this minimally invasive technology. With this insight, the present attention of abdominal, thoracic, and pelvic surgeons to laparoscopy can be viewed in its appropriate historical, economic, and social context. We can then perceive today's events not as a treatment digression of standard operative procedure but rather as a natural evolution in surgical intervention. This chapter focuses on those major developments that have advanced the capabilities and understanding of laparoscopy. Perhaps with this analysis we may even be able to glimpse the future.

Attempts to peer into the human body endoscopically can be traced to the initial developments of endourology in the beginning of the nineteenth century. Bozzini of Frankfort constructed a thin silver funnel that was illuminated by reflected candlelight held within its stand (Fig. 1–1).[1,2] The "Lichtleiter" was presented to the Faculty of Medicine in Vienna in 1805 for viewing of the human urethra. Unfortunately, the intended use of the instrument was considered an unnatural act, and Bozzini was censured by this scientific body, despite no evidence that this device was ever used on a human subject. Although the instrument would have proved cumbersome, inefficient, and painful for both operator and patient, it is recognized today as the first major foray into endoscopy.

Although Segalas of France refined the urethroscope in 1826 with an introductory cannula and mirrors for light reflection, it was Desormeaux, his fellow countryman, who presented the first serviceable endoscope to the Academy of Paris in 1853 (Fig. 1–2).[2,3] This major development included an illumination source of increased intensity, using the reflected light from an alcohol lamp. With this instrument he reported numerous investigations of the urethra and bladder. Clearly an intellectual milestone had been reached, for he was awarded a portion of the Argenteuil Prize for his achievement.[4]

The next major innovation would be the development of a light source that could be transported into the body cavity. Bruck, a dentist of Breslau, heralded the development of internal illumination in 1867 with his use of a platinum wire loop heated by an electric current.[5] This modality met with greater success in the mouth than his technique of diaphanoscopy—with the bladder transilluminated by a rectally placed coil (Fig. 1–3). Despite its being water-cooled, the technique was still dangerous and rather ineffective. Nitze, of Germany, successfully applied this illumination source to his cystoscope, apparently unaware of

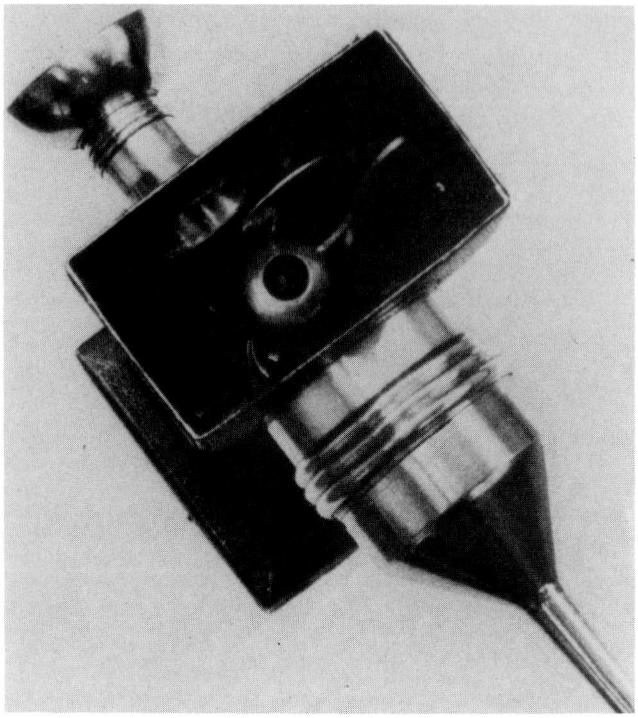

Figure 1–1. The Bozzini Lichtleiter, 1806. Apical view demonstrates mirror inspection eyepiece and spring-loaded candle. (From Gow, JG; Hopkins, HH: Handbook of Urologic Endoscopy. Edinburgh, Churchill Livingstone, 1978.)

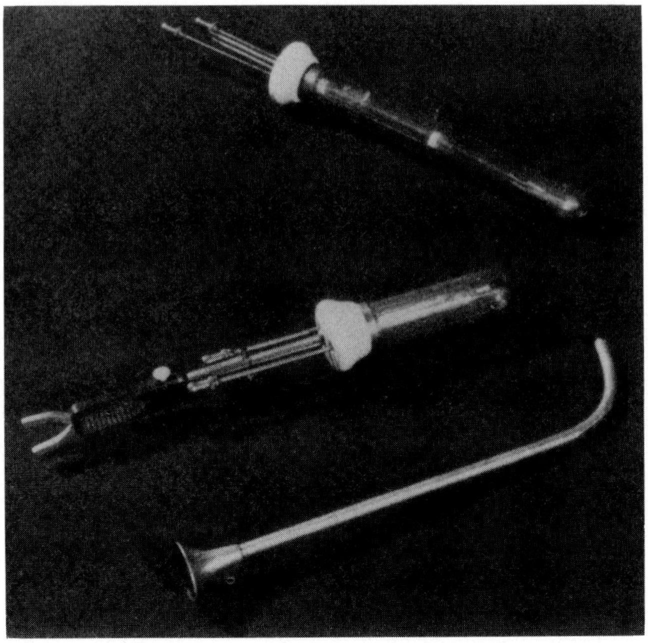

Figure 1–3. The Julius Bruck diaphanoscope elements. (From Gow, JG; Hopkins, HH: Handbook of Urologic Endoscopy. Edinburgh, Churchill Livingstone, 1978.)

Bruck's earlier attempts (Fig. 1–4). Nitze, compelled by the concept of an internal light source, stated succinctly, "In order to light up a room, one must carry a lamp into it."[5] He brought his ideas to Diecke, an instrument maker in Dresden, and together they were able to manufacture their first cystoscope in 1877.[1] This instrument was still rather bulky and unreliable and underwent subsequent improvements when Nitze teamed up with Leiter, a renowned instrument maker in Vienna. The Nitze-Leiter cystoscope, presented in 1879, used an electrically heated platinum wire light source placed behind a quartz shield (Fig. 1–5).

Despite these marked advances, the heat generated within the bladder required a bulky water-cooling device, and the electrical apparatus that created the necessary current for the platinum wire was difficult to maintain (Figs. 1–6 and 1–7). Further progress

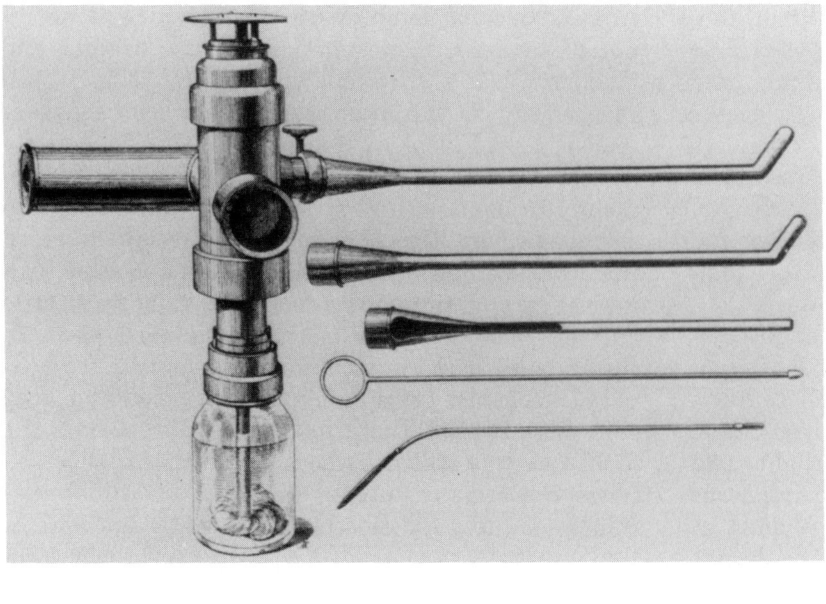

Figure 1–2. The Antonin Desormeaux alcohol lamp endoscope, 1853. (From Herman, JR: Development of the cystoscope. In Herman, JR, ed.: Urology: A View Through the Retrospectroscope. Hagerstown, MD, Harper & Row, 1973.)

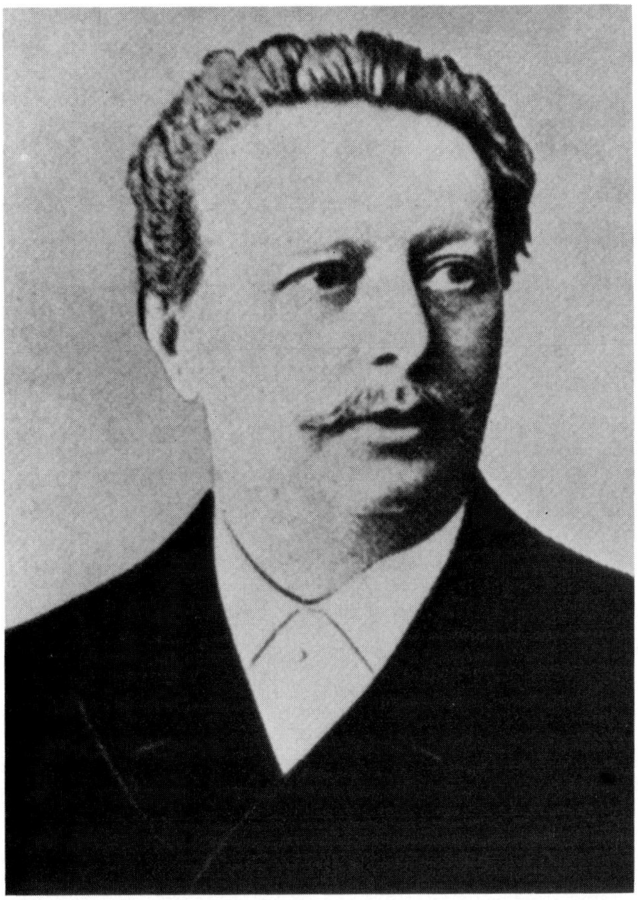

Figure 1–4. Maximillian Nitze. (From Bauer, KM: Cystoscopic Diagnosis: Technique and Typical Findings. Philadelphia, Lea & Febiger, 1969.)

awaited Edison's invention of the incandescent lamp in 1880. This landmark development provided increased illumination and alleviated the need for the water-cooling apparatus. More of the scope could then be dedicated to the optical lens system, resulting in better visualization with improved light delivery.[2] The incandescent bulb was applied by many endoscopists, including David Newman (1883), followed by Nitze (1887), Leiter (1887), and Dittel (1887).[1] More dependable illumination was made available with this bulb's refinement to the mignon lamp by Preston in 1898 (Fig. 1–8).[2] It produced a bright light requiring low-amperage current, becoming the primary light source for endoscopy until the development of adequate external light delivery systems fifty years later.

Such was the advancing technical state of the art when Ott, a famous Petrograd gynecologist, introduced *ventroscopy* for the inspection of the abdominal cavity.[6] His published works in 1901, 1902, and 1903 described the use of a head mirror to reflect light into a speculum introduced through a small anterior abdominal wall incision.[7,8] Although his technique was primitive, the concept of closed diagnostic inspection of intraperitoneal contents was thus conceived. It was Kelling of Germany who demonstrated more "modern" technique with the use of the Nitze cystoscope for inspection of the abdominal viscera. He performed this on a dog at the 73rd Congress of German Naturalists in 1901, terming the procedure *celioscopy* in his paper published the subsequent year.[9] Although Kelling's advanced work was particularly notable in that

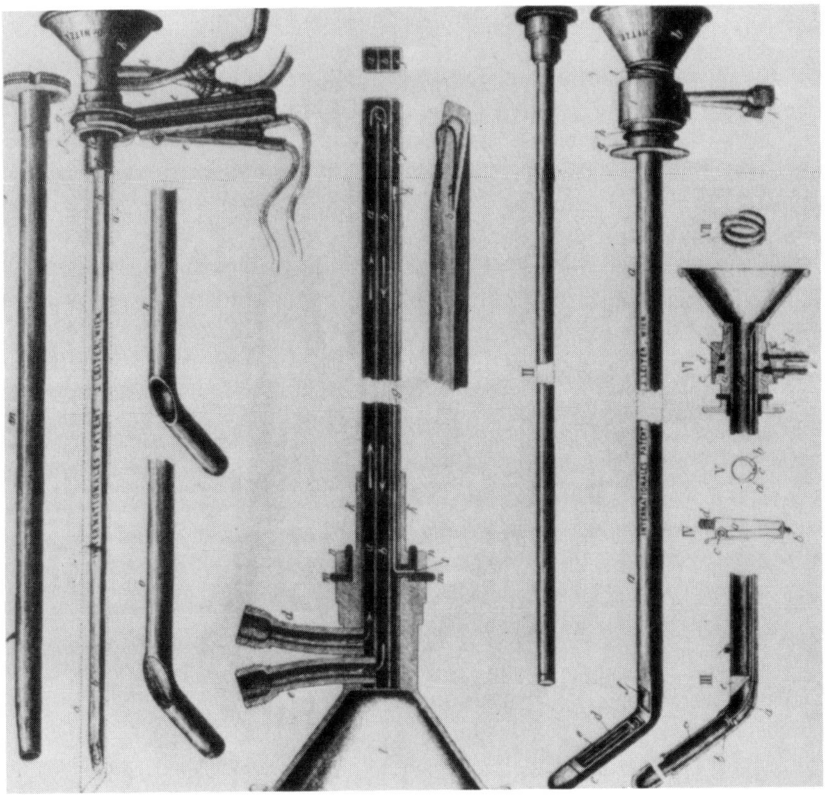

Figure 1–5. The Nitze-Leiter cystoscope. (From Lyons, A: Medicine—An Illustrated History. New York, Harry Abrams, 1978.)

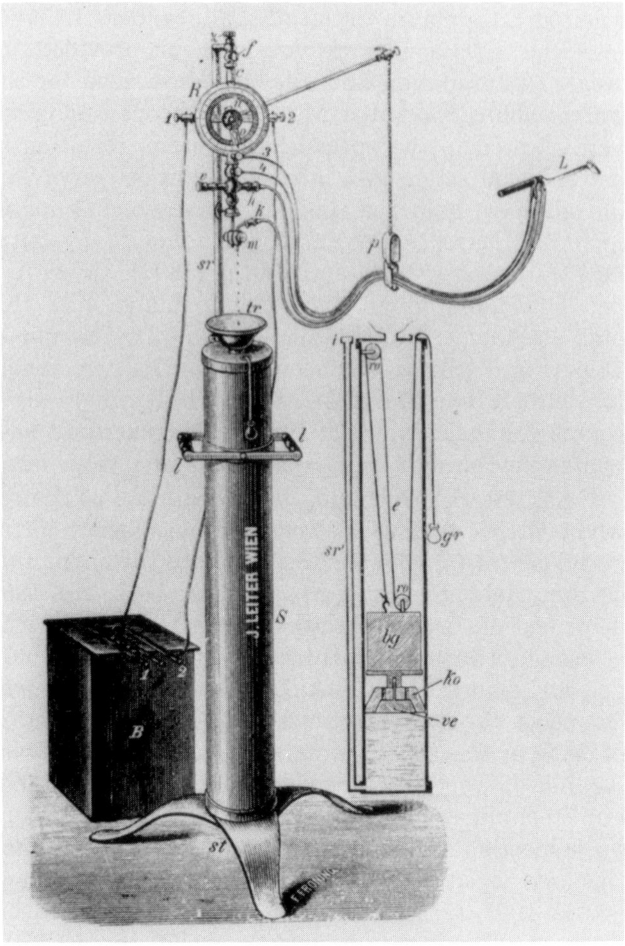

Figure 1–6. The Nitze water-cooling device. (From Gow, JG; Hopkins, HH: Handbook of Urologic Endoscopy. Edinburgh, Churchill Livingstone, 1978.)

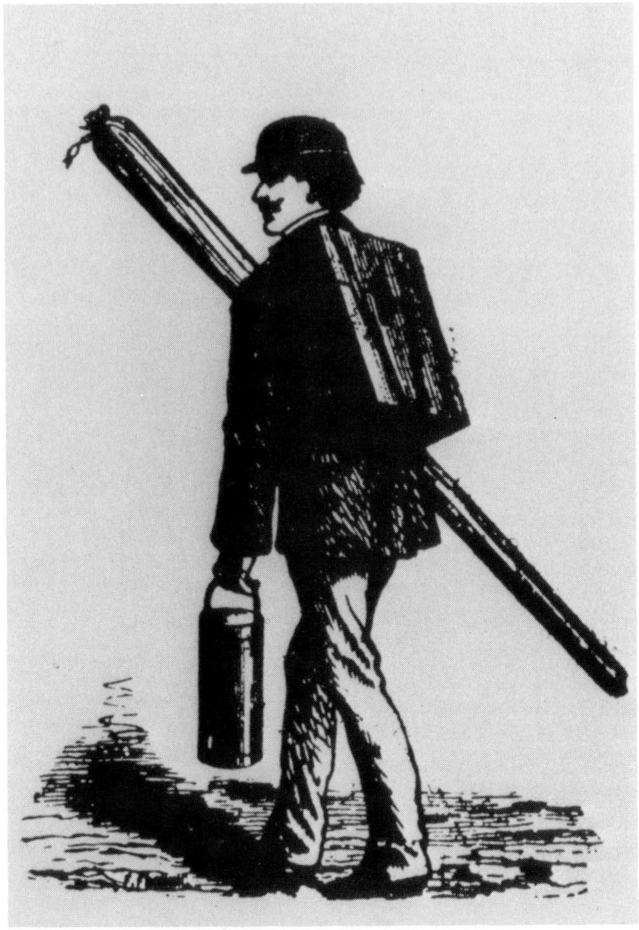

Figure 1–7. A well-equipped cystoscopist in the era of the early Nitze-Leiter equipment, burdened with the tools of his trade. (From Gow, JG; Hopkins, HH: Handbook of Urologic Endoscopy. Edinburgh, Churchill Livingstone, 1978.)

he used a separate needle to produce the pneumoperitoneum, he failed to publish his reported work on humans or the technical refinements he developed in a timely fashion. Jacobaeus, of Sweden, did publish on both human laparoscopy and thoracoscopy in 1910, stressing the benignity of the procedure despite using a single trocar both to produce the pneumoperitoneum and to provide endoscopic access (Fig. 1–9).[10] He documented his findings with 115 cases in subsequent reports by 1912.[11–13]

Additional reports followed from both Europe and the Americas with minor variations in equipment and technique.[14] In 1920 Orndorff, of the United States, devised a trocar with a pyramidal point along with developing an automatic cannula valve to prevent the escape of gas from the pneumoperitoneum.[15] Using these devices, he published his experience of laparoscopy incorporating the use of a roentgen screen. In 1924, Stone, also of the United States, described the fitting of the outer portion of the trocar with a rubber gasket to prevent the leakage of gas.[16] At the same time, Zollikofer, of Switzerland, introduced the use of

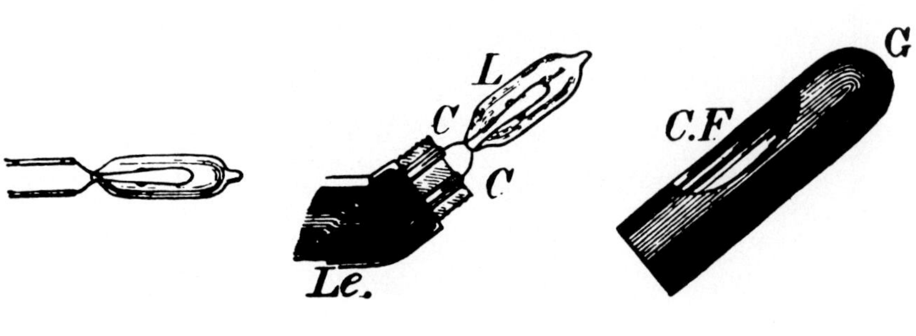

Figure 1–8. The mignon lamp, 1890. (From Gow, JG; Hopkins, HH: Handbook of Urologic Endoscopy. Edinburgh, Churchill Livingstone, 1978.)

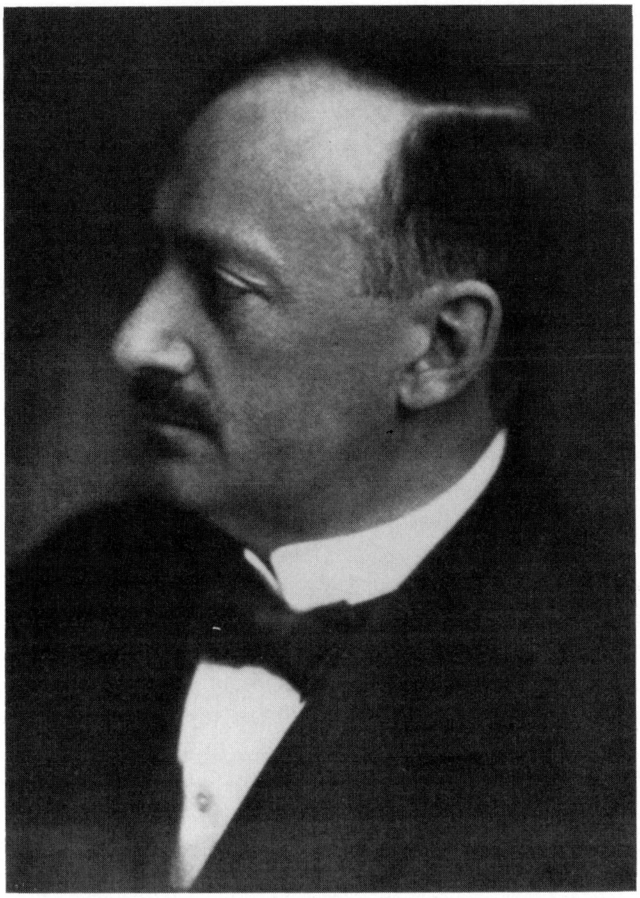

Figure 1–9. Hans Christian Jacobaeus. (From Brandt HG; Loddenkemper R; Mai J: Atlas of Diagnostic Thoracoscopy: Indications, Technique. Stuttgart, Georg Thieme, 1985.)

CO_2 for insufflation, appreciating its ease of absorption.[17] Previously filtered air, with its inherent risk of air embolism, was the primary medium. The automatic insufflation needle was developed by Goetze, of Germany, in 1918, minimizing the risks involved with initial abdominal puncture (Fig. 1–10).[18] This instrument was initially used with oxygen as the insufflating medium. Although the use of this gas had less problems of emboli formation in comparison with air, it became obsolete with the advent of electrocautery. In 1938, Verres, of Hungary, further refined the automatic needle initially used for the creation of pneumothoraces in the treatment of tuberculosis (Fig. 1–11).[19] We continue to use the instrument that bears his name, its now being the most frequently used device for creating pneumoperitoneum.

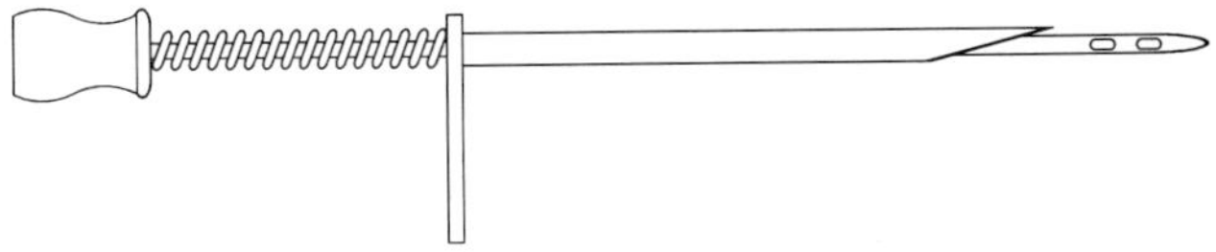

Figure 1–10. Goetze's pneumoperitoneum needle, 1918.

Many physicians renowned for their technical advances were also responsible for the teaching of laparoscopy as an accepted method. Kalk, of Germany, an outstanding proponent of "peritoneoscopy" throughout Europe, exemplified this pattern, (Fig. 1–12).[20–22] In addition to devising a foroblique (135-degree) viewing system, his teachings led to the widespread adoption of his methods. Having published some 21 papers in this burgeoning field between 1929 and 1959, he is often referred to as the "father of

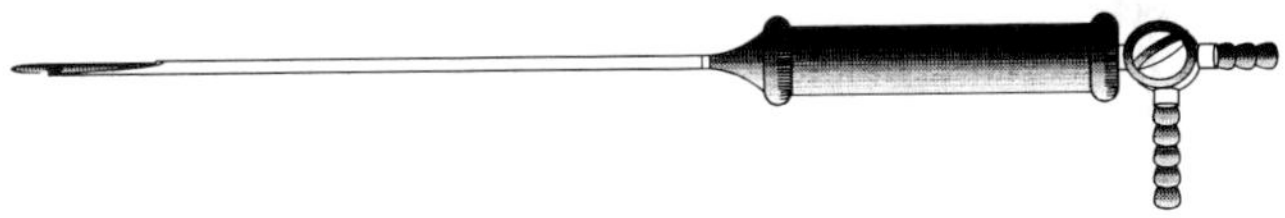

Figure 1–11. The Verres needle, 1938, originally introduced for the production of pneumothorax in the treatment of pulmonary tuberculosis.

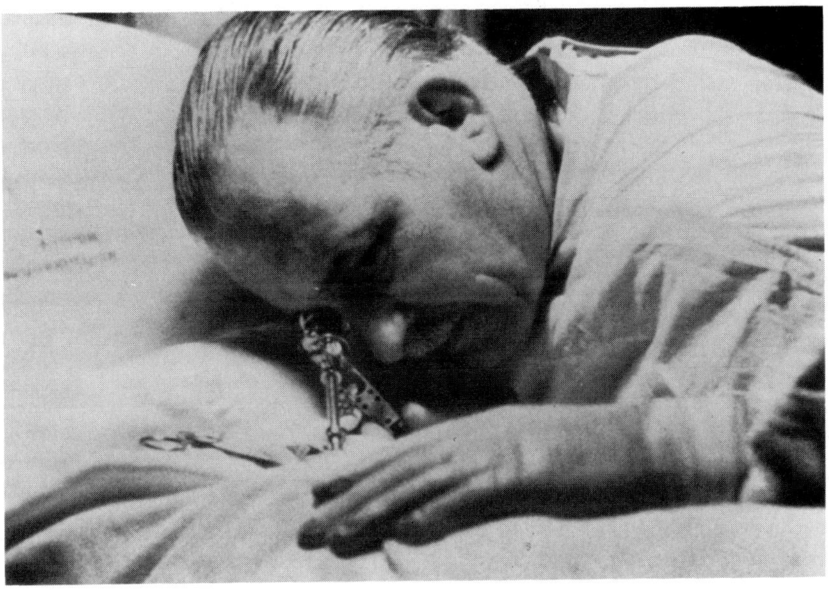

Figure 1–12. H. Kalk. (From Beck, K: Atlas der Laparoskopie. Stuttgart, F.K. Schattauer-Verlag, 1968.)

modern laparoscopy" for his work dealing with liver and gallbladder disease.[8] This was a considerable task given that the ability to convey the otherwise "closed" world of laparascopy was limited. Although multiple devices had been designed for photographing laparoscopic detail, most of the description was by illustration alone. These limitations continued until the introduction of the single-lens reflex camera for endophotography by Henning in 1931.[23] Kalk later published the first black and white and color photographic atlas in 1935.[23] This was followed by Caroli, Ricordeau, and Foures of France, who were the first to use an electronic flash intra-abdominally.[24] Further major advances in visual reproduction awaited the development of improved light transmission; lens systems; cinephotography; and, eventually, video technology.

Laparoscopy meanwhile made initial forays into the interventional realm. Fervers of Germany in 1933 burned abdominal adhesions and performed excisional biopsy, work advanced with modifications in high-frequency unipolar electrocautery.[25] Ruddock, of the United States, perfected not only his own peritoneoscope, pneumoperitoneum needle, and trocar but also ancillary biopsy instruments.[26–30] He published his initial series of 200 cases in 1934, followed by his subsequent experience with more than 2500 cases. Laparoscopic tubal sterilization using electrocautery was first introduced in 1935 by Boesch, of Switzerland, using a porcine model.[31] This procedure was later performed in 1941 on a human being by Power and Barnes, of the United States, with an interim published discussion of the technique by Anderson.[32,33] Donaldson, also of the United States, used the Ruddock peritoneoscope to perform a uterine suspension in 1942.[34] Further advancement in laparoscopic intervention awaited better provision for safe hemostasis in the closed abdominal cavity, made possible with improvements in electrocautery.

The United States during World War II turned its attention to culdoscopy, as introduced by Decker in 1944, which became the standard American gynecologic procedure for many years.[35–37] Meanwhile, Palmer, of France, greatly furthered gynecologic laparoscopy throughout Europe.[38,39] Interest was not rekindled in the United States until the publication of the first English laparoscopic text in 1967 by the British gynecologist Steptoe, who was influenced by his European contemporaries.[40] The resurrection of American laparoscopy occurred through the dissemination of contemporary experience and by the accompanying advances that had been made in optics, light transmission, insufflators, and ancillary materials. These largely European developments broadened the field's utility and better ensured patient safety.

In 1952 Fourestier, Gladu, and Valmiere, of France, developed a method for light transmission along a quartz rod that greatly improved the quality of light produced and removed the risk of electrical and heat injury that had plagued previous systems (Fig. 1–13).[41] The same year Hopkins and Kapany, of England, introduced fiber optics, initially developed for the fiberoptic gastroscope.[42] Hopkins was also responsible for the development of the quartz rod lens, which replaced prior lens systems in rigid endoscopes (Fig. 1–14).[43] Frangenheim incorporated many of these advances in laparoscopy, using diathermy for tubal sterilization in 1963, and fiber optics in 1965.[44] His extensive publishing on the subjects of anesthetic methods, pneumoperitoneum, tissue emphysema, air embolism, intestinal perforation, hemorrhage, burns, and cardiopulmonary problems, furthered the course of safe laparoscopic procedure.[45]

In the United States, Cohen, followed by Hulka, was at the forefront of laparoscopy through the late 1960s and early 1970s.[44–46] Through published experience, teachings, and texts, they were responsible for the widespread popularization of laparoscopy in the gynecologic community. Although its initial application was primarily diagnostic, the major proliferative force was its use for sterilization. These procedures were so widespread that the American Association of Gynecologic Laparoscopists was formed in 1972 by Phillips.[44] Its second annual meeting was held in 1973 in conjunction with the First International Congress of Gynecologic Laparoscopy with an attendance of 600. At that time approximately 500,000 laparoscopies were being performed annually in the United States. By 1981 laparoscopy had become a requirement of residency training in obstetrics-gynecology.[44]

Substantial pioneering work by Semm, of Germany, meanwhile had advanced the safety and range of laparoscopy.[4,31,47–51] Automatic control systems were developed for insufflation and maintenance of the pneumoperitoneum with CO_2. Further work in conjunction with Wissenschaftlicn Apparatbau (WISAP, Sauerlach, in what was then West Germany) led to the development of electronically controlled units through the 1970s. A history of prior laparotomy and adhesions, once a contraindication to laparoscopy, became safe ground with the development of the open trocar technique of Hasson, stemming from his work in 1971.[52,53]

Semms takes great note regarding the lack of safe hemostasis as additional impediment in the advancement of laparoscopic surgery.[31] The use of high-frequency monopolar cautery within the abdominal cavity had been historically fraught with the serious sequelae of bowel injury. Indeed, the second most frequent cause for lawsuits against obstetrician-gynecologists in the early 1970s was for laparoscopic bowel burns.[54] Therefore, a great deal of investigation was

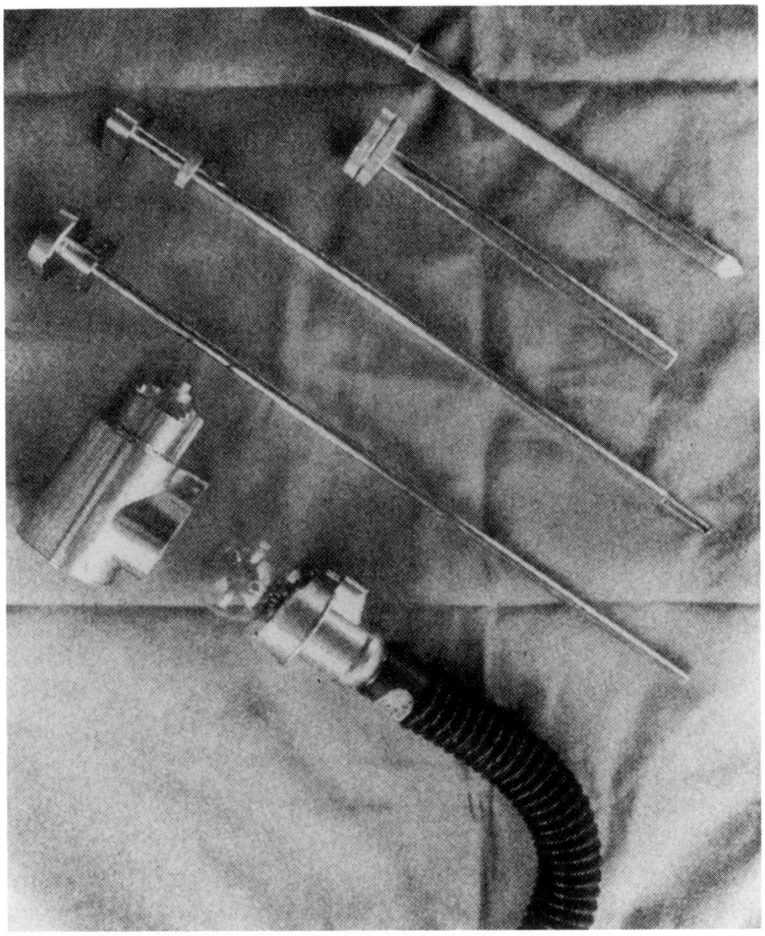

Figure 1–13. Components of a Fourestier, Gladu, and Valmiere quartz rod lens laparoscope. (From Saleh, JW: Laparoscopy. Philadelphia, WB Saunders, 1988.)

devoted to eliminating these dangers, particularly with the growing popularity of laparoscopic tubal disruption. The electrical shielding of instruments and current reduction were introduced to obviate these problems, along with the subsequent development of the 100°C endocoagulator. Hemostatic methods also included the use of "endoloop" and suturing devices for large blood vessel control. Semms further pushed the confines of laparoscopy with the development and bold use of a wide range of devices by 1982, describing techniques of appendectomy, lysis of adhesions, and bowel repair.[4,48,51]

Whereas historically laparoscopy had commonly been used to diagnose pathology of the liver and gall-

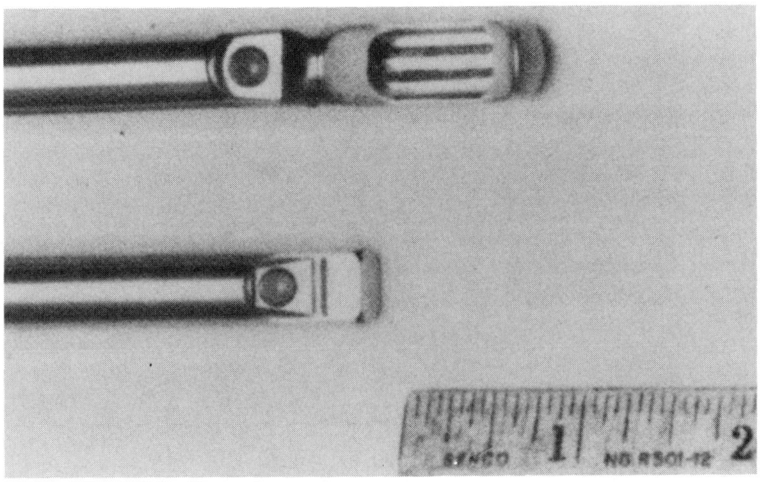

Figure 1–14. Laparoscope tips comparing prior distal bulb technology *(top)* to a fiber optic light source *(bottom)*. (From Phillips, JM: Laparoscopy. Baltimore, Williams & Wilkins, 1977.)

bladder in internal medicine, these uses became more infrequent as radiographic imaging moved to the forefront. Gynecologist Mouret, of France, first laparoscopically removed a diseased gallbladder in 1987 during a routine pelvic procedure.[42] McKernan and Saye, general surgeons in the United States, performed the next laparoscopic cholecystectomy in 1988, followed by Reddick in 1989.[42,55] Reddick's published series, along with those of Dubois, of France, documented the ability to reproduce this procedure that had been confined to open surgery.[56] These reports fueled such tremendous interest that the rapid dissemination of laparoscopy over a three-year period has led to the near replacement of elective open cholecystectomy in many centers.[42] This may be startling when viewed as an isolated event, but it is predictable when perceived within a broader framework.

The successful performance of complex intracorporeal procedures required more than the development of advanced mechanical instrumentation. It also relied on the ability to actively coordinate the efforts of more than a single operator. Standard laparoscopic practice had been for the surgeon to have sole benefit of viewing the operative field, his assistants' ability to substantially participate limited by their blind involvement. Additional eyepiece attachments had been developed but were incorporated only as learning tools, allowing the novice to gain the necessary skills to subsequently operate alone. Although the production of closed circuit television had been in existence since 1959, portable systems were not available until 1970.[44] The term *portable* should be applied sparingly, in that the initial cameras weighed some 10 pounds, coming equipped with an attachable ceiling harness. Their size, quality of image reproduction, and expense had relegated their use to rare and cumbersome teaching aids. It was not until the advent of microchip technology that practical real-time video imaging of the operative field could be performed (Fig. 1–15). Subsequent acceptance and use of video cameras became widespread throughout all areas of endoscopy, laying the groundwork for major laparoscopic intervention. With this visual "opening" of the closed abdominal cavity to the entire surgical team, more complex procedures could be undertaken with the aid of guided assistance.

The performance of novel techniques requires individual initiative, but these developments do not occur in a vacuum. The feasibility of these procedures must be determined, and the social and economic framework must be conducive for their development and success. These advanced technical capabilities were fostered in a realm of limited financial resources for health care. Procedures that minimized the requirements for expensive acute-care facilities had become a major focus, with greater use of ambulatory procedures together with limited hospital stays. Of additional importance was the indirect expense of open surgical procedures that removed patients from the work force for extended periods of convalescence. Thus techniques such as endoscopic and radiologic intervention, extracorporeal shock wave lithotripsy, and medical therapies, were pushed further into the forefront. In addition, patients had become more consumer-oriented in their involvement regarding health care decisionmaking, willing to question whether there were possible alternatives to the perceived "trauma" of surgery. Laparoscopy alleviated the morbidity of large abdominal incisions, providing a solution for economic and social considerations.

Although urologic laparoscopy has not yet had the same impact on surgical practice as did the develop-

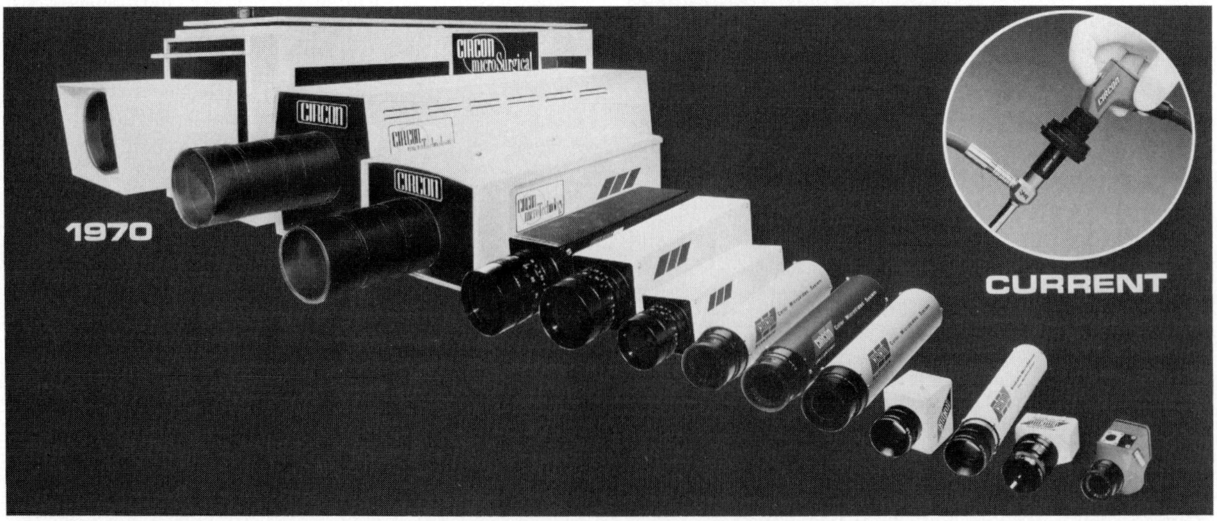

Figure 1–15. The progression of video camera technology over a 20-year span is demonstrated by this product line chronology of the CIRCON Corporation. (Courtesy of CIRCON Corporation, Santa Barbara, CA.)

ment of laparoscopic cholecystectomy, use of this technique has been on the periphery for some time. In 1976 Cortesi reported the use of the laparoscope to examine bilateral abdominal testes in an 18-year-old.[57] Since then cumulative experience of many authors has substantiated its use in cryptorchidism.[58–61] Other initial work was reported by Wickham, who in 1979 performed a laparoscopic ureterolithotomy by a retroperitoneal approach.[62] Additional stone manipulation was performed by Eshghi, who in 1985 laparoscopically monitored the percutaneous transperitoneal removal of staghorn calculi from a pelvic kidney.[63]

However, apart from its use in the pediatric population for cryptorchidism, urologic laparoscopy lacked a broad application in comparison with the general surgical population of patients with cholelithiasis. The inaccuracies of imaging techniques made pelvic lymphadenectomy a target laparoscopic procedure for staging of patients with prostate carcinoma.[64] Focused experimental work by Winfield described the performance of laparoscopic pelvic lymphadenectomy in 1989 using a porcine model.[65] Schuessler and associates performed this procedure in their human series with prostate cancer starting in 1989.[66] Reports of further experience with laparoscopy for pelvic lymph node dissection, as well as other procedures such as varicocele ligation, lymphocele peritonealization, bladder diverticulectomy, bladder neck suspension, partial cystectomy, and ileal conduit formation have since permeated the recent literature.[67–76]

Laparoscopic nephrectomy was first attempted by a retroperitoneal approach, as performed by Weinberg and Smith in 1988 using a porcine model.[77] Clayman and other authors have subsequently reported their results in human nephrectomy, using the transperitoneal approach.[78–80] This approach was initially performed in a patient with renal oncocytoma and followed by a series for benign disease and, subsequently, renal cell carcinoma. Although the first case required almost 8 hours to complete, later efforts reduced this time to as few as 4 hours. In addition nephroureterectomies have been performed for renal pelvic transitional cell carcinoma, along with attempts at radical prostatectomy.[81,82] The difficulties encountered in the latter procedure perhaps illustrate the inherent shortcomings of transferring learned methods from animal models to human subjects. However, this body of work does demonstrate that many of the traditional boundaries, once limiting these procedures to open surgery, have broken down under the expanding range of the laparoscope.

Conclusions

This review of the development of laparoscopic technique, with its potential to replace or augment standard surgical practice, should better prepare us for the future. We can expect a continued improvement of new instruments for the entire spectrum of laparoscopic intervention, many either currently in development or being produced. Minimally invasive capability will be in part determined by these advances in technical support along with our own ingenuity in incorporating laparoscopy, which will allow us better to meet the ongoing needs of our patients. The actual utilization of laparoscopic procedure still warrants further clarification, with careful investigation by the surgical specialties. Clinical trials defining the benefits of closed versus open procedure with comparisons of surgical outcome, morbidity, and cost remain to be performed. Despite these gaps, history demonstrates that the current stage of interest in laparoscopy is part of a coherent progression in surgical intervention. These advances should be viewed as only passing phenomena in the context that even less invasive technology will predictably arise to supplant them.

REFERENCES

1. Belt, AE; Charnock, DA: The history of the cystoscope. In: Cabot, H, ed. Modern Urology, Philadelphia, Lea & Febiger, 1936, p. 15.
2. Herman, JR: Development of the cystoscope. In: Urology: A View Through the Retrospectroscope, Hagerstown, MD, Harper & Row, 1973, p. 67.
3. Desormeaux, AJ: Transactions of the Societe de Chirurgie, Paris. Gazette Hop, 1865.
4. Semm, K: Endoscopic intraabdominal surgery in gynecology. Wien Klin Wochenschr 95:353, 1983.
5. Luys, G: History of cystoscopy. In: Wolbarst, AL, ed. A Treatise on Cystoscopy and Urethroscopy. (Trans from French) St. Louis, CV Mosby, 1918, p. 55.
6. Ott, DO: Die Beleuchtung der Bauchhöhle (Ventroskopie) als Methode bei Vaginaler Coeliotomie. Abl Gynäk 231:817, 1902.
7. Ott, DO: Ventroscopic illumination of the abdominal cavity in pregnancy. Zh Akushers Zhensk Bolezn 15:7–8, 1901.
8. Wittman, I: Peritoneoscopy. Budapest, Publishing House of the Hungarian Academy of Sciences. 1966, pp. 3–5.
9. Kelling, G: Ueber Oesophagoskopie, Gastroskopie und Koelioskopie. Munch Med Wochenschr 49:21, 1902.
10. Jacobaeus, HC: Üeber die Möeglichkeit, die Zystoskopie bei Untersachung seröser höhlungen anzuwenden. Münch Med Wochenschr 57:2090–2092, 1910.
11. Jacobaeus, HC: Kurze Übersicht über mei Erfahrungen mit der Laparothorakoskopie. Münch Med Wochenschr 58:2017, 1911.
12. Jacobaeus, HC: Laparo-thorakoskopie. Hygiea (Stockholm) 74:1070, 1912.
13. Jacobaeus, HC: Über Laparo- und Thorakoskopie. Beitr Klin Tuberk 25:183, 1912.
14. Nadeu, OE; Kampmeier, OF: Endoscopy of the abdomen: Abdominoscopy. A preliminary study, including a summary of the literature and a description of the technique. Surg Gynecol Obstet 41:259, 1925.
15. Orndoff, RH: The peritoneoscope in diagnosis of diseases of the abdomen. J Radiol 1:307, 1920.
16. Stone, ZE: Intra-abdominal examination with the aid of the peritoneoscope. J Kans Med Soc 24:63, 1924.
17. Zollikofer, R: Zur Laparoskopie. Schweiz Med Wochenschr 54:264, 1924.
18. Goetze, O: Die Röntgendiagnostik bei gasgefüllter Bauchhöhle; eine neue Methode. Münch Med Wochenschr 65:1275, 1918.

19. Verres, J: Neues Instrument zur Aüsfuhung von Brust oder Bauchpunktionen. Dtsch Med Wochenschr 1938, 41:1480–1481.
20. Kalk, H: Erfahrungen mit der Laparoskopie (Zugleich mit Beschreibung eines neuen Instrumentes). Z Klin Med 111:303, 1929.
21. Kalk, H: Laparoskopie. (Die Besichtigung der Bauchhöhle am Lebenden Menschen.) Ges Krankenh 5:97, 1935.
22. Kalk, H; Bruhl, W; Sieke, E: Die Gezielte Leberpunktion. Dtsch Med Wochenschr 69:693, 1943.
23. Saleh, JW: Indications and limitations. In Saleh, JW, ed. Laparoscopy. WB Saunders, Philadelphia, 1988, p. 1.
24. Caroli, J: La laparophotographie en couleurs par l'endographe de Foures. Rev Int Med 5:951, 1955.
25. Fervers, C: Die Laparoskopie mit dem Cystoskop. Ein Beitrag zur Vereinfachung der Technik und zur Endoskopischen Strangdurchtrennung in der Bauchhöhle. Med Klin 29:1042, 1933.
26. Ruddock, JC: Application and evaluation of peritoneoscopy. Calif Med 71:110, 1949.
27. Ruddock, JC: Peritoneoscopy. South Surg 8:113, 1939.
28. Ruddock, JC: Peritoneoscopy. Surg Gynecol Obstet 65:623, 1937.
29. Ruddock, JC: Peritoneoscopy. West J Surg 42:392, 1934.
30. Ruddock, JC: Peritoneoscopy: A critical review. Surg Clin North Am 37:1249, 1957.
31. Semm, K: History. In: Sanfilippo, JS; Levine, RL, eds. Operative Gynecologic Endoscopy. New York, Springer-Verlag, 1989.
32. Anderson, ET: Peritoneoscopy. Am J Surg 35:136, 1937
33. Power, FH; Barnes, AC: Sterilization by means of peritoneoscopic tubal fulguration. Am J Obstet Gynecol 41:1038, 1941.
34. Donaldson, JK; Sanderlin, JH; Harrell, WB, Jr: A method of suspending the uterus without open abdominal incision. Am J Surg 55:537, 1942.
35. Decker, A: Culdoscopy: Its diagnostic value in pelvic disease. JAMA 140:378, 1949.
36. Decker, A; Cherry, T: Culdoscopy: A new method in diagnosis of pelvic disease. Am J Surg 64:40, 1944.
37. Decker, A: Culdoscopy. Am J Obstet Gynecol 63:654, 1952.
38. Palmer, R: La coelioscopie par là vois transvaginale. CR Soc Franc Gynécol 17:229, 1947.
39. Palmer, R: La coelioscopie. Brux méd 28:305, 1948.
40. Steptoe, PC: Laparoscopy in Gynecology. Edinburgh, E & S Livingston, 1967.
41. Fourestier, N; Gladu, A; Vulmiere, J: Perfectionnements à l'endoscopie medicale. Realization bronchoscopique. Presse Med 60:1, 1952.
42. Gaskin, TA; Isobe, JH; Mathews, JL; et al: Laparoscopy and the general surgeon. Surg Clin North Am 71:1085, 1991.
43. Gow, JG; Hopkins, HH: Handbook of Urologic Endoscopy. Edinburgh Churchill Livingstone, 1978, p. 1.
44. Gunning, JE: The history of laparoscopy. In: Phillips, JM, ed. Laparoscopy. Baltimore, Williams & Wilkins, 1977.
45. Cohen, MR: Historical background. In: Laparoscopy, Culdoscopy and Gynecography, Philadelphia, WB Saunders, 1970, p. 6.
46. Cohen, MR: Culdoscopy vs. peritoneoscopy. Obstet Gynecol 31:310, 1968.
47. Semm, K: Change in the classic gynecologic surgery: Review of 3,300 pelviscopies in 1971–1976. Int J Fertil 24:13, 1979.
48. Semm, K: Endoscopic appendectomy. Endoscopy 15:59, 1983.
49. Semm, K: New methods of pelviscopy (gynecologic laparoscopy) for myomectomy, ovariectomy, tubectomy and adenectomy. Endoscopy 11:85, 1979.
50. Semm, K: Tissue-puncher and loop-ligation — new aids for surgical-therapeutic pelviscopy (laparoscopy) = endoscopic intraabdominal surgery. Endoscopy 10:119, 1978.
51. Semm, K; Mettler, L: Technical progress in pelvic surgery via operative laparoscopy. Am J Obstet Gynecol 138:121, 1980.
52. Hasson, HM: Open laparoscopy: A report of 150 cases. J Reprod Med 12:234, 1974.
53. Hasson, HM: A modified instrument and method for laparoscopy. Am J Obstet Gynecol 110:886, 1971.
54. Hulka, JF: Textbook of Laparoscopy. Orlando, FL: Grune & Stratton, 1985, pp. 1–5.
55. Reddick, E; Olsen, D: Laparoscopic laser cholecystectomy: A comparison with minilaparoscopic cholecystectomy. Surg Endosc 3:131, 1989.
56. Dubois, F; Card, P; Berthelot, G, et al: Coelioscopic cholecystectomy: Preliminary report of thirty-six cases. Ann Surg 211:60, 1990.
57. Cortesi, N; Ferrari, P; Zambarda, E; et al: Diagnosis of bilateral abdominal cryptorchidism by laparoscopy. Endoscopy 8:33, 1976.
58. Das, S; Amar, A: The impact of laparoscopy on modern practice. Urol Clin North Am 15:537–540, 1988.
59. Duckett, JW: Laparoscopy for cryptorchidism. Dialog Pediatr Urol 11:6, 1988.
60. Elder, JS: Laparoscopy and Fowler-Stephens orchiopexy in the management of the impalpable testis. Urol Clin North Am 16:399, 1989.
61. Weiss, RM; Seashore, JH: Laparoscopy in the management of the nonpalpable testis. J Urol 138:382, 1987.
62. Wickham, JEA: The surgical treatment of renal lithiasis. In: Urinary Calculus Disease. New York, Churchill Livingstone, 1979, pp. 145–198.
63. Eshghi, AM; Roth, JS; Smith, AD: Percutaneous transperitoneal approach to a pelvic kidney for endourological removal of staghorn calculus. J Urol 134:525, 1985.
64. Griffith, DP; Schuessler, WW; Nickell, KG; Meaney, JT: Laparoscopic pelvic lymphadenectomy for prostatic adenocarcinoma. Urol Clin North Am 19:407, 1992.
65. Winfield, HN; Ryan, KJ: Laparoscopy — new urological applications. Presented at the American Urological Association 84th Annual Meeting, May 7, 1989.
66. Schuessler, WW; Vancaillie, TG; Reich, H; Griffith, DP: Transperitoneal endosurgical lymphadenectomy in patients with localized prostate cancer. J Urol 145:988, 1991.
67. Chapple, CR; Osborne, JL: Laparoscopic colposuspension — a new procedure. Presented at the American Urological Association 87th Annual Meeting, May 11, 1992.
68. Das, S: Laparoscopic bladder diverticulectomy. Presented at the American Urological Association 87th Annual Meeting, May 13, 1992.
69. Donovan, JF; Winfield, HN: Laparoscopic varix ligation. J Urol 147:77, 1992.
70. Kavoussi, LR; Clayman, RV: Organ entrapment system for removing nodal tissue during laparoscopic pelvic lymphadenectomy. J Urol 147(3, Pt 2):879, 1992.
71. Kozminski, M; Partamian, K; Moeller, R; Remis, R: The laparoscopic formation of an ileal loop conduit. Presented at the American Urological Association 87th Annual Meeting, May 13, 1992.
72. Lowe, BA; Novy, MJ; Strang, E: Laparoscopic segmental cystectomy. Presented at the American Urological Association 87th Annual Meeting, May 13, 1992.
73. Parra, RO; Andrus, C; Boullier, J: Staging laparoscopic pelvic lymph node dissection: Comparison of results with open pelvic lymphadenectomy. J Urol 147:875, 1992.
74. Vancaillie, TG; Schuessler, W: Laparoscopic bladderneck suspension. J Laparoendosc Surg 1:169, 1991.
75. Waples, MJ; Wegenke, JD; Vega, RJ: Laparoscopic management of lymphocele after pelvic lymphadenectomy and radical retropubic prostatectomy. Urology 39:82, 1992.
76. Winfield, HN; Donovan, JF; Loening, SA; Williams, RD: Urological laparoscopic surgery. J Urol 146:941, 1991.

77. Weinberg, JJ; Smith, AD: Percutaneous resection of the kidney: Preliminary report. J Endourol 2:355, 1988.

78. Clayman, RV; Kavoussi, LR: Laparoscopic procedures: Nephrectomy. Technique and results. Presented at The Society for Minimally Invasive Therapy Third International Meeting, Nov. 12, 1991.

79. Clayman, RV; Kavoussi, LR; Soper, NJ; et al: Laparoscopic nephrectomy: Initial case report. J Urol 146:278, 1991.

80. Copcoat, M; Joyce, A; Rassweiler, J; Popert R: Laparoscopic nephrectomy: The Kings clinical experience. Presented at the American Urological Association 87th Annual Meeting, May 13, 1992.

81. Clayman, RV; Kavoussi, LR; Figenshau, RS; et al: Laparoscopic nephroureterectomy: Initial clinical case report. J Laparoendosc Surg 1:343, 1991.

82. Schuessler, WW; Kavoussi, LR; Clayman, RV; Vancaillie, TG: Laparoscopic radical prostatectomy: Initial case report. Presented at the American Urological Association 87th Annual Meeting, May 10, 1992.

SECTION II

PHYSIOLOGY AND ANATOMY

CHAPTER 2

Physiologic Considerations in Laparoscopy

Marshall L. Stoller, MD
J. Stuart Wolf, Jr, MD

Laparoscopy is an exciting development in urology. It is a significant step forward in the evolution of minimally invasive surgery. Laparoscopy is associated with decreased postoperative pain, shortened convalescence, and lower global costs. Enthusiasm, however, must not overshadow the limitations of laparoscopy. One of the most important considerations is the large set of physiologic alterations associated with laparoscopy. Instilling a physiologically active gas (CO_2) at a pressure of 20 mm Hg into the peritoneum of a patient placed in unusual positions can have significant effects.

Fortunately, urologists are accustomed to dealing with operative techniques that have unique physiologic effects. The most obvious example is transurethral resection. Early in training surgeons are taught about fluid absorption, hyponatremia, hemolysis and so forth. Consideration of the physiology of transurethral resection soon becomes an integral part of the procedure. Urologists think as much about potential extravasation as they do about where to place the electrocautery loop.

Laparoscopy should be no different. The cardiac and pulmonary effects of the technique are in many ways more profound than those associated with open surgery. Performing laparoscopic procedures without an awareness of what is being done to the patient's physiologic condition is as negligent as performing transurethral resection with no regard to perforation.

INSUFFLANT AND PULMONARY CONSIDERATIONS

Long before laparoscopy enjoyed widespread use, pneumoperitoneum was applied for diagnostic radiography and therapy for tuberculosis and chronic pulmonary emphysema.[1–3] Early investigations of the pulmonary effects of pneumoperitoneum focused on the mechanical aspects.[4,5] More recently, following the adoption of CO_2 for insufflation and the realization that hypercapnia has significant physiologic effects, investigators have considered the role of gas absorption during laparoscopy. The discussion of the insufflant and pulmonary considerations in laparoscopy begins with a description of the principles of gas absorption.

Gas Equilibria

The gas-filled peritoneal cavity is a closed, collapsible space.[6] The sum total of gas flux is always directed out of such a space. The *direction* of individual gas movement is determined by partial pressure gradients. The *rate* of movement is determined by the permeability of the surrounding blood-tissue to the gases.[7] The term *blood-tissue* refers to the tissue (peritoneum) surrounding the cavity and the medium (blood) flowing around it. The former limits gas absorption by diffusion and the latter limits absorption by perfusion.[8] The diffusibility and solubility coefficients of each gas, in conjunction with the nature of the tissue and degree of perfusion surrounding a cavity, determine the tissue permeability of the gas. Table 2–1 lists the solubility, diffusibility and tissue permeation (in subcutaneous tissue) for selected gases.

Tissues are highly permeable to CO_2, approximately 20 times more permeable than O_2. Figure 2–1 outlines the partial pressure differences driving the gas equilibria during CO_2 pneumoperitoneum. Carbon dioxide moves out of the cavity because of a very large gradient, whereas N_2 and O_2 diffuse in the opposite direction. Tissue permeation of O_2 and N_2 is low compared with CO_2, so that their movement is relatively slow. The primary effect is rapid diffusion of CO_2 into the blood stream.

The absolute rate of CO_2 absorption from the peritoneal cavity in humans has not been conclusively determined, but an estimate based on published figures can be derived. Collins[9] found nitrous oxide (N_2O) to be absorbed from the peritoneal cavity of piglets at a rate of 294 ml/hour. He estimated the rate in humans to be twice as high. The absorption rate of N_2O from the human peritoneal cavity thus would be 9.8 ml/minute and by extrapolation from Table 2–1, that of CO_2 would be 13.6 ml/minute. This seems to be a small amount of CO_2 compared with the basal metabolic production of CO_2 (150 to 200 ml/minute). The impact of CO_2 absorption during laparoscopy can be much greater in the clinical setting, however.

Carbon dioxide is transported in the blood in several forms.[10] The hydration of CO_2 to carbonic acid occurs slowly without a catalyst, but in the presence of carbonic anhydrase, the reaction accelerates. Once carbonic acid is formed, it ionizes almost completely to bicarbonate ion and hydrogen ion.

$$CO_2 + H_2O \leftrightarrow H_2CO_3 \rightarrow HCO_3^- + H^+$$

Table 2–1. PHYSICAL PROPERTIES OF SELECTED GASES

Gas	Solubility (relative to N_2)	Diffusion (relative to N_2)	Tissue Permeability (relative to N_2)
N_2	1.0	1.0	1.0
He	0.7	2.7	1.3
H_2	1.3	1.9	1.8
O_2	1.9	0.9	1.8
Argon	2.2	0.9	2.0
N_2O	33.0	0.9	28.0
CO_2	47.0	0.9	39.0

Sources: Data collected and extrapolated from references 7, 9, 174, 176, 178, and 179.

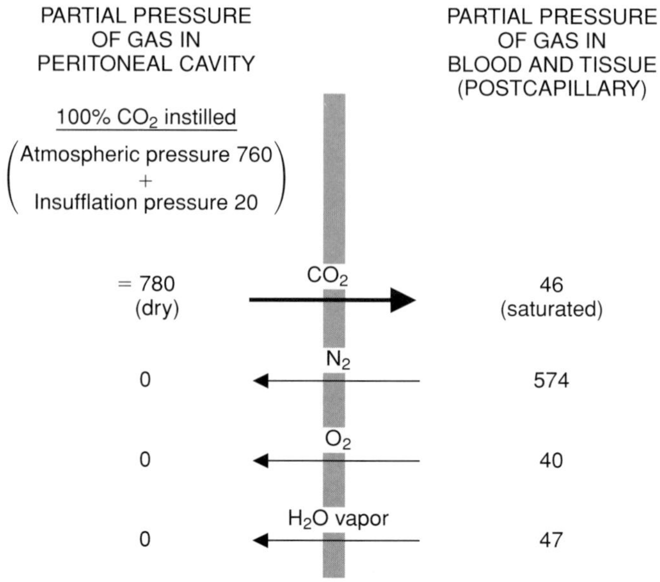

Figure 2–1. Gas equilibria during CO_2 pneumoperitoneum. Values are partial pressures in mm Hg.

Bicarbonate is the largest fraction of CO_2 in the blood, about 90%. The hydrogen ions produced are buffered by plasma proteins and reduced hemoglobin. On oxidation of hemoglobin in the alveolar capillaries, the hydrogen ions are released to drive the reverse reaction, and CO_2 is expired. Dissolved CO_2 and other minor forms constitute the remaining fraction of CO_2 in blood. Cell membranes permit rapid diffusion of CO_2 but are relatively impervious to hydrogen ion. CO_2 can diffuse across a membrane and if carbonic anhydrase is present, can rapidly disassociate to bicarbonate and hydrogen ions. Hydrogen ions are trapped by the membrane, but bicarbonate exchanges with chloride ions across the membrane.

The total amount of CO_2 in the human body is 120 L.[10] Most is stored in the bone and fat compartment, which equilibrates slowly (weeks) and is not important in a consideration of acute effects during laparoscopy. The rapid (primarily blood) and medium-speed (primarily skeletal muscle) compartments play a significant role in the response to CO_2 absorption during laparoscopy. These compartments buffer changes in CO_2 content so as to maintain the arterial CO_2 ($PaCO_2$) at a relatively constant pressure. Experimental estimates of the short-term (minutes to 1 to 2 hours) storage capacity average 1 ml/mm Hg/kg.[11,12] If CO_2 is the insufflating gas, and it is absorbed at a rate of 14 ml/min, the $PaCO_2$ should rise at a rate of 0.2 mm Hg/min in a 70-kg man. Over the course of a one-half hour procedure, 420 ml of CO_2 would be absorbed—enough to raise the $PaCO_2$ 6 mm Hg if ventilation is not increased.

This degree of $PaCO_2$ elevation is based on only

peritoneal absorption and does not take into account the effects of positioning, anesthesia, increased intra-abdominal pressure, and extraperitoneal gas. For example, CO_2 storage increases with decreasing cardiac output, decreasing alveolar ventilation, and increasing pulmonary deadspace.[10,13] These additional hemodynamic and respiratory changes have impact on CO_2 absorption as demonstrated by the variability of $PaCO_2$ and expired CO_2 found during clinical studies of laparoscopy.

Carbon Dioxide Absorption

Carbon dioxide production, the sum of metabolic CO_2 and absorbed CO_2, can be estimated by the product of expired CO_2 and minute ventilation. Despite its limitations, it is the best available measure of CO_2 absorption. The resting CO_2 production of an anesthetized patient is 100 to 200 ml/minute. Reported values of the increase of CO_2 production over baseline during laparoscopy range from 14 ml/minute to approximately 48 ml/minute.[14-17] One group reported that CO_2 production increased 60% in patients undergoing CO_2 laparoscopy.[18] No investigators have found a decrease in CO_2 production, and only one study reported no change.[19] In general, these findings indicate somewhat higher CO_2 production during clinical laparoscopy than is predicted based on experimental physiology. The findings of Sosa and associates[20] might explain part of this discrepancy. They reported that of eight patients with $PaCO_2$ over 50 mm Hg during laparoscopic pelvic lymphadenectomy, seven had subcutaneous emphysema. None of the eight patients with $PaCO_2$ less than 50 mm Hg had subcutaneous emphysema. Although subcutaneous gas is absorbed more slowly than peritoneal gas,[9] if the area and volume of subcutaneous emphysema are extensive, significant quantities of CO_2 may be absorbed.[21]

Table 2–2 summarizes the findings of three studies comparing N_2O insufflation with CO_2 insufflation in patients under general anesthesia with controlled respiration at a fixed minute ventilation. These investigations are especially valuable because any differences in $PaCO_2$ between the two groups should directly reflect CO_2 absorption. The average increase in $PaCO_2$ was 0.5 mm Hg in the N_2O group and 10.7 mm Hg in the CO_2 group. The duration of insufflation was less than one-half hour in all three studies. This increase in $PaCO_2$ is greater than that previously calculated, confirming the impression that CO_2 production during clinical laparoscopy is higher than expected.

Table 2–2. COMPARISON OF $PaCO_2$ CHANGES DURING N_2O AND CO_2 LAPAROSCOPY

Study	Change in $PaCO_2$ in mm Hg	
	N_2O group (No. of Patients)	*CO_2 group (No. of Patients)*
Alexander and Brown[50]	−1.4 (15)	+8.6 (15)
Magno[46]	0 (11)	+9.5 (13)
El-Minawi et al[51]	+1.9 (25)	+12.5 (25)
Average	+0.5 (51)	+10.7 (53)

Patients in all three studies were under general anesthesia with ventilation controlled at a fixed rate.

In clinical practice, however, patients are not managed with fixed ventilation rates. With the capacity to monitor end-tidal CO_2 by capnography, the anesthesiologist can increase ventilation to keep up with CO_2 absorption. The $PaCO_2$ should rise less than in patients managed with fixed ventilation. Among 40 patients in two studies managed with controlled respiration using variable minute ventilation, the average increase in $PaCO_2$ was 6.3 mm Hg.[22,23] The duration of pneumoperitoneum exceeded 30 minutes in both studies. Increasing minute ventilation will usually prevent dangerous hypercapnia. In a recent series of 250 laparoscopic cholecystectomies, including 10 in patients rating American Society of Anesthesiology (ASA) class 3, no case was aborted because of hypercapnia.[24] Wittgen and associates[23] converted two of 30 laparoscopic cholecystectomies to open procedures because of hypercapnia, both in patients classified as ASA 2 or 3. The experience at our institution has generally been that hypercapnia can be controlled, but we have converted one laparoscopic pelvic lymphadenectomy to an open procedure because of hypercapnia associated with extensive subcutaneous emphysema.

Several reports indicate that $PaCO_2$ or CO_2 production or both can remain persistently elevated after desufflation of the abdomen.[15,17,25,26] This is consistent with the concept of CO_2 storage. As more CO_2 is absorbed and stored in skeletal muscle, the longer it will take for a steady state to be achieved following desufflation. As laparoscopic procedures become more extensive and operative time increases, it is reasonable to expect this phenomenon of postlaparoscopy CO_2 elevation to be seen more frequently. Close monitoring in the recovery room is mandatory.

Mechanical Effects

Under general anesthesia, functional reserve capacity (FRC) and respiratory compliance are decreased, and pulmonary deadspace and shunt are increased.[27] Significant ventilation and perfusion mismatch may occur. The application of positive end-expiratory pressure (PEEP) may help counteract some of these adverse effects. PEEP reduces pulmonary shunt and increases FRC at the expense of decreasing cardiac output, as confirmed in a study of laparoscopic patients managed with 3.7 mm Hg of PEEP.[28]

Pelvic laparoscopy is often performed in a 15° to 25° Trendelenburg, or head-down tilt, position. The head-down tilt position elevates the diaphragm and decreases vital capacity. These effects are minimal in healthy patients and can easily be managed with controlled ventilation, but in patients with elevated left-sided heart pressures the concurrent increase in central pressure may lead to pulmonary edema.[29]

The increase in intra-abdominal pressure during gas insufflation has ventilatory effects similar to head-down tilt position. An intra-abdominal pressure of 4 mm Hg is equivalent to 25° head-down tilt in terms of pressure on the diaphragm, estimated to be 1 to 2 kg.[28] Scott[30] derived a greater figure of 50 kg of total force with 25 mm Hg intra-abdominal pressure. During 20 mm Hg intra-abdominal pressure, impedance measurements have demonstrated elevation of the diaphragm beyond that produced by 20° head-down tilt alone.[31] The increased intra-abdominal pressure is reflected by increased intrathoracic pressure, which necessitates an elevated airway pressure to maintain ventilation.[32] Lung capacity is reduced by intra-abdominal pressure, with worsening of ventilation and perfusion mismatch.[33] Reduction of capacity increases alveolar deadspace but decreases anatomic deadspace,[17] so that the combined effect on physiologic deadspace is unclear. Physiologic deadspace is one of the determinants of the arterial and end-tidal $PaCO_2$ gradient ($P[a/ET]CO_2$).[34]

Capnography

During laparoscopy the noninvasive measurement of expired (end-tidal) CO_2 with capnography is extremely useful for monitoring the effects of CO_2 absorption. Lee and associates[35] reported the end-tidal CO_2 to be elevated 8.3 mm Hg during CO_2 laparoscopy. For capnography to be a reliable indicator of CO_2 homeostasis, however, it must correlate with $PaCO_2$. In a resting patient, the $P(a/ET)CO_2$ gradient is 1 to 2 mm Hg. It generally rises to 3 to 4 mm Hg during general anesthesia. Brampton and Watson[36] noted a $P(a/ET)CO_2$ gradient of 3.3 mm Hg during laparoscopy, but they did not obtain baseline measurements for comparison. Most investigators have found no difference or a slight increase in $P(a/ET)CO_2$ during laparoscopy in healthy patients, compared with values obtained under anesthesia but before gas insufflation.[17–19,22,37–39] Wittgen and associates[23] in an extremely important study comparing ASA class 1 to ASA class 2 and class 3 patients undergoing laparoscopic cholecystectomy with CO_2 insufflation, found an increase in $PaCO_2$ and $P(a/ET)CO_2$ in both groups. The elevation of $PaCO_2$ was greater in the ASA 2 and 3 patients (14.1 mm Hg) than among the ASA 1 patients (5.9 mm Hg). End-tidal CO_2 rose less than $PaCO_2$, so that the $P(a/ET)CO_2$ gradient increased from 2.1 to 5.9 mm Hg in the ASA 1 patients and from 2.6 to 11.3 mm Hg in the ASA 2 and 3 patients. A significant correlation between $P(a/ET)CO_2$ and $PaCO_2$ has been confirmed in another laparoscopic study.[39]

$P(a/ET)CO_2$ is also increased by decreasing cardiac output, decreasing alveolar ventilation, and increasing pulmonary deadspace.[34] Because all these changes may occur with laparoscopy, especially with the longer procedures in older urologic oncology patients, the $P(a/ET)CO_2$ gradient may increase even more. This, combined with the thorough study by Raemer and associates[40] that demonstrated the extreme variability of $P(a/ET)CO_2$ between patients and even within patients over time, would argue that periodic arterial blood gas sampling is indicated in most patients undergoing extensive laparoscopic surgical procedures. Capnography remains useful for its real-time capability. Any unexpected trend or sudden change is an indication for arterial blood gas sampling.

Acid-Base Changes

Laparoscopy and CO_2 absorption cause a mild acidosis. Since patients may be hyperventilated during the procedure, the pH values during laparoscopy range from 7.25 to 7.50, with most reported values between 7.35 and 7.40.[41–44] A few investigators have reported bicarbonate values as well as pH and $PaCO_2$. A relative respiratory acidosis secondary to accumulation of CO_2 has been seen in all studies. Minimal trends towards metabolic alkalosis[22,37] or metabolic acidosis[38,45,46] have been noted. If artificial ventilation cannot keep up with the CO_2 accumulation either because of rapid CO_2 absorption or pulmonary disease, blood pH can drop precipitously.

It is interesting to acknowledge the acidic changes noted in fluid from the pouch of Douglas during CO_2 laparoscopy for oocyte retrieval or transfer procedures. Mean pHs of 6.69 and 6.99 have been reported.[22,47] One group of investigators also included patients in whom air was used for insufflation; the pH of pouch of Douglas fluid was normal at 7.40.[22] These findings confirm the supposition that CO_2 insufflation produces carbonic acid in the peritoneal cavity. The carbonic acid is thought to be responsible for increased pain with CO_2 compared with N_2O used for insufflation under local anesthesia.

Oxygenation

Laparoscopy can impair oxygenation by several mechanisms. Arterial oxygen pressure (PaO_2) is primarily increased by raising the inspired O_2 concentration. Certain hemodynamic conditions may blunt this effect. Decreased cardiac output, increased pulmonary shunt, worsened ventilation and perfusion mismatch, decreased alveolar ventilation, and acidosis—all of which may occur during laparoscopy—will decrease PaO_2.[48] Most clinical studies have indicated that PaO_2

tends to decrease during laparoscopy, but the change is not always statistically significant. Corall and associates[49] found the mean PaO_2 to fall from 163.1 to 146.5 mm Hg (not statistically significant) during N_2O laparoscopy in 10 patients. These investigators did note that two patients, both heavy smokers, experienced a drop in PaO_2 to less than 100 mm Hg. Among three groups of investigators comparing PaO_2 values during CO_2 and N_2O pneumoperitoneum, the only statistically significant change was a decrease from 274 to 231 mm Hg in the CO_2 group in one study.[46,50,51] Any theoretical risk of diffusion hypoxia secondary to N_2O absorption is not supported clinically. Baratz and Karis[41] recommended that inspired gas mixtures during laparoscopy should contain at least 50% O_2. Other investigators have also reported minimal to moderate decreases in PaO_2 during laparoscopy.[17,23,37,44,50] A few reports have noted no change in PaO_2 or even a slight increase.[18,42,43] In general, there is a tendency for PaO_2 to fall during laparoscopy. A higher inspired O_2 concentration than would be required during open surgery may be needed; using a concentration over 50% would provide an adequate margin of safety in most cases.

Extraperitoneal Gas

Laparoscopy is something of a misnomer. *Peritoneoscopy* was the medical subject heading used by the National Library of Medicine through 1992. It is more descriptive; the physician visualizes (*skopein* Greek, to look at) the peritoneal cavity (*periteinein* Greek, to stretch over). The term reminds us of the site of insufflation as originally intended. *Laparoscopy* (*lapara* Greek, flank) is actually more descriptive of direct extraperitoneal insufflation for retroperitoneal surgery, procedures to which the term *retroperitoneoscopy* has also been applied.[52] Direct extraperitoneal pelvic visualization through an endoscope has been appropriately referred to as *pelviscopy* (*pelvis* Latin, a basin).[53] Nonetheless, we continue with the term *laparoscopy* for the general description of examining pelvic, abdominal, or retroperitoneal organs through a gas-filled cavity.

Semantics aside, extraperitoneal gas insufflation, whether inadvertent or purposeful, carries additional physiologic considerations. The anatomically intact peritoneal cavity contains no openings except for the ends of the fallopian tubes. During ideal laparoscopy, insufflated gas should remain intraperitoneal except for that absorbed through the peritoneum or lost during instrument changes. However, the total volume of gas insufflated during a procedure is much more than can be accounted for by these mechanisms. Leakage around the trocar site is probably responsible for most of this excess gas loss. If the gas remains under the skin, subcutaneous emphysema ensues. When minimal, this is not of concern, since the CO_2 is rapidly absorbed. But if subcutaneous emphysema becomes pronounced, there may be significant adverse effects. The associated increased CO_2 absorption has been discussed earlier.

Extraperitoneal gas—whether subcutaneous, preperitoneal, or retroperitoneal—can dissect along planes and produce pneumomediastinum. As the mediastinal gas moves laterally along the visceral pleura of the pulmonary vasculature, rupture into the pleural space can cause pneumothorax.[54] Fatalities associated with both pneumomediastinum and pneumothorax secondary to pneumoperitoneum have been reported.[54,55] A less likely mechanism of pneumothorax, but one that has been suggested based on pathologic findings, is that of a diaphragmatic defect allowing passage of peritoneal gas directly into the pleural space.[56-58] The progression of subcutaneous emphysema to pneumomediastinum to pneumothorax is supported by the large survey of Brühl.[59] Among 63,845 laparoscopies, the complications of subcutaneous emphysema, pneumomediastinum, and pneumothorax were reported in 366, 50, and 18 cases, respectively. Although the passage of gas directly into the pleural cavity through a diaphragmatic defect can not be excluded, it would not explain the frequent concurrence of subcutaneous emphysema and pneumomediastinum with pneumothorax. Clayman and associates[60] initially reported that pneumothorax complicated the only laparoscopic nephrectomy performed by their group with a direct extraperitoneal insufflation technique; none of the transperitoneal nephrectomies resulted in pneumothorax. Retroperitoneal laparoscopy with direct extraperitoneal insufflation does not always meet with this complication.[52] There has been one case report of combined subcutaneous emphysema, pneumomediastinum, bilateral pneumothorax, and pneumopericardium following laparoscopy.[61]

Subcutaneous emphysema can be minimized by securing the trocars in place with sutures. The initial puncture with the Verres needle may also be the source of extraperitoneal gas. Care must be taken to ensure proper placement. Use of the Hasson cannula for open insertion will obviate the risk of initial extraperitoneal insufflation, but too large a fascial incision will allow gas to escape around the trocar. High intra-abdominal pressure contributes to subcutaneous emphysema. At least one case of subcutaneous emphysema has been attributed to a malfunctioning CO_2 insufflator that delivered excessive pressure.[62] If subcutaneous emphysema is noted, the patient must immediately be examined for evidence of pneumothorax such as hypotension, increased airway pressure, or decreased breath sounds. Needle thoracentesis is indicated if the patient's condition is unstable. Chest radiographs should be obtained when the diagnosis is in question. The end-tidal CO_2 tracing should be inspected and blood gas sampling should be considered to evaluate for hypercapnia. If a clinically small pneumothorax is subsequently detected, observation may be elected since rapid absorption of the CO_2 pneumothorax is expected.[63,64]

Gas Embolism

Venous gas embolism is the intravenous passage of gas bubbles into the heart and pulmonary circulation, resulting in circulatory restriction or blockage. It can be a dramatic laparoscopic complication, with several deaths reported.[65–69] The incidence of venous air embolism during neurosurgical procedures in the sitting position was 25% in one series.[70] It occurs infrequently during laparoscopy but remains a feared complication. Large surveys of laparoscopy report the incidence of gas embolism to be between 1.5 and 15.9 per 100,000 cases.[59,68,71] Gas embolism during pneumoperitoneum was recognized as early as 1921, and it was first noted during laparoscopy in 1951.[65] The recent literature contains many case reports of venous gas embolism associated with laparoscopy.

Most commonly, gas enters the venous system during initial insufflation, either with the Verres needle or the first trocar. Presence of blood on the initial test aspiration, pulsation of the gas flow monitor, and lack of abdominal distention are warning signs of intravascular needle placement. Laparoscopic punctures of the liver,[72] omental vessels,[73] and uterine fundus,[74,75] leading to gas embolism have been documented. Gas embolism has occurred during laparoscopic cholecystectomy following puncture of the liver with an air-cooled laser.[76] The actual site of venous puncture is often difficult to determine. Transvaginal insufflation seems to carry a higher risk.[77,78] Parenthetically, gas embolism occurs much more frequently during CO_2 hysteroscopy with an incidence of 5% reported by one group.[79]

Gas embolism rarely occurs beyond the first few minutes of the procedure. Brantley and Riley[80] reported two cases of cardiovascular collapse during laparoscopic tubal ligation, both occurring during manipulation of the fallopian tubes. They conjectured that CO_2 embolism might have been responsible, but severe vagal reaction is more consistent with the case reports. Although McKenzie[66] thought that CO_2 might enter a vein that has been ruptured by the elevated intra-abdominal pressure, and Kleppinger[81] reported a case thought to be due to entry through a bleeding mesosalpingeal vessel, it is likely that the emptied cephalad portion of an open vein will collapse under the elevated intra-abdominal pressure and prevent embolization by this route. If the venous laceration is minimal, however, allowing enough blood flow through the vessel to keep it open cephalad to the injury, then a CO_2 bolus could possibly enter the circulation in this manner. Root and associates[67] described a case of death secondary to gas embolism in which clinical deterioration was not noted until after laparotomy was performed, following a diagnostic laparoscopy. Postmortem films and autopsy demonstrated gas in the cerebral vessels, pulmonary artery, aorta, heart, inferior vena cava, and portal venous system. They postulated that CO_2 had entered the portal system through an undetected venous laceration and was trapped there for a period of time before embolizing centrally.

The pathophysiologic effects of gas embolism have been well described. A large bolus of gas entering the right atrium will cause an "air lock" of the right side of the heart's outflow track, effectively halting all cardiac output and leading to complete cardiovascular collapse. A smaller bolus will pass through the right side of the heart into the pulmonary vasculature, where it may cause reflexive vasoconstriction and directly block the pulmonary microcirculation. The result is intrapulmonary shunting around the blocked vessels and an increase in pulmonary artery pressure. The shunting causes increased alveolar deadspace which, disregarding for the moment the increase in CO_2 exchange which may occur if the embolized gas is CO_2, will diminish the amount of CO_2 expired. Nonhydrostatic pulmonary edema may occur secondary to leukocyte and platelet activation and aggregation.[82,83] As pressure rises on the right side of the heart and falls on the left side, the gradient for coronary artery flow is diminished. Additionally, if the right-sided heart pressure exceeds that of the left side, a probe-patent foramen ovale, present in 20% to 25% of the population, may open and allow paradoxical embolization into the arterial tree. Theoretically, arterial gas could also be the result of passage through the pulmonary circulation.[84] Arterial gas has been described by several investigators, the most serious effects being due to cerebral and coronary occlusion; it is often noted in fatal cases.[65,67,69,83–85]

The nature of the gas has an important role in determining the outcome of embolism. Air (~80% nitrogen) is resorbed slowly in blood. As Table 2–1 indicates, CO_2 is 47 times more soluble than nitrogen. Graff and associates[86] found the lethal dose of CO_2 in 50% of subjects (LD_{50}) to be five times that of air when injected intravenously in dogs. In humans, approximately 1200 ml of CO_2 or 240 ml of air therefore would be lethal. The rate of injection is also important, as slow injection of gas is well tolerated.[87] Using CO_2 for insufflation provides the greatest margin of safety should embolization occur.

The differential diagnosis of circulatory collapse during laparoscopy includes arrhythmia secondary to hypercapnia, vasovagal reaction, decreased venous return resulting from increased intra-abdominal pressure, pneumothorax, hemorrhage, pulmonary thromboembolism, or gas embolism. Physical findings consistent with gas embolism include hypotension, cyanosis, and arrhythmia. Cardiovascular collapse during insufflation is highly suggestive of gas embolism. Inspection of the ECG tracing may reveal a widened QRS complex and right-sided heart strain pattern.[88] The only absolute diagnostic criteria for gas embolization is aspiration of gas from the circulation. Noninvasive methods, however, are used for intraoperative monitoring. A precordial or esophageal stethoscope may reveal the classic "millwheel" murmur. In general, even a small pulmonary arterial occlusion can be detected by monitoring the *fall* in expired CO_2 that occurs when ventilated alveoli are deprived of pulmonary blood flow.[89] If the embolus is a CO_2 bubble, however, most investigators have reported that the end-tidal CO_2 transiently increases.[83,90,91] This is due to rapid dissolution of smaller CO_2 bubbles and increased amounts of CO_2 available for gas exchange in those alveoli that continue to receive pulmonary blood flow. Since a *decrease* in end-tidal CO_2 has also been reported with CO_2 embolism,[78] monitoring for acute changes of the capnograph tracing in either direction will alert the anesthesiologist to the possibility of gas embolism. Precordial Doppler ultrasonography or transesophageal echocardiography is exquisitely sensitive for gas embolism, but their expense is not justified, given the low incidence of gas embolism during laparoscopy.[92]

Treatment of gas embolism must be rapid. The inspired gas should be switched to 100% oxygen and the patient should be ventilated manually. Inspired N_2O will enlarge a bubble of air, because N_2O diffuses into the bubble faster than the air diffuses out. This does not occur with a CO_2 bubble, because CO_2 diffuses faster than does N_2O. The reason for the switch to 100% O_2 is simply to treat the concurrent hypoxia. Rapid manual ventilation speeds expiration of the resorbed CO_2 and provides a partial-pressure gradient for further dissolution. The abdomen should be desufflated, and the patient should be placed in a head-down and left lateral position. This position has been shown experimentally to allow continuity of blood flow past the "air lock" in the right side of the heart.[93] Aspiration of gas from the right side of the heart may be attempted but can be a difficult maneuver. Even under controlled conditions, it takes more than 6 minutes to pass a catheter to the right atrium and into the proper position for aspiration.[94]

Hyperbaric oxygen has been used to treat CO_2 embolus,[83] but its value has appropriately been questioned since O_2 (theoretically) should not speed the resorption of CO_2 (as it will with the N_2 bubbles that occur during diving accidents).[95] In fact, if treatment of a CO_2 embolus is delayed, enough O_2 can diffuse into the bubble—despite its lower solubility—to prolong its resorption.[96] Cardiac bypass has been used to treat laparoscopic gas embolism.[91] Most patients will recover with the rapid institution of head-down and left lateral position, 100% oxygen with manual ventilation, and cardiac resuscitation. Attempts at catheter aspiration are reasonable as long as positioning is not delayed.

Choice of Insufflant

Several of the preceding sections address the properties of different insufflating gases. Here we briefly outline the advantages and disadvantages of the ones most commonly employed during laparoscopy. The pioneers of laparoscopy used pneuma vulgaris (room air) to produce the pneumoperitoneum. The problems of air embolism and extremely slow absorption of air led to the search for alternative substances. Oxygen is not much more soluble than N_2, and carries the additional risk of supporting explosive combustion, as discovered by one unfortunate laparoscopist.[97] Carbon dioxide has been the gas primarily used during laparoscopy for several decades. Its advantages include inability to support combustion and rapid absorption. Its disadvantages are the irritating effects of CO_2 on the peritoneum and the potential for hypercapnia. Nitrous oxide was employed by many laparoscopists in the 1970s and 1980s. Its advantage is greatest in the patient undergoing laparoscopy with local anesthesia because of the decreased discomfort compared with CO_2 noted by most (but not all) investigators.[98–100]

Nitrous oxide will support combustion. In a series of letters in the British Medical Journal in 1975 and 1976 the explosive hazard of N_2O pneumoperitoneum was debated. One group argued that N_2O combined with methane and hydrogen, which might also be present in the peritoneal cavity either because of diffusion or bowel injury, was dangerously explosive and precluded any use of N_2O insufflation together with electrocautery.[101–104] The other group maintained that the risk of explosion was exaggerated and that electrocautery could safely be used in the presence of N_2O.[105–107] Not addressed in this exchange was the increased solubility of CO_2 over N_2O (a factor of 1.5). The extra margin of safety provided by CO_2 might be enough to prevent cardiovascular collapse should gas embolism occur.

Currently, CO_2 is the standard insufflating gas for operative laparoscopy. Most laparoscopists would rather confront the known effects of hypercapnia than risk an intra-abdominal explosion or exacerbation of gas embolism. For diagnostic procedures under local anesthesia, N_2O would be a good choice. It might also be preferred when a patient has pulmonary disease and there is concern regarding the ability of the patient to adequately expire an increased CO_2 load. The use of air is still reported,[108] but in general this is to be avoided if N_2O or CO_2 is available. Despite theoretical advantages and disadvantages, the admonition of Uhlich[109] merits attention: "The choice of the proper gas, although important, must always remain secondary to the proper technique for placing the pneumoperitoneum needle."

Clinical Implications

The additional burden on the respiratory system during laparoscopy is significant. Given generally good pulmonary function, the respiratory effects of laparoscopy are well tolerated by healthy patients. Alterations in pulmonary mechanics can be managed with intubation and artificial ventilation. The hypercapnia secondary to CO_2 absorption is usually controllable with increased minute ventilation—provided there is good gas exchange in the lungs, adequate circulation to prevent excessive CO_2 storage, no extensive subcutaneous emphysema, and no excessive intra-abdominal pressure. Capnographic monitoring is advised. Acid-base changes are minimal without hypercapnia. Hypoxia is not a problem with O_2 supplementation.

When considering older patients, however, the higher incidence of baseline pulmonary compromise may accentuate the impact of laparoscopy. Cardiovascular dysfunction may potentiate pulmonary problems. Hypercapnia can become significant, to the point at which the procedure must be converted to an open one. Operative times become prolonged with the more complicated laparoscopic procedures, further increasing the risk of pulmonary complications. Pulmonary function tests and consultation with anesthesiologists and pulmonologists should be considered in the patient with suspected respiratory disease. Patients with significant pulmonary disease poorly tolerate *any* procedure under general anesthesia, but there may be a subset of patients whose pulmonary reserves are adequate for an open procedure but insufficient for a prolonged laparoscopic one. Until more information is available, significant pulmonary disease should be considered a relative contraindication to laparoscopy.

Regardless of patient condition, pulmonary complications such as pneumomediastinum and pneumothorax may occur, necessitating emergent treatment. Extraperitoneal gas insufflation must be regarded as investigational at this point, as the risks of hypercapnia and pneumothorax may be increased. Finally, gas embolism is a rare but dramatic laparoscopic complication. The surgeon and anesthesiologist must be vigilant in monitoring the patient, especially during the critical initial insufflation.

Table 2–3. CARDIOVASCULAR EQUATIONS

Cardiac output = Heart rate × stroke volume

Arterial pressure = Cardiac output × arterial resistance

$$\text{Venous return} = \frac{\text{Systemic venous pressure} - \text{central venous pressure}}{\text{Venous resistance}}$$

CARDIOVASCULAR CONSIDERATIONS

Cardiovascular pathophysiology involves complex interrelationships. The equations listed in Table 2–3 reveal the primary relationships between cardiac performance and the peripheral vascular system. They appear deceptively simple. Using them to predict the hemodynamic effects of a given physiologic alteration can be difficult. Additionally, neural and hormonal feedback loops regulate the system continuously and alter the level of responsiveness to direct actions. Figure 2–2 is a simplified representation of some of the cardiovascular interrelationships.

The next topic headings describe the cardiovascular effects of positioning, CO_2, and intra-abdominal pressure, following which the integrated cardiovascular response to laparoscopy is presented. Both the authors and the readers must resist the temptation to oversimplify. It must be remembered that every patient comes into the operating room with a different blood volume, different baroreceptor sensitivity, different cardiac reserve, and so forth. No amount of preparation can allow prediction with certainty of the physiologic response of the individual patient to laparoscopy; there is no substitute for careful physical assessment and monitoring.

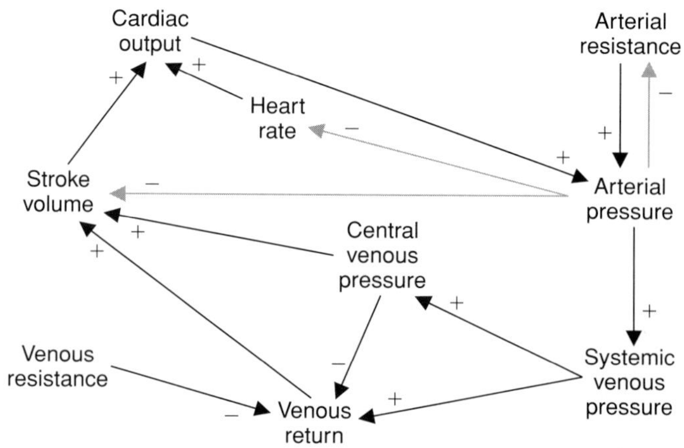

Figure 2–2. Simplified representation of cardiovascular interrelationships. The shaded arrows indicate baroreceptor feedback.

Effects of Positioning

The most common adult urologic laparoscopic procedures, pelvic lymphadenectomy and spermatic varicocelectomy, are performed with the patient in 15° to 20° head-down tilt position to improve access to the pelvic viscera. This position has several hemodynamic effects. It increases intracranial pressure while decreasing cerebral vascular flow.[29] These changes may be accentuated during laparoscopy as a result of increased intrathoracic venous pressure and hypercapnia. Patients with cerebral metastases may suffer dangerously elevated intracranial pressures.[110] Patients with marginal cerebral flow may experience ischemia.[29] A marked increase in ocular pressure with head-down tilt has been demonstrated in patients with poorly controlled glaucoma.[111] Myocardial oxygen demand is increased 15% by the head-down tilt position.[112] Patients with cerebral mass lesions, significant cerebral vascular disease, or glaucoma should not be placed in the head-down tilt position for prolonged periods.

In the normovolemic and normotensive healthy person, the hemodynamic alterations induced by head-down tilt are generally favorable, albeit minimal. Reich and associates[113] found that stroke output, arterial pressure, and cardiac output increased 6% to 13% with head-down tilt positioning in anesthetized cardiac patients. Findings were similar in a group of elderly postoperative patients.[114] The response of hypotensive patients to the head-down tilt position may be related to volume status. Two studies evaluating both normotensive and hypotensive subjects found cardiac output to be slightly increased in the former group but decreased in the latter.[115,116] Importantly, these hypotensive patients were apparently normovolemic. Considering hypovolemic shock, Zippe and associates[117] found that head-down tilt position in dogs maintained cardiac output despite a 24% blood volume loss. Detailed studies of hemorrhagic shock in humans treated with the head-down tilt position have not been reported in the literature.

The beneficial impact of the head-down tilt position during laparoscopy has been confirmed in several studies. Torrielli and associates[118] found that cardiac output fell 13% with pneumoperitoneum alone, but returned to baseline with addition of the head-down tilt position. An increase in cardiac output and arterial pressure was noted by Johannsen and associates[119] among patients with pneumoperitoneum after increasing head-down tilt from 15° to 30°. Kelman and associates[120] studied two groups of patients undergoing laparoscopy, one group in the horizontal position and the other in a 25° head-down tilt position. The latter group demonstrated higher baseline cardiac output. The head-down tilt position counteracts many of the adverse effects of increased intra-abdominal pressure.

Effects of Carbon Dioxide

Carbon dioxide, either by way of direct effects or by alterations in pH, is an important factor in normal cardiovascular regulation. It acts at several different sites in the body, often with opposing effects (Fig. 2–3). The direct effects of CO_2 primarily inhibit the cardiovascular system. In isolated or denervated preparations, CO_2 decreases the heart rate, cardiac contractility, and vascular resistance.[121,122] Counteracting these direct effects, however, is the stimulation of the sympathetic nervous system by CO_2. Sympathetic efferents and circulating catecholamines increase heart rate, cardiac contractility, and vascular resistance. If CO_2 rises to the point of acidosis, parasympathetic effects may be enhanced as well.[121] The overall result of moderate hypercapnia in the intact anesthetized patient is an increase in cardiac output and blood pressure. With a persistent, high elevation of CO_2, however, the cardiodepressive effects predominate, and hypotension may be fatal.[123] Total vascular resistance is decreased primarily because of alteration in the cerebral and cardiac circulations.[121] Stimulation by hypercapnia increases cardiac oxygen demand.[124]

Cardiac arrhythmias, primarily ventricular extrasystoles and tachycardia, may occur with hypercapnia and are caused by both sympathetic activation and direct effects of CO_2.[121] Scott[30] initially reported a 27% incidence of arrhythmias during laparoscopy. Later, in a study comparing CO_2 and N_2O for insufflation, the same investigator noted an incidence of arrhythmias of 17% with the former but only 4% with the latter.[125] Another group comparing CO_2 and N_2O found the incidence to be 50% and 0%, respectively.[126] These arrhythmias are usually benign, but fatal conduction disturbances can occur with marked $PaCO_2$ elevation. Laparoscopy with CO_2 insufflation less often causes

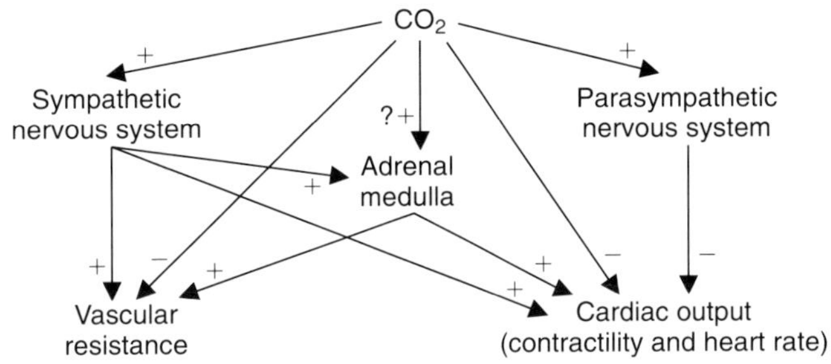

Figure 2–3. Cardiovascular effects of CO_2. (From Nunn, JF: The effects of changes in the carbon dioxide tension. In: Nunn, JF: Applied Respiratory Physiology. London, Butterworths, 1987, p. 461.)

bradyarrhythmias.[127,128] This is due to vagal stimulation by peritoneal stretch[129] combined with parasympathetic potentiation by hypercapnia. A case of asystolic cardiac arrest secondary to CO_2 pneumoperitoneum has been reported.[130] Premedication with atropine to prevent excessive vagal reaction, especially in patients undergoing laparoscopy with local anesthesia, has been recommended by some authors.[129,131]

When comparing the hemodynamics of N_2O and CO_2 pneumoperitoneum, El-Minawi and associates[51] found the increases in blood pressure and heart rate to be greater in the CO_2 group. Marshall and associates[132,133] also compared CO_2 and N_2O insufflation, and demonstrated that cardiac output was elevated 7% in the CO_2 group but decreased 27% in the N_2O group. Using N_2O or O_2 for insufflation, McKenzie and associates[134] noted cardiac output to decrease markedly, in contradistinction to the findings of other investigators using CO_2. The effects of CO_2 in patients undergoing laparoscopy are qualitatively similar to those of the head-down tilt position — increased cardiac output, increased arterial pressure, and decreased vascular resistance — but are somewhat greater in magnitude.

Effects of Increased Intra-abdominal Pressure

Hemodynamic alterations by increased intra-abdominal pressure have been extensively investigated. Animal models have played an important role in our understanding of the pathophysiology of increased intra-abdominal pressure. Unfortunately, almost all human studies have been in healthy young women undergoing diagnostic laparoscopy or laparoscopy with minimal manipulation. Investigations of patients similar to those undergoing urologic laparoscopy, who often are older and have multiple medical problems, are sorely needed. The hemodynamic impact of pneumoperitoneum can be broken down into the effects on cardiac output, vascular resistance, and vascular pressure. The alterations are often in opposing directions, so that the overall effect may be difficult to predict. We first describe a generalized model and then go on to explain how specific inputs can change the final outcome.

An important distinction is that between low-pressure and high-pressure pneumoperitoneum. As intra-abdominal pressure increases beyond a certain point, veins collapse, and overall blood flow becomes markedly impaired because of the great increase in resistance. At lower intra-abdominal pressure, the vessels are compressed, but collapse does not occur. Venous pressure is increased, but the change in resistance is much less than when the vessels are collapsed.[135] The balance between pressure changes and resistance changes is central to understanding the effects of pneumoperitoneum.

Arrhythmias resulting from CO_2 and pneumoperitoneum have been discussed earlier. Elevation of the diaphragm with pneumoperitoneum causes the heart to lie more transversely and to rotate slightly. Electrocardiographic morphology changes include left axis deviation and flattening or inversion of the T_3 wave.[175] Heart rate is generally elevated by increased intra-abdominal pressure, even in the absence of CO_2. At intra-abdominal pressures less than approximately 10 mm Hg, stroke volume is augmented, probably as a result of "autotransfusion" from partially emptied abdominal capacitance vessels.[28,120,140] At intra-abdominal pressures above this, stroke volume falls because the collapse of veins decreases venous return.[137–139,141] The result is that with extremely low intra-abdominal pressure ($\leq$10 mm Hg) cardiac output is modestly increased. At higher intra-abdominal pressure cardiac output tends to fall, depending on the balance between increased heart rate and decreased stroke volume. Any increase in intra-abdominal pressure generally causes an increase in arterial and venous resistance.[118,119,134,135,137,141–143] Compression forces blood out of the splanchnic vascular bed and sequesters it in the lower extremities.[144] Vasopressin release during laparoscopy may also play a role in increasing vascular tone.[145] If cardiac output is elevated, however, reflexes tend to relax vessel walls, and resistance may stay the same or even drop slightly.[28,140]

The balance between cardiac output and arterial resistance at intra-abdominal pressure $\leq$20 mm Hg tends to elevate arterial pressure.* At higher intra-abdominal pressure, particularly over 40 mm Hg, arterial pressure tends to fall as cardiac output decreases more than arterial resistance rises.[120,139,146] Lee[147] reported a case of acute hypotension during CO_2 laparoscopy with an intra-abdominal pressure of 40 mm Hg. After release of pneumoperitoneum, the blood pressure returned to normal and the procedure was successfully completed with an insufflation pressure of 15 to 20 mm Hg. Similar instances have been reported by others.[14] Occasionally, even the recommended levels of intra-abdominal pressure can cause hypotension. Lew and associates[148] reported the case of a 44-year-old healthy man who suffered hemodynamic instability near the end of a 2.5-hour laparoscopic cholecystectomy performed with a 20 mm Hg insufflation pressure. Death thought to be due to peritoneal overdistention and hemodynamic depression during laparoscopy has been reported.[149]

Central venous pressure, as measured by a trans-

*References 28, 32, 37, 118–120, 132, 133, 136, 138, 140, 141.

ducer within the right atrium, is the sum of intracardiac (transmural) and intrathoracic (pleural) pressures. The former reflects venous return and the ability of the heart to accept and pump blood. It is the effective cardiac-filling pressure. Intrathoracic pressure impedes venous return. The rise in central venous pressure usually seen during laparoscopy is primarily a consequence of increased intrathoracic pressure.[120,135,136,141] Intrathoracic pressure increases because of diaphragmatic elevation as a result of pneumoperitoneum. The transmural central venous pressure (measured central venous pressure minus intrathoracic pressure) rises with increasing intra-abdominal pressure up to approximately 20 mm Hg intra-abdominal pressure; with intra-abdominal pressure above this level, transmural central venous pressure falls. With excessive insufflation, the net effect on measured central venous pressure is to drop back to the baseline or lower as the decrease in transmural central venous pressure becomes greater than the increase in intrathoracic pressure. Measured central venous pressure is therefore not a good indicator of cardiac filling unless intrathoracic pressure is taken into account. Increases in airway pressure are reflective of diaphragmatic elevation by intra-abdominal pressure and can be used to help correct for transmural central venous pressure.

Systemic venous pressure, as measured by femoral vein pressure, rises in parallel with intra-abdominal pressure.[120,136,137,140,150] It is the driving force for venous return. For a given intra-abdominal pressure, the balance between systemic venous pressure, venous resistance, and transmural central venous pressure is dependent on the volume status of the patient. Kashtan and associates[135] constructed venous return curves based on experiments in dogs involving graded elevation of right atrial pressure with a Starling resistor. They demonstrated that at low right atrial pressure (analogous to hypovolemia in their model), a small increase of intra-abdominal pressure to 5 mm Hg caused an increase in venous return. Intra-abdominal pressure above this level decreased venous return. At normal right atrial pressure (2.6 mm Hg in their study), the point at which venous return started to drop occurred at higher intra-abdominal pressure. With elevated right atrial pressure (analogous to hypervolemia), venous resistance rose little because the capacitance vessels and smaller veins were too full to collapse; venous return was therefore augmented at intra-abdominal pressure up to 40 mm Hg. In a less complicated canine model, Toomasian and associates[150] found the adverse hemodynamic effects of pneumoperitoneum to be accentuated by graded hemorrhage.

Summarizing, an intra-abdominal pressure of less than 20 mm Hg (disregarding the effect of positioning or CO_2) modestly decreases stroke volume, cardiac output, and venous return while increasing heart rate, vascular pressure, and vascular resistance. Increasing intra-abdominal pressure beyond this, and certainly at pressures upward of 40 mm Hg, causes a substantial fall in cardiac output and less marked decrease in arterial pressure. The recommendation of limiting insufflation pressure to 15 to 20 mm Hg during laparoscopy has wide support in both clinical and experimental research.

Integrated Cardiovascular Response

The effects of positioning, CO_2, and intra-abdominal pressure on cardiovascular performance having been reviewed, the integrated response to laparoscopy can now be described. Table 2–4 summarizes the cardio-

Table 2–4. CARDIOVASCULAR RESPONSE TO LAPAROSCOPY

Function	Head-down tilt	IAP ≤ 20 mm Hg	IAP ≥ 40 mm Hg	Hypercapnia	Head-down tilt + IAP ≤ 20 mm Hg with CO_2	Head-down tilt + IAP ≥ 40 mm Hg with CO_2
Heart rate	O or ↓	↑	↑	↑	↑	↑
Stroke volume	↑	↓*	↓↓	↑	↓	↓
Cardiac output	↑	↓	↓↓	↑	↑ or O or ↓	↓
Arterial resistance	O or ↓	↑	↑	↓	↑	↑
Arterial pressure	O or ↑	↑	O or ↓	↑	↑	O or ↓
Systemic venous pressure	O or ↑	↑	↑	↑	↑	↑
Central venous pressure	↑	↑	O or ↓	↑	↑	O or ↓
Venous resistance	O or ↓	↑	↑↑	↓	↑	↑
Venous return	↑	↓	↓↓	↑	↑ or O or ↓	↓
References (human)	118, 119, 120	118, 132, 136	120, 136	51, 132, 134	32, 37, 120, 132, 137, 138	120, 137

*Note: At IAP < 10 mm Hg, stroke volume and cardiac output may increase and vascular resistance decrease.[28, 120, 140]
IAP, intra-abdominal pressure.

vascular effects of the head-down tilt position, CO_2 elevation, intra-abdominal pressure ≤20 mm Hg, intra-abdominal pressure ≥40 mm Hg, and the combined situations. It must be emphasized that just as with the pulmonary effects of laparoscopy, the response of any given patient may differ markedly from the generally expected results. At the recommended level of 15 to 20 mm Hg insufflation pressure, with use of CO_2 and the patient in the head-down tilt position, heart rate will generally increase. Stroke volume falls proportionally, so that cardiac output is more or less maintained. Given these parameters, the effect on cardiac output by laparoscopy in healthy patients ranges from a decrease of 19% or 17%[119,138] to no net change[118,120,137] to an increase of 7%.[132] Lower intra-abdominal pressure leads to increased cardiac output by 4% to 15%,[28,120,140] whereas intra-abdominal pressure in excess of 30 to 40 mm Hg decreases cardiac output.[120,137]

Changes in arterial pressure are similar, laparoscopy with use of CO_2 and the head-down tilt position causing a modest increase if the intra-abdominal pressure is limited to 20 mm Hg. Arterial pressure returns to baseline or lower at excessive intra-abdominal pressure. If another gas is used, the stimulatory effects of CO_2 are lost, and cardiac output falls even with an intra-abdominal pressure of 20 mm Hg.[133,134] Cardiac output is higher during laparoscopy with the patient in the head-down tilt position than when the horizontal position is used.[118,120]

Clinical Implications

The cardiovascular insult of laparoscopy is generally greater than that of open surgery. Nevertheless, it is usually well tolerated by healthy patients as long as insufflation pressures are limited to 15 to 20 mm Hg. Cardiovascular complications are rarely reported in this group without a technical error or equipment failure. The alteration in cardiac output and blood pressure are well tolerated, cardiac stimulation and increases in intracranial pressure remain within acceptable limits, and serious arrhythmias are unusual. In older patients, however, the cardiovascular burden of laparoscopy may pose a greater risk. For example, in a patient with poorly controlled hypertension and ischemic heart disease accompanied by a poor cardiac reserve or borderline heart failure, the advantages of laparoscopy may be outweighed by the cardiovascular risk of the procedure; an open operation might be safer for the patient. The risks must be openly addressed when contemplating a laparoscopic procedure in elderly patients or those with cardiovascular disease. Significant cardiovascular disease, especially heart failure or ischemic heart disease, should currently be considered a relative contraindication for laparoscopy until further experience is gained.

CONSIDERATIONS IN THE USE OF ANESTHETICS

The anesthetic management of a laparoscopic procedure can often be more difficult than that of an open one. The capnograph must be monitored closely, hemodynamic responses may vary from minimal to profound, and a whole new set of acute complications need to be considered. Postoperative monitoring must be vigilant until hypercapnia has cleared. Just as during transurethral resection, the urologist needs to be knowledgeable about the unique pathophysiology of the operation in order to advise the anesthesiologist regarding technique.

Local Anesthesia

In adults diagnostic laparoscopy or minimally manipulative operative laparoscopy has long been routinely performed under local anesthesia.[151] Intravenous agents such as narcotics, benzodiazepines, or propofol are used to augment the local action of lidocaine or bupivacaine administered subcutaneously and at the site of operative manipulation.[177] Although laparoscopic varicocelectomy using local anesthesia has been reported,[108] most urologists feel more comfortable, at least initially, using general anesthesia. In the future, the use of local anesthesia may become more widespread during urologic laparoscopy because of the rapid recovery, minimal risk, and lessened postoperative nausea.

Regional Anesthesia

The experience with regional anesthesia during laparoscopy is limited.[19,152–154] Investigators have reported good outcomes, but no detailed hemodynamic assessment has been performed. Schoeffler and associates[155] point out that an evaluation of the hemodynamic effects of sympathetic block combined with pneumoperitoneum has not been reported. Based on current knowledge, the loss of vascular tone associated with regional anesthesia may potentiate the adverse effects of elevated intra-abdominal pressure. Peritoneal anesthesia and abdominal relaxation require a block to the T4 level. Respiratory function may be impaired with this degree of neuromuscular blockade. Subdiaphragmatic pain is not relieved until the block reaches the cervical level,[131] so that some use of intravenous sedation would still be required for cases more extensive than a minimally manipulative procedure. Regional anesthesia cannot be recommended at this time for routine use during urologic laparoscopy.

General Anesthesia

General anesthesia is the technique most widely used for laparoscopic urologic surgery. Advantages include complete analgesia, patient amnesia, and a quiet and controlled operating room.[156] The airway is protected. Ventilation can be assisted to eliminate absorbed CO_2. Greater head-down tilt is tolerated, and intra-operative vagal reactions are minimized. The importance of muscle relaxation is frequently underestimated. Loveday[157] pointed out that the muscle tone of the conscious patient limits the "ballooning out" of the abdominal wall until higher intra-abdominal pressures are achieved. A paralyzed abdominal wall is much more compliant, allowing the surgeon more room to work (volume) with less insufflation (pressure). Muscle relaxants should be administered only after obtaining access to the peritoneal cavity, however. A more rigid abdomen is extremely helpful when inserting the Verres needle. Disadvantages of general anesthesia include the risks associated with intubation and mechanical ventilation, a prolonged and sometimes unpleasant recovery, and weakness and muscle pains following muscle paralysis. With improved anesthetic techniques, these ill effects are diminished. The relatively new anesthetic agent propofol reduces recovery time and side effects in laparoscopic patients.[158] Short-acting muscle relaxants such as atracurium or vecuronium are associated with more rapid neuromuscular recovery.[159]

Inhalational Agents

Although total intravenous anesthesia can be used for general anesthesia during laparoscopy,[160] inhalational agents are most commonly employed. Halothane should be avoided because it predisposes to hypercapnia-induced arrhythmias. Enflurane and isoflurane are acceptable, but enflurane will lower cardiac output.[155] The use of N_2O for inhalational anesthesia has been the subject of much debate. Nitrous oxide is a safe and pleasant inhalational agent, popular with anesthesiologists because it reduces the requirement for other anesthetics. Generally it has been the impression of laparoscopic surgeons that N_2O causes bowel distention that interferes with visualization. This is based in part on experimental work demonstrating that air-filled intestinal loops doubled in size within two hours with N_2O anesthesia.[161] In one blind study during open colonic surgery, surgeons reported that the bowels were empty in 11 of 20 cases in which 70% air was respired but in none of the 20 patients in which 70% N_2O was respired.[162] A study of 50 laparoscopic cholecystectomies yielded different results.[163] Again comparing N_2O to air and using a similar blind technique, surgeons did not detect any bowel distention and were unable to determine whether air or N_2O had been used. Despite the finding of this latter study, our bias is that bowel distention is increased with N_2O inhalation, particularly during long cases, and that it should not be employed during laparoscopic procedures. The blood content of N_2O when it is used for anesthesia is much higher than when it is used for peritoneal insufflation. Bowel distention has not been reported to be a problem with N_2O pneumoperitoneum.[50]

Fluid Management

The fluid requirements during laparoscopy are quite a bit less than during comparative open procedures. A maintenance fluid rate of 3 to 5 ml/kg/hour is sufficient once it is ascertained that the patient is well hydrated.[164] Since the adverse effects of increased intra-abdominal pressure are accentuated by hypovolemia, adequate volume status must be attained before pneumoperitoneum is created. Increasing blood volume to the point of moderate hypervolemia may improve the hemodynamic response to laparoscopy, as suggested by experimental data.[135] This cannot be done in patients with a tendency to heart failure.

Monitoring

Routine intraoperative monitors include capnograph, pulse oximeter, automated blood pressure cuff, electrocardiograph, and precordial or esophageal stethoscope. For the usual urologic laparoscopic procedure, these are sufficient. If advanced laparoscopy is being performed, an arterial catheter should be placed for blood pressure monitoring and blood gas sampling. When there is concern regarding the patient's cardiopulmonary function, an arterial line and central venous catheter are indicated to allow for accurate hemodynamic assessment. Postoperative monitoring after laparoscopy is similar to that in patients after any procedure under general anesthesia, except that capnography or blood gas sampling should be used to monitor those patients with marked hypercapnia to ensure resolution of this problem.

MISCELLANEOUS PHYSIOLOGIC CONSIDERATIONS

Lateral Position

Laparoscopic nephrectomy is performed with the patient in the lateral position, which is often combined with moderate head-up tilt. The lateral position creates more of a ventilation and perfusion mismatch in the anesthetized patient than does the head-down tilt position.[27] This can be managed effectively with controlled ventilation. The primary hemodynamic effect of the lateral position is to decrease vascular resistance. Venous return and cardiac output may fall when the table is also placed in a head-up position or if the patient's legs are jackknifed to a dependent position.[165] Compression of the vena cava can impair venous return if the kidney rest is elevated cephalad to the iliac crest or if the table is flexed excessively.[166]

With the fall in vascular resistance and possible decrease in cardiac output associated with the lateral and head-up position, arterial pressure drops. These effects are distinct from the increase in cardiac output and arterial pressure that occur with the head-down tilt position. When combined with pneumoperitoneum, it might be surmised that cardiac output would have more of a tendency to fall in the lateral and head-up position compared with the head-down tilt position. Since there is as yet no published data on this subject, the only recommendation is for close monitoring during laparoscopic procedures in the lateral position.

Pediatrics

The history of urologic laparoscopy is longer in the pediatric population than in adults. The physiologic response to laparoscopy is somewhat different in the pediatric population. Children seem to be more prone to extraperitoneal emphysema and CO_2 absorption, but they are also better able to expire the excess CO_2 and are somewhat more resistant to the effects of hypercapnia. Significant CO_2-related complications are unusual in pediatric patients. In terms of hemodynamics, several animal studies have shown the newborn to be exquisitely sensitive to elevated intra-abdominal pressure, with decreased cardiac output even at low pressure.[142,143,167,168] These studies were performed with insufflation of air or placement of gas-filled bags to increase intra-abdominal pressure, so the concurrent effects of CO_2 are unknown. The applicability of these studies to pediatric laparoscopy is uncertain. Clinically, pediatric patients seem to tolerate the hemodynamic alterations of pneumoperitoneum very well.

Obesity

The weight of abdominal fat is similar to an unrelaxed abdominal wall; less volume of pneumoperitoneum is achieved with a given insufflation pressure. The length of subcutaneous tissue that must be traversed makes correct placement of the initial needle less certain and increases the amount of subcutaneous emphysema that may go undetected. The adverse effect of head-down tilt position on pulmonary mechanics is accentuated in the obese patient. Nonetheless, less morbidity and mortality are noted among obese patients undergoing laparoscopy than those managed with laparotomy.[169] The technical difficulty and possible increased risk of cardiopulmonary complications must be considered carefully in this patient group.

Hypothermia

Ott[170] has calculated that the core temperature falls 0.3°C for every 50 L of CO_2 instilled into the peritoneal cavity. Since several hundred liters can be used during a long procedure, this may be of concern. Warming of the CO_2 before instillation,[171] or use of a heating blanket will obviate the problem.

Deep Vein Thrombosis

Lower extremity venous stasis occurs during laparoscopy as a result of the transmitted pressure from the abdomen. In addition to predisposing to metabolic acidosis, the risk of deep vein thrombosis is increased. Application of intermittent compression devices to the legs is the most direct way to reduce the risk of lower extremity stasis in this situation. We have not employed minidose heparin at our institution.

Argon-Beam Coagulator

The argon-beam coagulator delivers electrical energy in a controlled spray through a jet of argon gas. It provides excellent electrothermal hemostasis. Its usefulness for open partial nephrectomy has been demonstrated.[172] The device has recently been adapted for laparoscopic use. The authors have employed it during one laparoscopic renal cyst resection and two cases of laparoscopic excision of a stone-containing anterior calyceal diverticulum. In all patients, hemostasis was excellent and there were no urine leaks. The amount of argon gas propelled from the tip of the instrument is surprisingly high. Intra-abdominal pressure must be carefully monitored when this device is in the abdomen. We have found it necessary to open a trocar when the argon-beam coagulator is used to vent off the excess gas and to prevent excessive intra-abdominal pressure.

Argon is safe for use in humans. There are no physiologic effects even at a partial pressure of 600 mm Hg.[173] Argon's solubility and tissue permeability are only twice that of N_2. Based on animal studies, the rate of absorption of subcutaneous argon is approximately 1 ml/hour.[9,174] Subcutaneous emphysema of 200 ml volume will take more than 8 days to reabsorb. Indeed, one of the patients in whom we used the laparoscopic argon-beam coagulator still had a crepitant area over his rib cage 6 days following the procedure.

REFERENCES

1. Case, JT: A review of three years' work and articles on pneumoperitoneum. AJR 8:714–721, 1921.
2. Kory, RC; Roehm, DC; Meneely, GR; Goodwin, RA, Jr: Pulmonary function and circulatory dynamics in artificial pneumoperitoneum. I. Studies on patients with pneumoperitoneum therapy for pulmonary tuberculosis. Dis Chest 13:595–607, 1953a.
3. Kory, RC; Roehm, DC; Meneely, GR; Goodwin, RA, Jr: Pulmonary function and circulatory dynamics in artificial pneumoperitoneum. II. Studies on patients with pneumoperitoneum as a therapeutic measure in pulmonary emphysema. Dis Chest 13:608–620, 1953b.
4. Wright, GW; Place, R; Princi, F: The physiological effects of pneumoperitoneum upon the respiratory apparatus. Am Rev Tuberculosis 60:706–714, 1949.

5. Leiner, GC; Abramowitz, S: Spirometric studies in pneumoperitoneum. Am Rev Tuberculosis 65:465–476, 1952.
6. Piiper, J: Physiological equilibria of gas cavities in the body. In: Fenn, WO; Rahn, H, eds: Handbook of Physiology, Sec 3: Respiration, Vol 2. Washington, DC, American Physiological Society, 1965, pp. 1205–1218.
7. Loring, SH; Butler, JP: Gas exchange in body cavities. In: Fishman, AP, ed: Handbook of Physiology, Sec 3: The Respiratory System, Vol 4. Bethesda, MD: American Physiological Society, 1987, pp. 283–295.
8. Piiper, J: Various models for analysis of the absorption of inert gases from gas cavities in the body. Respir Physiol 9:74–85, 1970.
9. Collins, JM: Inert gas exchange of subcutaneous and intraperitoneal gas pockets in piglets. Respir Physiol 46:391–404, 1981.
10. Nunn, JF: Carbon dioxide. In: Applied Respiratory Physiology. London, Butterworths, 1987, pp. 207–234.
11. Fowle, ASE; Campbell, EJM: The immediate carbon dioxide storage capacity of man. Clin Sci 27:41–49, 1964.
12. Farhi, LE; Rahn, H: Dynamics of changes in carbon dioxide stores. Anesthesiology 21:604–614, 1960.
13. Farhi, LE: Rahn, H: Gas stores of the body and the unsteady state. J Appl Physiol 7:472–484, 1955.
14. Seed, RF; Shakespeare, TF; Muldoon, MJ: Carbon dioxide homeostasis during anesthesia for laparoscopy. Anaesthesia 25:223–231, 1970.
15. Lewis, DG; Ryder, W; Burn, N; et al: Laparoscopy—an investigation during spontaneous ventilation with halothane. Br J Anaesth 44:685–691, 1972.
16. DeSousa, H; Tyler, IL: Can absorption of the insufflation gas during laparoscopy be hazardous? Anesthesiology 67:A476, 1987.
17. Puri, GD; Singh, H: Ventilatory effects of laparoscopy under general anaesthesia. Br J Anaesth 68:211–213, 1992.
18. Brown, DR; Fishburne, JI; Roberson, VO; Hulka, JF: Ventiltory and blood gas changes during laparoscopy with local anesthesia. Am J Obstet Gynecol 124:741–745, 1976.
19. Ciofolo, MJ; Clergue, F; Seebacher, J; et al: Ventilatory effects of laparoscopy under epidural anesthesia. Anesth Analg 70:357–361, 1990.
20. Sosa, RE; Weingram, J; Stein, B; et al: Hypercarbia in laparoscopic pelvic lymph node dissection. J Urol 147:246A, 1992.
21. Kent, RB III: Subcutaneous emphysema and hypercarbia following laparoscopic cholecystectomy. Arch Surg 126:1154–1156, 1991.
22. Verbessem, D; Camu, F; Devroey, P; Steirteghem, AV: Pneumoperitoneum-induced pH changes in follicular and Douglas fluids during laparoscopic oocyte retrieval in humans. Hum Repro 3:751–754, 1988.
23. Wittgen, CM; Andrus, CH; Fitzgerald, SD; et al: Analysis of the hemodynamic and ventilatory effects of laparoscopic cholecystectomy. Arch Surg 126:997–1001, 1991.
24. Dashow, L; Friedman, I; Kempner, R; et al: Initial experience with laparoscopic cholecystectomy at the Beth Israel Medical Center. Gynecol Obstet 175:25–30, 1992.
25. Brady, CE III; Harkleroad, LE; Pierson, WP: Alteration in oxygen saturation and ventilation after intravenous sedation for peritoneoscopy. Arch Intern Med 149:1029–1032, 1989.
26. Tolksdorf, W; Strang, CM; Schippers, E; et al: The effects of the carbon dioxide pneumoperitoneum in laparoscopic cholecystectomy on postoperative spontaneous respiration (in German). Anaesthetist 41:199–203, 1992.
27. Nunn, JF: Respiratory aspects of anaesthesia. In: Applied Respiratory Physiology. London, Butterworths, 1987, pp 350–378.
28. Ekman, LG; Abrahamsson, J; Biber, B; et al: Hemodynamic changes during laparoscopy with positive end-expiratory pressure ventilation. Acta Anaesthesiol Scand 32:447–453, 1988.
29. Prentice JA; Martin JT: The Trendelenburg position. Anesthesiologic considerations. In Martin, JT, ed: Positioning in Anesthesia and Surgery. Philadelphia, WB Saunders, 1987, pp. 127–145.
30. Scott, DB: Some effects of peritoneal insufflation of carbon dioxide at laparoscopy. Anaesthesia 25:590, 1970.
31. Alexander, GD; Noe, FE; Brown, EM: Anesthesia for pelvic laparoscopy. Anesth Analg 48:14–18, 1969.
32. Youssef, A-RM; Ibrahim, MM; Abdel-Alim, MS; Ahmed, YA: Some physiological changes during anesthesia for laparoscopy. Middle East J Anaesthiol 6:219–225, 1982.
33. Hodgson, C; McClelland, RMA; Newton, JR: Some effects of the peritoneal insufflation of carbon dioxide at laparoscopy. Anaesthesia 25:382–390, 1970.
34. Nunn, JF: Distribution of pulmonary ventilation and perfusion. In: Applied Respiratory Physiology. London, Butterworths, 1987, pp. 140–183.
35. Lee, CY; Huang, SJ; Yeh, FC; Chang, CL: The rate of end-tidal CO_2 elevation after intraabdominal insufflation in laparoscopy. Ma Tsui Hsueh Tsa Chi 28:425–428, 1990.
36. Brampton, WJ; Watson, RJ: Arterial to end-tidal carbon dioxide tension difference during laparoscopy. Anaesthesia 45:210–214, 1990.
37. Pillalamarri, ED; Bhangdia, P; Rudin, RS; et al: Effect of CO_2 pneumoperitoneum during laparascopy on ABGs, end-tidal CO_2 and cardiovascular dynamics. Anesthesiology 59:A424, 1983.
38. Liu, SY; Leighton, T; Davis, I; et al: Prospective analysis of cardiopulmonary responses to laparoscopic cholecystectomy. J Laparoendosc Surg 1:241–246, 1991.
39. Yusa, T; Sasara, T; Shimabukuro, T; Higa, Y: Arterial to end-tidal carbon dioxide difference during laparoscopy (in Japanese). Masui Japanese Journal of Anesthesiology 41:232–237, 1992.
40. Raemer, DB; Francis, D; Philip, JH; Gabel, RA: Variation in Pco_2 between arterial blood and peak expired gas during anesthesia. Anesth Analg 62:1065–1069, 1983.
41. Baratz, RA; Karis, JH: Blood gas studies during laparoscopy under general anesthesia. Anesthesiology 30:463–464, 1969.
42. Montalva, M; Das, B: Carbon dioxide homeostasis during laparoscopy. South Med J 69:602–603, 1976.
43. Diamant, M; Benumof, JL; Saidman, LJ; et al: Laparoscopic sterilization with local anesthesia: Complications and blood-gas changes. Anesth Analg 56:335–337, 1977.
44. Kenefick, JP; Leader, A; Maltby, JR; Taylor, PJ: Laparoscopy: Blood-gas values and minor sequelae associated with three techniques based on isoflurane. Br J Anaesthesiol 59:189–194, 1987.
45. Desmond, J; Gordon, RA: Ventilation in patients anaesthetized for laparoscopy. Can Anaesth Soc J 17:378–387, 1970.
46. Magno, R; Medegård, A; Bengtsson, R; Tronstad, S-E: Acid-base balance during laparoscopy: The effects of intraperitoneal insufflation of carbon dioxide on acid-base balance during controlled ventilation. Acta Obstet Gynecol Scand 58:81–85, 1979.
47. Degueldre, M; Puissant, F; Camus, M; et al: Effects of carbon dioxide insufflation at laparoscopy on the gas phase in oocyte recovery fluids. J In-Vitro Fertilization Embryo Transfer 1:106, 1984.
48. Nunn, JF: Oxygen. In Applied Respiratory Physiology. London, Butterworths, 1987, pp. 235–283.
49. Corall, IM; Knights, K; Potter, D; Strunin, L: Arterial oxygen tension during laparoscopy with nitrous oxide in the spontaneously breathing patient. Br J Anaesth 46:925–928, 1974.
50. Alexander, GD; Brown, EM: Physiologic alterations during laparoscopy. Am J Obstet Gynecol 105:1078–1081, 1969.
51. El-Minawi, MF; Wahbi, O; El-Bagouri, IS; et al: Physiologic changes during CO_2 and N_2O pneumoperitoneum in diagnostic laparoscopy: A comparative study. J Reprod Med 26:338–346, 1981.

52. Gaur, DD: Laparoscopic operative retroperitoneoscopy: Use of a new device. J Urol 148:1137–1139, 1992.
53. Shafik, A: Extraperitoneal laparoscopic lymphadenectomy in prostatic cancer: a preliminary report of a new approach. J Endourol 6:113–116, 1992.
54. Sivak, BJ: Surgical emphysema: Report of a case and review. Anesth Analg 43:415–417, 1964.
55. Horwitz, ST: Laparoscopy in gynecology. Obstet Gynecol Surv 27:1–13, 1972.
56. Fitzgerald, TB; Johnstone, MW: Diaphragmatic defects and laparoscopy. Br Med J 2:604, 1970.
57. Doctor, NH; Hussain, Z: Bilateral pneumothorax associated with laparoscopy. Anaesthesia 28:75–81, 1973.
58. Whiston, RJ; Eggers, KA; Morris, RW; Stamatakis, JD: Tension pneumothorax during laparoscopic cholecystectomy. Br J Surg 78:1325, 1991.
59. Brühl, W: Complications of laparoscopy and liver biopsy under vision: The results of a survey. German Med Month 12:31–32, 1967.
60. Clayman, RV; Karoussi, LR; Soper, NJ; et al: Laparoscopic nephrectomy: Review of the initial ten cases. J Endourol 6:127–132, 1992.
61. Pascual, JB; Baranda, MM; Tarrero, MT; et al: Subcutaneous emphysema, pneumomediastinum, bilateral pneumothorax, and pneumopericardium after laparoscopy. Endoscopy 22:59, 1990.
62. Bard, PA; Chen, L: Subcutaneous emphysema associated with laparoscopy. Anesth Analg 71:101–102, 1990.
63. Murray, DP; Rankin, RA; Lackey, C: Bilateral pneumothoraces complicating peritoneoscopy. Gastrointest Endosc 30:45–46, 1984.
64. Heddle, RM; Platt, AJ: Tension pneumothorax during laparoscopic cholecystectomy. Br J Surg 79:374, 1992.
65. Jernstrom, P: Air embolism during peritoneoscopy. Am J Clin Pathol 21:573–575, 1951.
66. McKenzie, R: Laparoscopy. N Z Med J 74:87–91, 1971.
67. Root, B; Levy, MN; Pollack, S; et al: Gas embolism death after laparoscopy delayed by "trapping" in portal circulation. Anesth Analg 57:232–237, 1978.
68. Brown, JAC; Chamberlain, GVP; Jordan, JA; et al: Gynaecological laparoscopy: The report of the working party of the confidential enquiry into gynaecological laparoscopy. Br J Obstet Gynaecol 85:401–403, 1978.
69. Gomar, C; Fernandez, C; Villalonga, A; Nalda, MA: Carbon dioxide embolism during laparoscopy and hysteroscopy. Ann Fr Anesth Reanim 4:380–382, 1985.
70. Chang, JL; Chestnut, JR; Carroll, RG; et al: Air embolism. Anesthesiology 46:307, 1977.
71. Phillips, J; Keith, D; Hulka, J; Keith L: Gynaecological laparoscopy in 1975. J Reprod Med 16:205–217, 1976.
72. Bradfield, ST: Gas embolism during laparoscopy. Anaesth Intens Care 19:474, 1991.
73. Clark, CC; Weeks, DB; Gusdon, JP: Venous carbon dioxide embolism during laparoscopy. Anesth Analg 56:650–652, 1977.
74. Nichols, SL; Tompkins, BM: Probable carbon dioxide embolism during laparoscopy: Case report. Wis Med J 80:27–29, 1981.
75. De Plater, RMH; Jones, ISC: Non-fatal carbon dioxide embolism during laparoscopy. Anaesth Intens Care 17:359–361, 1989.
76. Greville, AC; Clements, EAF; Erwin, DC; et al: Pulmonary air embolism during laparoscopic laser cholecystectomy. Anaesthesia 46:113–114, 1991.
77. Morison, H; Riggs, JRA: Cardiovascular collapse in laparoscopy. Can Med Assoc J 111:433–437, 1974.
78. Ostman, PL; Pantle-Fisher, FH; Faure, EA: Circulatory collapse during laparoscopy. J Clin Anesth 2:129–132, 1990.
79. Crozier, TA; Luger, A; Dravecz, M; et al: Gas embolism with cardiac arrest during hysteroscopy. A case report on 3 patients (in German). Anasthesiologie Intensivmedizin Notfallmedizin Schmerztherapie 26:412–415, 1991.
80. Brantley, JC III; Riley, PM: Cardiovascular collapse during laparoscopy: A report of two cases. Am J Obstet Gynecol 159:735–737, 1988.
81. Kleppinger, RK: One thousand laparoscopies at a community hospital. J Reprod Med 13:13–20, 1974.
82. Desai, S; Roaf, E; Liu, P: Acute pulmonary edema during laparoscopy. Anesth Analg 61:699–700, 1982.
83. McGrath, BJ; Zimmerman, JE; Williams, JF; Parmet J: Carbon dioxide embolism treated with hyperbaric oxygen. Can J Anaesth 36:586–589, 1989.
84. Marquez, J; Sladen, A; Gendell, H; et al: Paradoxical air embolism without an intracardiac septal defect. J Neurosurg 55:997–1000, 1981.
85. Ivankovich, AD; Albrecht, RF; Zahed, B; Bonnet, RF: Cardiovascular collapse during gynecological laparoscopy. Illinois Med J 145:58–61, 1974.
86. Graff, TD; Arbegast, NR; Phillips, OC; et al: Gas embolism: A comparative study of air and carbon dioxide as embolic agents in the systemic venous system. Am J Obstet Gynecol 78:259–265, 1959.
87. Richardson, HF; Coles, BC; Hall, GE: Experimental gas embolism: I. Intravenous air embolism. Can Med Assoc J 36:584–588, 1937.
88. Durant, TM; Long, J; Oppenheimer, MJ: Pulmonary (venous) air embolism. Am Heart J 33:269–281, 1947.
89. Carroll, GC: Capnographic trend curve monitoring can detect 1 mL pulmonary emboli in humans. J Clin Monitor 8:101–106, 1992.
90. Shulman, D; Aronson, HB: Capnography in the early diagnosis of carbon dioxide embolism during laparoscopy. Can Anaesth Soc J 31:455–459, 1984.
91. Diakun, T: Carbon dioxide embolism: Successful resuscitation with cardiopulmonary bypass. Anesthesiology 74:1151–1153, 1991.
92. Wadhwa, RK; McKenzie, R; Wadhwa, SR; et al: Gas embolism during laparoscopy. Anesthesiology 48:74–76, 1978.
93. Oppenheimer, MJ; Durant, TM; Lynch, P: Body position in relation to venous air embolism and the associated cardiorespiratory changes. Am J Med Sci 225:362–373, 1953.
94. Mongan, P; Peterson, RE; Culling, RD: Pressure monitoring can accurately position catheters for air embolism aspiration. J Clin Monitor 8:121–125, 1992.
95. Etches, RC: Hyperbaric oxygen and CO_2 embolism. Can J Anaesth 37:270–271, 1990.
96. Stauffer, HM; Durant, TM; Oppenheimer, MJ: Gas embolism. Radiology 66:686–692, 1956.
97. Fervers, C: Die Laparoskopie mit dem Cystoskop. Medizin Klinik 29:1042–1045, 1933.
98. Sogge, MR; Goldner, FH; Butler, ML: Pain response comparison between carbon dioxide and nitrous oxide in peritoneoscopy. Gastrointest Endosc 26:78, 1980.
99. Minoli, G; Terruzzi, V; Spinzi, GC; et al: The influence of carbon dioxide and nitrous oxide on pain during laparoscopy: A double-blind, controlled trial. Gastrointest Endosc 28:173–175, 1982.
100. Sharp, JR; Pierson, WP; Brady, CE III: Comparison of CO_2- and N_2O-induced discomfort during peritoneoscopy under local anesthesia. Gastroenterology 82:453–456, 1982.
101. Robinson, JS; Thompson, JM; Wood, AW: Laparoscopy explosion hazards with nitrous oxide. Br Med J 3:764–765, 1975a.
102. Robinson, JS; Thompson, JM; Wood, AW: Laparoscopy explosion hazards with nitrous oxide. Br Med J 4:760–761, 1975b.
103. Robinson, JS; Thompson, JM; Wood, AW: Laparoscopy explosion hazards with nitrous oxide. Br Med J 1:1277, 1976.

104. Steptoe, P: Laparoscopy explosion hazards with nitrous oxide. Br Med J 1:833, 1976.
105. Corall, IM; Elias, JA; Strunin, L: Laparoscopy explosion hazards with nitrous oxide. Br Med J 4:288, 1975.
106. Drummond, GB; Scott, DB: Laparoscopy explosion hazards with nitrous oxide. Br Med J 1:586, 1976a.
107. Drummond, GB; Scott, DB: Laparoscopy explosion hazards with nitrous oxide. Br Med J 1:1531, 1976b.
108. Matsuda, T; Horii, Y; Higashi, S; et al: Laparoscopic varicocelectomy: A simple technique for clip ligation of the spermatic vessels. J Urol 147:636–638, 1992.
109. Uhlich, GA: Laparoscopy: The question of the proper gas. Gastrointest Endosc 28:212–213, 1982.
110. Schiller, WR: The Trendelenburg position. Surgical aspects. In Martin, JT, ed: Positioning in Anesthesia and Surgery. Philadelphia, WB Saunders, 1987, pp. 117–126.
111. Gartner, S; Beck, W: Ocular tension in the Trendelenburg position. Am J Ophthalmol 59:1040–1043, 1965.
112. Kubal, K; Komatsu, T; Sanchala, V; et al: Trendelenburg position used during venous cannulation increases myocardial oxygen demand. Anesth Analg 63:239, 1984.
113. Reich, DL; Konstadt, SN; Raissi, S; et al: Trendelenburg position and passive leg raising do not significantly improve cardiopulmonary performance in the anesthetized patient with coronary artery disease. Crit Care Med 17:313–317, 1989.
114. Gentili, DR; Benjamin, E; Berger, SR; Iberti, TJ: Cardiopulmonary effects of the head-down tilt position in elderly postoperative patients: A prospective study. South Med J 81:1258–1260, 1988.
115. Taylor, J; Weil, MH: Failure of the Trendelenburg position to improve circulation during clinical shock. Surg Gynecol Obstet 124:1005–1010, 1967.
116. Sibbald, WJ; Paterson, NAM; Holliday, RL; Baskerville, J: The Trendelenburg position: Hemodynamic effects in hypotensive and normotensive patients. Crit Care Med 7:218–224, 1979.
117. Zippe, C; Burchard, KW; Gann, DS: Trendelenburg versus PASG application in moderate hemorrhagic hypoperfusion. J Trauma 25:923–932, 1985.
118. Torrielli, R; Cesarini, M; Winnock, S; et al: Hemodynamic changes during celioscopy: A study carried out using thoracic electric bioimpedance (in French). Can J Anaesth 37:46–51, 1990.
119. Johannsen, G; Andersen, M; Juhl, B: The effect of general anaesthesia on the haemodynamic events during laparoscopy with CO_2 insufflation. Acta Anaesthesiol Scand 33:132–136, 1989.
120. Kelman, GR; Swapp, GH; Smith, I; et al: Cardiac output and arterial blood–gas tension during laparoscopy. Br J Anaesth 44:1155–1162, 1972.
121. Price, HL: Effects of carbon dioxide on the cardiovascular system. Anesthesiology 21:652–663, 1960.
122. Richardson, DW; Wasserman, AJ; Patterson, JL Jr: General and regional circulatory responses to change in blood pH and carbon dioxide tension. J Clin Invest 40:31–43, 1961.
123. Nunn, JF: The effects of changes in the carbon dioxide tension. In: Applied Respiratory Physiology. London, Butterworths, 1987, pp. 460–470.
124. Rasmussen, JP; Dauchot, PJ; DePalma, RG; et al: Cardiac function and hypercarbia. Arch Surg 113:1196–1200, 1978.
125. Scott, DB; Julian, DG: Observations on cardiac arrhythmias during laparoscopy. Br Med J 1:411–413, 1972.
126. Cimino, L; Petitto, M; Nardone, G; Budillon, G: Holter dynamic electrocardiography during laparoscopy. Gastrointest Endosc 34:72, 1988.
127. Groover, JR; Bierfeld, JL: Cardiac arrhythmias during peritoneoscopy under local anesthesia. Digest Dis 21:465–467, 1976.
128. Myles, PS: Bradyarrhythmias and laparoscopy: A prospective study of heart rate changes with laparoscopy. Aust NZ J Obstet Gynaecol 31:171–173, 1991.
129. Carmichael, DE: Laparoscopy-cardiac considerations. Fertil Steril 22:69–70, 1971.
130. Shifren, JL: Adlestein, L; Finkler, NJ: Asystolic cardiac arrest: A rare complication of laparoscopy. Obstet Gynecol 79:840–841, 1992.
131. Borten, M: Choice of anesthesia. In: Laparoscopic Complications. Toronto, BC Decker, 1986b, pp 173–184.
132. Marshall, RL; Jebson, PJR; Davie, IT, Scott, DB: Circulatory effects of carbon dioxide insufflation of the peritoneal cavity for laparoscopy. Br J Anaesth 44:680–684, 1972a.
133. Marshall, RL; Jebson, PJR; Davie, IT: Scott, DB: Circulatory effects of peritoneal insufflation with nitrous oxide. Br J Anaesth 44:1183–1187, 1972b.
134. McKenzie, R; Wadhwa, RK; Bedger, RC: Noninvasive measurement of cardiac output during laparoscopy. J Reprod Med 24:247–250, 1980.
135. Kashtan, J; Green, JF; Parsons, EQ; Holcroft, JW: Hemodynamic effects of increased abdominal pressure. J Surg Res 30:249–255, 1981.
136. Smith, I; Benzie, RJ; Gordon, NLM; et al: Cardiovascular effects of peritoneal insufflation of carbon dioxide for laparoscopy. Br Med J 13:410–411, 1971.
137. Motew, M; Ivankovich, AD; Bieniarz, J; et al: Cardiovascular effects and acid-base and blood gas changes during laparoscopy. Am J Obstet Gynecol 115:1002–1012, 1973.
138. Lenz, RJ; Thomas, TA; Wilkins, DG: Cardiovascular changes during laparoscopy. Anaesthesia 31:4–12, 1976.
139. Diamant, M; Benumof, JL; Saidman, LJ: Hemodynamics of increased intra-abdominal pressure: Interaction with hypovolemia and halothane anesthesia. Anesthesiology 48:23–27, 1978.
140. Versichelen, L; Serreyn, R; Rolly, G; Vanderkerckhove, D: Physiopathologic changes during anesthesia administration for gynecologic laparoscopy. J Reprod Med 29:697–700, 1984.
141. Ivankovich, AD; Miletich, DJ; Albrecht, RF; et al: Cardiovascular effects of intraperitoneal insufflation with carbon dioxide and nitrous oxide in the dog. Anesthesiology 42:281–287, 1975.
142. Masey, SA; Buck, JR; Koehler, RC; et al: Effects of increased intra-abdominal pressure on regional blood flow in newborn lambs. Anesthesiology 59:A425, 1983a.
143. Masey, SA, Buck JR, Koehler RC; et al: Cardiovascular and metabolic effects of increased intra-abdominal pressure in newborn lambs. Anesthesiology 59:A426, 1983b.
144. Borten, M: Circulatory changes. In: Laparoscopic Complications. Toronto, BC Decker, 1986, pp. 185–195.
145. Punnonen, R; Viinamäki: Vasopressin release during laparoscopy: Role of increased intra-abdominal pressure. Lancet 1:175–176, 1982.
146. Richardson, JD; Trinkle, JK: Hemodynamic and respiratory alterations with increased intra-abdominal pressure. J Surg Res 20:401–404, 1976.
147. Lee, CM: Acute hypotension during laparoscopy: A case report. Anesth Analg 54:142–143, 1975.
148. Lew, JKL; Gin, T; Oh, TE: Anaesthetic problems during laparoscopic cholecystectomy. Anaesth Intens Care 20:91–92, 1992.
149. Arthure, H: Laparoscopy hazard. Br Med J 4:492–493, 1970.
150. Toomasian, JM; Glavinovich, G; Johnson, MN; Gazzaniga, AB: Hemodynamic changes following pneumoperitoneum and graded hemorrhage in the dog. Surg Forum 29:32–33, 1978.
151. Alexander, GD; Goldrath, M; Brown, EM; Smiler, BG: Outpatient laparoscopic sterilization under local anesthesia. Am J Obstet Gynecol 116:1065–1068, 1973.
152. Burk, RK: Spinal anesthesia for laparoscopy: A review of 1063 cases. J Reprod Med 21:59–62, 1978.

153. Caceres, D; Kim, K: Spinal anesthesia for laparoscopic tubal sterilization. Am Obstet Gynecol 219–220, 1978.
154. Bridenbaugh, LD; Soderstrom, RM: Lumbar epidural block anesthesia for out-patient laparoscopy. J Reprod Med 23:85–86, 1979.
155. Schoeffler, P; Henry, C; Monteillard, C: Anesthesia. In: Bruhat, M; Mage, G; Pouly J-L; et al, eds: Operative Laparoscopy. New York, McGraw-Hill Book Co., 1992, pp. 33–38.
156. Lucas, LF; Rigor, BM: Anesthesia. In: Sanfilippo, JS; Levine, RL, eds: Operative Gynecologic Endoscopy. New York, Springer-Verlag, 1989, pp 162–178.
157. Loveday, R: Laparoscopy hazard. Br Med J 1:348, 1971.
158. Randel, GI; Levy, L; Kothary, SP; Pandit, SK: Propofol versus thiamylal-enflurane anesthesia for outpatient laparoscopy. J Clin Anesth 4:185–189, 1992.
159. Kong, KL; Cooper, GM: Recovery of neuromuscular function and postoperative morbidity following blockade by atracurium, alcuronium, and vecuronium. Anaesthesia 43:450–453, 1988.
160. Baile, R; Craig, G; Restall, J: Total intravenous anesthesia for laparoscopy. Anaesthesia 44:60–63, 1989.
161. Eger, EL II; Saidman, LJ: Hazards of nitrous oxide anesthesia in bowel obstruction and pneumothorax. Anesthesiology 26:61–66, 1965.
162. Scheinin, B; Lindgren, L; Scheinin, TM: Perioperative nitrous oxide delays bowel function after colonic surgery. Br J Anaesth 64:154–158, 1990.
163. Taylor, E; Feinstein, R; White, PF; Soper, N: Anesthesia for laparoscopic cholecystectomy. Is nitrous oxide contraindicated? Anesthesiology 76:541–543, 1992.
164. Sosa, RE; Weingram, J; Poppas, D; Lyons, J: Physiological considerations in laparoscopic surgery in urology. J Endourol 6:85–87, 1992.
165. Lawson, NW: The lateral decubitus position. Anesthesiologic considerations. In: Martin, JT, ed: Positioning in Anesthesia and Surgery. Philadelphia, WB Saunders, 1987, pp. 155–179.
166. Kropp, KA: Unusual positions. Urology: Surgical aspects. In: Martin JT, ed: Positioning in Anesthesia and Surgery. Philadelphia, WB Saunders, 1987, pp. 241–247.
167. Lynch, FP; Tomoshige, O; Scully, JM; et al: Cardiovascular effects of increased intra-abdominal pressure in newborn piglets. J Pediatr Surg 9:621–626, 1974.
168. Wesley, JR; Drongowski, R; Coran, AG: Intragastric pressure measurement: A guide for reduction and closure of the silastic chimney in omphalocele and gastroschisis. J Pediatr Surg 16:264–270, 1981.
169. Loffer, FD; Pent, D: Laparoscopy in the obese patient. Am J Obstet Gynecol 125:104–107, 1976.
170. Ott, DE: Laparoscopic hypothermia. J Laparoendosc Surg 1:127–131, 1991a.
171. Ott, DE: Correction of laparoscopic insufflation hypothermia. J Laparoendosc Surg 1:183–186, 1991b.
172. Hernandez, AD; Smith, JA, Jr; Jeppson, KG; Terreros, DA: A controlled study of the argon beam coagulator for partial nephrectomy. J Urol 143:1062–1065, 1990.
173. Rinfret, AP; Doebbler, GF: Physiological and biochemical effects and applications. In: Cook, GA, ed: Argon, Helium, and the Rare Gases, Vol 2. New York, Interscience Publishers, 1961, pp. 727–764.
174. Piiper, J; Canfield, RE; Rahn, H: Absorption of various inert gases from subcutaneous gas pockets in rats. J Appl Physiol 17:268–274, 1962.
175. Elwood, BJ; Piltz, GF; Potter, BP: Electrocardiographic observations on pneumoperitoneum. Am Heart J 19:206–217, 1940.
176. Kety, SS: The theory and application of the exchange of inert gas at the lungs and tissues. Pharmacol Rev 3:1–41, 1951.
177. Monk, TG; Weldon, BC: Anesthetic considerations for laparoscopic surgery. J Endourol 6:89–94, 1992.
178. Nunn, JF: Diffusion and alveolar/capillary permeability. In: Applied Respiratory Physiology. London, Butterworths, 1987, pp. 184–206.
179. Van Liew, HD: Coupling of diffusion and perfusion in gas exit from subcutaneous pocket in rats. Am J Physiol 214:1176–1185, 1968.

CHAPTER 3

Anatomic Perspectives During Laparoscopy

Louis R. Kavoussi, MD
Craig A. Peters, MD

Operative urologic laparoscopic surgery is a relatively new technique being applied to treat pathologies that have been approached for centuries with open surgical intervention. Its minimally invasive nature has great appeal to patients who benefit from decreased discomfort, shorter hospital stay, and a more rapid convalescence.[1–3] However, it is a distinctly different approach from traditional treatment of surgical diseases and requires a significant degree of training. One of the primary differences between laparoscopic and open surgical technique is the way in which the surgeon gains anatomic information related to the operative site.

With any surgical procedure, a firm understanding of basic anatomy is key to a successful outcome. Although actual anatomic relations do not change whether one is approaching an organ by an incision or a laparoscopic port, alteration in perspective can be extremely disorienting. The normal three-dimensional wide field of view is replaced during laparoscopy by a limited, fixed angle, flat field image. Moreover, tactile and proprioceptive information is blunted by instrumentation. These differences can cause familiar anatomic relationships to appear unusual.

The purpose of this chapter is to review the mechanisms that alter anatomic perspective compared with the surgeon's accustomed view during open surgery. Based on current technology, recommendations are made to help the operating physician compensate for perceived differences. The unique laparoscopic perspective may be used to our advantage, and with experience, a clear three-dimensional mental vision of abdominal and pelvic anatomy can be achieved.

ALTERATION IN ANATOMIC PERSPECTIVE

During any interventional procedure, the surgeon uses several cognitive tools to formulate and evolve an operative plan. First, he or she uses a basic knowledge of surgical anatomy along with an understanding of how each disease process affects normal anatomic relationships. The surgeon also draws from experience on how different tissues behave when manipulated (i.e., cut, coagulated, sutured) to perform an operation. Moreover, he or she accounts for variation in a given patient's anatomy through preoperative imaging studies. Finally, the surgeon uses "real-time" data to assess what is occurring in the operative field.

Real-time data is obtained through the senses, primarily in the form of visual and tactile information. There is great contrast in how the real-time anatomic data are delivered to the surgeon during open compared with laparoscopic procedures.

VISUAL IMAGE

Information obtained through visual images is markedly altered during laparoscopy. The primary difference compared with open procedures is that the surgeon is not directly observing the operative field but is basing operative decisions on reconstructed visual images that are subject to the limitations of current optical and video technology. Moreover, the angle at which the operative field is viewed is restricted by the location of the laparoscope. Finally, the pneumoperitoneum can alter the relationship between structures and impact on the visual information received by the surgeon.

Video Image

Laparoscopes are constructed of a rod-lens system consisting of an objective lens, rod lenses, an eyepiece lens and a fiber optic light cable (Fig. 3–1). The fiber optic cable runs through the endoscope in a concentric pattern around the lens system. It delivers noncoherent light that illuminates the surface of exposed organs.

Reflected light falls on the objective lens, which inverts and focuses the image on the end of the rod-lens system. The rod lenses are a series of glass lenses separated by air that reverse and transmit the image to the eyepiece. The eyepiece lens magnifies the image and presents it to the camera. The camera scans the incoming image and converts it to a series of electronic signals. Color, contrast, luminance, and synchronism information are all encoded on a composite signal that is carried by coaxial cable to the video monitor.

The quality of the image is dependent on the type of video system, light system, and laparoscope used. The visual image is created from reflected light; thus the quality of light greatly affects the reconstructed image. Light is not evenly distributed throughout the peritoneal cavity, since it is being produced at a point source (Fig. 3–2). If insufficient light enters the peritoneal cavity or if light is absorbed by dark surfaces (i.e., blood), the visual image is dark. On the other hand, when too much light is delivered or in instances when the lens is extremely close to the operative field, color may be washed out (Fig. 3–3).

The optical clarity varies with the resolution of the camera and the monitor. The resolution of the video image is defined as the number of horizontal lines that are encoded in the video signal to produce an image (Fig. 3–4). The greater the number of lines, the sharper the video image. Most available systems provide from 350 to 750 lines of resolution. High-definition televisions are being developed that have double the amount of resolution currently available.

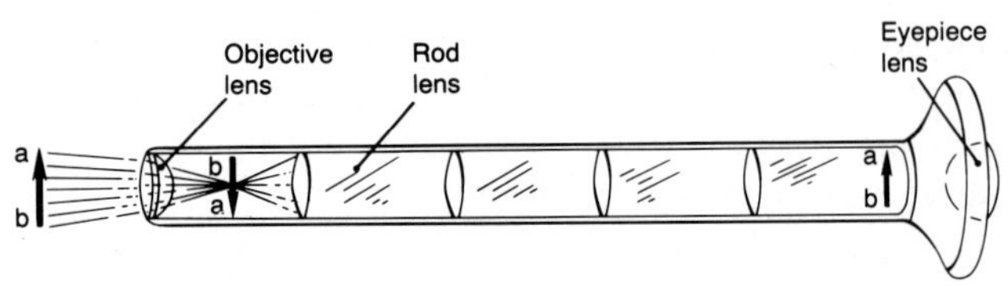

Figure 3–1. Diagram depicting construction of basic endoscope. Reflected light gathered by the objective lens produces an image that is magnified and inverted by the rod lenses.

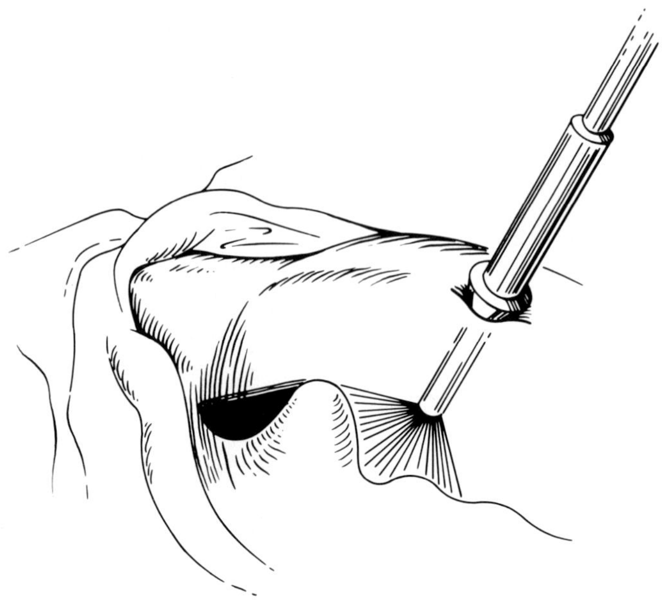

Figure 3–2. The endoscope in the peritoneal cavity acts as a point source of light. The irregular contour of abdominal organs causes light to be distributed unevenly and produces shadowing.

Color information transmitted by the camera depends on several factors. There is variability in color reproduction among manufactured video cameras. Most light sources cannot produce light containing wavelengths available from natural light. Consequently, the light available for reconstruction of the image color is altered. Current video systems can only encode video information in an analog manner; thus image color is always somewhat distorted.

The type of laparoscope used also affects the image obtained. During open surgery, the operating physician uses binocular vision to gauge distances between structures. In contrast, during laparoscopy a solitary lens gathers data. This monocular vision provides only a two-dimensional picture of three-dimensional structures, and thus normal depth perception cannot be obtained.

Image size is limited by the diameter of the laparoscopic lens and its distance to the operative field. The finite size of the objective lens restricts the amount of light collected. As the tip of the endoscope is moved closer to the operative field, light from a smaller area is collected and more detail is obtained. When the lens is pulled back to obtain a panoramic view, light from a wider area is recovered so image clarity and depth are

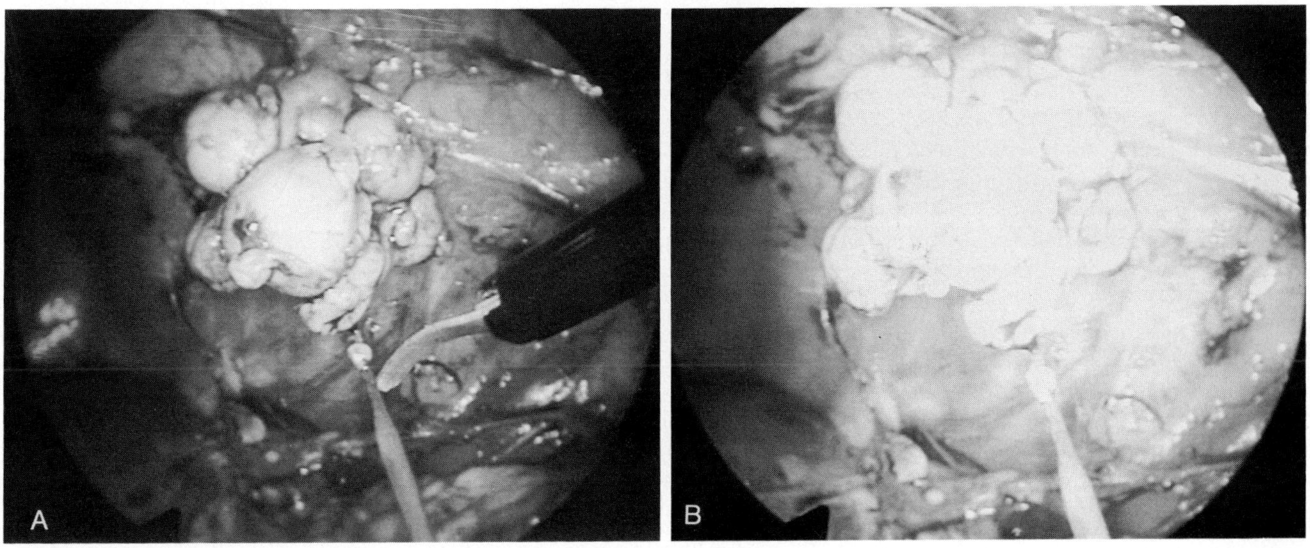

Figure 3–3. These photographs demonstrate differences in image quality secondary to lighting. *A*, Normal light. *B*, The glare produced in the center of the visual field when too much light is utilized. See also Color Plate 1.

lost. Consequently, only a limited amount of information from the operative field is available at any given moment. Smaller laparoscopes provide both decreased light-carrying ability and a smaller lens system, resulting in a more limited reconstructed image.

Debris on the lens can significantly obscure the image. Moisture can condense on the objective lens if a cold laparoscope is placed in the confines of the warm, humid peritoneal cavity. Blood, fat, and tissue debris can also collect on the lens. Smoke from electrocautery can accumulate in the pneumoperitoneum, inhibiting view of the operative field.

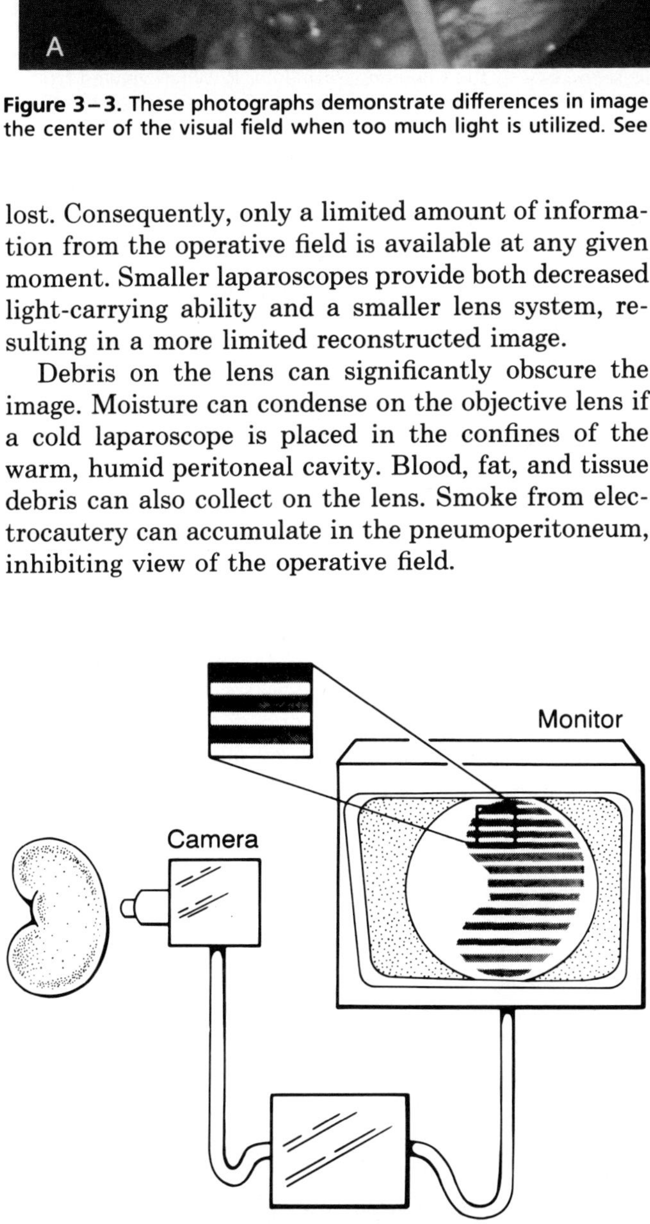

Figure 3–4. Each video picture is produced by converting optical data from the operative field to electronic signals that reconstruct the image as a series of horizontal lines.

Angle of View

During open surgery, one is able to view a specific location in the operative field from a vast variety of angles. The wide visual field obtained through the incision allows the surgeon to quickly become oriented to the anatomy. In contrast, during laparoscopy, the location in which trocars are placed dictates the perspective at which anatomic structures are viewed. The fixed number and location of trocars limit the potential views to a finite number.

Several effects result when observing anatomy from a fixed site with monocular vision. Structures can appear closer together than they actually are. Moreover, if one is viewing a structure at an oblique angle, it will seem foreshortened (Fig. 3–5). Also anatomic structures immediately behind the operative field may not be readily visualized.

The video image is fixed relative to the camera head. As the camera head is rotated, the entire image turns on the video monitor. Attempts at instrument manipulation in such a visual field are difficult, since hand motions do not correspond to the direction in which instruments are moving in the operative field. This discordance between hand and instrument movement also occurs when the surgeon is operating opposite the direction the laparoscope is facing or if instruments are entering behind the plane of the operative field (Fig. 3–6). In these circumstances, manipulated instruments will behave as if one were operating on a mirror image.

Effects of Pneumoperitoneum on Anatomy

The pneumoperitoneum can cause alterations in normal anatomy. Pliable structures can be compressed and have a different appearance from that seen during

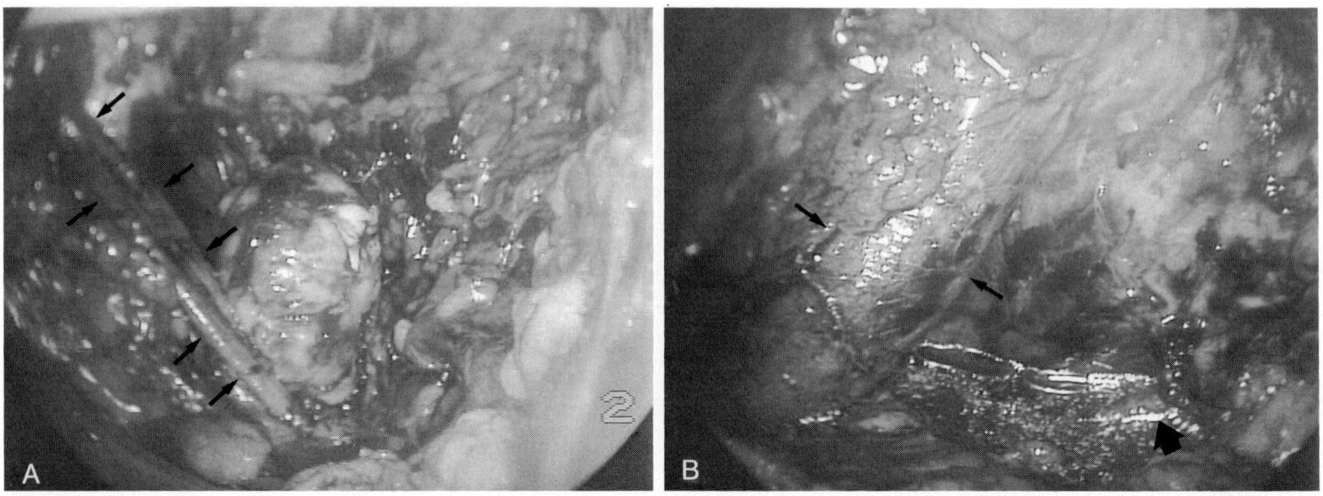

Figure 3–5. *A,* Picture demonstrating laparoscopic view of iliac vein *(arrows)* during laparoscopy from the umbilical trocar site. Note the enlarged lymph node in center and flattened vein. The vein is flattened secondary to the pneumoperitoneum. *B,* When viewed from a trocar site in the left lower quadrant, the full extent of the vein is now seen. The large arrow depicts the obturator nerve. See also Color Plate 1.

open surgery. The normal central venous pressure is approximately 7 mm Hg. When intra-abdominal pressure exceeds central venous pressure, veins are occluded. The maximal allowable intra-abdominal pressure is set at 15 mm Hg for most laparoscopic procedures. During the operation, intra-abdominal pressure will intermittently exceed central venous pressure. This can cause veins to alternatively appear flattened or filled as intra-abdominal pressure fluctuates.

In certain instances, the elevated abdominal wall can distort anatomic relationships. Structures adherent to the abdominal wall may be put on traction by the pneumoperitoneum. The peritoneum or bowel adherent to a hernia sac may bulge out of a defect in the fascia (Fig. 3–7).

The pneumoperitoneum is necessary in order to give the surgeon room to observe and work in the operative field. If there is inadequate pneumoperitoneum, structures tend to fall together, and tissue planes become less apparent. Also, overlying tissue can move into the operative field and obscure the view.

TACTILE INFORMATION

Tactile information is extremely important to the surgeon during open surgical intervention. Anatomic structures can be palpated to ascertain size, position, and consistency. For example, when not readily apparent, arteries can be located by feeling for a pulsation. The texture of tissue planes can be identified to facili-

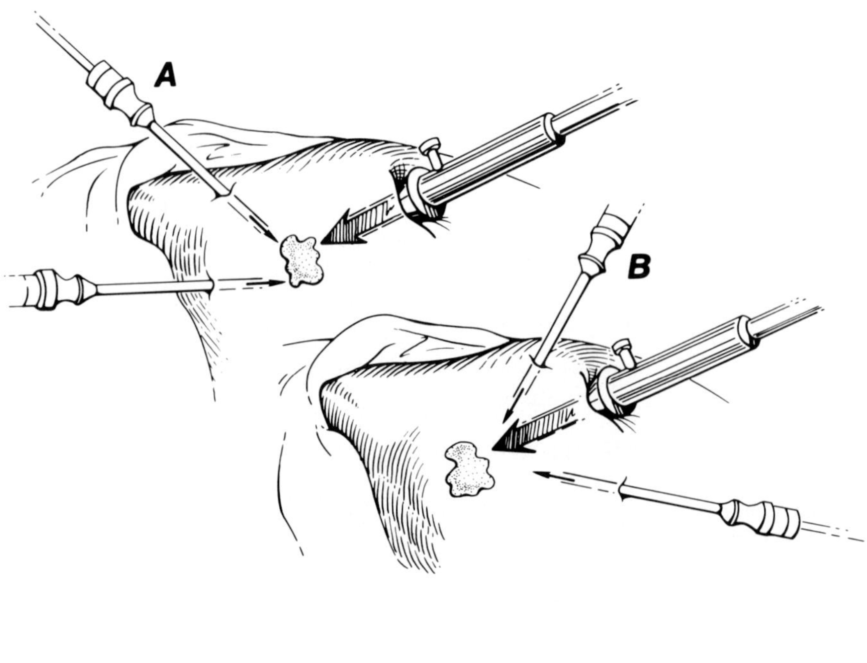

Figure 3–6. This diagram depicts the directions instruments enter the operative field relative to the laparoscope. *A,* Manipulating instruments placed in trocar sites behind the operative field can be awkward. *B,* Instruments should be placed so that they face the same direction as the laparoscope.

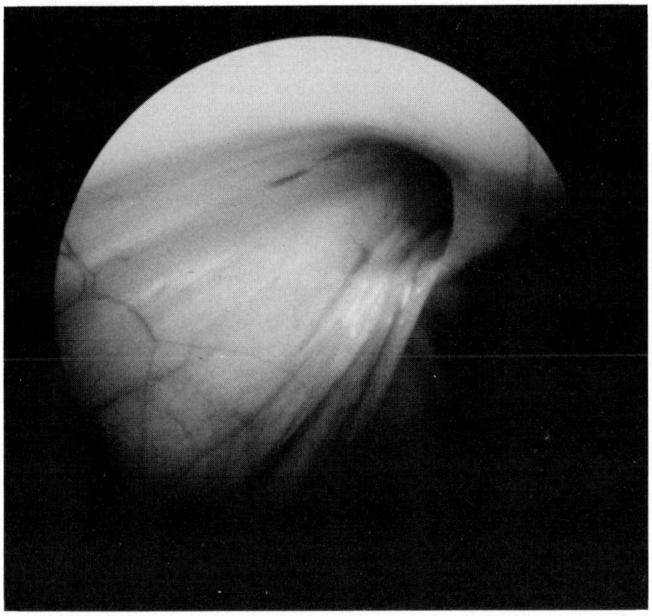

Figure 3–7. Endoscopic view of a hernia sac bulging out of the peritoneum.

tate dissection, and sites of fibrous attachments can be recognized.

During laparoscopic dissection, tactile sensation is blunted. Information regarding tissue composition is transmitted through rigid instruments which are fixed to the abdominal wall at the trocar site. Thus only gross differences in tissue consistency can be ascertained.

Proprioception is completely absent. Information regarding the location of an instrument relative to the operative field can be obtained only through visual images.

OTHER SENSES

Auditory information is usually obtained from ancillary personnel and staff in the operating room. For example, anesthesia gives data regarding the patient's overall status during a procedure. This does not change during laparoscopy except that additional information such as end-tidal CO_2 measurements are closely monitored.

The scrub technician and circulating nurse can let the surgeon know what equipment is available and how it is functioning in the environment of the operating room. Again, the information obtained from the staff varies from what one is accustomed to during open surgery because of equipment differences.

During laparoscopy all operating room personnel have access to the same image as the surgeon. An assistant may see the operative field from a different perspective and can give information to facilitate dissection. Auditory clues from the staff (unsolicited advice) may be helpful but can sometimes be misleading, especially if they are inexperienced.

Occasionally, the olfactory sense is helpful during an open operation. When one is dealing with an abscess, the odor of certain bacteria (i.e., *Pseudomonas*) is distinct. Moreover, if an unprepared bowel is opened, the feculent odor can be identified. Because of the closed nature of laparoscopic surgery, the molecules that stimulate the olfactory system are contained in the peritoneal cavity and thus this information is lacking.

COMPENSATORY MECHANISMS

In order for a laparoscopic procedure to be accomplished safely and successfully, the surgeon must understand the limitations of laparoscopic surgery previously noted. He or she must use alternative cognitive and technical skills to compensate for differences between open and endoscopic procedures.

Preoperatively, the surgeon must have a clear understanding of the pathology being approached. The anatomy of the operative site should be thoroughly reviewed. Structures that are not normally seen during open surgery may become important anatomic landmarks. For example, during the laparoscopic pelvic lymph node dissection (LPLND), the medial umbilical ligament (obliterated umbilical artery) must be identified throughout the dissection. Likewise, the inguinal ring and spermatic vessels, rarely seen with open node dissection, are essential to orientation during the LPLND.

A firm definition of each patient's pathology must be obtained through physical examination and radiographic studies. Indeed, when approaching disease entities laparoscopically, preoperative radiographic images not ordinarily obtained can prove helpful in planning an approach. When considering laparoscopic renal cyst ablation, for example, an abdominal computed tomographic (CT) scan is invaluable in giving precise anatomic orientation of the cyst relative to the parenchyma, collecting system, and vascular structures. All radiographic studies should be in the operative suite for intraoperative reference.

Choosing proper equipment, including insufflator, video system, and instruments is essential. The light source must be very bright and capable of producing wavelengths similar to sunlight. Currently, xenon light sources have the most desirable characteristics. The largest diameter endoscope available (10 mm) should be used to optimize visual information. One should use a high-resolution camera matched to a monitor of similar capabilities.

A thorough understanding of all equipment is mandatory. The surgeon must be able to interpret any intraoperative technical problems. Equipment needs to be checked to ensure that it is properly functioning before initiating a procedure. The camera should be focused to give a sharp image and white-balanced to provide the best color reproduction. The CO_2 tanks should be full, and a backup tank should be readily available in the operating suite.

Patient positioning is crucial, since this can alter the angle at which pathology is viewed and approached. Positioning is invaluable in exposing pertinent surgical anatomy. One may use gravity to move bowel or fluid out of the operative field by rotating or tilting the patient.

A variety of other techniques can be used to help identify anatomic structures. Vascular structures can be located with a laparoscopic Doppler probe.[4] The probe can be passed down a 5-mm port and will give an audible signal of blood flow through an artery or vein. Alternatively, when attempting to identify venous structures that may be flattened by the pneumoperitoneum, one may consider lowering the intra-abdominal pressure to allow the veins to fill.

The bladder wall can be more easily identified by instilling saline into the Foley catheter after the pneumoperitoneum is achieved. To locate the ureter, it is helpful to place an external ureteral stent. The firm stent can be palpated by sweeping a grasper across the operative field. The external portion of the stent can also be manipulated by an assistant to localize the ureter while the endoscopist inspects the operative field. The vaginal wall can be identified by having an assistant place a finger in the prepared vagina. Likewise, the rectum can be seen endoscopically by placing a finger into an O'Connor sheath positioned at the beginning of the procedure. A laparoscopic ultrasound probe has become available that gives real-time intraoperative images of anatomic structures 4 to 5 cm deep to the operative field (Fig. 3–8). Vascular structures, calculi, tumors, and visceral organs can be identified with this unit.

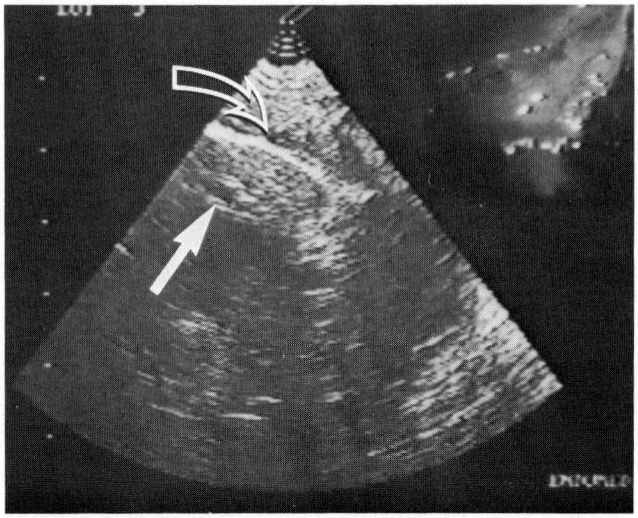

Figure 3–8. Intraoperative image of pancreas *(curved arrow)* taken through the mesentery by Laparoscan. Note the pancreatic duct *(solid arrow)*. See also Color Plate 1.

Precise trocar placement is important, because their locations determine the angles from which the operative field is viewed. When choosing trocar sites, it is important not to place a working port between the camera port and operative field. In this instance, the working port obscures the view (Fig. 3–9). Trocars should not be positioned close together, since this inhibits manipulation of instruments. In general, when working in the pelvis, a horseshoe or fan configuration allows adequate operative and visual access to pathology (see Chap. 13, Fig. 13–6). Similarly, when working on the kidney or the upper urinary tract, a diamond or trapezoidal configuration gives the most flexibility (see Chap. 13, Fig. 13–7).

Clear visualization of the operative field facilitates identification of anatomic structures. Since one is working within a confined space, it is helpful to keep the abdominal cavity maximally distended to optimize

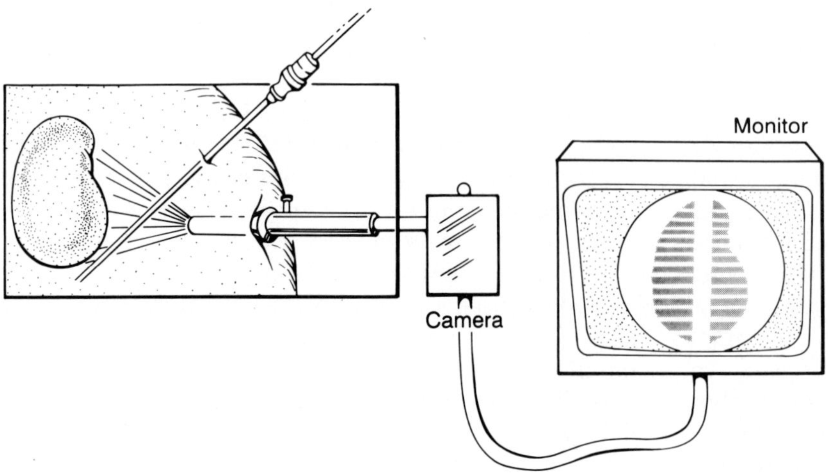

Figure 3–9. A working port placed in line with the laparosope and operative field will obstruct vision.

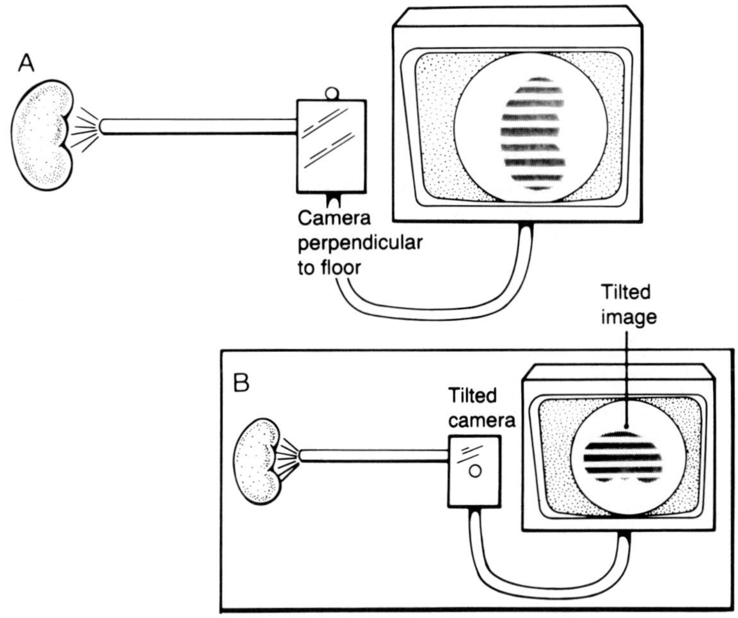

Figure 3–10. *A,* The camera should be oriented so that the image is perpendicular to the floor, not the patient. *B,* If the camera is tilted, the image on the video monitor will be turned.

visualization. Fogging of the image because of moisture condensing on the lens can be prevented by preheating the lens in a warmer or cleansing with hot water just before laparoscopy. Alternatively, a commercially available solution can be applied to the lens. Insufflating through a port other than the camera port minimizes the cooling effect of the insufflant gas on the camera lens, thus reducing fogging. For optimal view of the operative field, the laparoscope tip should be cleaned whenever blood or debris accumulates on the lens. If visualization is impaired as a result of smoke produced during electrocautery, a trocar valve may be opened to allow smoke to escape. There are commercially available insufflators that continually filter and recirculate the pneumoperitoneum to prevent an obscured view from smoke.

One of the most crucial factors in facilitating laparoscopic dissection is proper orientation of the camera. In order for the surgeon to maintain orientation, the camera holder must understand correct positioning of the laparoscope. The laparoscope must always be held so that the image is upright relative to the floor, not the operating table (Fig. 3–10). Appropriate alignment of the laparoscope, surgeon, and video monitor relative to the operative field is imperative. With the laparoscope aimed at the operative field, the surgeon should be stationed to face the same direction as the laparoscope (Fig. 3–11). The video monitor should be

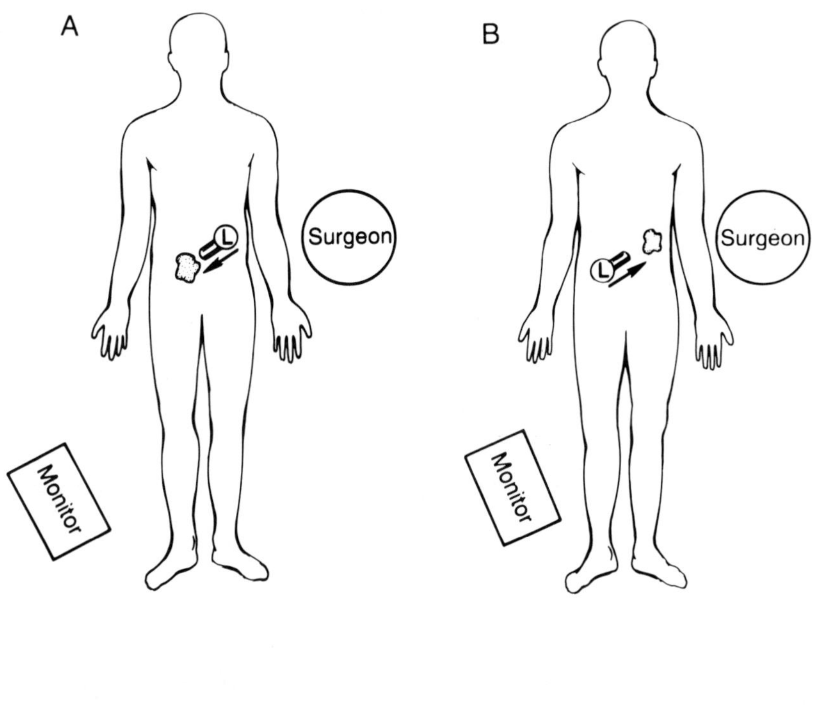

Figure 3–11. This diagram depicts a proper video system and surgeon's alignment during laparoscopy. The surgeon, camera, operative field, and video monitor should all be positioned as shown.

placed across the table, in line with the surgeon, laparoscope, and operative field. This positioning gives the most natural view and at the same time avoids operator strain.

Manipulation of instruments is awkward from the side opposite the direction of the camera's view. This usually occurs if trocars are positioned behind the vertical plane of the operative field or if the surgeon is operating from the direction opposite that which the camera is facing. In these instances, instruments behave as if one were operating on a mirror image (i.e., hand motion to the left would cause instruments to pivot at the skin).

Since a wide view is not available for observation, the surgeon must make an effort carefully to survey the intra-abdominal cavity and operative field. All landmarks for each operation outlined in this book should be identified, and the surgeon should make sure that all assistants are oriented to the anatomy. Because of the limitations of modern endoscopic images, dynamic manipulation of the laparoscope is necessary to gain the maximal amount of visual information. The camera should constantly be shifted in and out of the operative field to give the surgeon adequate information about how the procedure is progressing. The variable magnification of the laparoscope can be used to the surgeon's advantage. The endoscope can be brought close to an object when detail is desired. This also gives the surgeon information regarding the relative depth of structures in the operative field. Moving the camera back from the operative field gives a wider picture with less detail; however, this is most helpful in keeping orientation during a dissection.

Lighting can change markedly when the laparoscope is moving back and forth. Light decreases when the endoscope is pulled back from the operative field. Further deterioration of light quality occurs if blood pools in the abdominal cavity. Intermittent irrigation with a heparin-containing solution (5000 units of heparin/L of normal saline) and aspiration are useful in preventing clot formation.

When the lens is brought close to the operative field, a glare may be observed from the reflected bright light. To avoid glare, camera systems that have an automatic iris are available. These cameras measure light intensity in the center of the visual field and automatically adjust the amount of light entering the peritoneal cavity. Alternatively, a light source can be placed by a separate port to obtain a more even lighting that does not change with camera position.

Tactile information is markedly limited during laparoscopy and is primarily obtained through visual clues. Some tissue, such as bone, can be easily palpated through laparoscopic instruments; however, in most instances only gross differences can be discerned. The consistency of a structure may be ascertained by delicate ballottement with an instrument. Alternatively, tissue may be gently tugged, or an instrument may carefully be swept across its surface.

CONCLUSIONS

The difference between laparoscopic and open anatomy is the manner in which sensory information is presented to the operating physician. Laparoscopic surgeons rely heavily on modified visual data to successfully complete an operation. Unfortunately, the primary method of gaining a thorough understanding of laparoscopic anatomy is through experience. Just as residency training has prepared surgeons for open surgical approaches, only practice can train the laparoscopist's eye to appreciate subtle differences presented on the video screen. It is to be hoped that the laparoscopic learning curve will become less steep with improvements in imaging technology such as the development of practical three-dimensional video systems and intraoperative real-time radiographic imaging modalities.

REFERENCES

1. Winfield, HN; Donovan, JF; See, WA; et al: Urological laparoscopic surgery. J Urol 146:941, 1991.
2. Schuessler, WW; Vancaillie, TB; Reich, H; Griffith, DP: Transperitoneal endosurgical lymphadenectomy in patients with localized prostate cancer. J Urol 145:988, 1991.
3. Clayman, RV; Kavoussi, LR; Albala, DM; et al: Laparoscopic nephrectomy: Initial clinical series. J Urol 147:432A, 1992.
4. Loughlin, KR; Brooks, DC: The use of a Doppler probe to facilitate laparoscopic varicocele ligation. Surg Gynecol Obstet 174:326, 1992.

SECTION III

ANESTHESIA, SET-UP, AND ACCESS

CHAPTER 4

Anesthetic Considerations for Laparoscopic Urology

Terri G. Monk, MD
B. Craig Weldon, MD

Laparoscopic techniques have gained increasing popularity during the past two decades as illustrated by the fact that laparoscopy is the most frequently performed gynecologic procedure in North America.[1] Of late, there has been a dramatic increase in the indications for diagnostic and therapeutic laparoscopic urologic surgery. Many of these procedures are still evolving and are being evaluated to establish their effectiveness and superiority over conventional surgical techniques.[2] As laparoscopic procedures become more widely accepted and practiced, urologists must become familiar with their potential intraoperative complications (Table 4–1) as well as some general principles of anesthetic management.

This chapter reviews the pathophysiologic events that precede intraoperative complications and discusses their diagnosis and treatment. Although there is no single anesthetic technique for all laparoscopic procedures, the selected technique should maximize safety and provide adequate amnesia, analgesia, and muscle relaxation.[3] Laparoscopic surgery is associated with minimal postoperative pain and short hospital stays; therefore the anesthetic technique must also facilitate a rapid postoperative recovery. This chapter describes several anesthetic approaches presently used for laparoscopic surgery.

INTRAOPERATIVE COMPLICATIONS

The overall complication rate for laparoscopy approximates 4% with a mortality rate of 0.03%.[4] Intraoperative complications are often related to the laparoscopic technique itself (e.g., Trendelenburg position, abdominal insufflation, trocar insertion). Thus a thorough understanding of the "pathophysiology of laparoscopy" will aid in the early diagnosis, management, and prevention of these complications.

Cardiovascular Complications

Dysrhythmias

Cardiac rhythm disturbances are the most commonly recognized cardiovascular alterations during laparoscopy.[5–8] Dysrhythmias do not invariably cause serious cardiovascular compromise but frequently indicate that a potentially dangerous situation is developing. Bradycardias, tachydysrhythmias, and premature ventricular contractions constitute the majority of dysrhythmias seen during laparoscopy.

Bradycardia is often associated with CO_2 insufflation and manipulation of pelvic structures.[5] Intense surgical stimulation (i.e., peritoneal distention or visceral traction) produces a profound vagal reflex in lightly anesthetized patients.[9] In some patients, the

Table 4–1. POTENTIAL INTRAOPERATIVE COMPLICATIONS DURING LAPAROSCOPIC SURGERY

Cardiovascular
Dysrhythmias
Hypotension
Hypertension
Venous gas embolus
Pulmonary
Hypoxemia
Hypercapnia
Aspiration
Barotrauma/extraperitoneal gas migration
Pneumothorax
Pneumomediastinum
Pneumopericardium
Miscellaneous
Vascular injury
Visceral perforation
Peripheral nerve damage
Oliguria

heart rate may drop precipitously and on rare occasions, cardiac arrest may occur.[7,9–11] The differential diagnosis of bradycardia during laparoscopy also includes anesthetic overdose, hypoxemia, and venous gas embolus. Hypoxemia and venous gas embolus are discussed in detail later in this chapter. These two problems can be readily diagnosed if pulse oximetry and capnometry are used to monitor the patient under anesthesia. The initial treatment of bradycardia should be directed at eliminating the surgical stimulus by decompressing the pneumoperitoneum and releasing visceral traction. If these maneuvers do not result in a prompt increase in heart rate, atropine should be administered intravenously. The anesthetic should be discontinued and cardiopulmonary resuscitation initiated if severe hypotension or cardiac arrest develops. Vagotonic bradycardia may be prevented or blunted by ensuring an adequate depth of anesthesia before abdominal insufflation or visceral manipulation.

Tachydysrhythmias and premature ventricular contractions are often associated with either systemic absorption of CO_2 from the peritoneal cavity or hypoventilation, both of which result in hypercapnia. Carbon dioxide stimulates the sympathetic nervous system, causing tachycardia and predisposing the heart to premature ventricular contractions, ventricular tachycardia, and ventricular fibrillation. An inadequate level of anesthesia may cause sympathetic activation and tachycardia but is distinguished from hypercapnia by the monitoring of end-tidal CO_2 levels. Hypovolemia, hypoxemia, and venous air embolus can also cause sympathetic stimulation and tachydysrhythmias. Most tachydysrhythmias can be prevented by maintaining normocapnia following the establishment of the pneumoperitoneum and by providing adequate anesthesia during periods of surgical stimulation.

Hypotension

The hemodynamic changes that accompany the creation of a pneumoperitoneum and Trendelenburg position during laparoscopy have been studied in both animals and humans.[10,12–15] In these studies, hypotension rarely occurred solely as a result of abdominal insufflation. Ivankovich and colleagues[14] found that mean arterial pressure actually increased during intraperitoneal insufflation of CO_2 in dogs despite a decrease in inferior vena caval flow, stroke volume, and cardiac output. This was the result of a substantial increase in systemic vascular resistance during insufflation. Other animal studies have shown that arterial blood pressure remains stable during abdominal insufflation, whereas reductions are seen in cardiac output and inferior vena caval flow when intra-abdominal pressures exceed 20 mm Hg.[13,15]

Human studies examining the cardiovascular effects of increased intra-abdominal pressure during insufflation have largely confirmed the animal data.[12,16] Blood pressure appears to be maintained or increased in the anesthetized patient during intra-abdominal insufflation with concomitant decreases in venous return, stroke volume, and cardiac output. Thus elevated intra-abdominal pressure alone does not cause hypotension during laparoscopy. Instead, the changes in cardiovascular function that accompany abdominal insufflation, especially at intra-abdominal pressures above 20 mm Hg, make patients more susceptible to the hypotensive effects of anesthesia, positioning, and hypovolemia.

Anesthesia may cause hypotension by blunting the compensatory autonomic reflexes that normally maintain blood pressure. Baroreceptor function, myocardial contractility, and basal autonomic tone may be adversely effected by general anesthesia, resulting in hypotension.[17]

Changes in the position of a patient during surgery can also have significant effects on the blood pressure of anesthetized patients. The Trendelenburg, or head-down, position increases venous return from the lower extremities and is usually associated with an increase in cardiac output and blood pressure in normovolemic patients.[18,19] Conversely, the head-elevated position produces hypotension in anesthetized humans.[20] When increased intra-abdominal pressure is combined with anesthesia, hypovolemia, or the head-up position, hypotension is a predictable consequence. Hypotension may also result from hemorrhage secondary to a vascular injury, severe bradycardia, hypoxia, venous gas embolism, or tension pneumothorax.

Prophylactic measures for preventing hypotension include gradual intra-abdominal insufflation to pressures less than 20 mm Hg, avoidance of severe head-elevated positioning and anesthetic overdose, and the maintenance of normal circulating blood volume throughout surgery. When significant hypotension develops, treatment should include immediate release of the pneumoperitoneum, placement of the patient in the Trendelenburg position, decrease in anesthetic depth, rapid delivery of intravenous fluid, and vasopressor therapy. If auscultation of the chest indicates a pneumothorax, immediate tube thoracostomy is necessary.

Hypertension

Increased intra-abdominal pressure during insufflation is frequently associated with an increase in systemic vascular resistance and occasionally blood pressure. The differential diagnosis of hypertension during laparoscopy also includes inadequate anesthesia, hypoxia, and hypercapnia secondary to absorption of CO_2 from the abdominal cavity via the splanchnic circulation. Capnometry readily indicates the development of hypercapnia. Likewise, hypoxemia is easily detected by a drop in oxygen saturation on pulse oximetry. The initial management of hypertension should be directed at improving the patient's ventilation or oxygenation, as appropriate, and increasing the depth of anesthesia.

Venous Gas Embolus

Currently, CO_2 is the gas most commonly used to establish the pneumoperitoneum during laparoscopic surgery. Its high solubility in the blood allows it to be rapidly absorbed into the circulation and exhaled through the lungs. In addition, CO_2 does not support combustion, and electrosurgical instruments can be safely used in its presence.[3] Nitrous oxide is also highly soluble in blood (68% of the solubility of CO_2), but it supports combustion and is therefore rarely used during laparoscopy.[21]

Venous gas embolism is a well-recognized cause of cardiovascular collapse during laparoscopy.[22–30] If the Verres needle is inadvertently placed in a highly vascular organ or a blood vessel, CO_2 can reach the right side of the heart and pass into the pulmonary outflow tract. These CO_2 bubbles can impede circulation in the pulmonary artery or can cause acute pulmonary vasospasm.[31] This situation produces pulmonary hypertension, the development of acute right-sided heart failure, and a catastrophic drop in cardiac output. The clinical diagnosis of gas embolus is suspected when a "mill-wheel" murmur is associated with cardiac dysrhythmias, severe hypoxemia, and hypotension. Capnometry, with continuous monitoring of end-tidal CO_2, will show a rapid decrease to zero, signaling a sudden loss of pulmonary perfusion (Fig. 4–1).[32] However, a small volume of embolized CO_2 may not cause total cessation of pulmonary blood flow and may demonstrate only a transient increase in end-tidal CO_2 without the abrupt drop.[33]

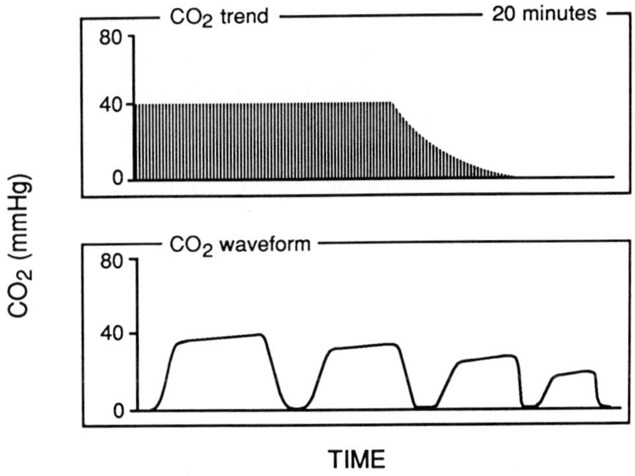

Figure 4–1. Rapid decrease of end-tidal CO_2 on capnogram. This pattern usually signals a catastrophic event—that is, pulmonary gas embolus or cardiopulmonary arrest. (Modified from See, WA; Monk, TG; Weldon, BC: Complications of laparoscopy: Strategies for prevention and treatment. In: Clayman, RV; McDougall, EM, eds: Laparoscopic Urology. St Louis, Quality Medical Publishing, 1993, pp. 183–206.)

The initial treatment of a gas embolism consists of resuscitative efforts to improve cardiac output and restore circulation as well as immediate release of the pneumoperitoneum, discontinuation of the anesthetic, and placement of the patient in a steep, head-down (Trendelenburg), left lateral decubitus position. This change in position will place the pulmonary outflow tract inferior to the right ventricle which should prevent the gas embolus from advancing further into the heart.[31] When a central venous pressure (CVP) catheter is in place, gas can be removed by aspirating through the catheter. In cases in which a pulmonary artery (PA) catheter is used, it is logical to attempt to aspirate gas through both the CVP and PA ports. However, aspiration of embolized gas through a PA catheter is reported to be less successful than aspiration through a CVP catheter.[34]

If traditional resuscitative efforts are unsuccessful in restoring cardiac activity, one case report suggests that the emergency institution of cardiopulmonary bypass be considered.[30] Cardiopulmonary bypass provides temporary circulatory support while the heart is emptied of gas. Additionally, if an intracardiac shunt exists, venous gas bubbles can enter the arterial circulation, resulting in a paradoxical gas embolus. McGrath and associates[35] report that early hyperbaric oxygen therapy can dramatically improve the neurologic outcome in such cases.

Pulmonary Complications

The respiratory effects of laparoscopic surgery are a subject of continuing investigation for both anesthesiologists and surgeons. The influences of anesthesia, patient positioning, and increased intra-abdominal pressure combine in complex ways, making it difficult to attribute specific effects to a single pathophysiologic mechanism. Nevertheless, a number of intraoperative complications involving the respiratory system have been studied and are reviewed here.

Hypoxemia

The cause of hypoxemia during laparoscopy may be multifactorial. This problem is often attributed to ventilation-perfusion ($\dot{V}/\dot{Q}$) mismatching that occurs as a direct consequence of the laparoscopic technique. Ventilation-perfusion mismatching causes an increase in intrapulmonary shunt whenever perfusion is maintained to an area of poorly ventilated lung.[36] In anesthetized patients, positioning and increased intra-abdominal pressure play an important causative role in $\dot{V}/\dot{Q}$ mismatching.

During laparoscopy, the Trendelenburg (head-down) position places the weight of the abdominal contents on the patient's diaphragm.[37] Anesthetized humans in the head-down position demonstrate a decrease in lung volumes that in turn contributes to the development of atelectasis and hypoxemia.[38,39] Elderly, obese, or debilitated patients are particularly susceptible to this effect of Trendelenburg positioning. In addition, the head-down position increases blood flow to the dependent (partially collapsed) portions of the lung.[40] Finally, the Trendelenburg position can displace the lungs and trachea in a cephalic direction while the endotracheal tube remains stationary, thereby creating the potential for movement of the endotracheal tube into a main-stem bronchus.[39]

The creation of a pneumoperitoneum with its increase in intra-abdominal pressure (IAP) may contribute to the $\dot{V}/\dot{Q}$ abnormalities seen with anesthesia and patient positioning. An IAP of 25 mm Hg exerts a force of approximately 30 g/cm^2, or a total pressure of 50 kg, against the diaphragm, which restricts lung expansion, decreases pulmonary compliance, and promotes the development of atelectasis and hypoxemia.[41]

Hypoxemia may also develop as a consequence of less common intraoperative events such as venous gas embolus, pneumothorax, pulmonary aspiration, or pulmonary edema. The development of $\dot{V}/\dot{Q}$ abnormalities is suspected when the patient develops a decrease in oxygen saturation on pulse oximetry or requires increasing inflation pressures to maintain pulmonary ventilation at a constant level.[42] Therapeutic maneuvers to improve oxygenation include increasing the inspired oxygen concentration, elimination of the Trendelenburg position, and release of the pneumoperitoneum. The chest should also be auscultated to verify the position of the endotracheal tube and to rule out a pneumothorax.

Hypercapnia

Hypercapnia has long been recognized as a common complication of laparoscopy.[3,4,10,42–44] Hypercapnia is often due either to systemic absorption of insufflated CO_2 or to hypoventilation.[3,42,43,45] Seed and co-workers documented the systemic absorption of CO_2 from the peritoneal space and suggested that the increase in $PaCO_2$ could be easily compensated by increasing minute ventilation.

Hypoventilation may account for occasional episodes of hypercapnia during laparoscopy. Patients who receive local or epidural anesthesia for laparoscopy are usually able to increase their minute ventilation to maintain normocapnia.[46,47] However, during general anesthesia, arterial carbon dioxide levels are significantly higher in spontaneously ventilating patients compared with patients who are mechanically ventilated.[42]

Hypercapnia and the accompanying respiratory acidosis predispose to dysrhythmias, sympathetic nervous system activation, and myocardial dysfunction. Capnometry will detect the gradual increase in end-tidal CO_2 ($ETCO_2$) (Fig. 4–2). It therefore is advantageous to use capnometry during general anesthesia and to adjust the minute ventilation to maintain the $ETCO_2$ between 30 and 40 mm Hg. This generally ensures a $PaCO_2$ of less than 50 mm Hg.

Monitoring $ETCO_2$ during laparoscopy can make patient management much easier if several caveats are remembered: (1) The $ETCO_2$ is only a reflection of the $PaCO_2$. No absolute determinations of $PaCO_2$ can be made without arterial blood gas analysis. (2) The normal relationship between $ETCO_2$ and $PaCO_2$ is altered

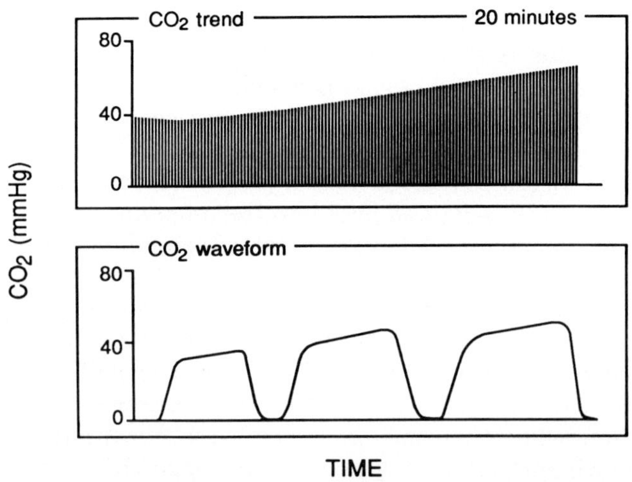

Figure 4–2. Gradual increase in end-tidal CO_2. This may be associated with hypoventilation, absorption of CO_2 during insufflation, or partial airway obstruction. (Modified from See, WA; Monk, TG; Weldon, BC. Complications of laparoscopy: Strategies for prevention and treatment. In: Clayman, RV; McDougall, EM, eds: Laparoscopic Urology. St. Louis, Quality Medical Publishing, 1993, pp. 183–206.)

in patients with an unusually large amount of dead-space ventilation (i.e., patients with chronic obstructive pulmonary disease [COPD] or certain forms of cyanotic heart disease). In these patients, the $ETCO_2$ to $PaCO_2$ gradient may be quite large, and the $ETCO_2$ may grossly underestimate the $PaCO_2$. (3) Monk and colleagues[48] have shown that the $ETCO_2$ to $PaCO_2$ difference increases during the course of prolonged laparoscopic procedures, making the $ETCO_2$ a less reliable predictor of $PaCO_2$ over time.

Aspiration

Regurgitation and aspiration of gastric contents have been reported to occur during laparoscopy.[45,49,50] Both Trendelenburg positioning and increased intra-abdominal pressure predispose patients to silent regurgitation under anesthesia. Aspiration frequently occurs when regurgitation or vomiting takes place after anesthetic induction but before tracheal intubation can be accomplished. Clinical signs suggesting aspiration include wheezing, tachycardia, hypotension, and hypoxemia. In awake patients, severe coughing, tachypnea, and shortness of breath may also be prominent findings. Radiographic evidence of aspiration includes fluffy infiltrates or lobar consolidation (the right lower lobe is the most common location). However, a retrospective study revealed that 10 to 15% of chest radiographs following a documented aspiration episode are initially read as normal.[51]

The risk of aspiration during general anesthesia can largely be eliminated by intubating the patient's trachea. It should be noted, however, that Kurer and Welch[52] found that young, nonobese women undergoing brief (<20 minutes) laparoscopic procedures did not have an increased risk of aspiration. Unfortunately, most laparoscopic surgeries last longer than 20 minutes and are not performed on healthy, nonobese patients. Thus tracheal intubation is recommended for the majority of procedures done under general anesthesia.

If aspiration occurs, supportive therapy includes supplemental oxygen, positive pressure ventilation, and positive end-expiratory pressure. These therapies should alleviate the hypoxemia and may help prevent the formation of atelectasis. The decision to continue or postpone surgery must be based on the patient's underlying medical condition, the severity of the pulmonary dysfunction induced by the aspiration, and the urgency of the planned operation. Treatment of aspiration pneumonitis with antibiotics or steroids may be detrimental and is not recommended.[53]

Barotrauma and Extraperitoneal Gas Migration

Pneumothorax, pneumopericardium, and pneumomediastinum may occur during laparoscopy as a direct consequence of pulmonary barotrauma or the extraperitoneal migration of insufflated gas.[54–58] Subcutaneous emphysema may also result from either mechanism and may involve the abdominal wall, thorax, head and neck, or the penis and scrotum.[59]

Pulmonary barotrauma is usually associated with high peak airway pressures in mechanically ventilated patients with chronic lung disease, reduced pulmonary compliance, or high airway resistance.[60] During laparoscopic procedures, there is a decrease in pulmonary compliance following the establishment of the pneumoperitoneum, resulting in an increase in peak airway pressure.[48,61] Patients exhibiting high peak airway pressures (≥50 cm) following abdominal insufflation therefore are at increased risk for pulmonary barotrauma. The careful monitoring of airway pressures is essential to safely conducting mechanical ventilation during laparoscopy.

The extraperitoneal migration of insufflated gas during laparoscopy may result in pneumothorax, pneumomediastinum, pneumopericardium, and subcutaneous emphysema.[3,54–58,62] Defects in the diaphragm allow gas under pressure to dissect along the tissue planes adjacent to vascular structures and into the mediastinum. This gas may eventually reach the pericardial space or, more commonly, dissect into the subcutaneous tissues of the thorax, neck, and head.[56] Frequently, the gas is trapped in the mediastinal tissues and ruptures directly into the thoracic cavity, creating a pneumothorax. Alternatively, a pneumothorax may occur if a trocar is placed above the 12th rib during retroperitoneoscopy.[63]

The diagnosis of pneumothorax is suspected when hypoxemia and escalating peak airway pressures develop following abdominal insufflation. These clinical signs may also be accompanied by tracheal deviation, a unilateral decrease in breath sounds, wheezing, and subcutaneous emphysema. A chest radiograph can confirm the diagnosis when the clinical picture is unclear. When profound hypoxemia and hypotension accompany the other clinical signs of pneumothorax, a "tension" pneumothorax is said to exist. This can occur if the intrapleural gas is under enough pressure to collapse the ipsilateral lung and impair systemic venous return to the heart. A tension pneumothorax represents a potentially life-threatening complication.

Pneumothoraces of less than 20% can usually be followed expectantly. However, if the patient exhibits any signs of physiologic instability, a chest tube should be placed immediately. In addition, the surgeon should release the pneumoperitoneum, and the anesthesiologist should terminate the administration of nitrous oxide, because this gas readily diffuses into a closed space and may expand the pneumothorax. If a tension pneumothorax is suspected, an 18-gauge needle should be placed through a high anterior interspace to convert the tension pneumothorax to a simple pneumothorax. Once cardiovascular stability is restored, a tube thoracostomy can be performed.[64]

Isolated pneumomediastinum is generally a radiologic diagnosis with no associated clinical manifestation. The diagnosis can also be inferred by other clinical signs of extraperitoneal gas migration such as subcutaneous emphysema. No treatment is required, but the patient's respiratory status should be monitored closely to ensure the early detection of an evolving pneumothorax.

Pneumopericardium is a relatively rare complication of laparoscopy. In a recent case report, pneumopericardium was not suspected clinically but was found when a postoperative chest radiograph was obtained to rule out a pneumothorax.[65] This patient did not require treatment, and the pneumopericardium resolved spontaneously. Although there are no reports of a clinically significant pneumopericardium associated with laparoscopy, the potential exists for serious cardiovascular compromise.

Miscellaneous Complications

Vascular Injury

Vascular injury usually results from puncture by the Verres needle or the trocar placed blindly at the beginning of the laparoscopic procedure. These injuries range in severity from an insignificant abdominal wall hematoma to laceration of the abdominal aorta.[4,59,66] A review of the early experience with urologic laparoscopy by Evans and associates[59] found a 3% incidence of injury to major vessels requiring conversion to open laparotomy for the control of bleeding. When the aorta, inferior vena cava, or common iliac vessels are traumatized, bleeding is usually profuse, and the surgeon is immediately aware of the injury. However, retroperitoneal bleeding may not become clinically apparent until the patient develops hypotension or the enlarging hematoma interferes with the planned procedure. Vascular injuries associated with a rapid accumulation of blood in the peritoneal cavity or hypotension require immediate open surgical intervention. The penetrating instrument should be left in place to tamponade the bleeding and guide the surgeon to the site of injury.[4] Maintenance of the pneumoperitoneum before laparotomy also helps to tamponade bleeding and may reduce the risk of injury to other abdominal structures during initial stages of the open procedure.

Perforation of Intra-abdominal Organs

Intra-abdominal organs (stomach, intestines, bladder, liver) are at risk for injury by instruments that are either passed blindly (e.g., Verres needle, initial trocar) or manipulated blindly.[63,67] The risk of gastric perforation is increased when the stomach is distended.[68] Gastric distention is a common finding following positive-pressure mask ventilation or inadvertent esophageal intubation but is quickly remedied with the placement of a nasogastric or orogastric tube prior to instrument insertion. Likewise, a full bladder is also vulnerable to needle or trocar injury and should be drained with a Foley catheter before Verres needle insertion is attempted.

Peripheral Nerve Damage

Peripheral nerve damage has been reported during both Trendelenburg positioning and laparoscopy.[19,69] Shoulder braces used to restrain patients in the Trendelenburg position may cause the clavicle to be pushed into the retroclavicular space and thereby exert pressure on the brachial plexus.[19] One can avoid the use of shoulder braces for steep head-down positioning by securing the patient to the operating table with tape or straps at the level of the ankles, hips, and shoulders. Brachial plexus injury also occurs when the arm is abducted beyond 90° or the arm is externally rotated and abducted. Hershlag and co-workers[69] have observed that femoral nerve damage may result from abduction and extreme external rotation of the hip during laparoscopy in the dorsal lithotomy position.

Oliguria

Prolonged elevations in intra-abdominal pressure have been associated with oliguria and even anuria.[70,71] In these reports, decreased urine output occurred despite adequate cardiac output and the presence of ureteral catheters. Possible mechanisms for the decrease in urine output include vena caval or renal vein compression, neurohumoral dysfunction, and the redistribution of renal blood flow from the cortex to the medulla. As laparoscopic procedures become longer and more complicated, intraoperative oliguria may become more common.

ANESTHETIC CONSIDERATIONS

Patient Preparation

Prior to any planned laparoscopic procedure, the patient must be evaluated by an anesthesiologist. Preexisting medical conditions may significantly alter a patient's surgical or anesthetic risk. These problems should be elucidated before the anesthetic plan is finalized and should be discussed with the patient as a part of the informed consent process.

Laparoscopy is associated with an increased risk of regurgitation of gastric contents.[3,49,50] It has been traditionally recommended that all patients fast for at least 8 hours before surgery.[49] However, recent studies have shown that gastric fluid volumes are less in patients given 150 ml of water within 2 to 3 hours of the induction of anesthesia when compared with patients who have fasted.[72,73] Thus to stimulate gastric peristalsis and emptying, small volumes of clear liquids may be ingested until 3 hours before the scheduled surgery. The prophylactic administration of a histamine H_2 receptor antagonist (ranitidine, famotidine) can reduce the acidity of stomach contents. Metoclopramide, a dopamine antagonist, acts both centrally and peripherally to stimulate gastric emptying and increase lower esophageal sphincter tone.[74] O'Sullivan and co-workers[75] found that the most effective pharmacologic approach for reducing the risk of acid aspiration was the combination of an H_2 receptor antagonist and metoclopramide. Therefore it is advisable to administer oral ranitidine, 150 mg, in combination with oral metoclopramide, 10 mg, approximately 3 hours before surgery to all patients with diseases that increase their risk of aspiration (e.g., morbid obesity, hiatal hernia, diabetic gastroparesis).

During trocar or Verres needle insertion, injury to a major vessel or hollow viscus can occur. The risk of life-threatening hemorrhage, although small, mandates that all patients have a secure, large (>18 gauge) intravenous line and a type and screen for blood. To minimize the incidence of organ perforation, the bladder and stomach should be decompressed prior to abdominal insufflation.

The risk of peripheral nerve damage during laparoscopy can be improved by making sure that all bony points are padded and that the arms are never abducted beyond 90°. Additionally, the use of straps at the level of the ankles, hips, and shoulders will secure the patient on the operating table without the use of shoulder braces.

Intraoperative Monitoring

Routine intraoperative monitoring during laparoscopic procedures includes an electrocardiogram, stethoscope, noninvasive blood pressure, airway pressure, and temperature monitors. The use of pulse oximetry and capnography is strongly recommended to aid in the diagnosis of cardiopulmonary derangements during laparoscopy. Pulse oximetry provides a continuous, noninvasive assessment of the patient's oxygen saturation and alerts the anesthesiologist to the development of hypoxemia before cyanosis or organ dysfunction becomes clinically apparent. Capnography measures the exhaled CO_2 in each breath and aids in the early detection of hypercapnia.

Patients who have severe pre-existing pulmonary or cardiovascular disease and are undergoing laparoscopic procedures, should be considered candidates for invasive monitoring. However, the anesthesiologist must weigh the risks of placing these monitoring lines against the benefit of the information they can provide. In addition, the pressures obtained from a central venous or pulmonary artery catheter reflect not only transmural pressure but also pleural pressure. The existence of a pneumoperitoneum often increases the airway pressure required for ventilation during the procedure and increases the measured central venous and pulmonary artery pressures.[13] One cannot assume that these pressures accurately reflect venous return or cardiac performance. Accordingly, cardiac function should be directly assessed by measurement of cardiac output with a pulmonary artery thermodilution catheter or transesophageal echocardiography.

Anesthetic Techniques for Laparoscopy

All three major anesthetic techniques (i.e., local, regional, and general anesthesia) have been utilized during laparoscopic surgery. The choice of the technique should be based on the duration of the procedure and the medical condition of the patient as well as the preferences of both the patient and surgeon.

Local and Monitored Anesthesia Care

Numerous reports discuss the use of local anesthesia for brief laparoscopic (≤60 minutes) diagnostic and sterilization procedures.[3,47,76] Before surgery, the abdominal wall is infiltrated with local anesthesia at each potential trocar site. Once the abdomen is entered, the intra-abdominal structures are sprayed with local anesthesia before manipulation. The most commonly used local anesthetics are 1% lidocaine and 0.5% bupivacaine. The addition of epinephrine to these local anesthetic solutions increases their duration of action and also reduces systemic absorption of these drugs.

Patients often experience diffuse abdominal pain during laparoscopy as CO_2 gas combines with peritoneal fluid and forms carbonic acid.[59] Patients undergoing laparoscopy with local anesthesia often require intravenous analgesics to blunt the pain associated with peritoneal irritation. During monitored anesthesia care (MAC) techniques, the anesthesiologist administers additional sedative-hypnotic and analgesic medications to supplement the local anesthesia. Titration of midazolam or propofol and fentanyl is common during these procedures.[77,78] As with all anesthetic techniques, the doses of these intravenous sedative-hypnotic and analgesic medications should be titrated carefully to minimize cardiorespiratory depression and to permit a rapid postoperative recovery.

Local anesthetic techniques offer some advantages over general anesthesia, including avoidance of the risks of general anesthesia, a rapid postoperative recovery, and a decreased incidence of postoperative nausea and vomiting.[3,76] In addition, an awake patient can alert the anesthesiologist to the initial signs of developing problems. However, awake patients frequently experience intraoperative anxiety, dyspnea, shoulder pain, and abdominal pain from peritoneal irritation. Therefore, local anesthesia is best reserved for brief laparoscopic procedures that can be performed with a gentle surgical technique on cooperative patients.

Regional Anesthesia

Spinal or epidural anesthesia has not been widely employed for laparoscopy, in part because of concerns over patients' ability to tolerate the respiratory dysfunction and shoulder pain that accompany the CO_2 pneumoperitoneum.[3,79] Such concerns may be unwarranted in young, healthy patients as demonstrated by Bridenbaugh and Soderstrom, who studied 100 women scheduled for laparoscopic tubal ligation.[80] The short-acting local anesthetic chloroprocaine was used for the epidural block and met with nearly unanimous acceptance by surgeons and patients alike. Two advantages were identified for this regional technique: (1) a rapid recovery and (2) a low incidence of postoperative vomiting. One potential drawback of epidural anesthesia is the frequent occurrence of intraoperative shoulder pain, necessitating opioid supplementation. With this caveat acknowledged, epidural anesthesia can offer a safe, effective alternative to general anesthesia in young, healthy patients undergoing brief (≤60 minutes) laparoscopic procedures.

General Anesthesia

Many diagnostic and therapeutic laparoscopic procedures are carried out with the aid of general anesthesia. This technique affords the anesthesiologist more control of intraoperative cardiopulmonary derangements, patient pain and anxiety, and the operating environment. Ventilation is adjusted in response to positioning and insufflation-induced changes described earlier. The patient is rendered free of pain and anxiety and is amnestic for even prolonged procedures. With a motionless operative field and relaxed abdominal wall, visualization and manipulation of intra-abdominal organs are made easier. As discussed previously, patients undergoing laparoscopy with general anesthesia are at particular risk for aspiration and usually require tracheal intubation.

There is no evidence to suggest that a particular general anesthetic technique affects the incidence of major intraoperative complications during laparoscopy. Yet less severe postoperative problems (nausea, vomiting, headache, myalgia, shoulder pain, dizziness) may be strongly influenced by the choice of anesthetic agent.[81–83] Dhamee and co-workers [81] compared halothane, enflurane, and fentanyl-based anesthesia for laparoscopy and found that fentanyl was associated with more nausea and vomiting, whereas halothane-treated patients had the highest incidence of headache. This finding should come as no surprise, since the opioids have long been known to be emetogenic. When halothane, enflurane, and isoflurane were compared in laparoscopic procedures, postoperative headache was a common problem with isoflurane (44%) but less so with halothane (20%) and enflurane (12%).[83] De Grood and associates[84] compared the postoperative recovery profile and side effects of isoflurane inhalation anesthesia with those for total intravenous anesthesia (TIVA) using either propofol or etomidate. These investigators found that the propofol-based TIVA technique resulted in less nausea and vomiting and faster early postoperative recovery than the isoflurane technique but that long-term recovery was unaffected by anesthetic choice.

Nausea and vomiting is a postoperative complication of laparoscopy that warrants special attention simply because of its frequent occurrence and its impact on the quality and duration of recovery.[85] As described earlier, the use of propofol or regional anesthesia may reduce the likelihood of nausea and vomiting as may the avoidance of opioids.[80,84] However, pain is often implicated as a *cause* of postoperative nausea, making it unwise to completely eliminate opioid analgesics from the anesthetic regimen.

Antiemetic prophylaxis is frequently employed in emetogenic procedures such as laparoscopy. Droperidol, 0.625–1.25 mg IV, has been shown to provide effective antiemetic prophylaxis in a placebo-controlled study of outpatient laparoscopic surgical patients.[86] Droperidol's effectiveness, however, is limited by the drug's sedative effects, extrapyramidal symptoms, hypotension, and dysphoric reactions. Although free from major side effects when used in small doses, metoclopramide has not demonstrated reliable prophylactic efficacy in all patient populations studied. Rao and colleagues[87] recommend its use for laparoscopy-induced vomiting, but others have demonstrated no advantage of metoclopramide over placebo.[88] Recently, Monk and co-workers[89] compared metoclopramide and the serotonin-receptor antagonist ondansetron in patients undergoing urologic procedures. These investigators found that ondansetron provided excellent antiemetic prophylaxis whereas metoclopramide was no more effective than placebo.

An effective approach to the management of pain associated with laparoscopy must address several potential mechanisms: (1) incisional (somatic) pain, (2) diffuse abdominal pain (secondary to peritoneal irritation by CO_2 or carbonic acid), (3) visceral pain produced by manipulation and injury of intra-abdominal organs, and (4) referred shoulder pain secondary to diaphragmatic irritation from retained intraperitoneal CO_2. Traditional methods of pain control rely heavily on intraoperative and postoperative opioid analgesics, which may aggravate the emetic effects of laparoscopy, prolonging recovery time.[81] Thus several strategies have been developed to maximize postoperative pain control and minimize the need for opioid analgesics.

The peritoneal and diaphragmatic irritation caused by CO_2 insufflation may be ameliorated by thoroughly emptying the intraperitoneal space of gas at the end of surgery.[90] Local anesthesia may be injected intraperitoneally[91] or instilled into the peritoneal cavity in combination with incisional infiltration of local anesthetic.[92] Both of these techniques provide improved pain control, resulting in reduced opioid requirements in the early recovery phase when compared with controls. Likewise, topical anesthesia is effective in managing the postoperative pain associated with fallopian tubal ligation.[93] The use of topical anesthesia on other intra-abdominal organs (e.g., gallbladder) has not been investigated.

Non-opioid analgesics have recently become popular as part of a postoperative pain control regimen. With the introduction of nonsteroidal anti-inflammatory drugs (NSAIDs) with potent analgesic effects, opioids may be delegated to a minor role in the pain management of less painful procedures such as laparoscopy. Ibuprofen, given orally 1 hour before surgery to laparoscopy patients, was compared with fentanyl and found to provide a longer duration of analgesia and to reduce the need for opioids in the postanesthesia care unit (PACU).[94] The authors also found that patients who received ibuprofen suffered less nausea than those given fentanyl. Ketorolac is a parenterally administered NSAID with potent analgesic properties that are opioid-sparing.[95] When ketorolac was compared with fentanyl in women undergoing outpatient laparoscopy, a significant decrease in total opioid dose was observed in the ketorolac group. Interestingly, the opioid-sparing effect of ketorolac did not translate into fewer emetic symptoms in this group.[96] Further research is required to determine the possible role of ketorolac in laparoscopic surgery.

The use of nitrous oxide as a general anesthetic adjuvant for laparoscopic procedures is a controversial issue. One property of nitrous oxide recommending its use is its ability to act additively with both inhalational and intravenous agents, thereby reducing the need for these more potent (and potentially more toxic) drugs. Nitrous oxide's quick onset and short elimination time make it particularly useful in the induction of anesthesia and rapid emergence from anesthesia. One objection to the use of nitrous oxide is its propensity for diffusing into closed, gas-filled cavities in the body and expanding the existing gas volume in such spaces.[97] If a pneumothorax occurs during laparoscopy, nitrous oxide can contribute to the severity of the situation by expanding the volume of gas in the pneumothorax. There has also been concern that nitrous oxide might increase the gas volume of normal bowel, as it does in obstructed loops of bowel, and thereby interfere with laparoscopic procedures. Taylor and associates'[98] data suggest that this concern is unwarranted for laparoscopic cholecystectomy procedures. In this randomized study, surgeons unaware of the anesthetic techniques were asked at the end of surgery to predict which of their patients had been given nitrous oxide. Operative conditions were identical in both groups and the operating surgeons were unable to identify the patients who had received nitrous oxide. It remains to be seen whether longer laparoscopic procedures (e.g., nephrectomy and pelvic lymph node dissection) are affected by the use of nitrous oxide, since its diffusion into closed spaces is not instantaneous but takes place over time.[97]

Table 4–2. BASIC PRINCIPLES IN THE MANAGEMENT OF LAPAROSCOPIC SURGICAL PROCEDURES

Obtain a preoperative type and screen for blood on all patients
Insert a large (14- to 16-gauge) intravenous line
Monitor with all standard monitors and also with pulse oximetry and capnography
Have a laparotomy set-up available
Intubate with a cuffed endotracheal tube if general anesthesia is employed
Place an oral or nasogastric tube to decompress the stomach and a Foley catheter to drain the bladder prior to instrument insertion
Avoid intra-abdominal insufflation pressures greater than 20 mm Hg
Control ventilation and adjust ventilatory patterns carefully to compensate for intraoperative pulmonary abnormalities

CONCLUSIONS

As more is learned about the pathophysiology of laparoscopy and the effects of old and new anesthetic agents on patients undergoing laparoscopy, more specific recommendations regarding the safe use of anesthesia for this procedure can be made. At present, basic operative and anesthetic principles continue to guide us in providing appropriate anesthesia and physiologic support for patients as newer information is incorporated into our practice (Table 4–2).

Major intraoperative complications are most influenced by the care, skill, and experience of the laparoscopist and anesthesiologist. Close communication between these two individuals, especially during times of patient instability, plays an important role in the outcome of patients undergoing laparoscopic procedures. Many potentially serious events during laparoscopy can be either anticipated or identified before they become life-threatening. Some complications can be successfully managed with early recognition and cooperative intervention, while others can be avoided altogether utilizing careful surgical techniques.

REFERENCES

1. Taylor, PJ; Gomel, V: Introduction. In: Taylor, PJ: Laparoscopy and Hysteroscopy in Gynecologic Practice. Chicago, Year Book Medical Publishers, 1986, pp. 1–6.
2. Stroumbakis, N; Hernàndez-Graulau, JM: The future of laparoscopy in urologic surgery. Semin Urol 10:141–145, 1992.
3. Fishburne, JI; Keith, L: Anesthesia. In: Laparoscopy. Baltimore, Williams & Wilkins, 1977, pp. 69–85.
4. Winfield, HN; Donovan, JF; See, WA; et al: Urological laparoscopic surgery. J Urol 146:941–948, 1991.

5. Myles, PS: Bradyarrhythmias and laparoscopy: A prospective study of heart rate changes with laparoscopy. Aust NZ J Obstet Gynaecol 31:171–173, 1991.
6. Harris, MNE; Plantevin, OM; Crowther, A: Cardiac arrhythmias during anaesthesia for laparoscopy. Br J Anaesth 56:1213–1217, 1984.
7. Myles, PS: Arrhythmias during laparoscopy. Br J Anaesth 63:365, 1989.
8. Scott, DB: Some effects of peritoneal insufflation of carbon dioxide at laparoscopy. Anaesthesia 25:590, 1970.
9. Shifren, JL; Adlestein, L; Finkler, NJ: Asystolic cardiac arrest: A rare complication of laparoscopy. Obstet Gynecol 79:840–841, 1992.
10. Motew, M; Ivankovich, AD; Bieniarz, J; et al: Cardiovascular effects and acid-base and blood gas changes during laparoscopy. Am J Obstet Gynecol 115:1002–1012, 1973.
11. Doyle, DJ; Mark, PWS: Laparoscopy and vagal arrest. Anaesthesia 44:448, 1989.
12. Lenz, RJ; Thomas, TA; Wilkins, DG: Cardiovascular changes during laparoscopy. Anaesthesia 31:4–12, 1976.
13. Kashtan, J; Green, JF; Parsons, EQ; Holcroft, JW: Hemodynamic effects of increased abdominal pressure. J Surg Res 30:249–255, 1981.
14. Ivankovich, AD; Miletich, DJ; Albrecht, RF; et al: Cardiovascular effects of intraperitoneal insufflation with carbon dioxide and nitrous oxide in the dog. Anesthesiology 42:281–287, 1975.
15. Richardson, JD; Trinkle, JK: Hemodynamic and respiratory alterations with increased intra-abdominal pressure. J Surg Res 20:401–404, 1976.
16. Johannsen, G; Andersen, M; Juhl, B: The effect of general anaesthesia on the haemodynamic events during laparoscopy with CO_2 insufflation. Acta Anaesthesiol Scand 33:132–136, 1989.
17. Seagard, JL; Bosnjak, ZJ; Hopp, FA Jr; et al: Cardiovascular effects of general anesthesia. In: Covino, BG; Fozzard, HA; Rehder, K; Strichartz, G, eds: Effects of Anesthesia. Baltimore, Williams & Wilkins, 1985, pp. 149–177.
18. Ekman, LG; Abrahamsson, J; Biber, B; et al: Hemodynamic changes during laparoscopy with positive end-expiratory pressure ventilation. Acta Anaesthesiol Scand 32:447–453, 1988.
19. Prentice, JA; Martin, JT: The Trendelenburg position: Anesthesiologic considerations. In: Martin, JT, ed: Positioning in Anesthesia and Surgery, 2nd ed. Philadelphia, WB Saunders, 1987, pp. 127–145.
20. Martin, JT. The head-elevated positions: Anesthesiologic considerations. In: Martin, JT, ed: Positioning in Anesthesia and Surgery, 2nd ed. Philadelphia, WB Saunders, 1987, pp. 79–115.
21. Scott, DB; Julian, DG: Observations on cardiac arrhythmias during laparoscopy. Br Med J 1:411–413, 1972.
22. Östman, PL; Pantle-Fisher, FH; Faure, EA; Glosten, B: Circulatory collapse during laparoscopy. J Clin Anesth 2:129–132, 1990.
23. Brantley, JC; Riley, PM: Cardiovascular collapse during laparoscopy: A report of two cases. Am J Obstet Gynecol 159:735–737, 1988.
24. Clark, CC; Weeks, DB; Gusdon, JP: Venous carbon dioxide embolism during laparoscopy. Anesth Analg 56:650–652, 1977.
25. Bradfield, ST: Gas embolism during laparoscopy. Anaesth Intensive Care 19:474, 1991.
26. DePlater, RMH; Jones, ISC: Non-fatal carbon dioxide embolism during laparoscopy. Anaesth Intensive Care 17:359–361, 1989.
27. Root, B; Levy, MN; Pollack, S; et al: Gas embolism death after laparoscopy delayed by "trapping" in portal circulation. Anesth Analg 57:232–237, 1978.
28. Yacoub, OF; Cardona, I; Coveler, LA; Dodson, MG: Carbon dioxide embolism during laparoscopy. Anesthesiology 57:533–535, 1982.
29. Greville, AC; Clements, AF; Erwin, DC; et al: Anaesthesia 46:113–114, 1991.
30. Diakun, TA: Carbon dioxide embolism: Successful resuscitation with cardiopulmonary bypass. Anesthesiology 74:1151–1153, 1991.
31. Bedford, RF: Venous air embolism: A historical perspective. Semin Anesth 2:169–176, 1983.
32. Glenski, JA; Cucchiara, RF; Michenfelder, JD: Transesophageal echocardiography and transcutaneous O_2 and CO_2 monitoring for detection of venous air embolism. Anesthesiology 64:541–545, 1986.
33. Shulman, D; Aronson, HB: Capnography in the early diagnosis of carbon dioxide embolism during laparoscopy. Can Anaesth Soc J 31:455–459, 1984.
34. Shapiro, HM; Drummond, JC: Neurosurgical anesthesia and intracranial hypertension. In: Miller, RD, ed: Anesthesia. New York, Churchill Livingstone, 1990, pp. 1737–1789.
35. McGrath, BJ; Zimmerman, JE; Williams, JF; Parmet, J: Carbon dioxide embolism treated with hyperbaric oxygen. Can J Anaesth 36:586–589, 1989.
36. Benumof, JL: Respiratory physiology and respiratory function during anesthesia. In: Miller, RD, ed: Anesthesia. New York: Churchill Livingstone, 1990, pp. 505–549.
37. Inglis, JM; Brooke, BN: Trendelenburg tilt—an obsolete position. Br Med J 2:343–344, 1956.
38. Altschule, MD: The significance of changes in the lung volume and its subdivisions during and after abdominal operations. Anesthesiology 4:385–391, 1943.
39. Wilcox, S; Vandam, LD: Alas, poor Trendelenburg and his position: A critique of its uses and effectiveness. Anesth Analg 67:574–578, 1988.
40. Carmichael, DE: Laparoscopy—cardiac considerations. Fertil Steril 22:69–70, 1971.
41. Scott, DB: Some effects of peritoneal insufflation of carbon dioxide at laparoscopy. Anaesthesia 25:590, 1970.
42. Hodgson, C; McClelland, RMA; Newton, JR: Some effects of the peritoneal insufflation of carbon dioxide at laparoscopy. Anaesthesia 25:382–390, 1970.
43. Alexander, GD; Noe, FE; Brown, EM: Anesthesia for pelvic laparoscopy. Anesth Analg 48:14–18, 1969.
44. Marshall, RL; Jebson, PJR; Davie, IT; Scott, DB: Circulatory effects of carbon dioxide insufflation of the peritoneal cavity for laparoscopy. Br J Anaesth 44:680–684, 1972.
45. Seed, RF; Shakespeare, TF; Muldoon, MJ: Carbon dioxide homeostasis during anaesthesia for laparoscopy. Anaesthesia 25:223–231, 1970.
46. Ciofolo, MJ; Clergue, F; Seebacher, J; et al. Ventilatory effects of laparoscopy under epidural anesthesia. Anesth Analg 70:357–361, 1990.
47. Brown, DR; Fishburne, JI; Roberson, VO; Hulka, JF: Ventilatory and blood gas changes during laparoscopy with local anesthesia. Am J Obstet Gynecol 124:741–745, 1976.
48. Monk, TG; Weldon, BC; Lemon, D: Alterations in pulmonary function during laparoscopic surgery. (Abstract) Anesth Analg 76:S274, 1993.
49. Duffy, BL: Regurgitation during pelvic laparoscopy. Br J Anaesth 51:1089–1090, 1979.
50. Carlsson, C; Islander, G: Silent gastropharyngeal regurgitation during anesthesia. Anesth Analg 60:655–657, 1981.
51. Le Frock, JL; Clark, TS; Davies, B: Aspiration pneumonia: A ten-year review. Am Surg 45:305–313, 1979.
52. Kurer, FL; Welch, DB: Gynecological laparoscopy: Clinical experiences of two anaesthetic techniques. Br J Anaesth 56:1207–1211, 1984.
53. Wynne, JW; Modell, JH: Respiratory aspiration of stomach contents. Ann Intern Med 87:466–474, 1977.
54. Kalhan, SB; Reaney, JA; Collins, RL: Pneumomediastinum and subcutaneous emphysema during laparoscopy. Cleve Clin J Med 57:639–642, 1990.
55. Saleh, JW: Complications. In: Saleh, JW, ed: Laparoscopy. Philadelphia, WB Saunders, 1988, pp. 253–266.

56. Pascual, JB; Baranda, MM; Tarrero, MT; et al: Subcutaneous emphysema, pneumomediastinum, bilateral pneumothorax, and pneumopericardium after laparoscopy. Endoscopy 22:59, 1990.
57. Doctor, NH; Hussain, Z: Bilateral pneumothorax associated with laparoscopy. Anaesthesia 28:75–81, 1973.
58. Altman, AR; Johnson, TH: Pneumoperitoneum and pneumoretroperitoneum: Consequences of positive end-expiratory pressure therapy. Arch Surg 114:208–211, 1979.
59. Evans, RM; Hulbert, JC; Reddy, PK: Complications of laparoscopy. Semin Urol 10:164–168, 1992.
60. Haake, R; Schlichtig, R; Ulstad, DR; Henschen, RR: Barotrauma: Pathophysiology, risk factors, and prevention. Chest 91:608–613, 1987.
61. Puri, GD; Singh, H: Ventilatory effects of laparoscopy under general anaesthesia. Br J Anaesth 68:211–213, 1992.
62. Gabbott, DA; Dunkley, AB; Roberts, FL: Carbon dioxide pneumothorax occurring during laparoscopic cholecystectomy. Anaesthesia 47:587–588, 1992.
63. Yuzpe, AA: Pneumoperitoneum needle and trocar injuries in laparoscopy. J Reprod Med 35:485–490, 1990.
64. Koster, JK Jr; Sanders, JH Jr: Thoracic injuries. In: May, HL, ed: Emergency Medicine. New York, John Wiley & Sons, 1984, pp. 365–377.
65. Knos, GB: Sung, YF; Toledo, A: Pneumopericardium associated with laparoscopy. J Clin Anesth 3:56–59, 1991.
66. Baadsgaard, SE; Bille S; Egeblad, K: Major vascular injury during gynecologic laparoscopy. Acta Obstet Gynecol Scand 68:283–285, 1989.
67. Penfield, AJ: Trocar and needle injuries. In: Phillips, JM, ed: Laparoscopy. Baltimore, Williams & Wilkins, 1977, pp. 236–241.
68. Reynolds, RC; Pauca, AL: Gastric perforation, an anesthesia-induced hazard in laparoscopy. Anesthesiology 38:84–85, 1973.
69. Hershlag, A; Loy, RA; Lavy, G; De Cherney, AH: Femoral neuropathy after laparoscopy. J Reprod Med 35:575–576, 1990.
70. Smith, JH; Merrell, RC; Raffin, TA: Reversal of postoperative anuria by decompressive celiotomy. Arch Intern Med 145:553–554, 1985.
71. Richards, WO; Scovill, W; Baekhyo, S; Reed, W: Acute renal failure associated with increased intra-abdominal pressure. Ann Surg 197:183–187, 1983.
72. Sutherland, AD; Maltby, JR; Sale, JP; Reid, CRG: The effect of preoperative oral fluid and ranitidine on gastric fluid volume and pH. Can J Anaesth 34:117–121, 1987.
73. Maltby, JR; Koehli, N; Shaffer, EA: Gastric fluid volume, pH, and emptying in elective inpatients. Influences of narcotic-atropine premedication, oral fluid, and ranitidine. Can J Anaesth 35:562–566, 1988.
74. Gibbs, CP; Modell, JH: Management of aspiration pneumonitis. In: Miller, RD, ed: Anesthesia. New York, Churchill Livingstone, 1990, pp. 1293–1319.
75. O'Sullivan, G; Sear, JW; Bullingham, RES; Carrie, LES: The effect of magnesium trisilicate mixture, metoclopramide, and ranitidine on gastric pH, volume and serum gastrin. Anaesthesia 40:246–253, 1985.
76. Alexander, GD; Goldruth, M; Brown, EM; Smiler, BG: Outpatient laparoscopic sterilization under local anesthesia. Am J Obstet Gynecol 116:1065–1068, 1973.
77. Monk, TG; Weldon, BC: Anesthetic considerations for laparoscopic surgery. In: Clayman, RV; McDougall, EM, eds: Laparoscopic Urology. St. Louis, Quality Medical Publishing, 1993, pp. 19–27.
78. Zelcer, J; White, PF: Monitored anesthesia care. In: Miller, RD, ed: Anesthesia. New York, Churchill Livingstone, 1990, pp. 1321–1334.
79. Mulroy, MF: Regional anesthesia: When, why, why not? Prob Anesth 2:82–92, 1988.
80. Bridenbaugh, LD; Soderstrom, RM: Lumbar epidural block anesthesia for outpatient laparoscopy. J Reprod Med 23:85–86, 1989.
81. Dhamee, MS; Gandhi, SK; Callen, KM; Kalbfleisch, JH: Morbidity after outpatient anesthesia. A comparison of different endotracheal anesthetic techniques for laparoscopy. Anesthesiology 57:A375, 1982.
82. Collins, KM; Docherty, PW; Plantevin, OM: Postoperative morbidity following gynaecological outpatient laparoscopy. Anaesthesia 39:819–822, 1984.
83. Tracey, JA; Holland, AJC; Unger, L: Morbidity in minor gynaecological surgery: A comparison of halothane, enflurane, and isoflurane. Br J Anaesth 54:1213–1215, 1982.
84. De Grood, PMRM; Harbers, JBM; Van Egmond, J; Crul, JF: Anaesthesia for laparoscopy: A comparison of five techniques, including propofol, etomidate, thiopentone, and isoflurane. Anaesthesia 42:815–823, 1987.
85. Jacobs, BR; Silverman, DG: Postoperative nausea and vomiting. In: Corfman, RS; Diamond, MP; DeCherney, AH, eds: Complications of Laparoscopy and Hysteroscopy. Oxford, Blackwell Scientific Publications, 1993, pp. 5–10.
86. Wetchler, BV; Collins, IS; Jacob, L: The antiemetic effects of droperidol on the ambulatory surgery patient. Anesth Rev 9:23–26, 1982.
87. Rao, TLK; Madhavareddy, S; Chinthagada, M; El-Etr, AA: Metoclopramide and cimetidine to reduce gastric fluid pH and volume. Anesth Analg 63:1014–1016, 1984.
88. Korttilla, K; Kauste, A; Auvinen, J: Comparison of domperidone, droperidol, and metoclopramide in the prevention and treatment of nausea and vomiting after balanced general anesthesia. Anesth Analg 58:396–400, 1979.
89. Monk, TG; White, PF; Lemon, D: Ondansetron reduces nausea following outpatient lithotripsy. Anesthesiology 77:A19, 1992.
90. Shrivastav, P; Nadkarni, P: Prevention of shoulder pain after laparoscopy. Lancet 339:744, 1992.
91. Narchi, P; Benhamou, D; Fernandez, H: Intraperitoneal local anesthetic for shoulder pain after day-case laparoscopy. Lancet 338:1569–1570, 1991.
92. Helvacioglu, A; Weis, R: Operative laparoscopy and postoperative pain relief. Fertil Steril 57:548–552, 1992.
93. Kaplan, P; Freund, R; Squires, J; Herz, M: Control of immediate postoperative pain with topical bupivacaine hydrochloride for laparoscopic falope ring tubal ligation. Obstet Gynecol 76:798–802, 1990.
94. Rosenblum, M; Weller, RS; Conard, PL; et al: Ibuprofen provides longer lasting analgesia than fentanyl after laparoscopic surgery. Anesth Analg 73:255–259, 1991.
95. Buckley, MMT; Brogden, RN: Ketorolac: A review of its pharmacodynamic and pharmacokinetic properties and therapeutic potential. Drugs 39:86–109, 1990.
96. Ding, Y; Terkonda R; White, PF: Use of ketorolac and dezocine as alternatives to fentanyl during outpatient laparoscopy. Anesth Analg 74:S67, 1992.
97. Eger, EI; Saidman, LJ: Hazards of nitrous oxide in bowel obstruction and pneumothorax. Anesthesiology 26:61–66, 1965.
98. Taylor, E; Feinstein, R; White, PF; Soper, N: Anesthesia for laparoscopic cholecystectomy. Is nitrous oxide contraindicated? Anesthesiology 76:541–543, 1992.

CHAPTER 5

Laparoscopic Operating Room Setup, and Patient and Instrument Preparation

Raul C. Ordorica, MD
Michael E. Moran, MD

Despite the vast array of instruments available, the performance of complex laparoscopic procedures has inherent limitations. From the operator's standpoint, these may be defined as limitations in instrument manipulation. The dexterity experienced is mechanically defined as the ability to revolve, rotate, and advance an instrument from a specific site.[1] Since the fixed portals determine the degree of manipulation of any rigid instrument, the access to the nonuniform topography of the abdomen and pelvis from a given site is finite. As to equipment, there are defined capacities for instruments to execute predetermined functions. Additionally, the maintenance of the pneumoperitoneum places restrictions on the performance of required tasks, such as blood and smoke evacuation. Yet despite this relative decrease in capability and functional response time in comparison with that experienced in open procedures, laparoscopic procedures of increasing complexity can safely be performed, because these limitations can be counterbalanced by careful anticipation and preparation. The setup of the operating room should reflect that preparation, from the timing and availability of actual equipment to its position in relation to the operating team and patient. The equipment should be chosen to perform not only the actual planned procedure, but also in anticipation of the potential requirement for open technique with emergency maneuvers. The following discussion of preparation for laparoscopic procedure includes operating room setup, equipment availability, and team training. From this information, a specific routine can be designed to suit a surgeon's needs by removing those variables that can adversely affect outcome. This consistency provides for efficient functioning of the laparoscopic team.

OPERATING ROOM REQUIREMENTS

The operating suite should have the capability to fully support the performance of laparoscopic procedures.[2-6] This requires space and materials for multiple sterile tables, suction apparatus, video equipment, insufflation equipment, electrocautery apparatus, pressure irrigation equipment, and full anesthetic complement. A diagram exemplifying a typical preoperative setup is given in Figure 5-1. The support

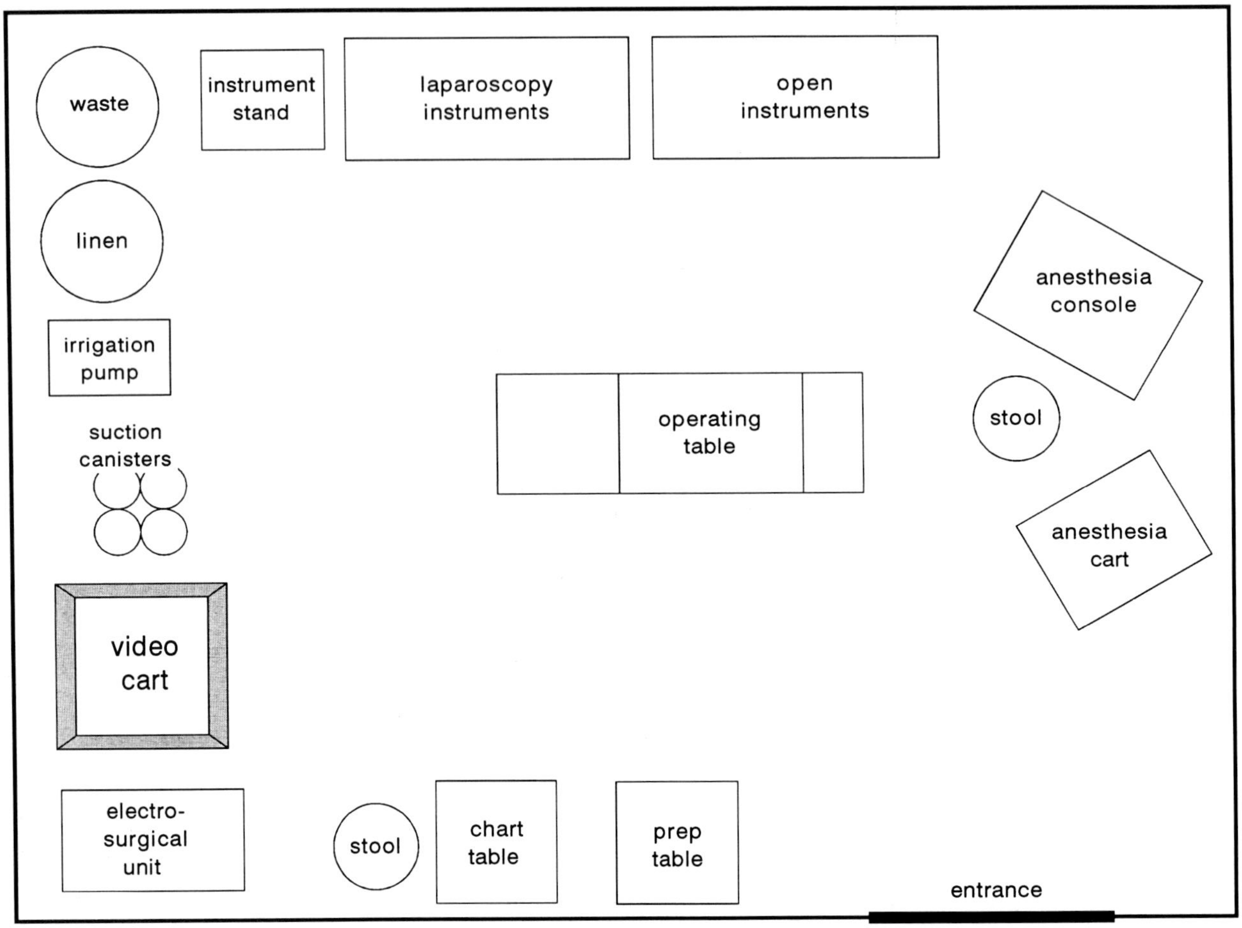

Figure 5–1. The setup of equipment for laparoscopy prior to patient entrance. Materials are readily available for rapid deployment as demonstrated in Figure 5–8.

should be no less than that provided for open abdominal procedures, which may ultimately be required in this setting. Therefore many ambulatory settings are perhaps ill-suited for laparoscopic procedures, despite the minimal recovery requirements of these patients.

Fluoroscopic capability can assist with imaging of the urinary tract, and support should be available in the form of portable equipment. Furthermore, the use of laser technology is generating increasing popularity during laparoscopic interventions.[1,3] These instruments have specific requirements to enable their function, and the manufacturer's advice should be followed regarding electrical supply, couplings, potential for water cooling, and safety precautions.[7] Although individual pieces of laparoscopic equipment are mobile, concentrating their use by several surgical services in select operating rooms may result in greater efficiency while adding to their longevity.

Operating Room Table

The performance of urologic laparoscopic procedures implies intervention in pelvic and retroperitoneal organs. These dependent areas require active retraction of intra-abdominal contents to allow visualization of the target organs and tissue. Patient positioning can alleviate some of the demands of retraction by moving the focused area out of a dependent, concealed position.[1,8] This ability to readily tilt the patient in multiple directions is best achieved with an electrically powered operating room table with controls that are easily accessible. Although alterations in table orientation may benefit the operator, they can produce further stress on the patient, including possible pressure injury and alterations in hemodynamic response and respiratory function.[9] Therefore proper patient padding and securing, along with intraoperative coordination between the surgical and anesthesia teams, are essential. Extremes in table tilting may result in patient slippage, which can be safeguarded against with the provision of padded shoulder braces in the case of Trendelenburg positioning and foot rests for the reverse position. In the case of pelvic surgery, elevation of the pelvis with additional padding can obviate some of these requirements.[8–10] The table should also enable placement of the patient in lithotomy and lateral positions.

Although the performance of laparoscopic biliary procedures often requires fluoroscopic imaging capability, this tool is infrequently used in current urologic laparoscopic practice.[11] Exceptions include the potential placement of a ureteral stent before ureteral surgery or nephrectomy. Any consideration of this necessity is best planned preoperatively, since the use of radiolucent portals should be considered for unobstructed imaging.

PATIENT EVALUATION AND PREPARATION

Evaluation of the patient should be performed in order to prevent complications and guide laparoscopic technique.[12–14] Significant history of chronic obstructive pulmonary disease (COPD) can alert the anesthetist regarding difficulties in CO_2 elimination. Hiatal hernia, abdominal wall hernia, and esophageal reflux are examples of conditions that may be exacerbated by the pneumoperitoneum and with extremes in patient positioning. A history of easy bruising may be consistent with a coagulopathy contraindicating laparoscopic technique. To clarify the condition, additional studies such as arterial blood gases and pulmonary function tests are indicated in the patient with COPD or hematologic studies in patients with bleeding diathesis.

Physical examination can offer basic information regarding potential difficulties in portal placement and subsequent dissection. Abdominal scars and hernias can guide the methods and sites of trocar placement and also alert the operator about possible underlying adhesions. Abnormal venous dilation on the abdominal wall may indicate portal hypertension and suggest possible coagulopathy. Palpable organomegaly may be indicative of underlying pathology, and caution should be exercised during trocar placement and laparoscopic instrumentation.

Basic preoperative laboratory assessment is similar to procedures requiring general anesthesia. Complete blood count; serum electrolyte, blood urea nitrogen, creatinine, and glucose levels; partial thromboplastin and prothrombin times; and urinalysis are routinely performed. A baseline electrocardiogram is advisable, particularly with the potential for hemodynamic alterations such as cardiac irritability secondary to hypercapnia, vasovagal responses with pneumoperitoneum, and compromises in venous return (see Chap. 4). Chest radiography is performed in those patients with significant pulmonary history.

Obtaining of patient consent should be thorough and should serve as a guide for perioperative expectations.[6,8,12,13,15] Particular note should be made regarding the potential for open procedure. Not only should the discussion include the possible requirement for emergency maneuvers, it should also note the possible inability to complete the task by laparoscopic means alone. Clear goals should thus be established for the procedure, with prior discussion of what would be acceptable alternative methods if endoscopy is not successful. Less significant details can take on exaggerated proportion if not also discussed beforehand, especially if the patient has preconceived notions regarding what may have been described as a "painless" procedure. Examples include the potential for abdominal wall discomfort, diaphragmatic irritation, scrotal emphysema, ileus, and urinary retention.[10] A review of laparoscopic complications can act as a rough guide in preparation for preoperative discussions with the patient, tailored to the individual situation.

Patient preparation in the perioperative setting varies slightly from that for open abdominal procedures. Those measures that may minimize bowel distention can be followed, and we routinely have our patient avoid dairy products for several days before laparoscopy. Additionally, we request that the anesthesia team avoid the use of nitrous oxide in prolonged procedures to prevent further intestinal distention. Nasogastric tubes with continuous suction also aid in this setting.[1,13,16] This is particularly true if gastric distention has occurred during anesthesia induction or for a pediatric patient in whom the stomach occupies a larger proportion of the peritoneal cavity compared with an adult. We do not routinely incorporate sterile bowel preparations for those procedures in which it is not indicated for open procedures. However, special consideration should be given to patients with a history of extensive abdominal surgery or peritoneal inflammation, in which dense bowel adhesions can be anticipated. Urethral catheterization is routinely performed to keep the bladder decompressed and thus to avoid inadvertent injury during Verres needle and trocar insertion.[6,8] In addition, the continuous monitoring of urinary output may alert the surgeon of bladder injury with the development of hematuria. Skin preparation includes clean shaving and sterile scrub performed at the time of surgery. The area incorporated should include those boundaries required for both laparoscopic and potential open exposure. It should be noted that the manometric pressure of the pneumoperitoneum will readily collapse the pelvic veins, compromising return of blood from the lower extremities.[16] We routinely incorporate pneumatic compression stockings for anti-embolic prophylaxis in this setting. Anticoagulants for deep vein thrombosis prophylaxis are not used.

PATIENT AND EQUIPMENT POSITIONING

Video Cart

Video monitoring equipment, high-intensity light sources, and automatic high-flow insufflators are best maintained on a single mobile cart. The light cord, video input, and insufflator tubing all stream to or near the laparoscope and its portal, allowing the organization of these cables and tubes from a single source for efficient maneuvering without cluttering the operating field. This arrangement also permits the team to easily observe both the monitor and insufflator throughout the procedure, for both provide important feedback regarding the status of the operating environment with video and manometric information. These carts can also contain video recording equipment and hard-copy color laser or thermal printers.[1] This allows accurate documentation of the surgical procedure on a scale beyond routine written operative record keeping.[17]

Besides permitting coordination of the operating team, the video monitor frees the surgeon from relying on direct visualization through the laparoscope.[1,3] With monitor placement allowing comfortable viewing by the operating team, fatigue is avoided during potentially lengthy and complex procedures.[2] Subsequent positioning of an individual team member and corresponding monitor is determined by the area focused on for the procedure. Primary surgeon positioning should best ensure forehand instrument manipulation with unobstructed monitor viewing. The portals should remain within peripheral view for ready observation during instrument exchange as required. For pelvic procedures such as varicocelectomy, lymphadenectomy, or others involving the lower urinary tract, the operator, laparoscope camera manipulator, and potential assistant are situated alongside the upper abdomen and chest of the patient. The team's orientation is caudal, and those using a two-monitor system have them placed opposite each operator, and beside the patient's legs, whereas those using a single monitor have it placed at the patient's feet (Figs. 5–2 and 5–3). This placement affords equally comfortable viewing with minimal fatigue for all assisting with the procedure.

Adequate operator mobility for proper instrument manipulation and monitor viewing is crucial for the performance of laparoscopic procedures. In the case of pelvic surgery, this often places the surgeon alongside the shoulders of the patient. A further demand in positioning is the requirement for the laparoscope manipulator to be "behind" the operator. Therefore the patient's arms are best tucked at his side to accommodate the team without the risk of brachial plexus injury from enthusiastic shoulder abduction.[6] The anesthetic team should be prepared for this request, since it isolates sources of peripheral access during the procedure. This encroachment into the traditional space reserved for anesthetic purpose can be minimized by using mechanical camera-holding systems. However, their utility as a nonfatiguing stationary aid must be evaluated in those procedures requiring frequent adjustment of the laparoscope.

The procedure may be focused on the upper abdomen as occurs during retroperitoneal lymphadenectomy, ureteral, renal, or adrenal surgery. Team and monitor positioning should reflect this orientation, demonstrated in Figures 5–4 and 5–5. Use of the low

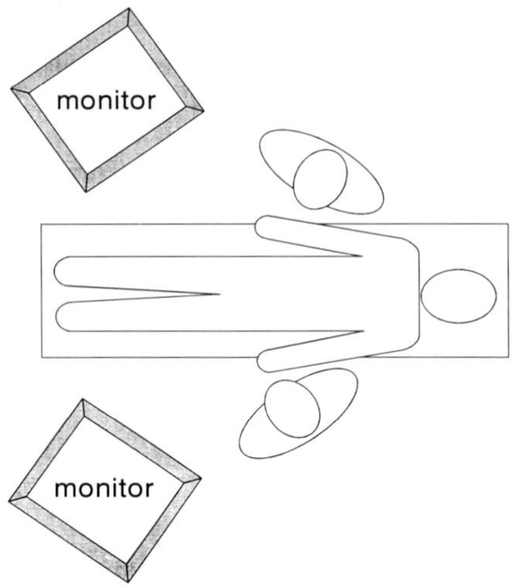

Figure 5–3. Double monitor and patient orientation for procedures focused in the pelvis. The monitor placement maximizes comfortable viewing for both operators.

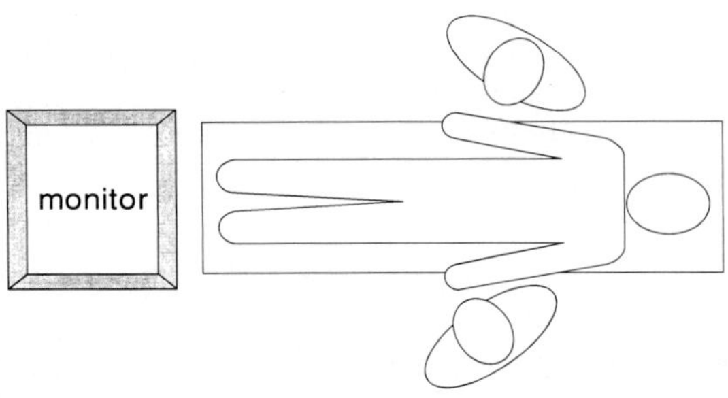

Figure 5–2. Single monitor and patient orientation for procedures focused in the pelvis. The monitor placement minimizes fatigue for both operators.

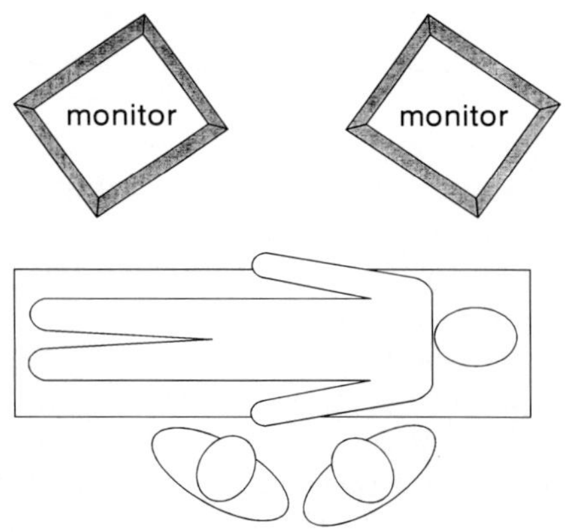

Figure 5–4. Double monitor and patient orientation for procedures focused in the midabdomen.

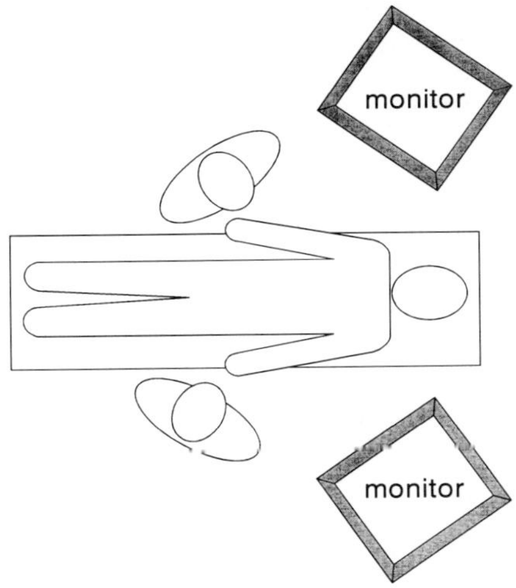

Figure 5–5. Double monitor and patient orientation for procedures focused in the upper abdomen.

lithotomy position can provide for additional operator space or access to the bladder if other than flexible instruments are required. This position is routinely used by gynecologic laparoscopists for vaginal access to pelvic organs, allowing intraoperative manipulation. Care must be exercised if cystoscopy is attempted in the presence of pneumoperitoneum, as filling of the bladder can be difficult because of the extravesical pressure exerted by the insufflated gas.

Placement of the patient in the lateral position has been advocated by some authors for adrenal and renal surgery, displacing bowel away from these typically dependent organs (Fig. 5–6).[18,19] Preparation for securing the patient in this position can be made with provision of an underlying bean bag. Axillary roll placement and flexion of the dependent leg with adequate padding will ensure against pressure injury. Table flexion can further elevate renal structures while providing greater abdominal wall surface area for cannula and instrument manipulation. Placement of initial portal sites can be performed with the patient supine, before this positioning. An alternative method of positioning is demonstrated in Figure 5–7, in which the patient is positioned on the table at a supported oblique angle. Subsequent lateral tilting of the table provides the necessary orientation for all stages of the procedure, without requiring complete repositioning of the patient.

It should be stressed that the alignment of the laparoscope and surgeons should be in the same direction, otherwise instrument orientation and motion will be reversed as viewed on the monitor.[13] Although this effect of operating through a "rear view mirror" can be mastered with patience, it is usually counterproductive in initial attempts at efficient manipulation.

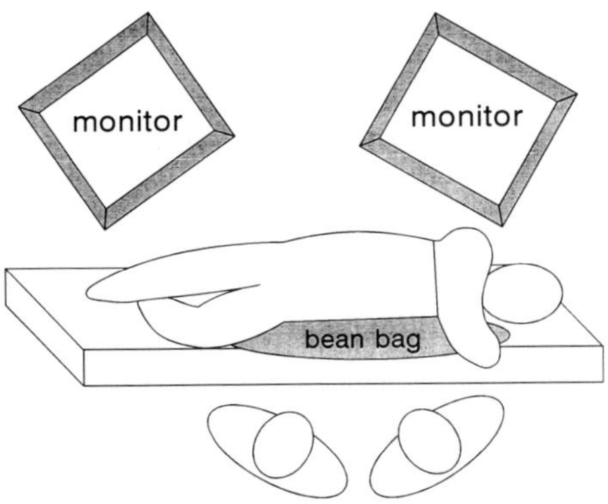

Figure 5–6. Double monitor and patient orientation for procedures focused in the retroperitoneum. Decubitus positioning with stabilization on a bean bag provides bowel displacement away from normally dependent structures. Pneumoperitoneum can be provided for prior to altering patient position. Monitors can also be placed as in Figure 5–5.

EQUIPMENT AND INSTRUMENT PREPARATION

Just as the necessary instruments are ready before anesthetic induction for open surgical procedures, laparoscopic equipment should also be available, tested, and poised for use.[20] Thus following positioning and sterile preparation of the patient, the monitor-insufflator cart, instrument stand, and instrument tables can be maneuvered into position without unnecessary

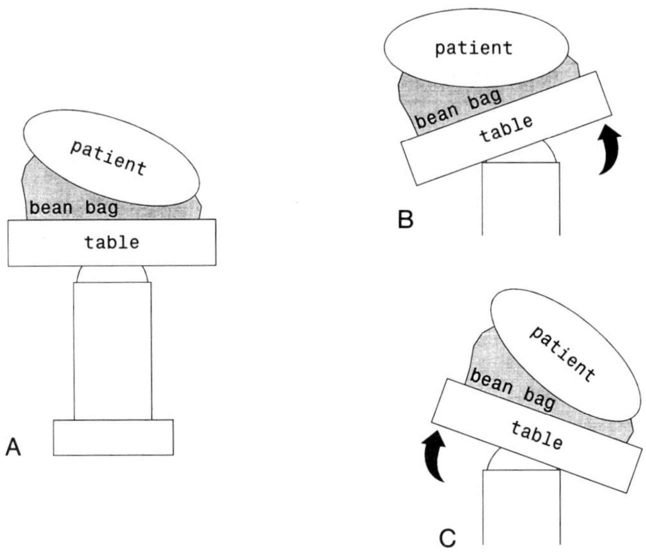

Figure 5–7. Alternative patient and table positioning prior to planned exposure of the retroperitoneum. *A*, Supported in a 20° lateral position by bean bag or padding, the patient has a range of 0° to 40° without slippage from the table or requiring repositioning. Lateral table tilting, as demonstrated in *B*, orients the patient in a supine position for pneumoperitoneum formation. This is followed by position *C*, which is more favorable for lateral trocar placement and dissection.

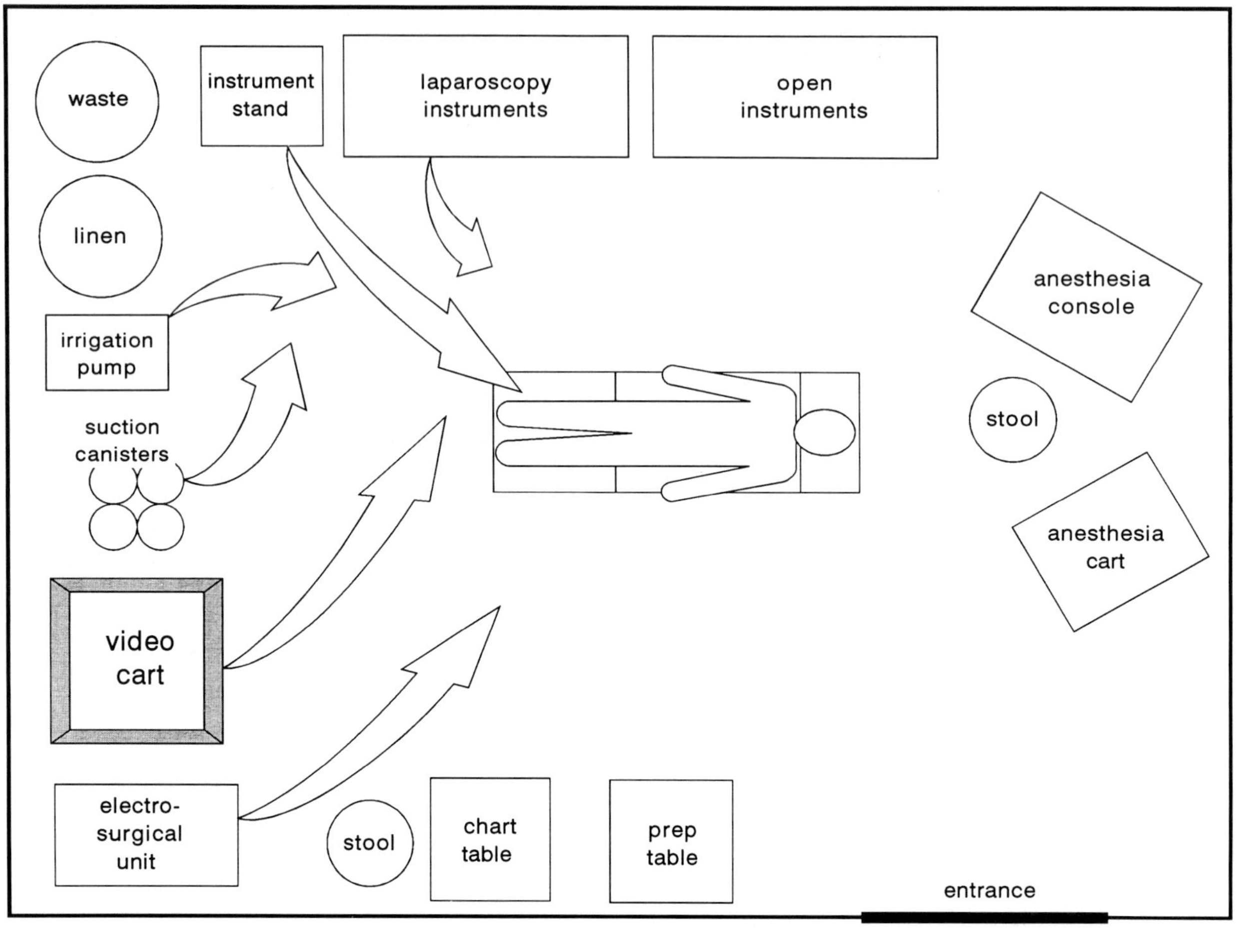

Figure 5–8. Deployment of equipment following patient positioning. Prior preparation allows for unobstructed equipment motion.

delay (Figs. 5–8 and 5–9). Table 5–1 illustrates a checklist for the preparation of the various instruments required for the establishment of the pneumoperitoneum and initial view of the abdomen. Because of space limitations immediately within reach of the surgeons, instruments should be organized on the laparoscopic table for ready access to economize effort and avoid confusion. The equipment available on the instrument stand should reflect the immediate task undertaken. An example of the initial setup is given in Table 5–2, the first tasks being the development of the pneumoperitoneum, insertion of the initial portal and laparoscope, and placement of additional portals. Subsequent tasks such as dissection and bulky tissue removal require equipment with specific designs and necessitate rotation of materials on the operating stand to make these readily available to the team.

Note, that an open set of instruments should be instantly available in case of a catastrophic emergency. Although this does not require an "opened" set for every contingency, a basic table equipped with scalpel, retractors, and vascular clamps would be considered adequate preparation for the potential hemorrhagic complication. The more common troublesome bleeding encountered during laparoscopic dissection is not the type that would mandate immediate emergency exploration. Rather, it is the bleeding of small arterial and venous branches that although not life-threatening, can pose unique problems in the closed abdominal cavity. The small, dependent confines of the pelvis and retroperitoneum can quickly fill with oozing from these small vessels that obliterates once easily recognized tissue planes and obscures areas that require careful identification. It is prudent to control meticulously all bleeding at every point in the dissection to preserve this anatomy. In addition, such bleeding may increase postoperatively when the compressive effects of the pneumoperitoneum are released on completion of the procedure. The availability from the outset of suction, irrigation, and cautery equipment is essential, since response time and capability is decreased in the closed abdominal cavity because of the limitations imposed by the necessary maintenance of the pneumoperitoneum. Therefore the irrigation and suction cannula should be tested as part of the opening steps of preparation, not urgently assembled following the commencement of bleeding. Such preparation can mean the difference between successful

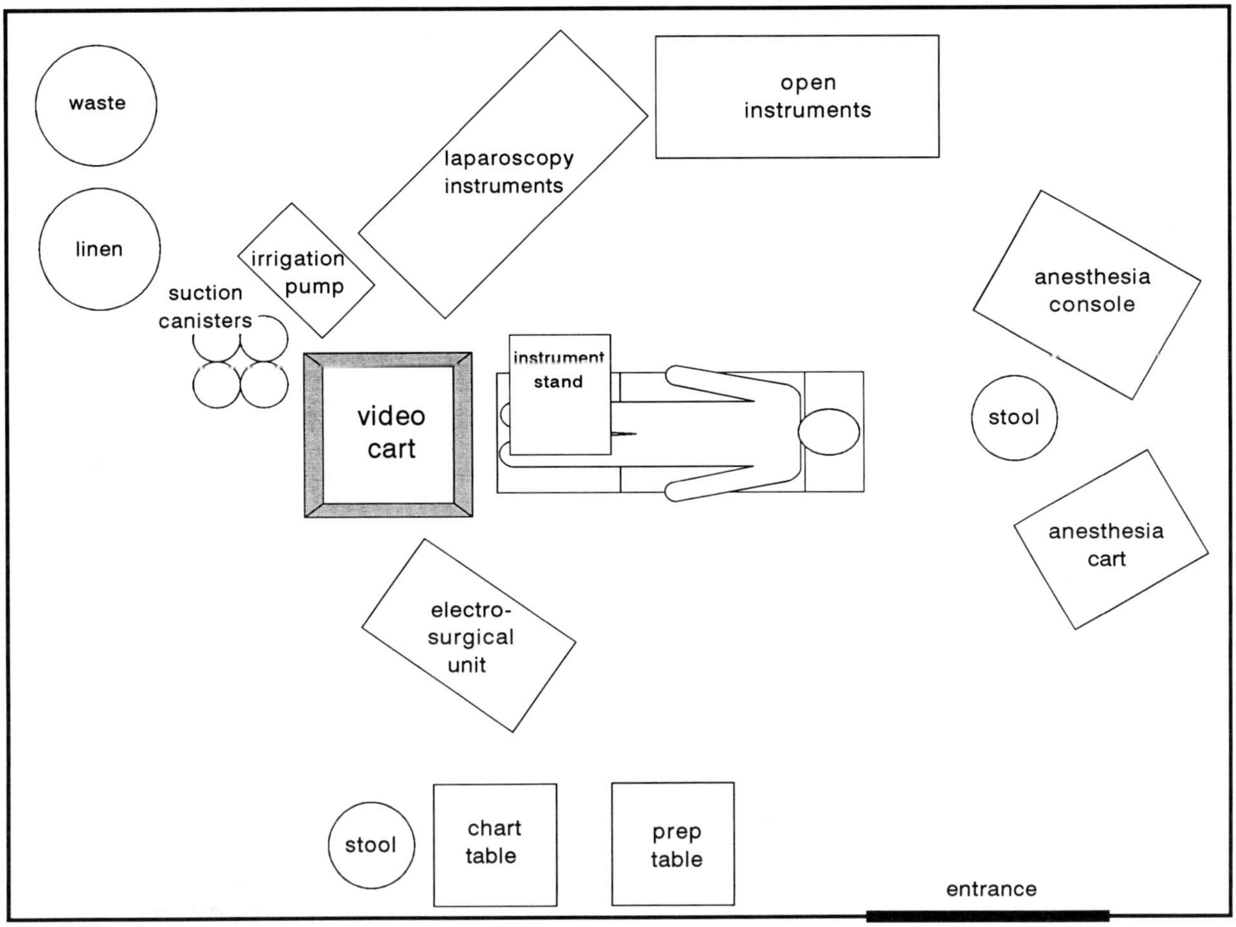

Figure 5–9. Equipment placement for performance of laparoscopy. Demonstrated monitor orientation is for procedures focused in the lower abdomen and pelvis.

completion of the proposed task and otherwise unsatisfactory results.

OPERATING ROOM PERSONNEL

The proper setup and care of the necessary laparoscopic equipment requires the support of a coordinated team.[1,3] Specialized training sets standards for usage and guides future continuity of experience among both operating room support staff and physicians. Guidelines for individual team members' responsibility and participation are presented in Table 5–3. Rapid development of new instrumentation requires frequent in-service training of staff, and a supervisor can be

Table 5–1. INITIAL EQUIPMENT PREPARATION

Verres Needle
- Safety cannula freely mobile with proper spring function
- Tip sharp
- Colored indicator ball freely mobile (where applicable)
- Patent
- Stopcock functional and open

Trocars
- Safety cannula freely mobile with proper spring and safety lock function (where applicable)
- Tips sharp
- Flap valve/trumpet valve functional
- Abdominal wall screws/retainers in place on sheath (where applicable)
- Stopcock turned off
- Variable size instrument gaskets/adapters available

Insufflator
- Adequate CO_2 for procedure (backup tank availability)
- Pressure setting
- Flow setting
- Volume setting
- Flow check

Image Reproduction
- Monitor function
- Light source check (verify replacement bulb or additional light source availability)
- Light cable and connectors check
- Laparoscope lens check
- "White" balance, focus
- Defog (warming of scope, defogging solution)

Irrigation and Suction
- Cannula patent
- Suction present
- Irrigation present
- Valve check (proper function without leak)

Table 5–2. EQUIPMENT TABLES

Pneumoperitoneum
- Verres needle
- 10-ml syringe
- # 15 blade skin knife
- Portals with abdominal wall screws/retainers (portals without retainer mechanisms should be sutured securely to the skin)
- Laparoscope
- Laparoscope cleanser/antifog solution
- 4 × 4 gauze
- Video camera attachment
- Towel clips*
- (Available but not open: Hasson-type trocar with appropriate suture)

Tissue Dissection/Manipulation
- Endosurgical scissors (may have electrocautery capability)
- Endosurgical tissue graspers (traumatic, nontraumatic)
- Endosurgical dissectors
- Suction/irrigation cannula
  (may have hydrodissection capability)
- Clip appliers
- Endosurgical needle drivers and suture*
- Stapling devices*
- Electrocautery applicator*
- Argon-beam coagulator*
- Laser probe*
- Doppler probe*

Tissue Removal†
- (Dependent on procedure should be available on main table)
- 10-mm spoon forceps
- Resectoscopes
- Tissue punch
- Isolation sack
- Morcellator

Closure
- Needle driver
- Skin retractors
- Skin forceps
- Suture
- Steri-Strips
- Gauze bandages

Hemostasis
- Mechanical systems: abdominal wall*
  - # 2 nylon suture swedged on large needle
  - High-capacity balloon catheter (Foley with plug)
- Mechanical systems (intra-abdominal)*
  - Cautery probes
  - Cryoprobe
  - Intra-abdominal suture device
    - Roeder loop
    - Endosurgical needle driver and suture
- Chemical systems*
  - Calcium-impregnated swabs
  - Endo-Avitene
  - Fibrin glue applicator (Tisseal)

Back Table: Prepared for Open Procedure
- #10 blade skin knife
- Abdominal wall retractors
- Tissue scissors
- Needle driver
- Suture scissors
- Vascular clamps
- Vascular forceps
- Tissue clamps
- Tissue forceps
- Sutures (including monofilament, nonabsorbable, for vascular repair)‡

*Depending on the procedure and the surgeon's preference.
†Depending on the procedure, these should be available on the main table.
‡Should be available in room but can remain unopened.

Table 5–3. LAPAROSCOPIC TEAM RESPONSIBILITIES

Laparoscopic Equipment Technician
- Familiarization with and maintenance of insufflator, light source, video monitor, and recording equipment
- Present for initial preparation and assurance of proper equipment function
- Immediately available for potential trouble-shooting
- Training of laparoscopic team regarding routine equipment operation

Scrub Nurse
- Familiarization with laparoscopic instrumentation, sterilization, and maintenance
- Inspection of laparoscopic instrumentation for wear or misuse
- Organization and provision of materials for step-wise application
- Preparation of Verres needles, trocars, suction/irrigation device
- Cleansing and preparation of laparoscope
- Organization of insufflation tubing, video, light source, and electrocautery cables
- Familiarization with open technique for major abdominal surgery

Circulating Nurse
- Assist with patient positioning and preparation
- Electrocautery pad placement
- Familiarization with basic controls for insufflator, light source, video monitor, recording equipment, and electrocautery apparatus
- Irrigation and suction canister maintenance
- Room lighting control
- Provision of materials for scrub team

selected to oversee equipment replacement and personnel training.[5] Such instruction and responsible use not only safeguard user and patient alike but also contribute to the longevity of expensive equipment.[21,22] This is particularly appropriate for video, cautery, and laser technologies, which not only represent the bulk of the laparoscopic budget but are also capable of delivering large amounts of potentially destructive energy if used improperly.[7]

CONCLUSIONS

Although the physician performing laparoscopy should ultimately be familiar with all the aspects of care outlined, a team approach allows the surgeon to focus on the successful completion of the assigned procedure. Given the use of laparoscopy in gynecologic, general, thoracic, and urologic surgery, having the required degree of focus in a segment of the operating room staff should be feasible even in small hospitals. This concentration is beneficial in order to maintain the equipment stressed through use by many operators with different specializations. Provision of dedicated personnel can be difficult to achieve in emergency settings during off-hours. However, this should not impact negatively on urologic practice, which normally confines the use of laparoscopy to scheduled routine procedures. With the proper care and preparation outlined, laparoscopic procedures should be performed safely and effectively for a wide range of urologic indications.

REFERENCES

1. Cuschieri, A; Berci, G: Instruments and basic operative techniques for laparoscopic surgery. In: Cuschieri, A; Berci, G. Laparoscopic Biliary Surgery. London, Blackwell Scientific Publications, 1990, pp. 15–37.
2. Murphy, AA: Technique and instrumentation in operative laparoscopy. In: Azziz, R; Murphy, AA, eds: Practical Manual of Operative Laparoscopy and Hysteroscopy. New York, Springer-Verlag, 1992, pp. 65–77.
3. Boyers, SP: Operating room setup and instrumentation. Clin Obstet Gynecol 34:373–386, 1991.
4. Hulka, JF: Facilities and equipment. In: Hulka, JF, ed: Textbook of Laparoscopy. Orlando, Grune & Stratton, 1985, pp. 45–54.
5. Corson, SL: Operating room preparation and basic techniques. In: Phillips, JM, ed: Laparoscopy. Baltimore, Williams & Wilkins, 1977, pp. 88–102.
6. Winfield, HN; Kavoussi, LR: Laparoscopic pelvic lymph node dissection. Surg Tech Urol 4:1–8, 1991.
7. Dorsey, JH: Operating room organization: Lasers and advanced operative laparoscopy. Obstet Gynecol Clin North Am 18:569–574, 1991.
8. Winfield, HN; Donovan, JF; Loening, SA; Williams, RD: Urological laparoscopic surgery. J Urol 146:941–948, 1991.
9. Schuessler, WW; Vancaillie, TG; Reich, H; Griffith, DP: Transperitoneal endosurgical lymphadenectomy in patients with localized prostate cancer. J Urol 145:988–991, 1991.
10. Griffith, DP; Schuessler, WW; Nickell, KG; Meaney, JT: Laparoscopic pelvic lymphadenectomy for prostatic adenocarcinoma. Urol Clin North Am 19:407–415, 1992.
11. Heerden, JA; Donohue, JH: Laparoscopic cholecystectomy. Prob Urol 6:373–380, 1992.
12. Borten, M: Informed consent and counseling. In: Borten, M, ed: Laparoscopic Complications: Prevention and Management. Toronto, BC Decker, 1986, pp. 415–428.
13. Dunn, DC; Watson, CJE: Pre-operative preparation. In: Dunn, DC; Watson, CJE, eds: Laparoscopic Cholecystectomy. London, Blackwell Scientific Publications, 1992, pp. 56–60.
14. Fishburne, JI, Jr: Anesthesia for laparoscopy: Considerations, complications, and techniques. In: Phillips, JM ed: Endoscopy in Gynecology: Proceedings of the Third International Congress on Gynecologic Endoscopy, San Francisco, American Association of Gynecologic Laparoscopists, 1977.
15. Semm, K: Patient preparation for endoscopic abdominal surgery. In Semm, K, ed: Operative Manual for Endoscopic Abdominal Surgery. (Translated and edited by Friedrich, ER.) Year Book Medical Publishers, Chicago, 1987, pp. 20–23.
16. Eshghi, M: Endoscopic surgery of the urinary tract, Part IV: Transitional cell carcinoma and laparoscopic surgery. Monogr Urol. 13:60–76, 1992.
17. Paz-Partlow, M: Documentation for laparoscopy. In: Berci, G; Cuschieri, A; eds: Practical Laparoscopy. London, Bailliere Tindall, 1986, pp. 19–32.
18. Clayman, RV; Kavoussi, LR: Laparoscopic procedures. Nephrectomy: Technique and results. Presented at The Society for Minimally Invasive Therapy Third International Meeting, Boston, Nov. 12, 1991.
19. Clayman, RV; Kavoussi, LR; Soper, MJ; et al: Laparoscopic nephrectomy: Initial case report. J Urol 146:278–282, 1991.
20. Gomel, V; Taylor, PJ; Yuzpe, AA; Rioux, JE: The technique of endoscopy. In: Gomel, V; Taylor, PJ; Yuzpe, AA; Rioux, JE; eds: Laparoscopy and Hysteroscopy in Gynecologic Practice. Chicago, Yearbook Medical Publishers, 1986, pp. 32–55.
21. Engel, T: Instrument maintenance and personnel training. In: Phillips, JM, ed: Laparoscopy. Baltimore, Williams & Wilkins, 1977, pp. 46–50.
22. Gregory, E; Simmons, D; Weinberg, JJ: Care and sterilization of endourologic Instruments. Urol Clin North Am 15:541–546, 1988.

CHAPTER 6

Laparoscopic Equipment and Instruments

Michael E. Moran, MD
Raul C. Ordorica, MD

No laparoscopic surgical procedure should be undertaken without a minimal working knowledge of the equipment, instruments, and their maintenance necessary to accomplish the operation without compromising safety. By design current laparoscopic instruments cannot provide the same constant performance that a surgeon expects with open instrumentation. Longer instruments with delicate mechanisms are necessary for laparoscopic surgeons. They are more difficult to clean, and corrosion is a major factor influencing the longevity of these devices. This may account to some degree for the popularity of disposable instruments in laparoscopic surgery. A disposable trocar, scissors, dissector, or grasper always has new mechanisms that will not catch or jam. The edges or points tend to be sharper, and the smaller interstices tend not to accumulate debris that can cause malfunction. Disposable instruments exact a price for these advantages, and there is no data to support any other claim of their superiority over the reusable instruments. In the long run, it becomes an issue of the surgeon's preference.

Before any specific discussion of laparoscopic instrumentation, a short digression into the theoretical characteristics of instrument design is appropriate. Laparoscopic instruments are long by necessity, the exact length required depending on the procedure being performed, the placement of the trocars, and the body habitus of the patient. Although heavy and long are not synonymous, shorter instruments tend to be lighter and create less magnification of movements, allowing better control. The ideal instrument for laparoscopic surgery should have the characteristics outlined in Table 6–1. A reticulated instrument is crucial for the fine manipulation at the distal tip with minimal exertion of the hand. This is a dominant feature on most disposable instruments but is evolving with newer reusable types. An instrument that is multifunctional has more utility than one with a single feature. During the course of laparoscopic surgery, considerable amounts of time are lost in exchanging one instrument for another. The addition of electrocautery to an instrument provides a dual function; irrigation and suction devices represent another example. Other features are always sought so that streamlined, coordinated movements are promoted. Finally, all too little attention has been given to the distal end of laparoscopic instruments. Classic, open surgical instruments have rings for stabilization during fine manipulations. The laparoscopic urologic surgeon is facing an entirely different operating environment in which the aids of the open procedure become the handicaps of the endoscopic one. Prolonged operating times, constraints of pelvic anatomy, limitations imposed by the anterior abdominal wall, and loss of mechanical advantage all increase the stress of functioning flawlessly. Stabilization of the laparoscopic instrument is a function of the working trocar. The

Table 6–1. LAPAROSCOPIC INSTRUMENT DESIGN: THEORETICAL IDEALS

Light weight
Capable of ambidextrous application
No entrapment of surgeon's fingers
Length proportional to surgery of interest
Malleable/curved
Multifunctional
Parallel profile low/stem axis tight
Long-lasting
Easy to clean and to maintain

rings that are in large measure present on most laparoscopic instruments are a hindrance to accomplishing the prolonged dissection and reconstruction that is necessary for urologic surgery. Ideally, the instrument should have a streamlined parallel axis that can be easily rotated in the surgeon's palm. Microscopic surgery has been using these principles for decades (Fig. 6–1). Mechanical assistance systems to increase the torque of these long, thin instruments would decrease the fatigue of the surgeon's hand. Now available are the beginnings of instruments designed for prolonged laparoscopic procedures in order to enhance, not hinder, the technical ability of the surgeon.

Laparoscopic urologic surgery is challenging even to experienced endoscopic surgeons. The constraints of operating in a closed environment with electronically mediated imaging has both advantages and disadvantages (Table 6–2). The major disadvantage lies in the surgeons' lack of acquaintance with the new equipment and techniques. As with any new operative technique there rightly exists some degree of skepticism.[1] Any new operative approach should be able to demonstrate substantial patient advantages before being considered standard practice. To this end there exists no urologic laparoscopic surgery, localization of the undescended testicle included, that meets this

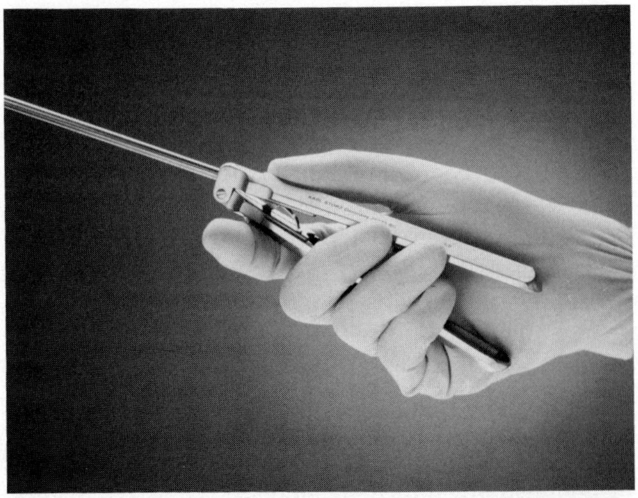

Figure 6–1. Idealized finger-tip controlled laparoscopic instrument.

Table 6–2. ADVANTAGES AND DISADVANTAGES OF ELECTRONIC IMAGING IN THE CLOSED LAPAROSCOPIC ENVIRONMENT

Advantages
Magnification (precision)
Electronic processing (education, documentation, teaching, patient interest)
Less physical straining
Disadvantages
New technology
Volume of technology
Magnification (clumsiness)
Lack of urology-specific instrumentation
Illumination
Mobility
Retraction

standard. Other disadvantages are also readily apparent: the genitourinary organs of interest are not easily accessed by laparoscopy. The overwhelming amount of technology necessary for laparoscopy may be perceived as a disadvantage. It is extremely difficult to keep abreast of all the new technology. This fosters the uneasiness felt by the clinician struggling to assess the role that laparoscopic surgery will play in the everyday practice of urology. Laparoscopic urologic surgery is complex, and the reliance on electronic video imaging is total.[2] Maneuvering instruments by electronic video control is a further skill that urologists have to master.[3] The electronic image is magnified. For neophytes, this produces an uncomfortable experience of disorientation, incoordination, and clumsiness. By careful and patient practice, by moving slowly and gradually into more and more difficult skills, the ability to perform complex tasks can be acquired. Instrumentation specific for laparoscopic urologic surgery is nonexistent. This represents the major disadvantage of laparoscopic urologic surgery. There is hope that manufacturers are becoming increasingly responsive to our clinical needs. Finally, there are the disadvantages inherent in operating in a closed environment. This should not foster the same degree of uneasiness in a urologist as it might in a general surgeon, because urologists have been removing organs endoscopically for more than 50 years.

There are clear advantages to laparoscopic urologic surgery. First and foremost is patient demand. When presented with a whole list of potential risks and no large clinical study documenting long-term followup, patients in increasing numbers are willing to sign informed consent for this type of surgery. There is credence to the statement that the suffering of the patient who has undergone an open operation directly parallels the suffering of the surgeon who is performing the laparoscopic equivalent. On closer inspection, however, the disadvantages may actually be advantages if we are trying to improve the way the surgery is performed. The magnification inherent in the laparoscope and electronic imaging equipment produces magnified visual images that reveal anatomic nuances not appreciated in open surgery without the use of a loupe. The electronic equipment is increasingly sophisticated. Digitalization of all electronic systems is certain to result in complete integration of every imaginable data acquisition device—ultrasound, infrared, ultraviolet, fluoroscopic, and so forth—to produce simultaneous imaging. Documentation of complex cases is already part of most video chains with laparoscopic systems. The patient is curious about the operation and now can receive photographs of the surgery. Resident and medical student education is enhanced by being able to observe these types of surgeries. Surgeons can review the recorded surgeries in order to learn from mistakes and to develop better methods of accomplishing the same result.

It is difficult to cover the breadth of technology available to the urologist for performing laparoscopic surgery.[4,5] The authors have elected to introduce this technology by dividing all the devices necessary to accomplish laparoscopic surgery into groups. Initially, the equipment necessary to establish and maintain the working environment for laparoscopic surgery is presented, next the instruments necessary to perform urologic laparoscopic surgery are covered. In this section, a large number of devices are described, and their urologic implications are discussed. The next chapter (Chap. 7) discusses operating room setup and patient positioning for urologic laparoscopic surgery.

LAPAROSCOPIC EQUIPMENT

Laparoscopes

The laparoscope is the fundamental instrument necessary to be able to visualize the abdominal viscera to perform this type of surgery. Rod-lens systems have been the primary optics of choice in the present era of laparoscopy.[6] The rod-lens systems is encased within a rigid endoscope that is passed into the body to guide the surgeon. The portal for entry must bridge the body and by its position, provide the correct orientation and allow zoom or panoramic viewing. Optical engineering has produced endoscopes with magnitudes of image superiority over what was available just one decade previously.[7,8] The compensating lens is such an endoscope (Fig. 6–2). By computer-enhanced interaction of the lenses, the problems of central clarity at the expense of peripheral image have been compensated. The result is an endoscope with a greater range of visual clarity.

Rigid laparoscopes are available in a variety of diameters, 2.7 to 12.0 mm (Fig. 6–3). The 10-mm endoscope is the workhorse for most clinical urologic laparoscopy because of the degree of illumination possible. The 10-mm laparoscope is similar in construction to the standard cystoscope. One feature available on some 10-mm laparoscopes is a detachable eyepiece interface (Fig. 6–4). This source of unintentional light loss can be removed, permitting direct coupling of the electronic camera to the endoscope. Some laparoscopes come with fixed endoscopic camera couplers (Fig. 6–5). The major advantage of the fixed systems is that no focusing is required, and the need for connection and disconnection is eliminated. The major drawback of these systems is that any problem with either the camera or the endoscope results in a lack of function of both. Scopes with removable eyepieces and direct coupling mechanisms maximize the current advantages and minimize the disadvantages.

Of the scopes available in other sizes, the largest is the operating laparoscope, which has a working channel through the endoscope similar to that of a nephroscope. This scope has substantial utility if the surgeon is trying to minimize the number of trocars needed for a given laparoscopic operation (Fig. 6–6). The major advantage of a working laparoscope is the addition of multifunctional capacity through a given portal, increasing the amount of work possible through a fixed area of access. The major drawback is that more space

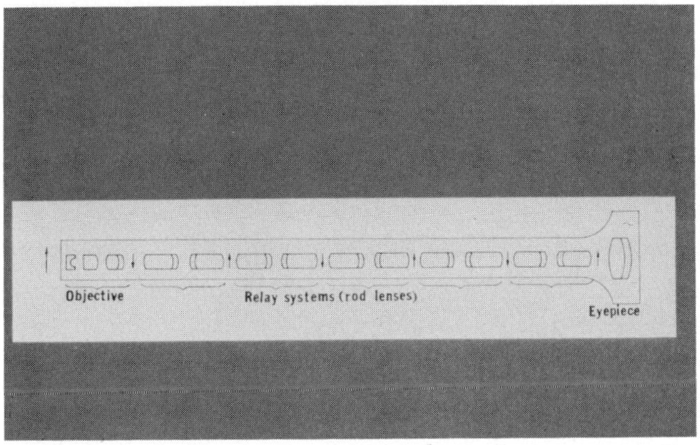

Figure 6–2. Cut-away view of the Olympus rod-lens system (compensating lens).

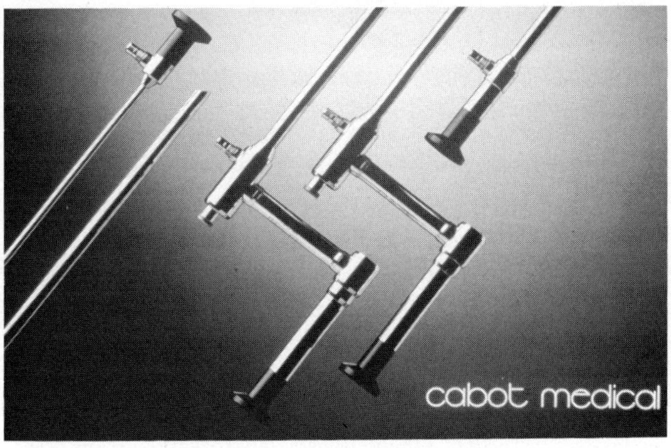

Figure 6–3. Variously sized and configured rigid laparoscopes.

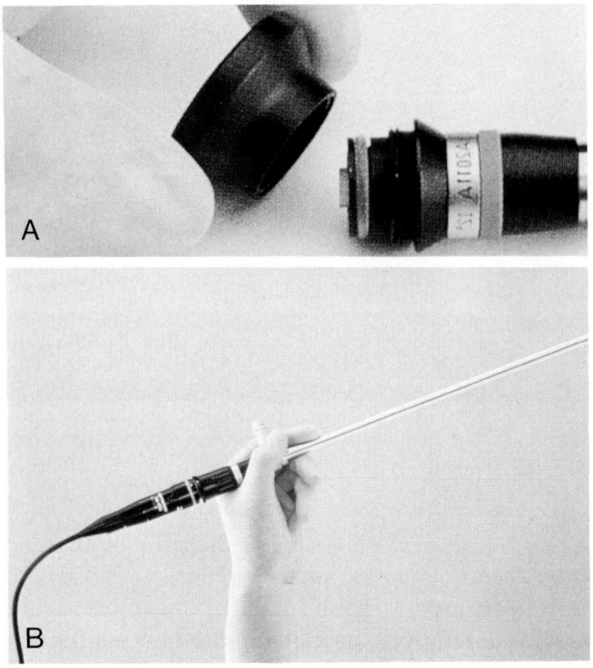

Figure 6–4. Detachable eye piece system for direct coupling of laparoscope to video camera. *A*, Detachable eye piece and *B*, direct coupling. (Courtesy of Olympus Corp.)

is taken up by instrumentation and less is available for light delivery and optics. Smaller laparoscopes are available as 8-mm, 7-mm, 5-mm, and 2.7-mm rigid rod-lens systems. The smaller the size, the worse the image. The smaller endoscopes have not become popular for complex endoscopic surgery. Angle of view is another consideration in selecting a laparoscope. A wide range of choice is available, depending on the size of the scope. Most complex laparoscopic urologic surgery should be done with an angled endoscope because of the broader field of view. Smaller movements of the imaging system are necessary to observe the operative

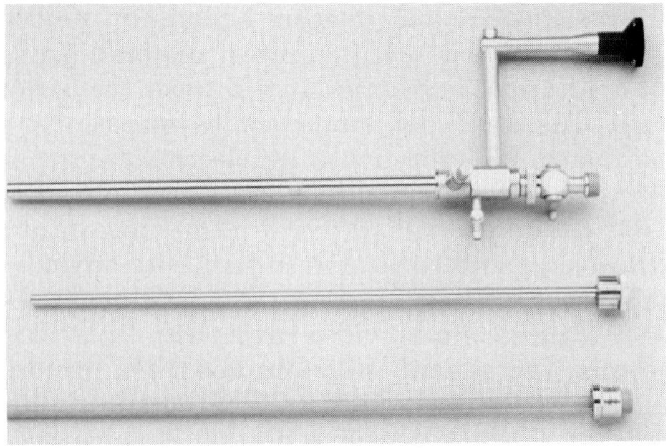

Figure 6–6. Operative laparoscope.

field. Finally, there are laparoscopes that have built-in self-cleaning and defog lens systems (Fig. 6–7).

Flexible laparoscopes are also available. Included in this category are some unique scopes that incorporate features of both the more typical rigid shaft along with the fiberoptics and flexible tip of a purely flexible endoscope (Fig. 6–8). The flexible laparoscope has the inherent advantage that it is steerable. Whereas the abdominal contents are largely a hindrance for the performance of urologic surgery by the transabdominal route, the flexible scopes allow the image to wrap around barriers to the target area of dissection. Although the image quality from fiberoptic scopes is not as good as rod-lens systems, it has significantly improved over the last 5 years.

Electronic Chain

The surgeon's ability to coordinate his or her efforts with those of the assistant and support people in the operating room is enhanced by incorporating advanced electronic image processing.[9,10,11] The founda-

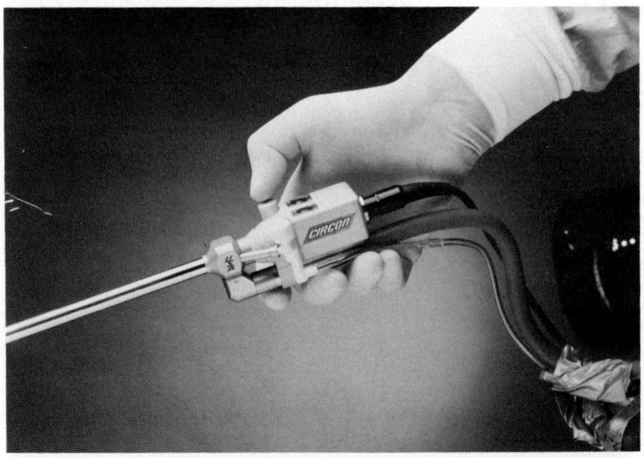

Figure 6–5. Digital video Hydro laparoscope. (Courtesy of Circon/ACMI.)

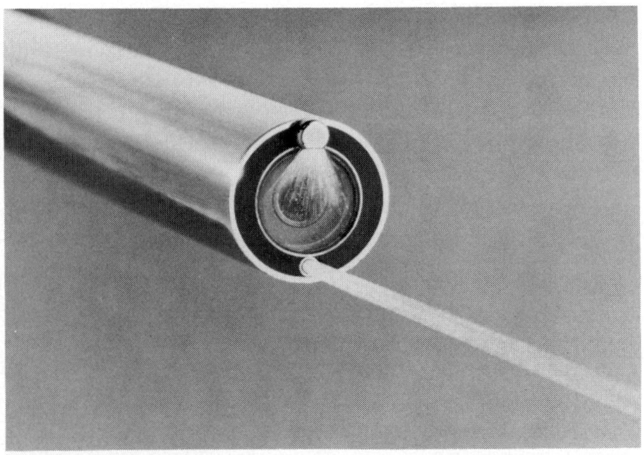

Figure 6–7. Hydro laparoscope tip with fluid actuation for in situ lens cleaning. Multipurpose system includes a lens warming system and the ability to irrigate in front of the lens. (Courtesy of Circon/ACMI.)

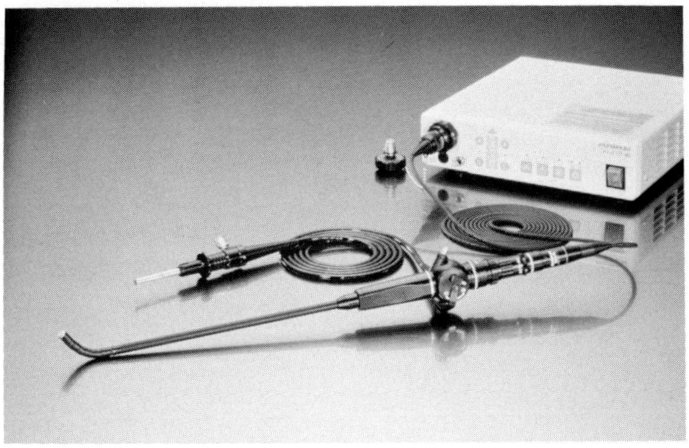

Figure 6–8. Semiflexible fiberoptic laparoscope. (Courtesy of Olympus Corp.)

Table 6–3. COMPONENTS OF THE ELECTRONIC IMAGING CHAIN

Basic*
High-intensity light source
Video camera (>400 lines)
Video monitor
Custom†
Auto-iris features, multiscope capable, flash RGB, 3-chip, 3-dimensional
High-resolution, HDTV
VCR (SVHS), professional editing
Video printer
Disc recorder
Video mixer
Video/audio editors

*Considered essential for basic laparoscopic surgery.
†Additions that improve image quality and performance—HDTV, high-definition television; RGB, red, green, blue; SVHS, super-VHS.

tion of image production and visualization is a small electronic chip called the charged coupling device, or CCD chip (Fig. 6–9). The ability to access and process an image is being replaced by electronics.[12] Every piece of data can be converted from analog (real-time image) to digital (electronic signals) that reproduce images to an extremely accurate degree. The ability to observe outside the human spectrum of sight can be incorporated into the image systems. Since the signals are electronically mediated, they can be processed by a wide range of output devices such as recorders and printers and can be integrated with other image systems (ultrasound, infrared [IR], ultraviolet [UV], and the like).[13]

To understand the electronic imaging system, it is crucial to be conversant with the basics of the electronic chain (Table 6–3), which is a group of electronic processors that accomplish a given task. For laparoscopic surgery, the standard features of the electronic chain include the video camera (CCD), the light source (often incorporated with auto-iris features), camera processor, and the output devices (video monitor[s], video recorders [VHS and S-VHS], video printers, digital storage devices, personal computers, and so forth).

The most expensive of the elements is usually the CCD video camera. Endoscopic cameras can have many features that the surgeon may find useful. First and foremost, the CCD chip itself should have resolution that exceeds 400 lines. The chip should be red, green, and blue (RGB)-capable. Other features can include direct-coupling mechanisms for attachment to the endoscope instead of an ocular lens. By adding two additional chips, each designated for one basic color, improved imaging in the red range is possible. By angling the CCD chip, the image can be perceived in 3-dimensions with special prismatic lenses. The electronic chip does not have to be limited to the visual spectrum. Imaging of UV and IR wavelengths are possible. The zoom feature of some endoscopic camera systems is helpful when electronic transition is needed from panorama to closeup. The zoom button can be accessible either on the camera (Fig. 6–10) or by remote control.

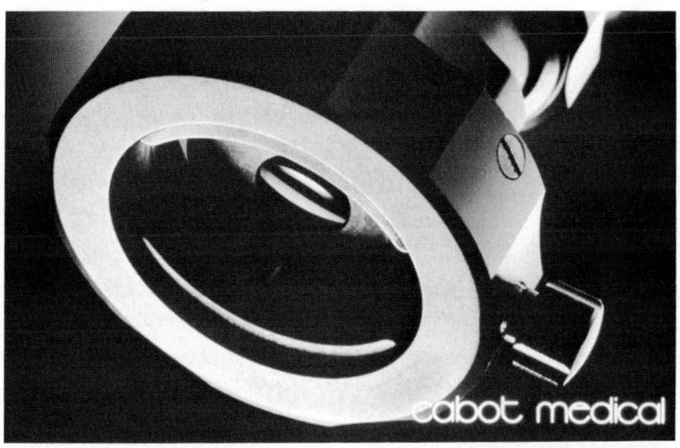

Figure 6–9. Close-up view of video camera system whose function is related to the microprocessor charged coupling device (CCD).

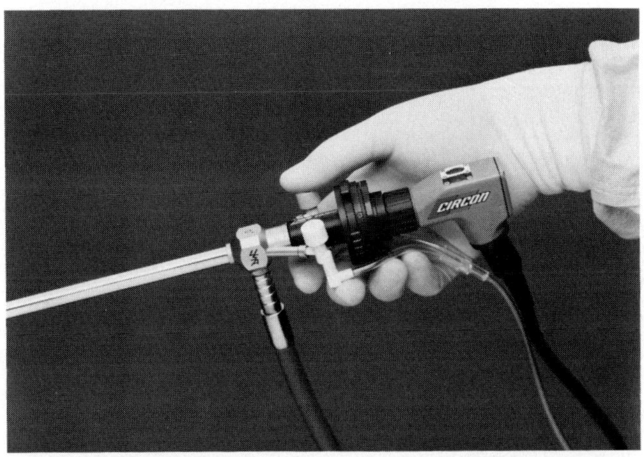

Figure 6–10. Zoom features on some video cameras may be directly on the camera, as demonstrated here, or may be remotely controlled. (Courtesy of Circon/ACMI.)

Light sources have substantially changed in the past decade. Halide element light sources produce much more light than the old tungsten units.[2] The ability to superheat this inert element results in light with less color distortion for the illumination through endoscopes.[6] Light sources are also available with multifunctional capacity, including insufflation and electrocautery. In addition, each light source should be able to integrate with available light cables and endoscopes. Most manufacturers have ancillary adapters for coupling to various endoscopes. Liquid light cables have the potential to provide as much as 20% more light than can be standard in fiberoptic cables.[2] Liquid cables tend to be heavier and less flexible. Illuminated fiberoptic cables have now been introduced. The ability to see the cable in darkened, ambient room lighting during these procedures can be a consideration (Fig. 6–11). The auto-iris feature is an electronic feedback circuit that enables the rapid automatic adjustment of light intensity, depending on the image being viewed. Since the intensity of light is inversely proportional to the distance from the laparoscope tip, camera motion can create marked fluctuations in image illumination. Whereas visceral structures reflect a large amount of light and diminish the need for high intensity output, bleeding demands greater intensity because of the light absorbed by the hemoglobin pigments. Finally, light systems that can adapt to many different types of endoscopes and provide flash capability for 35-mm cameras allow considerable flexibility. During a given laparoscopic procedure, switching from a rigid to a flexible instrument may be necessary, and the light source should be adaptable (Fig. 6–12).

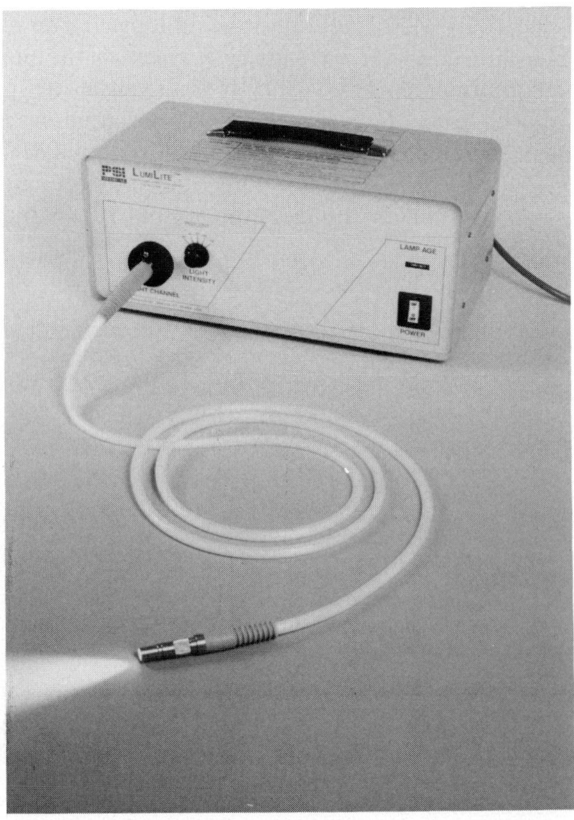

Figure 6–11. A luminescent light fiber bundle system.

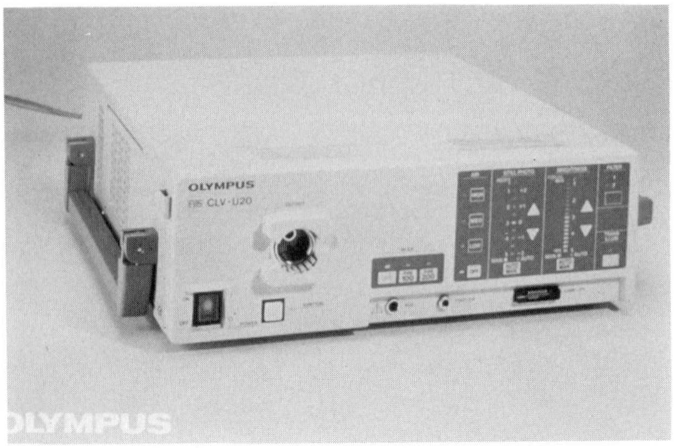

Figure 6–12. Multiscope light source with instant capability for video source utility or flash photography. It can switch from a fiberoptic to a rod-lens system. (Courtesy of Olympus Corp.)

Output devices are the most user-specific equipment necessary for urologic laparoscopy. These electronic converters can either produce an image or store and modify the image. Most systems use the analog (real-time image) from the endscopic video camera. There are increasing numbers of devices that can convert the national standard broadcast pattern (NTSC) to a digital image.[11] The most common output methods used for laparoscopic surgery include color monitors, video recorders, and thermal color printers. These devices allow the surgeon to visualize the endoscopic image larger than life without straining to see through the endoscope. Video monitors have a wide range of sizes with varied resolution. Larger color monitors are not necessarily better if resolution is sacrificed. Monitors range in size from 13 inches (measured diagonally) through 26 inches. Medical quality video monitors have industrial power cords and safety features not available on commercial televisions. A resolution of more than 400 lines should be available. High-definition television (HDTV) is the digital version of analog image processing (Fig. 6–13). Video recorders come in an exceptionally wide range of capability. Low-end recorders can capture the video signal on video tape for routine documentation. High-end super-VHS recorders (S-VHS) require special video tapes, and the image is not converted for replay by standard video recorders. The image is only about 10% better with these recording systems, and their primary advantage is when further video editing is required. Editing features can be added to the video recorder, increasing the utility and capability of these

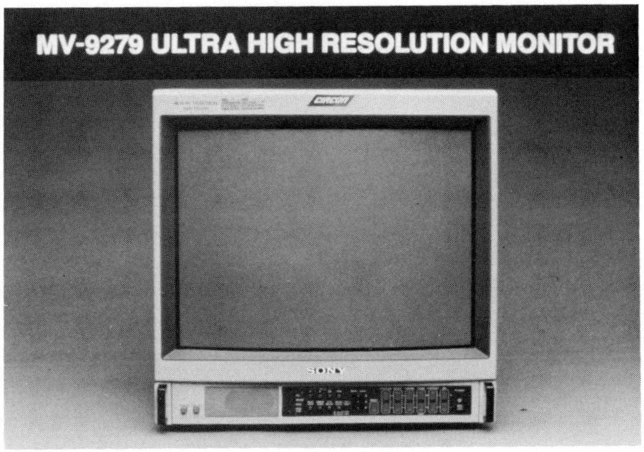

Figure 6-13. The first of several high-resolution television monitors for endoscopic surgical purposes. (Courtesy of Circon/ACMI.)

image-processing devices. A thermal color printer can be integrated into the electronic chain for the production of instant photographic documentation (Fig. 6-14).

Other electronic features can be added to the electronic chain to modify the image or add processing features. Fluoroscopic and ultrasound images are electronically processed to video monitors.[13] These images can be captured and manipulated for view on the same monitor by adding a video mixer to the chain (Fig. 6-15). Dual image camera systems can be obtained for similar purpose (Fig. 6-16). Disc recording devices produce a digital image that can be stored on computer disks. These have been advertised to produce images of the quality of still photographs and can be rapidly transferred for personal computer editing.

Finally, before leaving this section on electronic imaging equipment, mention should be made of video carts. Almost every endoscopy manufacturer has one, and they all have similar features (Fig. 6-17). Features that are desirable include a transparent, locking front door, adjustable shelves, vented rears with cable organizers, rustproof material, a solution and irrigant pole, extra storage capacity, and an adjustable monitor tray. There are distinct advantages to having all this

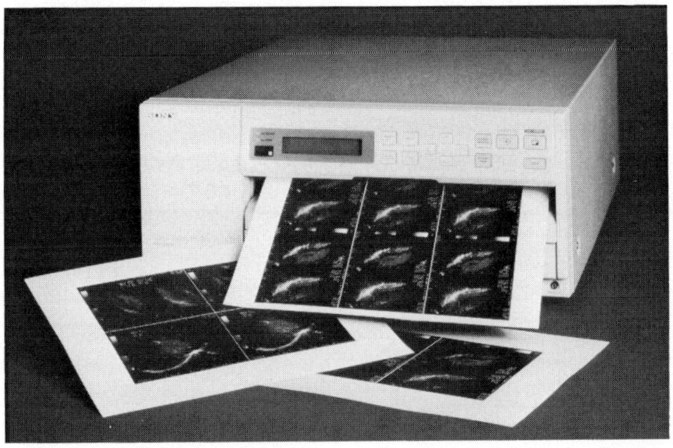

Figure 6-14. A high-resolution video printer capable of printing color, B & W and transparencies. (Courtesy of Sony.)

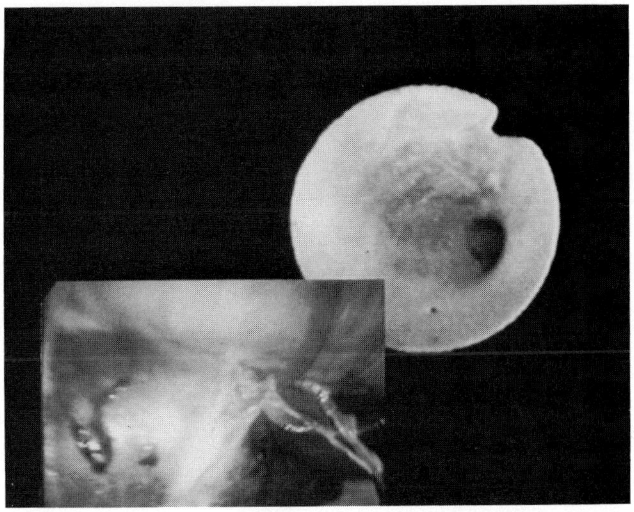

Figure 6-15. Image-on-image from the addition of a video mixer to the imaging chain.

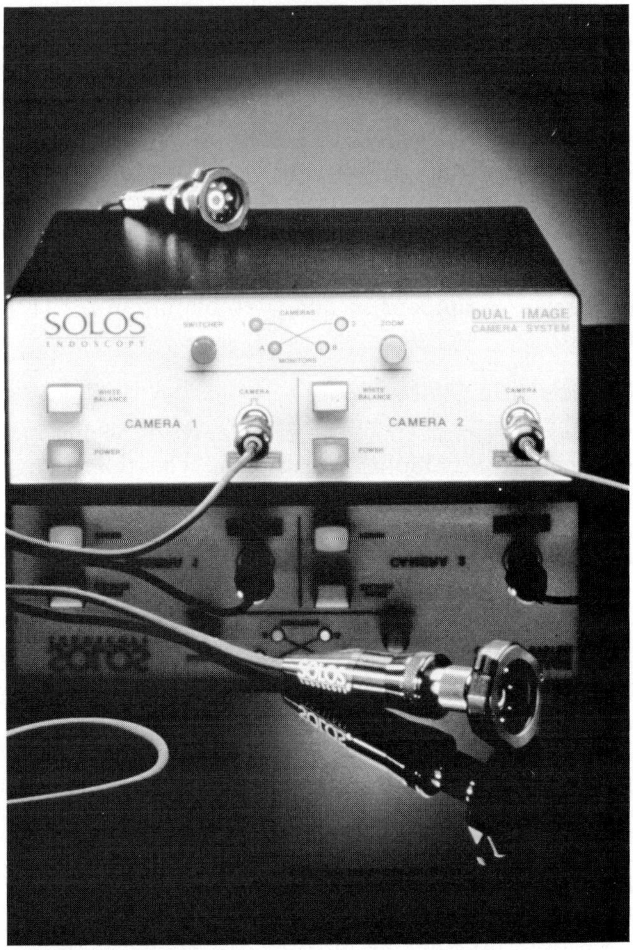

Figure 6-16. Dual-image camera system. (Courtesy of SOLOS.)

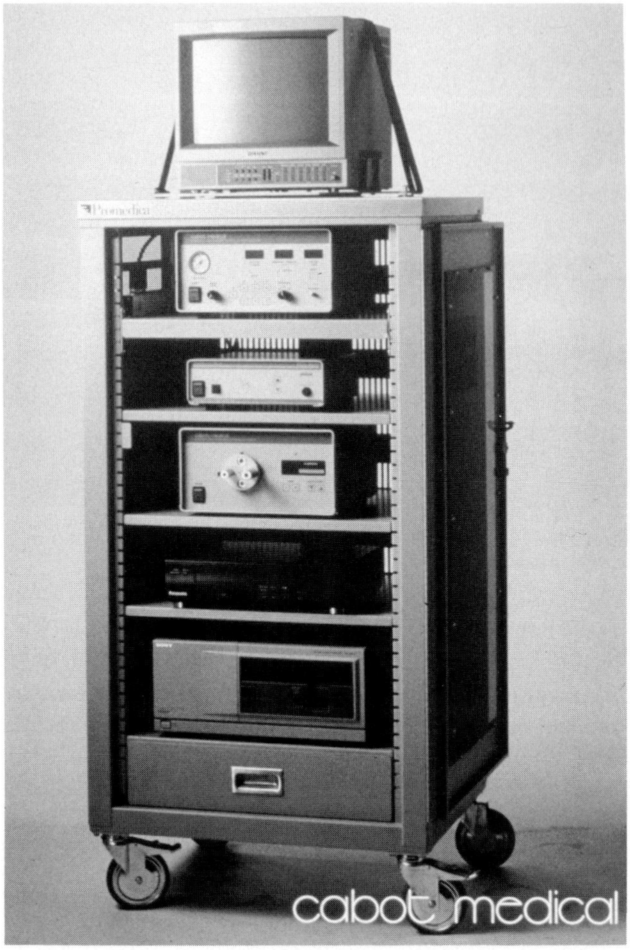

Figure 6–17. A standard configuration video cart system demonstrating the "stacked" organization of endosurgical hardware.

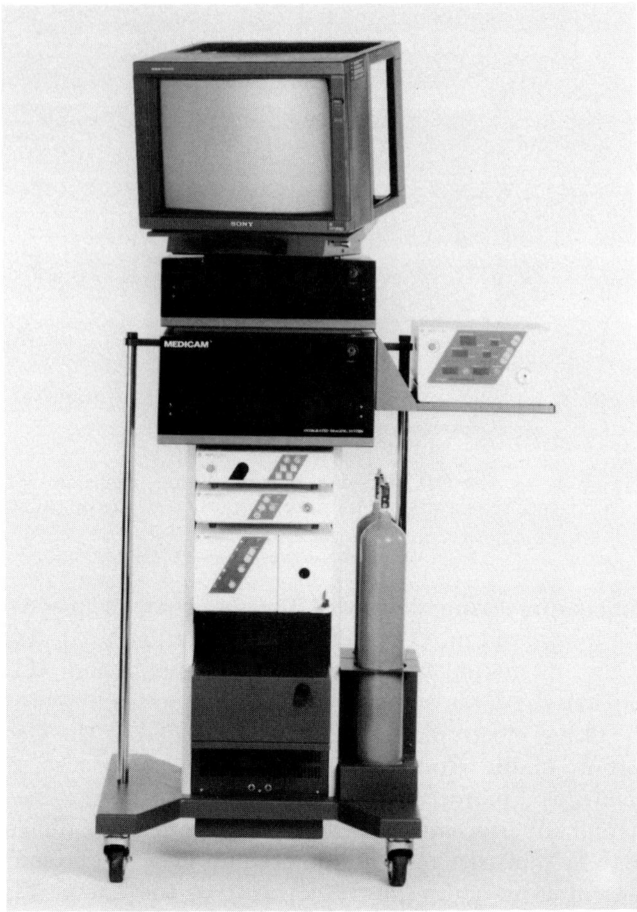

Figure 6–18. A contemporary design to achieve a streamlined yet practical solution. (Courtesy of MP Video.)

expensive equipment in one portable organizer (Fig. 6–18).

Hemostatic Systems

The laparoscopist should be familiar with the methods available to accomplish hemostasis. The closed environment of laparoscopy makes special demands on equipment that the open surgeon may take for granted because of the degree of control and clear visualization with an open abdomen. Contiguous structures and viscera can potentially be injured by electrocautery instruments and lasers with devastating consequences. The equipment necessary for achieving this purpose are available in everincreasing numbers and complexity. Table 6–4 lists methods that have been used for laparoscopic hemostasis. Radio-frequency monopolar electrocautery has been the standard method of controlling hemorrhage during laparoscopic urologic surgery. Modern solid state systems may achieve voltages as high as the older spark-gap systems, but wattage indicators are capable of providing feedback data to the surgeon so as to avoid dangers of high-voltage electrical injury. The higher the peak-to-peak voltage, the greater the chance of capacitive discharge and inadvertent injuries.[14] Electrosurgical generators operate between 500 kHz and 3 MHz. The frequency output can also affect current leakage, especially when associated with the high frequencies. Finally, impedance must be considered. The trocars themselves can potentiate the chance for thermal injury. Because the trocars are remote to the area of attention, the laparoscopic field, these injuries can easily go unnoticed.

Table 6–4. METHODS OF HEMOSTASIS AVAILABLE FOR LAPAROSCOPIC SURGERY

Pressure (clamp, probe, Kitner)
Ligature/suture
Clip/stapler
Thermal
Electrical (monopolar, bipolar, argon beam coagulator)
Laser
Microwave
Cryoprobes
Chemical
Systemic
Topical

The FDA has recommended that nonconductive trocars (most disposable) not be used if they are more than 7 mm.[15] That is because the nonconducting trocars and fascial screws insulate the cannulas and prevent dispersion of current that would normally occur through these portals to the abdominal wall and skin. Conduction through the instruments can thus produce inadvertent visceral injury. Granted that the FDA guidelines were prompted by injuries occurring primarily with surgery through a solitary portal, the physics still apply. Devices are available that are meant to solve the problems of inadvertent electrical current discharge. The Electroshield (Fig. 6–19) is a 7-mm shield that slides over 5-mm instruments and deactivates the cautery should a fault be detected. Specific concerns of monopolar electrocautery have been the degree of tissue necrosis caused by the discharge from these units and the unintended possibility for conduction and thermal injury to contiguous areas (insulation failure, direct coupling or capacitative). It is for these reasons that the Bureau of Devices of the FDA published standards for the safe utilization of electrocautery during laparoscopy.[16] Despite well-publicized concerns for electrothermal safety, large series of laparoscopic biliary surgical procedures have demonstrated little significant injury from this power source.[17]

Bipolar electrocautery systems are available, but the clinician should be aware that untoward injuries with these have also been reported. Bipolar instruments do not have the wide variety and multipurpose capability now available with monopolar instruments (Fig. 6–20).

There are those who have a preference for lasers.[18] Comparative studies are scarce, but no advantage has been documented for laser energy compared with monopolar electrocautery.[16] There are increasing concerns for the unskilled use of hemostatic laser energy secondary to unrecognized deep tissue necrosis possible from this modality. Microwave, cryoprobes, argon-beam coagulators, and chemical systems have all been infrequently used according to the urologic literature to date, but each has the potential for particular urologic surgical scenarios.

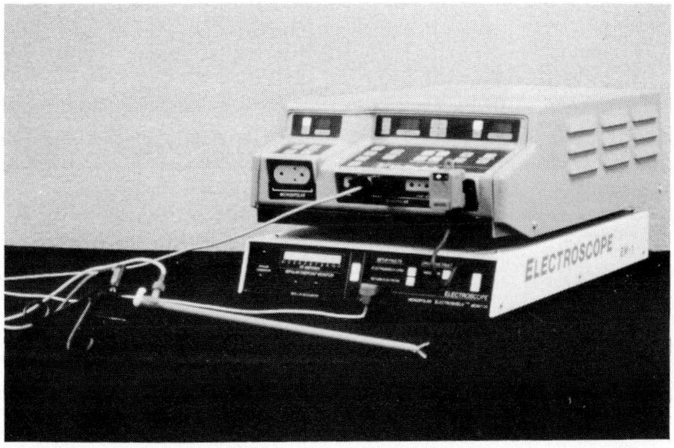

Figure 6–19. The Electroshield and monitor for utilization of controlled cautery.

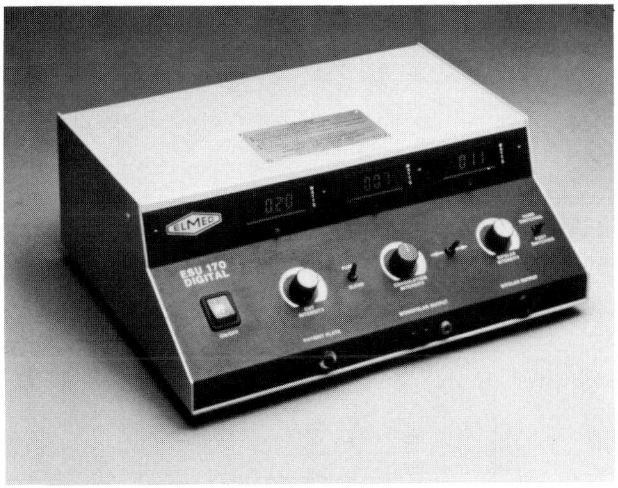

Figure 6–20. A digital radio-frequency electrocautery unit with both monopolar and bipolar capability.

Argon-beam coagulators (ABC) have been available for open surgery for several years.[19] The clinical utility to urologists for partial nephrectomy, radical prostatectomy, retroperitoneal lymphadenectomy, and cystectomy is also known. Low-flow units are approved for clinical laparoscopic use, but lack the power that a urologist is familiar with during open procedures. The ABC has specific utility for laparoscopic surgeons. The argon gas flow blows blood from the surface of the targeted area or organ, allowing the plasma to cauterize the region effectively. High-flow systems run the risk of producing tension pneumoperitoneum or pneumomediastinum. This risk can be overcome by cautious use and continuous venting while the system is being activated. The probes lacked the capacity for multifunctional use until recently. Currently, multipurpose probes are being investigated (Fig. 6–21). The most common combination is such a probe with a cautery electrode, thus combining the major advantages of both thermal energy sources. The ABC has other inherent advantages for the laparoscopic urologist. Complex laparoscopic bladder or bladder neck surgery requires the careful identification of tissue planes and mucosa for reconstruction. The limited depth of penetration with little tissue charring combined with the ability to achieve hemostasis make it an ideal tool for use in the lower urinary tract.

Chemical agents also have a definite capacity to augment hemostasis in the restricted environment of laparoscopy.[20] Microfibrillar collagen has this inherent property, based on its helical molecular structure of hemostatic activation. Its hydrophilic nature (stickiness), although a potential drawback, could be an

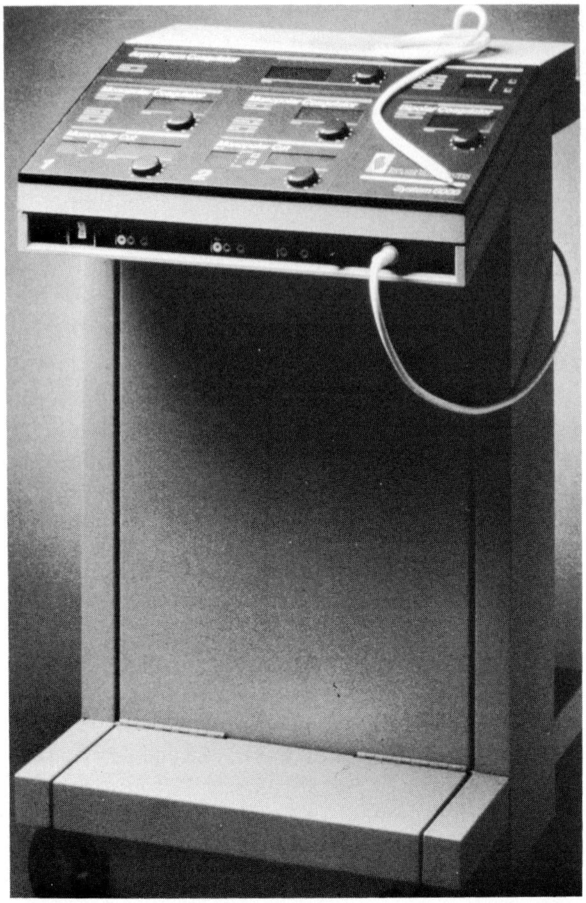

Figure 6–21. The argon beam coagulation unit with conventional electrocautery capacity. (Courtesy of Birtcher Medical.)

advantage if it could be delivered to the site without being handled unnecessarily. Endo-AviteneR is an endoscopic applicator for supplying collagen to the active bleeding site without the necessity to handle the fluff (Fig. 6–22). Studies with laparoscopic controlled tissue removal systems have documented the efficacy of Endo-AviteneR compared with pressure to stop significant hemorrhage within the liver of the pig.

Fibrin glue is another agent capable of endoscopic delivery.[21–23] There are potential risks of applying this material under pressure during laparoscopy, specifically thromboembolic events. Fibrin glue is formed from a combination of a solution of concentrated fibrinogen and Factor XIII with a solution of bovine thrombin and calcium. It may be applied topically or by atomized spray. An endoscopic delivery system is available (Fig. 6–23).

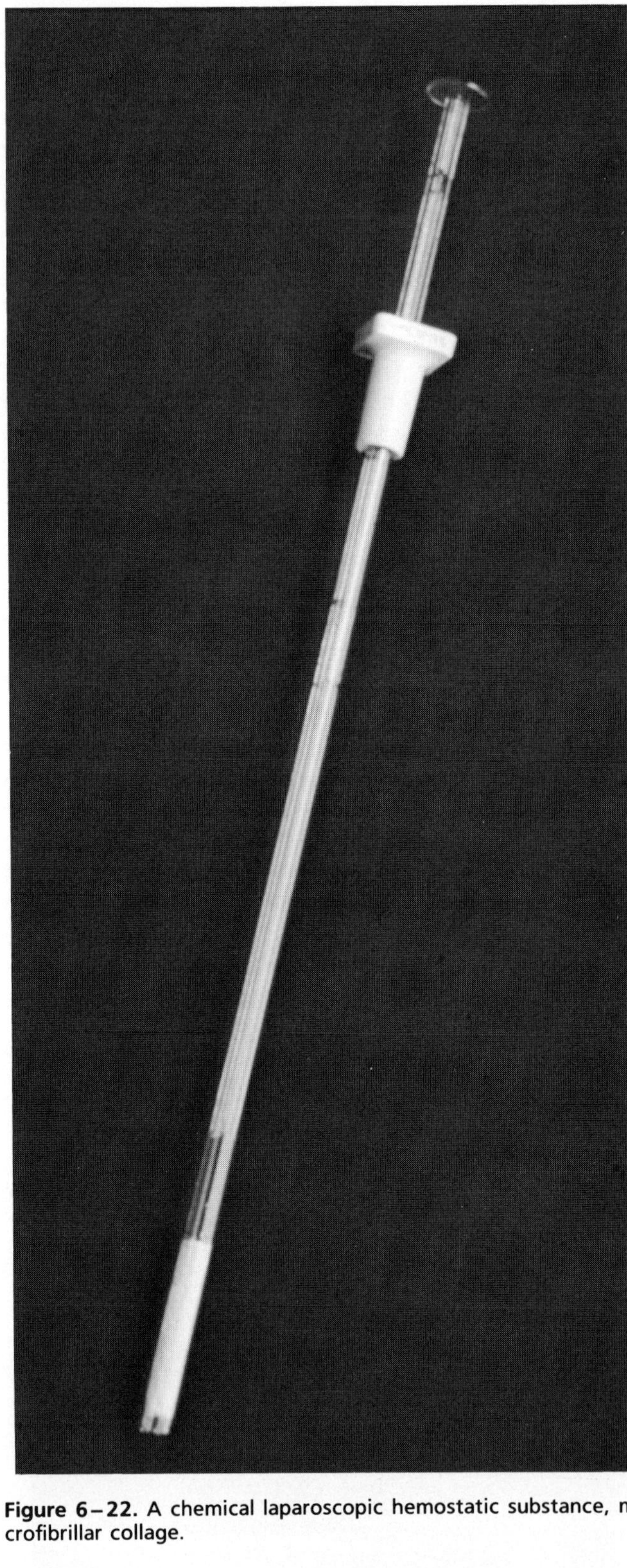

Figure 6–22. A chemical laparoscopic hemostatic substance, microfibrillar collage.

Insufflators

Once intraperitoneal access has been obtained by Verres needle insertion or open Hasson cannula placement, the next step is to insufflate the abdomen with a nontoxic gas. Understanding of the equipment designed to facilitate and monitor insufflation is necessary for the safe performance of operative laparoscopy. Systems now exist that provide immediate feedback of intra-abdominal pressure, the amount of gas in the cylinder, and the flow rate. The ability of

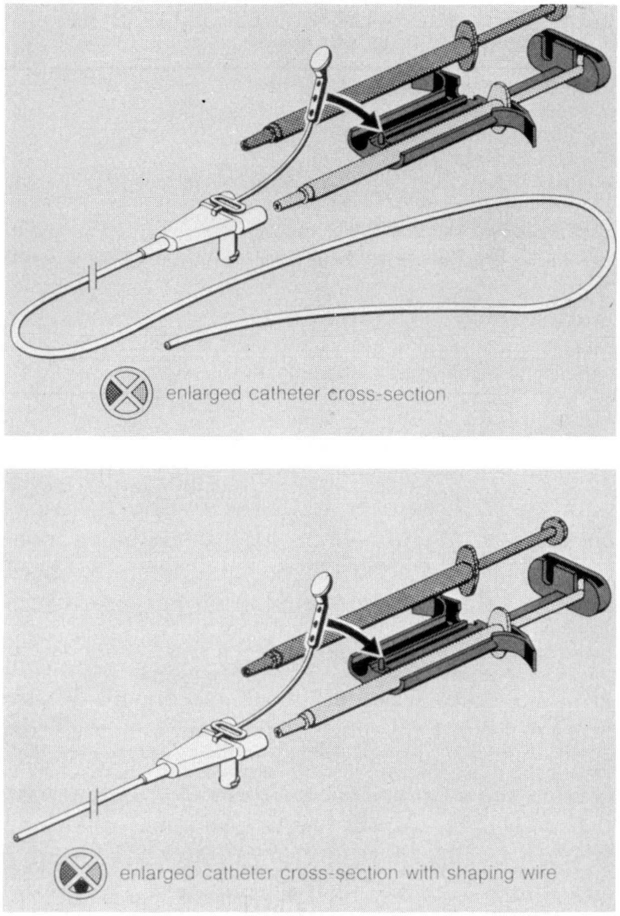

Figure 6–23. Topical fibrin glue spray gun for laparoscopic application.

the insufflator to output large volumes of insufflant is one of the major differences among the many available systems (Fig. 6–24). The manufacturers provide brochures on the safe performance of each device with scheduled performance checks. High-flow insufflators are more likely to be available if the system is being used jointly with the general surgeons. High-flow insufflation is necessary during complex surgical procedures. Longer, more difficult dissections require irrigation and aspiration instruments that will nonspecifically aspirate the insufflant unless the tips are carefully positioned below fluid levels. High-flow systems that achieve maximal flows above 6 L/minute are available. Increasingly, systems are available that deliver flows in excess of 10 L/minute.

The insufflator must display accurate, quick digital feedback of the internal pressures. The ability to confuse parameters can be minimized by the addition of simple graphic overlays available on some systems. The insufflation tubing can fill with irrigant fluid and blackflow into the insufflator, which results in destruction of the pressure and flow sensors in these electronic devices. It is recommended always to keep the insufflator above the patient in order to avoid this costly error. Fortunately, most video carts provide space for the insufflator at the higher levels within the "stack."

Laparoscopic surgery imposes many constraints on operating and maintaining visualization when irrigant aspiration must be used or vapor plumes from hemostatic systems are present. In order to overcome these problems and minimize the amount of pneumoperitoneal pressures needed and thereby decreasing the irritative exposure to CO_2 with the resultant respiratory and metabolic consequences, innovative investigators have begun performing gasless or minimal insufflant laparoscopy.[24–26] In order to achieve visualized distention of the abdomen, a variety of retraction systems have been developed to pull the anterior abdominal wall away from the parietes. First used by Mouret,[24] these abdominal wall suspension systems have many features in common. A perforating instrument is used to hook the anterior abdominal wall. In addition there is some mainframe retraction system that will attach to the "lift" (Fig. 6–25). The exact role these devices will serve in continuing develop-

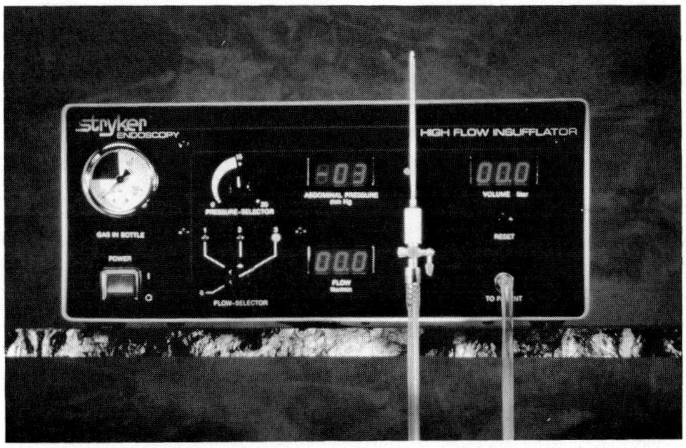

Figure 6–24. High-flow laparoscopic pneumoinsufflation device.

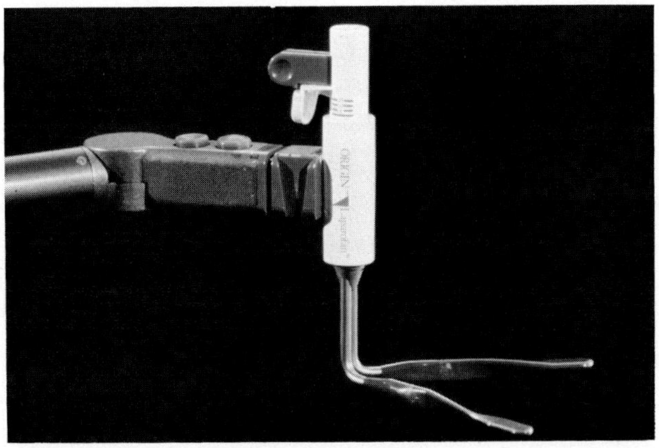

Figure 6–25. Abdominal wall–lifting system for gasless laparoscopy.

ment of laparoscopic urologic surgery remain to be seen, yet they offer expanded utility in the restricted endoscopic environment.

LAPAROSCOPIC INSTRUMENTS

Pneumoperitoneum Needles

Needle access and successful insufflation is the first hurdle in performing laparoscopic urologic surgery.[27] A variety of access needles have been described in the past for specialty applications and for use in pediatric laparoscopy.[28] The standard access needle in most surgeons' hands remains the Verres-type. The Verres needle is large (14-gauge) with an inner core, spring-loaded, blunt stylet. During blind passage through the anterior abdominal wall, this blunt stylet retracts to allow the outer sharp needle portion to cut through the fascia, muscles, and areolar tissue.[29]

The major determinant in choosing an access needle is the size of the patient, since various lengths are available (100, 120, and 150 cm). Another choice is whether to purchase reusable or disposable needles. Reusable laparoscopic needles amortize their costs over many procedures. However, advantages for disposable needles include an always sharp outer cutting edge, smoothly functioning spring safety stylet, no risk of weakening or breaking from repeated usage at the weakest spot (insufflation eyehole), lack of maintenance costs, and availability of various manufacturers innovations (Fig. 6–26).

Laparoscopic Portals (Trocars and Cannulas)

The trocar and cannula unit is the essential instrument through which laparoscopic urologic surgery is performed. These portals may be reusable or disposable and are made of a variety of materials. They are also available in differing lengths and diameters and can have ancillary features. Laparoscopic portals to date have had a limited functional requirement—i.e.,

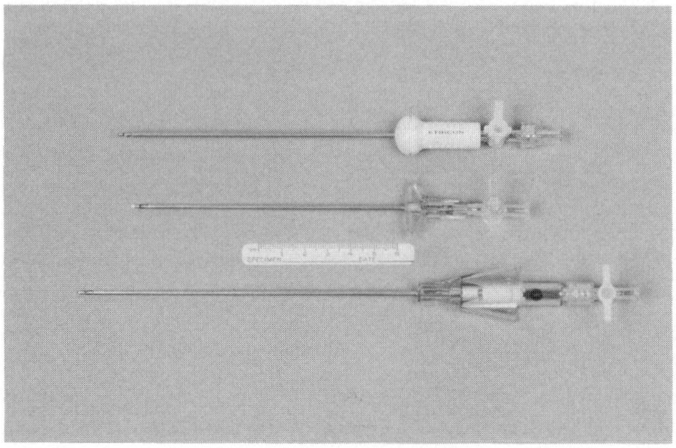

Figure 6–26. Various manufacturers' configuration of the Verres needle.

Table 6–5. CHARACTERISTICS OF THE IDEAL ACCESS PORTAL

Safe and expeditious insertion
Self-retaining
Low intra-abdominal profile
Low extra-abdominal profile
Capable of accepting a wide range of instruments without adapters (one-handed)
Access activated by tip of instrument
Maintenance of internal environment without spraying during access
Radiolucent material
Multifunctional
Flexible
Electrically safe for viscera, abdominal wall, and surgeon

to provide a pathway for performing intra-abdominal tasks. Environmental constraints should allow more flexibility of these portals in the future. Instead of rigid instruments, pliable prototypes are being investigated.[30] Multifunctional portals are also being sought to aid in retraction and other purposes (Table 6–5).[2]

The trocar is usually the inner, sharp, removable stylet that allows percutaneous placement. Hasson trocars are blunt for placement through a small incision, or celiotomy.[31] The major advantage of Hasson trocars is the avoidance of inadvertent, blind injury to blood vessels or viscera before pneumoinsufflation.[32] They can be placed away from previous incisions to avoid injury to areas with scarification and visceral adhesions.[29,33] Primary drawbacks are few, but some state that they delay entrance and increase the risk of gaseous leak (around the trocars), however, this has not been convincingly demonstrated. Detractors also state that more dissection is required with increased risks for patient discomfort, wound infection, and portal-site hernias. These also have not been demonstrated by groups routinely using open placement techniques.[34]

Sharp trocars can be conical, pyramidal, or needle-like to allow tissue penetrance (Fig. 6–27). The decision of which trocar type to use eventually becomes the surgeon's preference from experience and familiarity. Disposable trocars offer the added safety feature of automatic shielded covering of the cutting tip.[35] Some manufactures claim that by "floating" their trocar's cutting tip, stellate punctures are produced that are less traumatic to tissues. Safety shields vary from manufacturer to manufacturer. Careful comparison and clinical use should allow practitioners to chose which is right for them. One unique trocar is the Woodford spike. It utilizes a principle similar to the Verres needle; the trocar has an inner spring-tension safety with an outer cutting sheath.

Frequently, the trocar choice is determined by the cannula through which a surgeon wishes to work (Fig. 6–28). In any event, it behooves the laparoscopic surgeon to be familiar with the open trocar placement

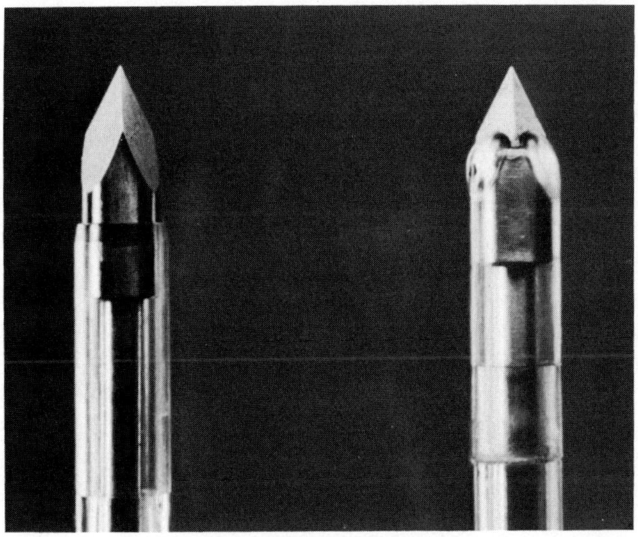

Figure 6–27. Disposable trocar tips demonstrating the pyramidal knife with varying safety shielding configurations.

techniques as these can be the only safe method of access at times.[34] Open reusable and disposable cannulas are available.[28] These are predominantly the Hasson type and are regaining popularity at many institutions. The primary purpose of these portals are for the secure maintenance of a pneumoperitoneum seal after being placed through a small open peritoneotomy. They all have a blunt, inner core, removable stylet, an olive-tipped sleeve to form the sealed wedge against the abdominal wall, and a suture wing to hold them into position. This trocar design has recently undergone another evolutionary step by incorporating a flexible shaft so that curved instruments may be introduced (Fig. 6–29). Another design to accomplish this is a disposable balloon portal system.

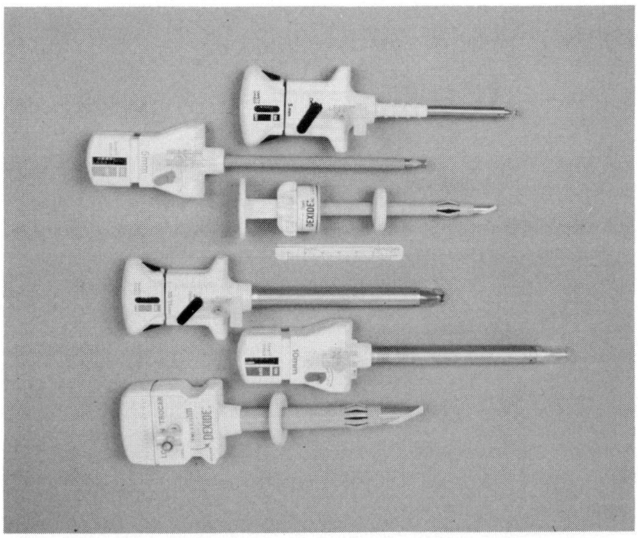

Figure 6–28. Various disposable trocar designs; 5-mm devices are shown above the ruler and 10-mm devices below.

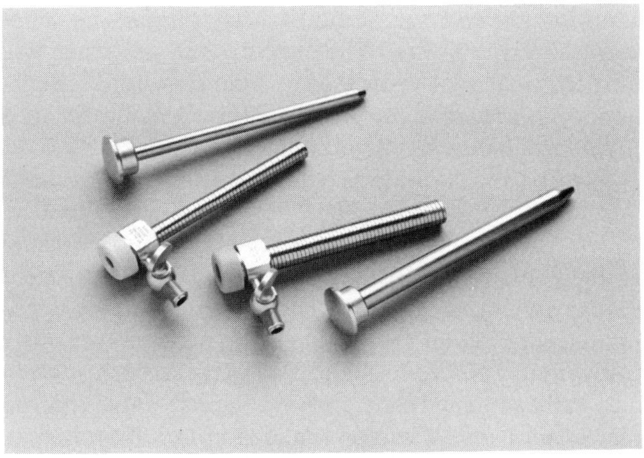

Figure 6–29. A contemporary design along the conventional theme of open trocar systems (Hasson). This is a flexible trocar system that allows the insertion of curved instruments.

The choice of cannula is becoming increasingly complex. That reflects the everincreasing variety and availability of differing designs that allow the laparoscopic urologist a number of options. Reusable cannulas are usually constructed of stainless steel. For complex laparoscopic urologic surgery this has a particular advantage beyond the cost issue of the reusable instrument. A noninsulated metal cannula greater than 7 mm in diameter does not promote output impedance from electrosurgical sources. By insulating the trocar, capacitive and direct coupling of the electric current through each metallic instrument or scope is possible, resulting in a risk of inadvertent electrical burns distant from the point of application. Cannula sleeves may also be constructed of plastic or Fiberglas to allow unimpeded radiographic and fluoroscopic imaging synchronously if necessary.

All cannulas usually have an insufflation line input valve, usually at the proximal housing area, and a small antisuction hole at their distal tips. Aside from these essential features, a good deal of variety remains. The trocar may be affixed to the abdominal wall to ensure stability during a given procedure. Fascial screws either can be fixed to the trocar or can be attachable. The major concern for the urologist should be adaptability of the cannula to meet the demands of the particular case. Restraints of operating laparoscopically in the pelvis make selection of the ideal cannula crucial. Because of a fixed pelvic inlet and morphometric limitations, the smaller the intrusion into the abdominal cavity by the distal cannula tip the better. Stability of trocar placement is also crucial. Retracting, flanged, locking trocars accomplish both of these theoretical advantages, providing a low intra-abdominal profile and a secured portal. The secure cannula is of more importance as the surgery becomes increasingly complex. The surgeon and assistant will find that optimal coordination requires fluid, single-handed instrument exchanges. Cannula malposition is the consequence unless stability is secured.

Finally, the cannula's sealing mechanism should be familiar to the urologist. The valvular mechanism allows the maintenance of intra-abdominal pressure as instruments are passed. These valves can prevent inadvertent spraying of peritoneal fluids during opening. Depending on the case-specific instruments used, the valvular mechanisms can impede smooth motion and damage equipment. Certain flapper-valve mechanisms can actually scrape the insulation off an instrument, thus promoting electroconductive injuries. Trumpet valves available on most reusable cannulas require careful maintenance to ensure smooth performance. These valves must be opened for instrument placement and thus require the use of two hands, an important consideration during tedious reconstructive efforts. A feature of all currently available cannulas is the mechanism of pressure maintenance using reduction sleeves or caps during placement of smaller instruments. A newer innovation is an iris valve–like device that should facilitate smoother instrument transfers along a wide range of sizes.

Cannulas range in size from 3 mm to as large as 30 mm (Fig. 6–30). Sizes above 10 mm increase the risk for access site hernias if the fascia is not carefully reapproximated. Access strategies that use Z-tract trajectories are touted as decreasing the risk.[36] Certainly, those trocar sites in the 20- to 30-mm range warrant careful fascial closure.

Cannulas of the future may overcome some or all of the drawbacks that have been highlighted during this brief discussion. Combinations of reusable and disposable features would be advantageous. An interactive access port that requires only one hand to change instruments would be ideal. Security of the portal plus a low profile are further requirements. Metallic conductance to the anterior abdominal wall would be important for at least some of the larger portals. A pliable material that would allow for maneuverability in a limited environment could also make the placement of other than round instruments possible.

Graspers and Forceps

A number of suitable graspers are available for laparoscopic surgeries. These instruments come in the usual disposable or reusable choices. Various grasping instruments tips are depicted in Fig. 6–31. Most are 5 mm in diameter. Atraumatic tissue manipulation is the primary concern during reconstructive surgery, whereas for laparoscopic pelvic lymph node dissection, the tissue graspers can have more of a biting tip. Classic Babcock and Allis configurations are available in either 5- or 10-mm sizes. Of note is the fact that locking or spring-tension mechanisms are available on some of these instruments. One-handed release is an important consideration when choosing this feature. These are important considerations if the grasper is to be used as a tissue retractor. The 10-mm Babcock clamp has successfully been used to retract the small and large colon for complex retroperitoneal urologic surgery such as nephrectomy, partial nephrectomy, retroperitoneal lymphadenectomy, and adrenalectomy.

Scissors

Laparoscopic scissors are probably the most unique instrument compared with the open surgical counterpart. This instrument allows the laparoscopic surgeon to control hemostasis synchronously and precisely during tissue dissection. Metzenbaum type scissors have been most used because the outer curved, blunt edges allow controlled spreading to separate tissue planes during the dissection. Potts or Geralds type instruments, which are needed to carefully divide the

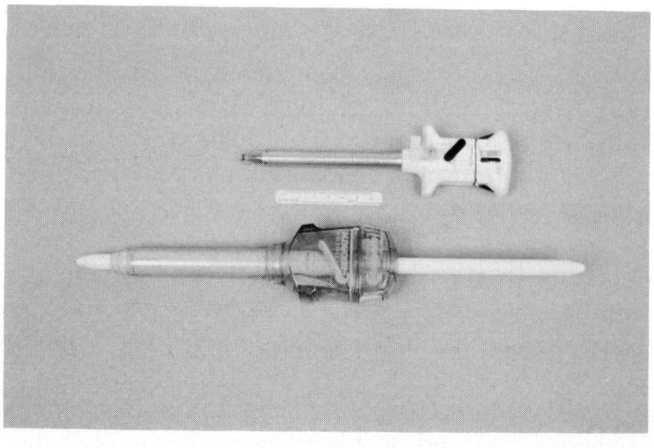

Figure 6–30. Larger trocars are increasingly utilized for extra-abdominal work through the trocar, utilization of larger instruments or delivering larger organs intact from the abdomen.

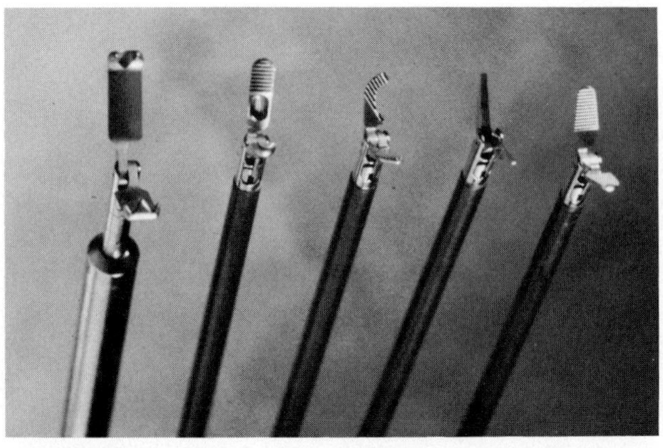

Figure 6–31. Reusable laparoscopic graspers viewed *en face*.

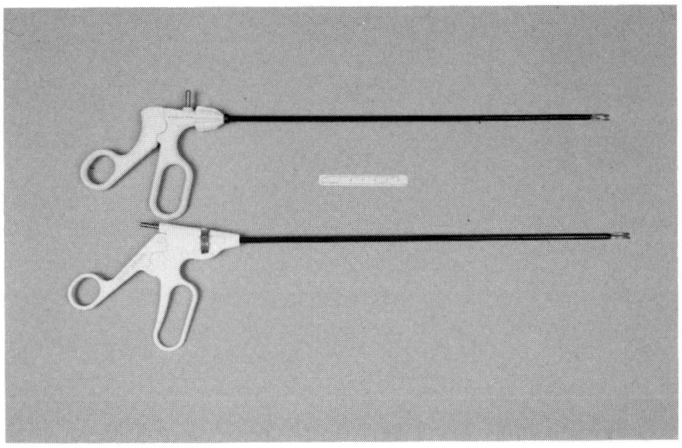

Figure 6–32. Laparoscopic disposable scissors with finger-tipped control features and adaptors for electrocautery.

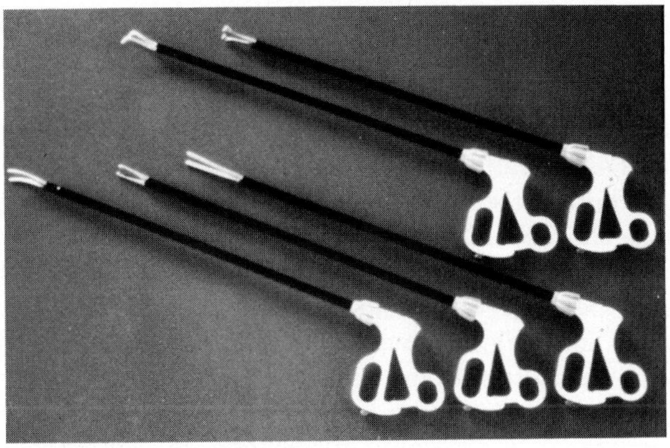

Figure 6–33. Finger-tipped control mechanisms are finding expanding use, since this means of instrument control allows precise instrument alignment.

smaller urogenital structures or to cleanly expose mucosa for precise mucosa-to-mucosa repair, are just beginning to become available. Most laparoscopic scissors have dual levering from both the thumb and back finger holes. Smaller, more precise movements can be obtained by going to a single-action mechanism. By incorporating a spring-assist release mechanism, the closure force can be accentuated. The currently available laparoscopic scissors are the best instruments available to the urologists (Fig. 6–32).

Disposable laparoscopic scissors have a major advantage over the reusable instruments because of the sharpness of the cutting edges. These small scissors have a tendency to become rapidly dull. In addition, the cautery insulation can easily wear during multiple passages of these instruments. Finger-tip control is another practical feature of the disposable scissors that give them greater utility for the laparoscopic surgeon.

Dissectors

Dual-capacity laparoscopic dissectors are available that are insulated for electrocautery application. Because this device does not require an ever-sharp cutting edge, the major impetus for disposability no longer applies. Finger-tip control mechanisms allow for precise placement and repositioning of the dissector's tips with one hand (Fig. 6–33). This feature, imparting dexterous manipulation, is increasingly available on both reusable and disposable dissectors.

Multiple dissector tip configurations have lacked one feature until recently. A right-angled tip has finally become available (Fig. 6–34). Sharper and duller tapered point configurations are also available. The continued increase in availability of such dissectors should allow the safe expansion of urologic laparoscopic procedures.

Suturing Instruments/Needle Drivers, Needles & Future

Laparoscopic suturing, knotting, and ligature placement is the topic of another chapter. The difficulty of these tactile maneuvers has prompted the most intense search for tools to diminish the frustration of the task.[37] Until recently, there has not been a specific set of instruments that allows the surgeon to use both hands synchronously to perform suturing with the ambidexterity of the open procedure surgeon. A concerted effort to eliminate the requirement for these difficult skills by automating or obviating the need to suture has been undertaken by investigators and manufacturers. Stapling has been the method most often considered for the solution. Many problems with both delivery and placement have yet to be overcome.[38] In addition, the metallic staple continues to provide the foreign-body problems that have been noted in the urologic literature.[39,40] Biologic gluing has been a sought-after alternative for decades. No adequate method yet avails itself for laparoscopic urologic sur-

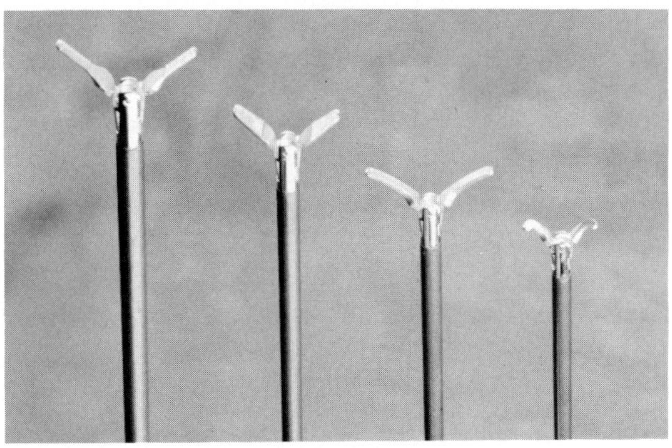

Figure 6–34. Reusable laparoscopic dissectors *en face* with variable degrees of curvature increasing from left to right.

gery. Finally, interest in laparoscopic laser welding of tissues represents another method of trying to avoid laparoscopic suturing. Recent studies suggest that with the addition of certain fluorescent dyes, the laser welds are capable of producing tissue reapproximation with burst strengths approaching that necessary to make this technique applicable. The instruments are extremely expensive, and the ability to laser weld must be currently considered experimental. That leaves suturing, although a complex task as yet, the remaining alternative.

A variety of sutured ligatures can be placed extracorporeally. Endoscopic placement of pretied slip-knot loops of various configurations are available.[41] In addition, with some practice a slip-knot loop can be fashioned in the operating room to achieve the same purpose.[42] A variety of suture materials are available for these slip loop ligatures, including chromic gut, plain gut, Vicryl, and silk. The method of laparoscopic placement is depicted in the illustration but requires the passage of a separate reducer sleeve during the deployment of the ligature. A wide variety of extracorporeal instruments are necessary if suturing and knotting are to be performed with external control.[43,44] Special suturing instruments that increase the mechanical force at the lever point (where the needle holder grips the needle) are available with variations of handle configurations (Fig. 6–35). They are limited in design, being unable to assist with tissue control and suture placement. Special devices exist to facilitate passage of the tied extracorporeal knot in the form of grooved or holed knot pushers.

Intracorporeal suturing and knotting obviates all the equipment necessary for extracorporeal suturing but increases the complexity of the skill necessary to successfully accomplish this task (Fig. 6–36).[44] Special instruments that approximate the utility of open needle holders and tissue forceps that can be interchangeable if necessary to allow ambidextrous passage

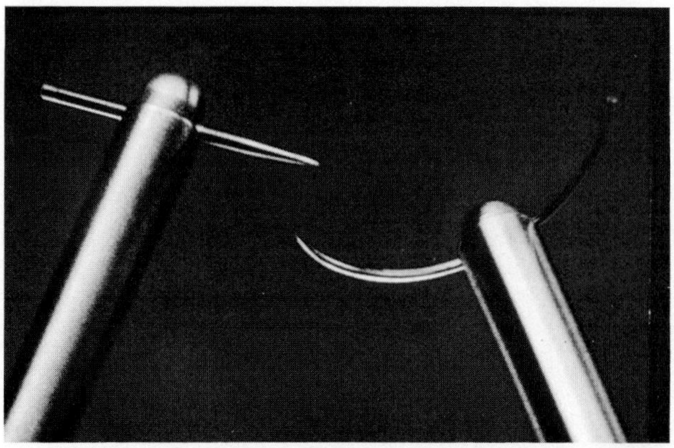

Figure 6–35. The pin-vise principle of needle driving is employed by several manufacturers to increase the mechanical advantage of the driver.

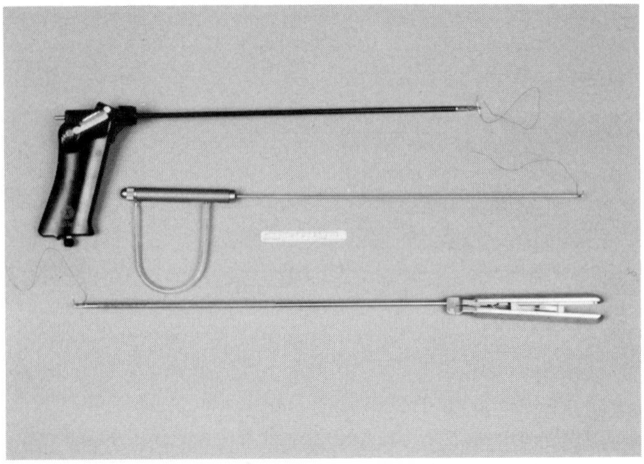

Figure 6–36. Various types of needle drivers shown together to demonstrate the wide variety available.

of the needle are ideal. One such set of instruments is the Szabo-Berci suturing set (see Fig. 6–1). Each instrument is 5 mm in diameter and is similar in conception to the Castroviejo instruments of microsurgery. There are no finger rings to restrain the hands from fine movements. There is a locking, ratcheting system that need not be used once the movements become fluid and confidence is gained with the intracorporeal skills. The parrot-jawed instrument is the primary device for needle driving. For a right-handed surgeon it is best held in the right hand. The flamingo-jawed instrument was designed principally for tissue handling and assistance. It can also be used to pass a stitch left-handed if necessary. Discussion of such instruments and their further application to urologic surgery can be found in Chapter 24.

Laparoscopic sutures and needles with specific features designed to enhance their endoscopic utility are becoming available.[45] Straight and ski needle designs have predominated. The specific needs of urologic reconstruction has received little attention until recently. In a series of modeling and small animal investigations, the application of several "custom" needle configurations has allowed laparoscopic urologic reconstruction with a variety of suture lines (e.g., running, interrupted, locking). Interrupted end-to-end anastomoses required three differing needle configurations for intracorporeal reconstructions. Long-running vascular suture lines that are not deep within the pelvis require more of the standard ski configurations. Endoscopic suture material for urologic reconstruction should be absorbable. Color-coordinated materials that would allow intracoporeal identification of individual sutures before tying have been investigated.

Retractors

Of all the instruments for laparoscopic urologic surgery, the one that has the most potential and is least available is the retractor.[46] The closed laparoscopic environment represents unique challenges for urologic surgery. The environment not only is closed, the access is limited and the ability to observe the retractor and what is being retracted is currently a severe limitation.

Despite such restrictions, a number of devices that allow limited retraction are available. Graspers with ratcheted tension control provide the ability to move visceral structures out of the surgical field (Fig. 6–37). Once the grasper has moved the targeted organ beyond the field of vision, minimal further manipulation should be performed. Injury from such clamps are possible, and in addition they take up limited access space. Another innovative method uses ureteroscopic alligator forceps to grasp tissue and lock into a fixed retraction position; this forceps takes up minimal access space.[46]

A number of simple mechanical devices also allow laparoscopic retraction. Almost all devices are variations of a fanlike system. Major differences are in the construction of the expansion mechanisms and the tips. Most of these instruments are 10 mm in diameter and require a lot of access space. Once positioned they also are off the camera. One investigation of mechanical retractors on different visceral structures demonstrated minimal contusions superficially but definite risks of the tips lacerating mesenteric attachments if undue leverage is applied. Laparoscopic balloon retractors have been used experimentally and offer some advantages over these mechanical devices. A broad, compliant, contiguous sweep allows the force of retraction to spread over the entire balloon surface (Fig. 6–38).

Vascular retractors are available from several manufacturers (Fig. 6–39). Currently all are 10-mm instruments because of physical limitations imposed by

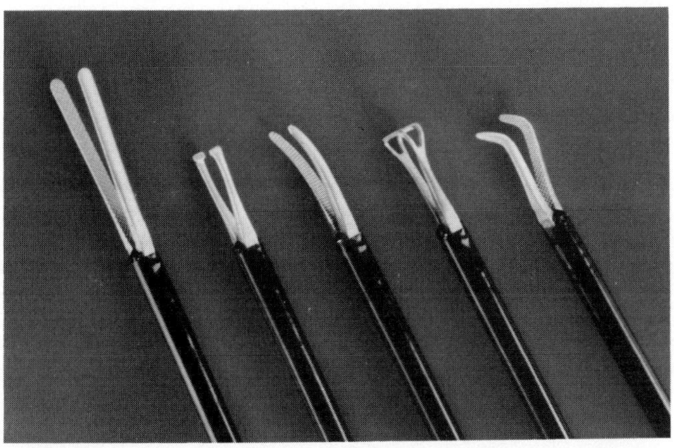

Figure 6–37. Bowel clamps are often employed for their ability to grasp the viscera atraumatically as a laparoscopic method of retracting. Injuries can still occur, especially since the field of view is elsewhere after retraction is accomplished.

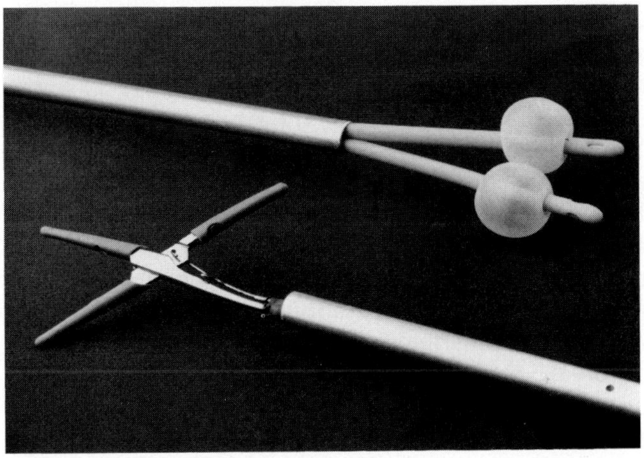

Figure 6–38. Innovative designs are essential to increase the laparoscopist's control over a closed environment. Two prototypic designs are demonstrated.

the curved lip of the retractor blade. Shape-memory metal constructed from nickel-titanium alloy offers a potential to overcome these problems.[30] These devices can be placed while straight, and the shape-memory, curved portion can be extruded once placed intra-abdominally. Each of these instruments relies on placement through rigid trocars, again representing waste of access space. Despite all the limitations there are possibilities that retractors can perform similarly in open surgery. Even with such limited capacity, advanced urologic surgeries are being accomplished, usually by gravity displacement of viscera.

Irrigators and Aspirators

The ability to maintain a clear view of tissue planes and the surgical target area relies on the ability to aspirate blood, bowel contents, or urine from the area of interest.[47] The problems with these devices from a laparoscopic viewpoint is that clotting can rapidly diminish the efficacy of these small instruments and that they can also aspirate the insufflant gas. Of

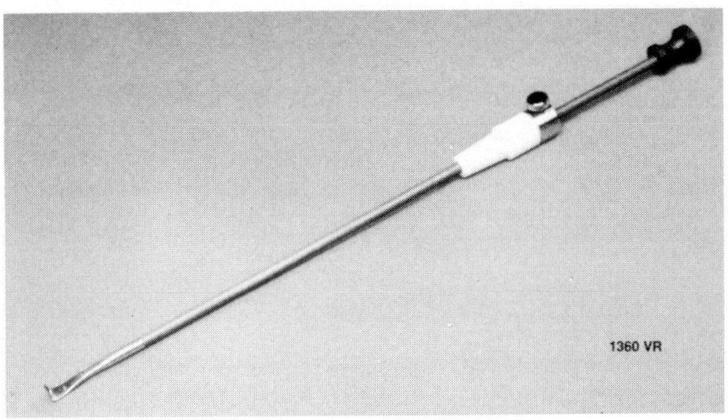

Figure 6–39. Retraction of vascular structures such as veins and arteries require different designs. Demonstrated is the WISAP vein retractor.

course, the best solution is to prevent the necessity for an irrigant or aspirator by meticulous attention to hemostatic detail; however, the availability of these devices is still obligatory.

There are the usual reusable/disposable considerations when choosing this instrument. The disposables have no advantage other than the convenience of not having to maintain and clean them. Almost all systems are 5 mm in diameter. The principle difference among the simple irrigation-aspiration devices is the activation mechanisms. Trumpet valves predominate, although cumbersome on-off switch mechanisms are also available. Most irrigant systems can and should allow for the addition of heparin to diminish the clotting that will obstruct the lumen of these devices. The construction should allow rapid cleaning if obstruction by clot does occur.

Multifunctional irrigator-aspirator-probe coagulators are available.[48] A final instrument in this group is the hydrodissector.[49] In addition to irrigation and aspiration it allows pressurized aquadissection (Fig. 6–40). The theoretical advantages include the ability to rapidly dissect in potential spaces and confined areas with little trauma.[50] Experimental application of such devices for pelvic lymphadenectomy, retroperitoneal lymphadenectomy, and renal pedicle dissection has prompted the authors to begin utilizing the device clinically. Potential adverse sequelae can result from clysis with the irrigant or disruption of small venules. Investigation of these potential problems has been encouraging, and none of these complications has been reported.

Clip Appliers and Staplers

Secure ligation is the key to vascular control during open and laparoscopic surgeries.[51] The limitations discussed previously during this chapter probably account for the immediate adaptation of metallic clip

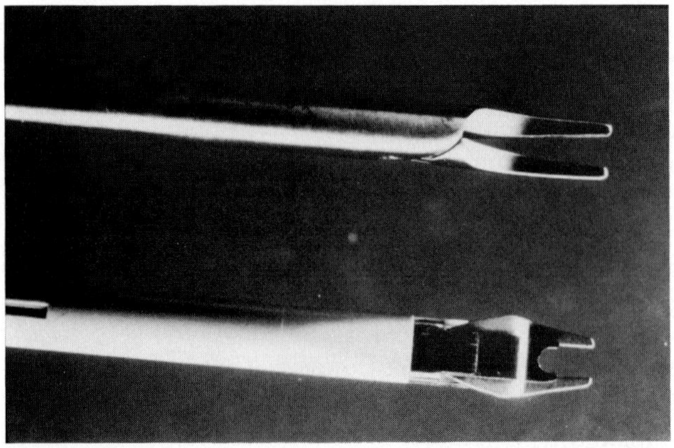

Figure 6–41. Laparoscopic clip application can be accomplished by reusable instruments (*top*) or by disposable automatic devices (*bottom*).

appliers for laparoscopic purposes. These instruments are available in reusable and disposable devices of 10-mm diameter (Fig. 6–41). Clip appliers can also be single-fire, reloadable, nondisposable, and multifire in reusable or disposable designs. The instruments usually contain 9-mm titanium clips.

Another laparoscopic clip device delivers staples with a biting, toothed configuration developed for herniorrhaphies. This clip applier incorporates an articulating head in order to angle the clip applier toward the stapler head, maximizing the angle of entrance upward to the anterior abdominal wall. These instruments have been described for reperitonealization following transabdominal laparoscopic pelvic lymphadenectomies and for the securing of pubobladder-neck slings in research studies.

Finally, the development of automatic mechanical stapling systems similar to those commonly utilized for open gastrointestinal reconstruction have been developed (Fig. 6–42).[52] These linear cutting devices apply six rows of stainless steel staples (vascular or bowel), three rows on either side of a cutting blade. The adaptation of this device for complex intracor-

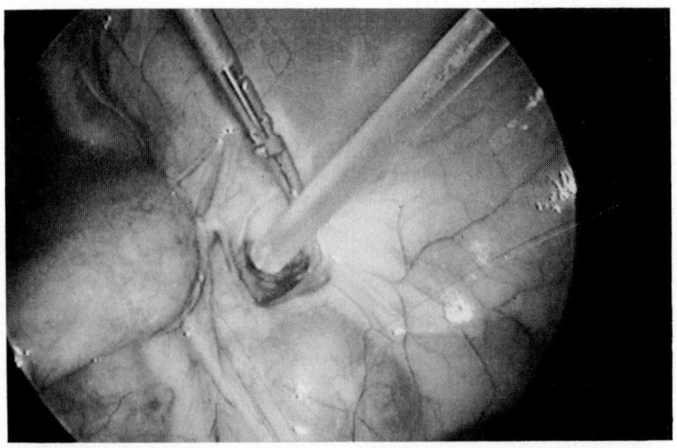

Figure 6–40. Suction-irrigation devices have also been modified by the addition of pulsatile pressure systems to provide the multifunctional capability of aqua dissectors.

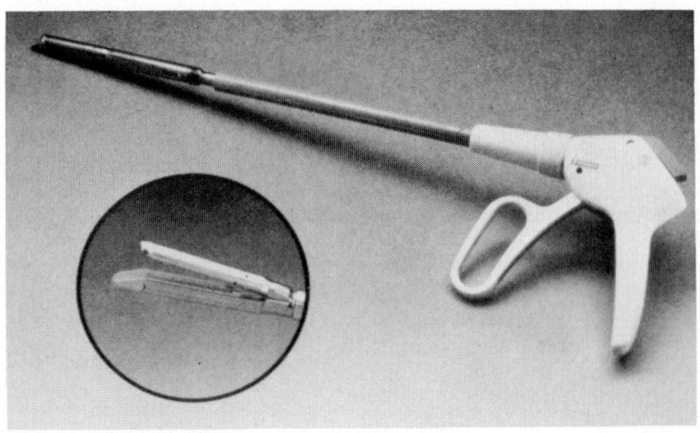

Figure 6–42. Automated staplers can deliver a variety of stapler sizes for hemostatic or reconstructive purposes. Demonstrated here is the 12-mm Endo-GIATM.

poreal bowel resection and anastomosis by a functional end-to-end technique has been described. Modifications of these techniques have led to the clinical performance of laparoscopic ileal conduit urinary diversion. The application of the device for renal pedicle ligation has also been investigated and clinically used.[53] In addition, the ability to perform distal ureterectomy with partial cystectomy for upper tract transitional cell carcinomas has been reported.[54,55]

Environmental Containment and Tissue Removal Systems

Urologic surgery can be perceived broadly as either reconstructive or extirpative. Most adult abdominal urologic surgery falls into the latter, extirpative category. That is, most genitourinary organs are removed for specific disease processes, e.g., cancer, infection, and so forth. In order for laparoscopy to accomplish the same goal, specific concerns, such as removing the targeted pathologic organ without further extending the access or risking contamination of sterile areas by the disease process, must be demonstrated. Unfortunately, large clinical series and long-term follow-up are lacking. Innovative methods for removal have been tried for laparoscopic nephrectomy, including transvaginal removal in females. But such intact organ removals are not always possible, and methods of reducing the visceral mass to an extractable dimension are required.[56] Once visceral integrity is compromised, the disease process is no longer confined. Hence, environmental containment is a requirement for tissue removal systems.

A variety of tissue bags are available for clinical utilization (Fig. 6–43). A clear sack allows the surgeon to visualize any manipulations of the tissue within. The LapSac has been most utilized for laparoscopic nephrectomies.[54] It has proven to be sturdy and nonpermeable. It is large by necessity and takes a good deal of space within the closed confines of the insufflated abdomen. Careful, coordinated assistance is required to place the kidney within this enclosure. The opposing squared and rounded edges help identify each side to aid in opening and the drawstring can be grasped to deliver the open end via the laparoscopic portal. Some laparoscopic containment sacks have no means of closing the opening and rely upon delivering the mouth via an access portal to limit contamination. Other systems provide an O-ringlike material to spring open the entrance to the sack.

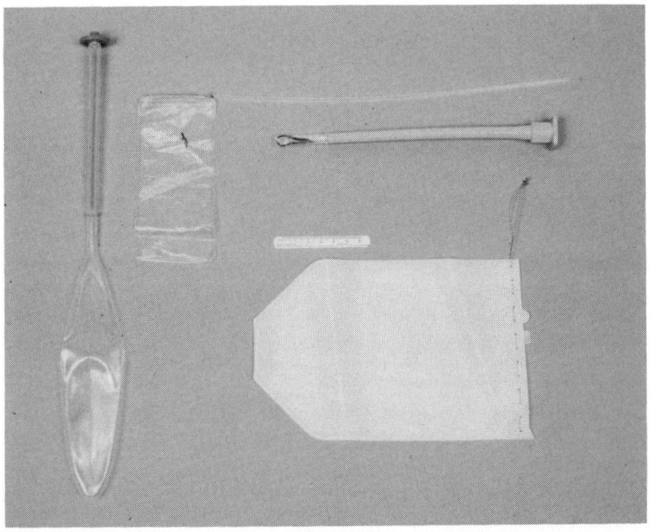

Figure 6–43. Environmental containment systems (ECS) can be used to isolate contaminated structures (inflamed, infected, or malignant) prior to their removal.

A number of mechanical devices are available to disrupt the organ once entrapped. The simplest method, using a pair of Mayo scissors, has been described by Copcoat and co-workers.[56] Tissue punches can remove large portions of tissue, up to 12 mm in diameter, but can take time if the organ is large, like the kidney.[41] This device requires some skill as it can grasp the environmental containment system and result in spillage of tissue. The Tissue Removal System, consisting of a sharpened, sealed outer sleeve and an inner corkscrew can reliably remove tissue of varying diameters. The major drawback is the amount of time required to remove large amounts of tissue. The proximal end of the sleeve is extremely sharp and can easily disrupt most sacks. The device was primarily designed for a biopsy type of tissue removal. Use of this system to obtain large samples of poorly differentiated retroperitoneal sarcomas or pelvic neoplasms and to sample solid visceral structures before morcellation is an option. Resectoscopes have also been used experimentally with some success.[57] Requirements for the cutting current can be overcome and hundreds of grams of tissue can be removed, but double-access environmental containment sacks were used (grounding, irrigation, and chip removal). The entire process is time-consuming.

Automated tissue removal systems are necessary to facilitate speedy organ ablation. Tissue shavers have been used by orthopedic surgeons for years. A robotic device to remove prostatic tissue (ELSA) has been modified for intracorporeal tissue removal.[56] The problem with these devices is that the activated disrupter is not specific to the organ. These devices are capable of quickly morcellating the entrapment sack. To overcome these problems, a laparoscopic electrical tissue morcellator was devised (Fig. 6–44). This system works on an extracorporeal electrical motor and suction after physically forcing tissue up the intracoporeal sleeve. It has been reported to facilitate rapid extraction of large-volume tissue (spleen and kidney).[54] The tissue extracted is ground, allowing

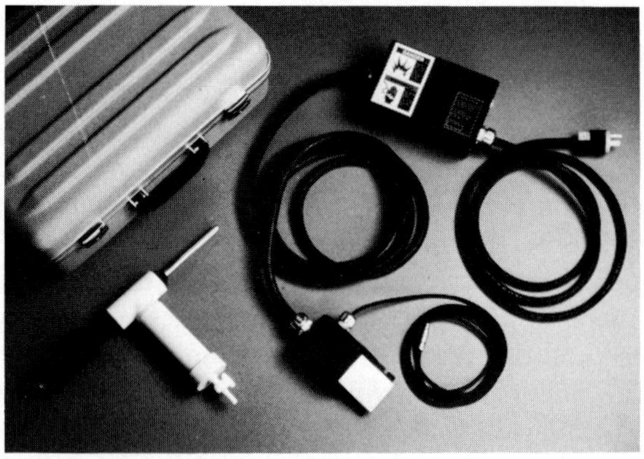

Figure 6–44. The electronic tissue morcellator. (Courtesy of Cook OB/Gyn, Cook Urological.)

histologic inspection but making pathologic interpretation of microcapsular penetration, identification of multifocal lesions, or quantification of pathologic tissue volume difficult or impossible.

Every laparoscopic removal of a malignant organ carries the potential for inadvertent tumor seeding. Reports that the LapSac is impermeable to cells is encouraging, but the surgical techniques themselves — subsequent morcellation and potential disruption of the environmental containment system (ECS) — reflect continued need for caution. In a study assessing risk of tumor spillage by using vital dye sham lesions, no inadvertent spillage could be identified at laparotomy if the ECS was intact and surgical margins around the kidney were maintained during the nephrectomy. The authors currently have begun to remove lymph nodes by ECS from patients with transitional cell carcinoma of the bladder or squamous carcinoma of the penis because of theoretical risks of seeding during manipulation of the nodal packets through cannulas.

Laparoscopic Doppler and Ultrasound Probes

Small doppler probes that provide auditory feedback regarding the location and position of blood vessels have been developed by a number of manufacturers (Fig. 6–45). They can be used during varicocele ligation to aid in the identification of small internal spermatic arteries. Pelvic lymphadenectomies can be aided by identification of the course of the iliac artery or the presence and proximity of the obturator artery, and the location of the lumbar arteries are identifiable during retroperitoneal lymphadenectomies. Usually, these structures are easily identified, however, without the necessity of Doppler confirmation. Recently, anterior pyelocaliceal diverticuli and cysts have been successfully unroofed and fulgurated laparoscopically. Identification and avoidance of small arterioles can be facilitated by such probes.

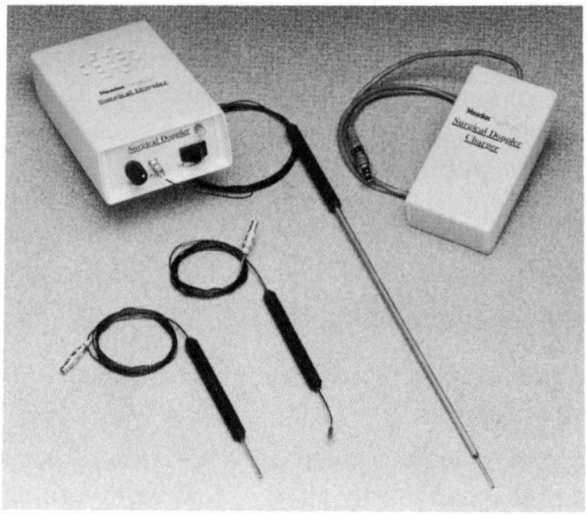

Figure 6–45. Laparoscopic Doppler system for identification of blood vessels.

Advances in catheter-based ultrasound probes allow much broader application than simpler Doppler devices. Ultrasound transducers are available with rotating or fixed piezoceramic elements using 7.5 to 50 MHz transducers (Fig. 6–46). Catheter size ranges from 1 to 5 mm and can provide tissue penetration from 2 to 4 cm. These probes can provide information about parenchymal lesions, surrounding vasculature, or the precise location of calculi. The small probes are easily introduced through a laparoscopic portal with aid of a reduction sleeve. They are not widely available, and the cost and expertise necessary for clinical application are limiting factors.

Robotic Assistants

A mechanical assist system such as Omnitract or Iron Intern has been available for open retraction assistance for years. The functional utility of these systems for laparoscopic camera portal assistance requires

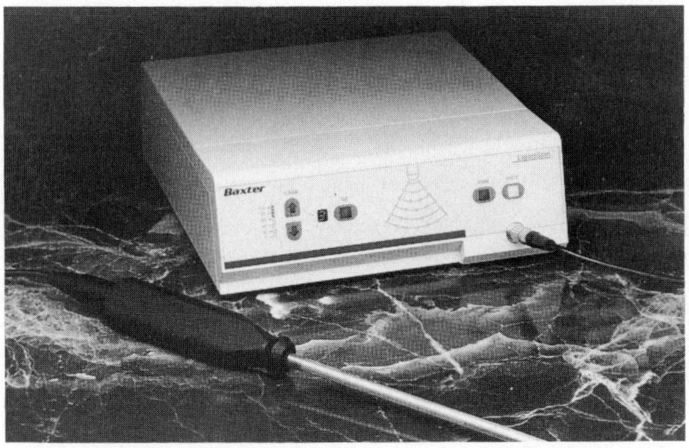

Figure 6–46. Laparoscopic 2-D Doppler system.

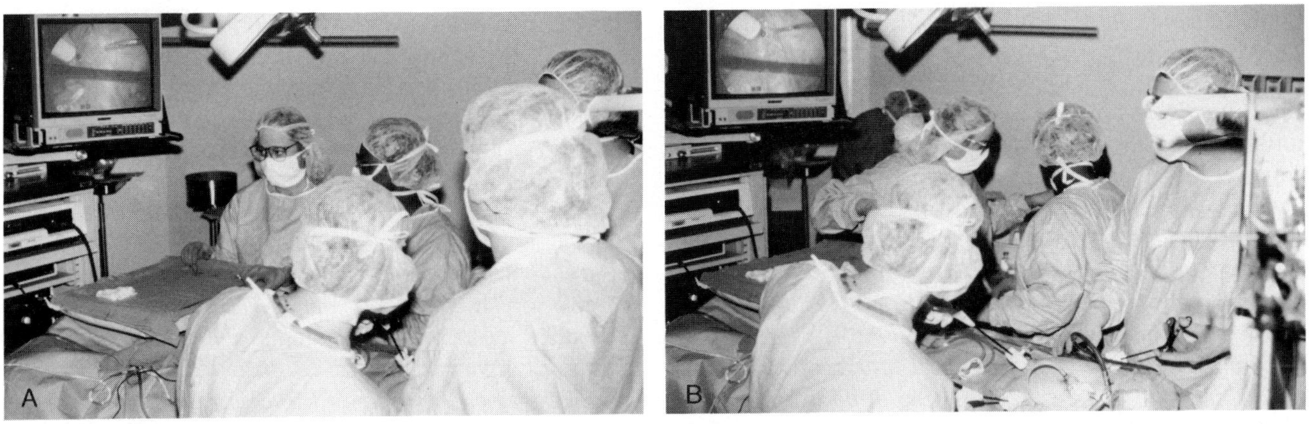

Figure 6–47. Demonstration of the room attainable during laparoscopic pelvic surgery by the deployment of a robotic arm assistant. *A*, to the left, is the standard configuration with a human assistant. *B* shows the same situation with the robotic assistant. Note the freedom for movement to the surgeon's right.

minor adaptations. As mentioned in various other instrument sections, space is a premium commodity during laparoscopic cases. This holds true in the extracorporeal environment as well. With tubes and cords running to multiple off-field sources, the anterior abdominal wall quickly becomes cluttered. The fewer hands and arms that limit portal movement further, the better. In addition, for laparoscopic urologic pelvic surgery, the lateral table margins become an area to which the surgeon and assistant need full access (Fig. 6–47). Therefore during the setup for most laparoscopic pelvic cases it is recommended that both the patient's arms be tucked at the sides to allow greater mobility for the surgeon and assistant. The absence of a dedicated human camera assistant frees more lateral mobility for the surgeon.[58]

Mechanical assistance devices can be broadly classified into static mechanical assistance systems (Fig. 6–48) or robotic arms (Fig. 6–49). The mechanical assistance systems have the potential advantage of lower costs. The robotic arms offer broader applications, servoassisted maneuverability, and, potentially, extracorporeally assisted intra-abdominal retraction.[2]

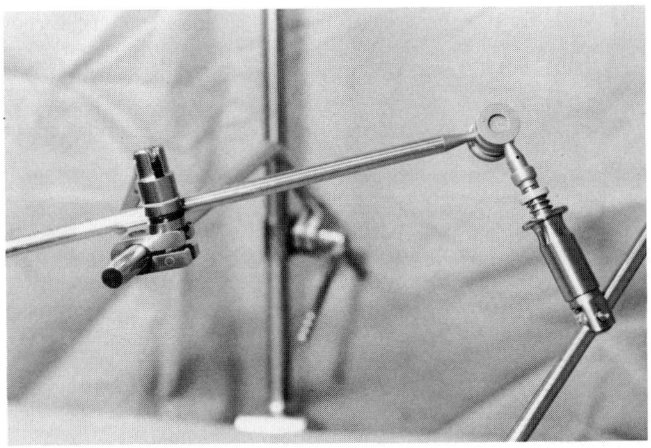

Figure 6–48. A simple mechanical arm for laparoscopic camera assistance. (Courtesy of Omnitract.)

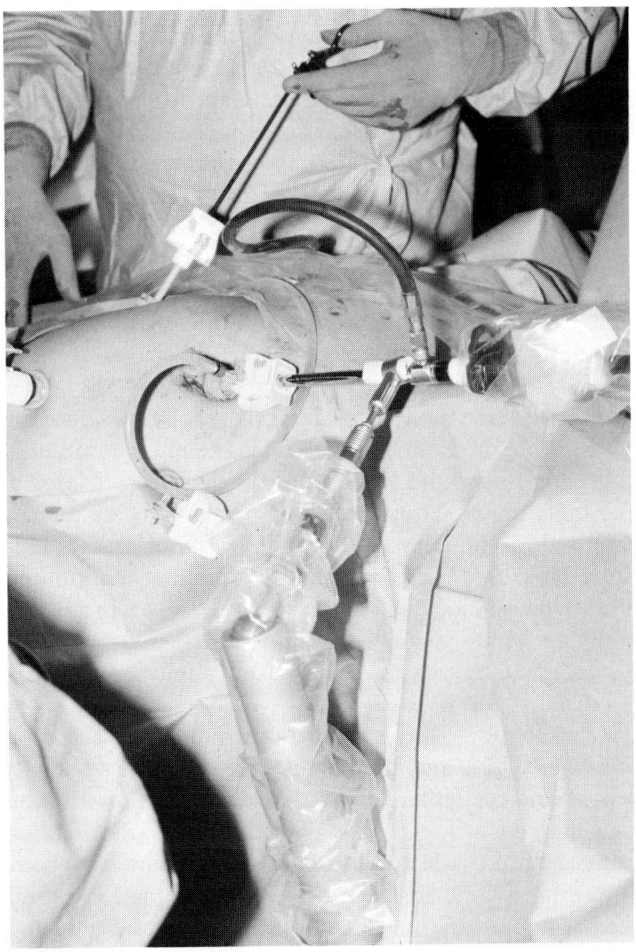

Figure 6–49. An electronically controlled pneumatic robotic arm camera assistant.

EQUIPMENT AND INSTRUMENT CARE, MAINTENANCE, AND STERILIZATION

Care and maintenance of laparoscopic equipment should follow the manufacturer's instructions.[59] Most manufacturers provide in-service, hands-on demonstrations of the equipment. Maintenance schedules and cleaning can be reviewed at that time. Most hospital operating rooms have mechanicians and engineers that routinely inspect power equipment and initiate repairs when necessary.[60] Communication with a designated laparoscopic team is vital in order to avoid elective surgery when crucial pieces of equipment are scheduled for maintenance.

Following every laparoscopic procedure, all of the nondisposable instruments should be dismantled and washed in mild detergent soap to remove gross debris. Ultrasonication can then be performed to remove smaller particulates, especially in the interstices of these fine instruments; then the instruments can be dried and prepared for resterilization.

Sterilization is the absolute lack of any microbe, including spores. It is important to distinguish this from disinfection, which is commonly employed for urologic equipment. High-grade disinfection usually destroys all microbials except bacterial spores. It is currently recommended that all laparoscopic instruments be sterile. Infectious complications from laparoscopic procedures to date have been infrequent. The American Association of Gynecologic Laparoscopists reported an incidence of only 0.3% from 117,000 cases. In a study specifically looking at methods of instrument preparation, there was no definite conclusion that high-level disinfection was any worse than sterilization with regard to wound infection or contamination.

Sterilization can be accomplished by gas, steam, irradiation, or chemicals. Steam is the most commonly available and rapid method of sterilization. Many of the instruments used for laparoscopic surgery can be steamed in the autoclave. Notable exceptions include most laparoscopes and electronic imaging equipment. The mechanical assistance systems except for Robotrac can be sterilized in the autoclave.

Chemical agents for sterilization include 2% stabilized hydrogen peroxide, time-released chloride dioxide, peracetic acid, and 2% glutaraldehyde. The first two agents are highly corrosive and are not generally acceptable for laparoscopic instruments. The 2% glutaraldehyde provides effective high-level disinfection but does not eradicate bacterial spores. The fumes are irritating to mucous membranes, and time exposures must be greater than 20 minutes. Peracetic acid has recently become more popular as the active ingredient for automated chemical sterilization systems. The closed system eliminates many of the operator-dependent drawbacks of previous chemical soaking processes. All of the data by the manufacturer indicates that it provides sterilization, not only high-level disinfection. The major drawback of the system is lack of long-term clinical experience in its use.

CONCLUSIONS

A great variety of laparoscopic equipment and instrumentation is required for the safe performance of complex laparoscopic urologic surgery. What works best for a given operation or surgeon may not work for someone else. Any attempt to cover the wide variety of such instrumentation cannot hope to fully detail the breadth of available products. In addition, new instruments are being produced at a remarkable rate, and the sales hyperbole surrounding them makes objective assessment difficult. The best method of deciding which instrument works best for any given problem requires familiarity with available alternatives. Despite the wide array of tools available for clinical laparoscopic urologist, there is room for more specialty-specific instruments. By understanding some of the principles of instrument design and application it is hoped that an interaction with the clinician and manufacturer can rapidly facilitate the development of this type of surgery.

BIBLIOGRAPHY

1. Berman, IR: Frontiers in general surgery: Pioneers, cowboys and desperados. Surg Endosc 6:82–83, 1992.
2. Cuschieri, A: Minimal access surgery and the future, or interventional laparoscopy. Am J Surg 161:404–407, 1991.
3. Jordan, GH; Robey, EL: Laparoscopy—laparoscopic surgery in urology. AUA Update Series 10:266–271, 1991.
4. Leadbetter, GW; Gillenwater, JY: Urology. JAMA 265:3175–3176, 1991.
5. Winfield, HN; Donovan, JF; See, WA; et al: Urologic laparoscopic surgery. J Urol 146:941–948, 1991.
6. Hopkins, HH: Optical principles of the endoscope. In: Berci, G, ed: Endoscopy. New York, Appleton-Century Crofts, 1976, pp. 3–27.
7. Berci, G; Paz-Partlow, M: Electronic imaging in endoscopy. Surg Endosc 2:227–233, 1988.
8. Demling, L; Hagel, HJ: Video endoscopy: Fundamentals and problems. Endoscopy 17:167–169, 1985.
9. Satava, RM: A comparison of direct and indirect video endoscopy. Gastrointest Endosc 33:69–72, 1987.
10. Satava, RM; Gooden, SM: The impact of video endoscopy on surgical training. Am Surg 55:263–266, 1989.
11. Schreiber, WF: What is image processing? In: Fundamentals of Electronic Imaging Systems. Some Aspects of Image Processing. New York, Springer-Verlag, 1991, pp. 1–20.
12. Schreiber, WF: Light and optical imaging systems. In: Fundamentals of Electronic Imaging Systems. Some Aspects of Image Processing. New York, Springer-Verlag, 1991, pp. 20–59.
13. Stoehlein, JR; Borroso, A; Glombick, A; Sachs, I: Documentation of fluoroscopic and endoscopic images using a color video printer. Gastrointest Endosc 36:392–394, 1990.
14. Voyles, CR; Tucker, RD: Education and engineering solutions for potential problems with laparoscopic monopolar electrosurgery. Am J Surg 164:57–62, 1992.

15. ECRI: Health devices. Electrosurg Laparosc 2:222, 1972.
16. U.S. Food and Drug Administration: Classification and Guidelines: Subcommittee on endoscopy. Federal Register 45:12701, 1980.
17. Hunter, JG: Laser or electrocautery for laparoscopic cholecystectomy? Am J Surg 161:345–349, 1991.
18. Reid, R: Physical and surgical principles of laser surgery in the lower genital tract. Obstet Gynecol Clin North Am 18:429–474, 1991.
19. Henderson, MR; Link, WJ; Incroperta, FR; Glover, GL: Gas transport resulting from plasma-scalpel surgery. Med Biol Eng 12:208, 1974.
20. Briggs, TP; Parker, C; Smith, C; Miller, RA: Augmented hemostasis: A review of the pharmacology of hemostasis in endoscopic surgery. Mini Invas Ther 1:7–11, 1991.
21. Dupunt, O; Waclawiczek, HW: Prevention and treatment of lymphatic fistulae following lymph node dissections by means of fibrin sealing. In: Waclawiczek, HW, ed: Progress in Fibrin Sealing, New York, Springer-Verlag, 1991, p. 65.
22. Levinson, AK; Swanson, D; Johnson, DE; et al: Fibrin glue for partial nephrectomy. Urology 38:314–316, 1989.
23. Rovsov, J: Fibrin glue: An effective hemostatic agent for nonsuturable bleeding. Ann Thorac Surg 38:409, 1984.
24. Mouret, P:L Le pneumopéritoine en suspension. Endomag 2:2–3, 1991.
25. Banting, S; Shimi, S; Velpen, GV; Cuschieri, A: Abdominal wall lift. Low-pressure pneumoperitoneum laparoscopic surgery. Surg Endosc 7:57–59, 1993.
26. Hashimoto, D; Nayeem, SA; Kajiwara, S; Hoshino, T: Laparoscopic cholecystectomy: An approach without pneumoperitoneum. Surg Endosc 7:54–56, 1993.
27. Lacey, CG: Laparoscopy: A clinical sign for intraperitoneal needle placement. Obstet Gynecol 47:625–627, 1976.
28. Oshinsky, GS; Smith, AD: Laparoscopic needles and trocars: An overview of designs and complications. J Laparoendosc Surg 2:117–125, 1992.
29. Dorsey, JH; Tabb, CR: Mini-laparoscopy and fiber-optic lasers. Obstet Gynecol Clin North Am 18:613–617, 1991.
30. Cuschieri, A: Variable curvature-shape memory spatula for laparoscopic surgery. Surg Endosc 5:179–181, 1991.
31. Hasson, HM: Open laparoscopy: A report of 150 cases. J Reprod Med 12:234–238, 1974.
32. Hasson, HM: Open laparoscopy vs closed laparoscopy: A comparison of complication rates. Adv Planned Parent 8:41–50, 1976.
33. Sigel B; Golub, RM; Loiacono, LA; et al: Technique of ultrasonic detection and mapping of abdominal wall adhesions. Surg Endosc 5:161–165, 1991.
34. del la Torre, R; Brooks, DC; Becker, JM: Open trocar insertion facilitates laparoscopic cholecystectomy and decreases morbidity. Surg Endosc 6:98, 1992.
35. Tews, G; Arzt, W; Bohavmilitzky, T; Fureder, R; Frolich, H: Significant reduction of operational risk in laparoscopy through the use of a new blunt trocar. Surg Gynecol Obstet 173:67–68, 1991.
36. Driscoll, GL; Tyler, JP; Simpson, P: Closure of laparoscopy incisions. Clin Reprod Fertil 1:241–242, 1982.
37. de Silva, EG: Suturoscope: A new device that allows endoscopic sutures to be performed with traditional threads. Surg Endosc 4:220–223, 1990.
38. Wheeless, CR: Use of absorbable staples for closure of proximal end of ileal loops. Obstet Gynecol 67:280, 1986.
39. Bisson, J; Vinson, RK; Leadbetter, GW: Urolithiasis from stapler anastomosis. Am J Surg 137:280, 1989.
40. Lieskovsky, G; Skinner, DG; Boyd, SD: Complications of the Kock pouch. Urol Clin North Am 15:195, 1988.
41. Mettler, L; Semm, K: Pelviscopic uterine surgery. Surg Endosc 6:23–31, 1992.
42. Marrero, MA; Corffman, RS: Laparoscopic use of sutures. Clin Obstet Gynecol 34:387–394, 1991.
43. Ko, ST; Airan, MC: Therapeutic laparoscopic suturing techniques. Surg Endosc 6:41–46, 1992.
44. Szabo, Z: Extra- and intracorporeal knotting and suturing techniques. Gastrointest Clin North Am (in press).
45. Reich, H; Clarke, C; Sekel, L: A simple method for ligating with straight and curved needles in operative laparoscopy. Obstet Gynecol 79:143–156, 1992.
46. Griffith, DP; Quesada, ET: Extracorporeal retraction of intracorporeal structures during laparoscopy. J Endourol 5:315–316, 1991.
47. Marshburn, PB; Hulka, JF: A simple irrigator-aspirator cannula for laparoscopy: The Stewart system. Obstet Gynecol 75:458–460, 1990.
48. Vara-Thorbeck, C; Gomez-Gamez, A: New endoscopic surgery instrument: Separator combined with sound for lavage and aspiration. Surg Endosc 6:80–81, 1992.
49. Popp, LW: Improvement in endoscopic hernioplasty: Transcutaneous aquadissection of the musculofascial defect and preperitoneal endoscopic patch repair. J Laparoendosc Surg 1:83–90, 1991.
50. Reich, H: Water works: An update on aquadissection. OBG Manag November 1990.
51. Steichen, FM; Ravitch, MM: Contemporary stapling instruments and basic mechanical suturing techniques. Surg Clin North Am 64:425–440, 1984.
52. Julian, TB: Closure of the urinary bladder with stainless steel and absorbable staples. Ann Surg 2044:186, 1986.
53. Kirker-Head, CA; Steckel, RR; Schwartz, A; Williams, R: Evaluation of surgical staples for ligation of the renal pedicle during nephrectomy. Urol Res 16:63, 1988.
54. Clayman, RV; Kavoussi, LR; Soper, NJ; et al: Laparoscopic nephrectomy: Initial case report. J Urol 146:278–282, 1991.
55. Figenshau, RS; Albala, DM; Clayman, RV; et al: Laparoscopic nephroureterectomy: Initial laboratory experience. Mini Invas Ther 1:93–97, 1991.
56. Copcoat, MM; Ison, KT; Wickham, JEA: Endoscopic tissue liquidization and surgical aspiration. J Endourol 2:321–331, 1988.
57. Weinberg, JJ; Smith, AD: Percutaneous resection of the kidney: Preliminary report. J Endourol 2:355–359, 1990.
58. Moran, ME: Robotic-assisted laparoscopic urologic pelvic surgery. J Laparoendosc Surg (in press).
59. Boyers, SP: Operating room setup and instrumentation. Clin Obstet Gynecol 34:373–386, 1991.
60. Dorsey, JH: Operating room organization. Lasers and advanced operative laparoscopy. Obstet Gynecol Clin North Am 18:569–573, 1991.

CHAPTER 7

Laparoscopic Entry and Exit

Gary S. Oshinsky, MD
Gopal H. Badlani, MD, FACS
Arthur D. Smith, MD, FACS

Minimal access surgery has emerged as a recognized means of performing therapeutic and diagnostic surgical procedures. Although gynecologists have utilized the laparoscope for several decades, only of late has laparoscopic surgery gained increased acceptance in the general surgical and urologic community. The number of laparoscopic procedures being performed routinely is now extensive and growing rapidly. The critical step in performing laparoscopic surgery is establishment of pneumoperitoneum and placement of the trocars. This initial part of the procedure, when performed properly, ensures safe and reliable access, allowing the procedure to commence. Difficulties with this part may preclude continuing with the operative procedure and more importantly may result in potentially severe injuries. Therefore a detailed discussion of the method of performing laparoscopic entry and exit provides the urologist with the essentials to perform safe and successful laparoscopy.

PATIENT PREPARATION

Patient preparation begins at the initial consultation for the urological procedure.[1] The patient should be fully informed of the nature of the procedure; risks, benefits, and alternatives to the planned procedure should be carefully explained to the patient. The patient must have a clear understanding that laparoscopic surgery, although minimally invasive, always presents a risk of laparotomy.

All patients should undergo routine preoperative laboratory testing, including complete blood count, Sequential Multiple Analyzer-7, prothrombin and partial thromboplastin times, urinalysis, chest x-ray, and electrocardiogram. Any abnormal result should be fully evaluated to determine the suitability of the patient for the laparoscopic procedure (Table 7–1).

CONTRAINDICATIONS TO LAPAROSCOPIC SURGERY

Major Contraindications

Multiple Laparotomies. Patients who have had several abdominal procedures represent an inappropriate level of risk for any laparoscopic procedure.[2] The potential presence of multiple abdominal wall adhesions almost certainly precludes safe laparoscopic entry. These patients are better served by laparotomy. The patient with one or two prior laparotomies may occasionally be managed laparoscopically through a modification of Verres needle insertion into an upper abdominal quadrant or through the use of the Hasson cannula.

Table 7–1. CONTRAINDICATIONS TO LAPAROSCOPIC SURGERY

Major Contraindications	
	Multiple laparotomies
	Coagulopathy
	Cardiac disease (severe)
	CHF
	COPD (severe)
	Peritonitis
	Inexperienced surgeon
Minor Contraindications	
	Generalized ileus or bowel obstruction
	Massive ascites
	Organomegaly
	Abdominal hernia
	Obesity
	Extremely thin patient

Coagulopathy. Any patient with a known coagulopathy should not undergo laparoscopic surgery. Laparotomy would be preferred in order to ensure meticulous hemostasis. However, the patient on anticoagulation may undergo laparoscopic surgery provided the coagulation parameters are corrected preoperatively and perioperatively.

Cardiac Disease. Any patient with a history of myocardial infarction within six months of the planned procedure is at an increased risk for recurrent infarction. Although invasive hemodynamic monitoring can probably allow a significant percentage of patients to safely undergo laparoscopic surgery, it is highly recommended that the elective procedure be deferred for 6 months. Severe cardiac dysfunction represents an absolute contraindication to laparoscopic surgery if the patient will not be able to tolerate the hemodynamic demands of the Trendelenburg or the supine position and pneumoperitoneum.

Severe Chronic Obstructive Lung Disease. The creation of pneumoperitoneum and the resultant elevation of the diaphragm may impair oxygenation and result in hypoxia. Additionally, hypercapnia may result from hypoventilation or from CO_2 absorption, leading to cardiac dysrhythmias. Mechanical ventilation may allow adequate compensation in many patients with less severe pulmonary disease.

Other. Another important contraindication is peritonitis in a patient. An inexperienced surgeon should not attempt laparoscopic surgery.

Minor Contraindications

Laparoscopic surgery for patients with generalized ileus or bowel obstruction, massive ascites, and organomegaly is generally not recommended.

Abdominal Hernias. At one time, the presence of hernias represented a contraindication to laparoscopy. However, as laparoscopic surgery has advanced, it is now possible to carry out elective herniorrhaphy in conjunction with the planned urologic procedure. Herniorrhaphy may be performed laparoscopically, using either an intraperitoneal or properitoneal approach. Several stapling devices and synthetic materials are available that facilitate sound repairs. In the presence of an umbilical hernia, a surgeon may elect to perform laparoscopy with a Hasson cannula followed by open herniorrhaphy.

Obesity. The obese patient may represent a challenge because of the massive bulk of the anterior abdominal parities. However, with modification in technique and experience, many of these patients can safely be offered laparoscopic surgery. A longer Verres needle and long trocars may be necessary for access, or one might consider using a Hasson cannula for open laparoscopy.

Extremely Thin and Cachectic Patients. Just as the obese patient may deviate from the usual anatomic landmarks and relationships, so too may the asthenic patient. It is necessary to be cognizant of the proximity of the great vessels to the skin and to allow appropriate caution. The use of a Hasson cannula should be considered.

It is evident that proper patient selection is equally important as the surgeon's expertise in accomplishing a successful outcome of the desired procedure.

PREOPERATIVE PREPARATION

All patients undergoing laparoscopy should undergo some form of bowel preparation, ranging from a colonic enema to a full mechanical bowel preparation with oral antibiotics. Dairy products are restricted for several days to minimize intestinal distention. One dose of broad-spectrum antibiotics is given parenterally 1 hour before the procedure. Shaving of the abdomen is performed in the operating room.

ANESTHESIA

Laparoscopic surgery should be performed under general anesthesia with muscular relaxation. This provides for optimal patient comfort and avoids complications resulting from attempting entry in an inadequately anesthetized patient. Reflex movements during intra-abdominal dissection may precipitate injury to the viscera and vessels.

Regional anesthesia with spinal or epidural anesthesia has been described in the literature, but has not received wide acceptance. However, in a patient with severe obstructive lung disease or cardiac insufficiency, regional anesthesia may prove useful.

Local anesthesia can be used but only for diagnostic procedures or procedures in which tissue manipulation will be at a minimum. A field block, using bupivacaine or lidocaine, can be performed at the trocar entry sites. The diaphragmatic and peritoneal irritation associated with CO_2 precludes its use, and nitrous oxide is preferred. However, nitrous oxide supports combustion and therefore should not be used with electrocautery.

PREPARATION FOR ENTRY

On induction of general anesthesia, a nasogastric tube is passed to decompress the stomach. Foley catheter placement facilitates bladder decompression and is always recommended in order to reduce the incidence of bladder injury.

The abdomen should be fully prepared from nipple to thigh as for a standard laparotomy. We use a fenestrated laparotomy drape and place an adhesive steri-drape over this to prevent contamination of the field when the table is rotated to extremes. It is important to tape or strap the patient securely so that he or she can be placed in varying degrees of the Trendelenburg, reverse Trendelenburg, or lateral tilt position as the procedure may warrant (Fig. 7–1). A bolster may be placed under the lower back to provide for better pelvic orientation. The patient is placed in 10° to 15° Trendelenburg to prepare for the Verres needle placement.

CREATION OF PNEUMOPERITONEUM

This is the most critical step in the performance of laparoscopic surgery. The correct placement of the Verres needle and proper insufflation of the peritoneal cavity allow for the safe insertion of the trocar and subsequent performance of the procedure.

VERRES NEEDLE

The Verres needle is used to establish pneumoperitoneum. It consists of a blunt-tipped inner stylet surrounded by a sharp outer needle. The inner stylet is spring-loaded, and when the needle is introduced through the abdominal layers, the stylet retracts and allows penetration. However, once the peritoneum is entered, the lack of tissue resistance allows the blunt stylet to protrude and therefore to prevent perforation of abdominal structures. A distally lateral hole on the stylet allows gas entry and creation of the pneumoperitoneum. The proximal end has a stopcock that is connected to the insufflator. The standard lengths of Verres needles are 100 mm, 120 mm, and 150 mm. A modified needle (Verres-Frangenheim) is double-barreled to allow simultaneous insufflation and measurement of intraperitoneal pressure.[3] However, the newer insufflators provide this with a standard Verres needle.

A Foures-Kuss needle has both fore and lateral holes that allow normal insufflation to continue when the distal end is embedded in the omentum. For transvaginal pneumoperitoneum, a Verres needle can be modified with a stop 3 cm proximal to the tip.[2] Verres needles are available as disposable and reusable systems. Disposable needles offer the advantage of consistent sharpness and do not require maintenance. Reusable needles have been used reliably for many years but may pose a small hazard from weakness occurring in the tip at region of the lateral hole. This can lead to bending with repeated use and difficulty in retraction during entry, or even loss of the tip in the abdomen.[4] Careful inspection of the instrument before use is essential for all types of needles.

Placement of the Verres Needle

The patient's abdomen should be examined for scars from prior surgery. The abdomen should be palpated for any organomegaly or intra-abdominal masses that must be avoided during laparoscopic access. One must

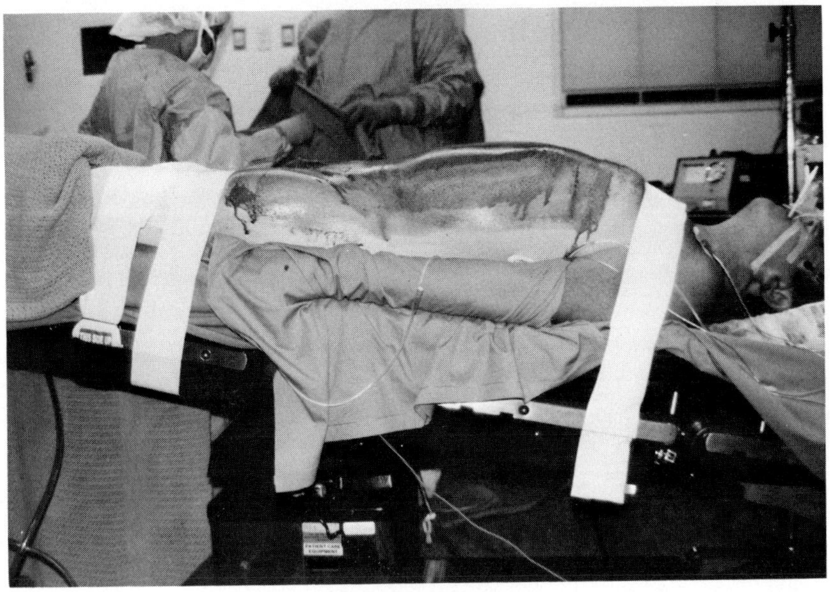

Figure 7–1. The patient must be adequately secured to the operating room table.

be cognizant of the relationship of the umbilicus to the great vessels if they are to be avoided. Careful vigilance at every detail during this stage of the procedure cannot be overemphasized.

Using a No. 15 or No. 11 scalpel blade, a 10-mm curvilinear or longitudinal skin incision is made in the lower edge of the umbilicus. The incision at the umbilicus is critical, because at this point, the distance between the skin and the peritoneum is the smallest with the least amount of properitoneal fat. Blunt dissection is performed to the level of the fascia. The Verres needle is then inserted through the fascia at this location. The Verres needle may also be inserted directly into the umbilicus and the incision may be made before placement of the trocar. The skin incision must be adequate for easy entry of the trocar with no restricting connective tissue bands and at the same time must allow for a good seal around the cannula.

Other sites of insertion include the midline between umbilicus and pubic symphysis, above the umbilicus in the midline, the lateral border of the rectus along the midclavicular line, or the left midclavicular line two fingerbreadths below the costal margin (Fig. 7–2). These alternative sites are used when entry at the umbilicus will be unsuccessful because of properitoneal or subcutaneous placement or when umbilical insertion is contraindicated, as with a prior midline incision. In a female patient, pneumoperitoneum can be effected transvaginally by introducing the Verres needle into the pouch of Douglas.

The Verres needle should be carefully inspected for patency and any defects. The spring mechanism should be tested against a firm surface. The needle is

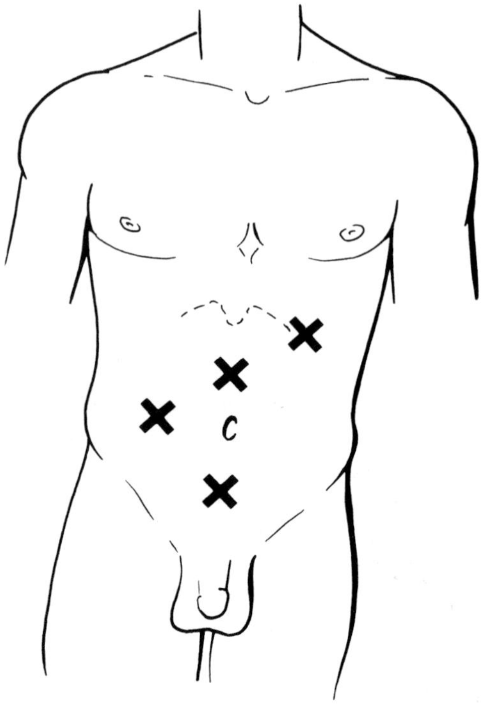

Figure 7–2. Alternative sites for placement of the Verres needle.

then connected to the insufflator to monitor the baseline pressures and to ensure that the insufflator is functional prior to the placement of the needle. The patient is now placed in a 10° to 20° Trendelenburg position.

The Verres needle is grasped by the dominant hand in a secure but comfortable grip (Fig. 7–3). The ulnar

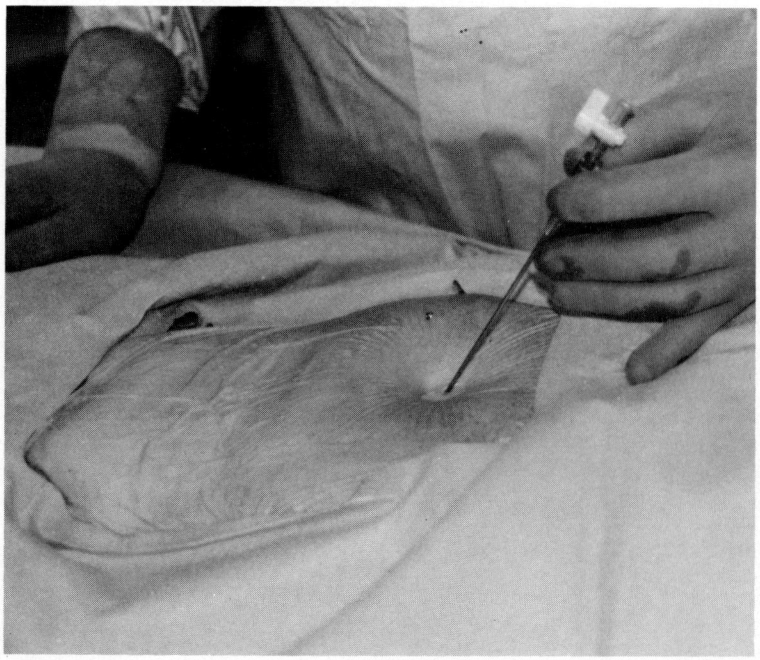

Figure 7–3. Proper entry technique for the Verres needle. Note that the needle may be placed without first incising the skin.

border of the hand is rested on the abdomen to act as a brake. The needle is then advanced at a 45° angle toward the hollow of the pelvis, thereby avoiding the bifurcation of the great vessels. In an obese patient, the angle should be more toward the vertical in order to traverse the thick subcutaneous layer. In a thin patient, the angle should be more toward the horizontal to compensate for proximity of the aorta to the abdominal wall. The entry movement is performed with slow and steady pressure exerted by the wrist, not the shoulder or arm. Overzealous, rapid entry may result in injury to the viscera or great vessels. On the other extreme, a tentative beginner may not advance the needle far enough to enter the peritoneal cavity. Two areas of resistance are encountered, one at the level of the linea alba and the other on penetration of the peritoneum. With experience, these two tactile sensations are readily recognized as is the perceived loss of resistance on entry into the peritoneum. On elevating the abdominal wall, the resulting negative pressure in the peritoneal cavity often causes an audible movement of air into the stopcock.

One may lift the abdominal wall with towel clips or with the nondominant hand. This maneuver is supposed to both lift and stretch the peritoneum. The result is compression of the properitoneal layer, thereby shortening the distance the needle must traverse to enter the peritoneum while increasing the distance between the skin and the great vessels and viscera. This maneuver is controversial; others claim that it does not lift the peritoneum and may actually make peritoneal insertion more difficult.[5] It has been proposed that a near-vertical insertion angle in all patients ensures traversing the shortest distance to the peritoneum. However, there is a risk of great vessel perforation in the asthenic patient. We do not routinely lift the abdominal wall either manually or with towel clips except in thin individuals.

The surgeon should be aware of the advantages and pitfalls of both techniques and should choose a technique with which he or she feels most comfortable. Only through experience does this essential step become second nature and ensure a smooth establishment of pneumoperitoneum.

CONFIRMATION OF NEEDLE PLACEMENT

A variety of tests must be performed to confirm adequate position of the Verres needle.[6] A 5-ml syringe is connected to the Verres needle and aspirated. There should be no return of blood, gastric contents, bowel contents, or urine. Any of these indicates improper placement and needs to be managed accordingly. Injection of 3 to 5 ml of air should not be met with resistance. Finally, 5 to 10 ml of sterile saline should be injected without resistance, and on aspiration there should be no return (Fig. 7–4). Additionally, if the saline is injected through the Verres needle and the syringe is then disconnected, elevation of the abdomen will create a negative pressure and pull the saline into the abdomen.

After these tests one should be reassured that the needle is in proper position; however, these tests are not totally accurate, and one should always proceed with caution.

INSUFFLATION OF THE ABDOMEN

The Verres needle is now connected to the insufflation tubing. The baseline intraperitoneal pressure should be noted. If this pressure is greater than 10 mm Hg one should suspect improper needle placement and

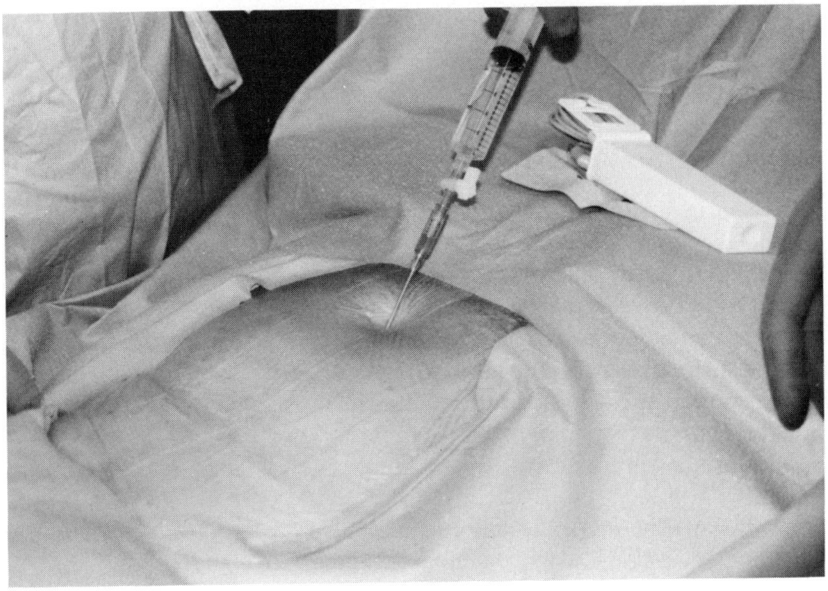

Figure 7–4. The saline should flow easily if the tip of the needle is intraperitoneal.

should consider localization tests and possibly repositioning the needle. If pressure rises suddenly to more than 20 mm Hg, a displaced needle or movement of a loop of bowel or the omentum over the needle tip, blocking the insufflating hole, should be suspected. Often by simply shaking the needle in a gentle fashion, the offending loop of bowel or omentum can be repositioned. If this is unsuccessful, needle reposition or removal and reinsertion is necessary. With flow set at 1 L/minute, within 1 minute loss of liver dullness can be demonstrated by percussion. If this does not occur, a preperitoneal insertion is likely, and the needle should be withdrawn and repositioned. If preperitoneal insertion is not recognized at this point, the preperitoneal space will eventually fill enough to cause loss of liver dullness.

At this time, others advocate testing for free rotation of the needle, consistent with placement within the peritoneal space, and monitoring the intraperitoneal pressure with insufflation at 1 L/minute. If intervening bowel or adhesions come in contact with the needle tip, the pressure will rise; therefore, one can determine if there is a free space for insertion of the trocar. Similarly, a spinal needle connected to a 10-ml syringe with 5 ml of saline can be advanced into the peritoneal space with slow aspiration, and the observation of gas bubbles will confirm placement, upon lateral excursions off midline, any loss of bubbling in the syringe will indicate intervening bowel or adhesions. Although these maneuvers may be of merit on occasion, it is our policy to immediately perform open laparoscopy whenever we encounter difficulty with insufflation or suspect adhesions to be present.

Insufflation at 1 to 3 L/minute is recommended, and the average adult patient requires 4 to 6 L of CO_2 to achieve an intraperitoneal pressure of 12 to 15 mm Hg, which is adequate for trocar insertion. Any further elevation in intraperitoneal pressure is of no benefit and can only lead to vascular and respiratory compromise. Once a sufficient pneumoperitoneum is obtained the Verres needle is removed.

CANNULAS AND TROCARS

Like the insertion of the Verres needle, the insertion of the trocar is a blind procedure. Therefore a thorough understanding of trocar design and operation is required for successful placement, use during the procedure, and removal at the end of the procedure.

The principal cannula and trocar unit is used for initial entry into the peritoneum and then primarily for operation of the laparoscope camera. The secondary cannula and trocar unit is mainly for instrumentation.

A feature common to all cannulas is a valve to prevent gas leakage when the laparoscope or any other instrument is removed from the abdomen. This may be a trumpet or flapper type of valve mechanism. The trumpet valve allows manual opening and closing. The flapper valve works automatically with a self-occluding mechanism. Virtually all cannulas have a lock valve allowing connection to the insufflator unit. An important feature on most cannulas is a small hole at the distal end. This prevents formation of a vacuum that can pull viscera into the cannula during removal of the trocar and cause herniation of viscera through the fascial puncture.[7] This hole also allows for insufflation if the end of the cannula becomes occluded by tissue. Cannulas with both oblique and flat distal end are available; it is questionable if one has an advantage over the other during penetration of the peritoneum.

Another important feature present on several cannulas is a mechanism to prevent the inadvertent removal of the cannula during the procedure. This is not an infrequent event and can be extremely irritating to the operator. Additionally, loss of the cannula during a critical part of the procedure can have potentially disastrous results. Self-retaining sleeves that can be threaded into the fascia are available and are quite effective (Fig. 7–5).[8] Moreover, they can be hemostatic and can possibly prevent abdominal wall bleeding. Adjustable threaded sleeves are desirable as the internal length of the cannula can be easily adjusted and secured (Fig. 7–6). One new product uses expandable arms that stabilize the cannula from within the peritoneum when combined with a locking screw at the skin level (Fig. 7–7). This arrangement provides for excellent retention; however, the possibility of fat or debris preventing easy removal of the cannula re-

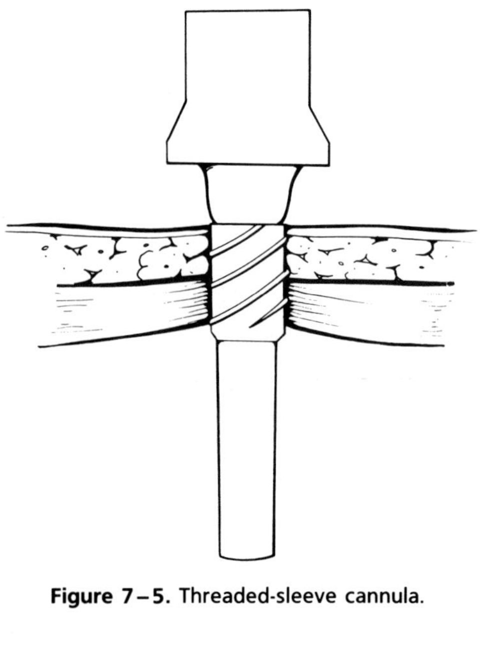

Figure 7–5. Threaded-sleeve cannula.

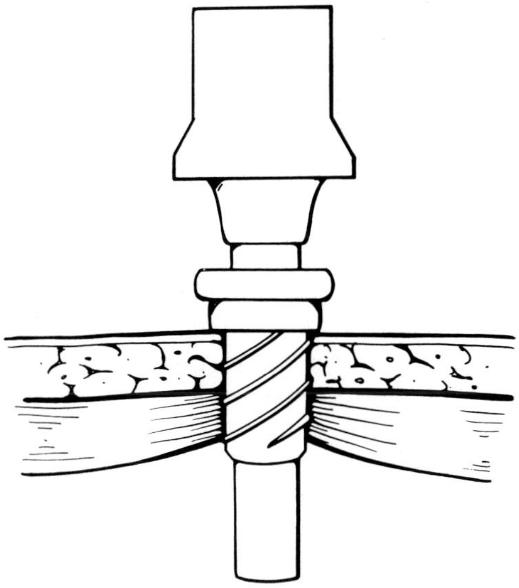

Figure 7–6. Adjustable threaded sleeve.

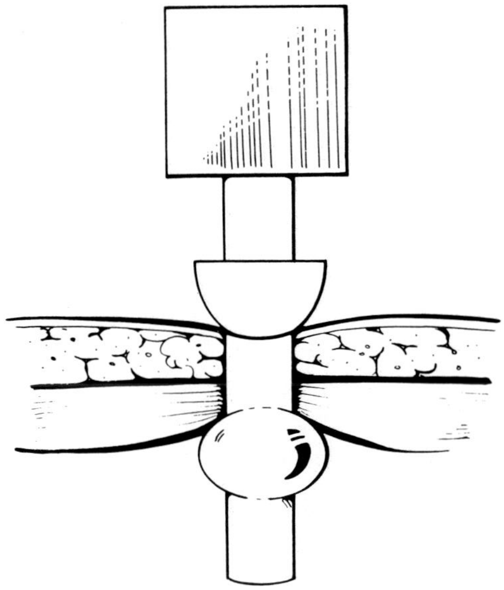

Figure 7–8. Inflatable balloon.

mains a concern. A cannula with an inflatable balloon that lies within the peritoneum is available and when combined with an outer ring, provides for good stabilization of the cannula (Fig. 7–8).

Regardless of the cannula used, we always place an anchoring suture through the skin and tie it around the cannula for additional security.

In patients with prior abdominal surgeries, it is prudent to consider the use of a Hasson cannula (Fig. 7–9). This device consists of a blunt-tipped trocar and a cannula with an outer gasket. The peritoneum is opened, and the cannula is positioned under direct vision (Fig. 7–10). Peritoneal and fascial sutures are secured to the wings of the cannula. The gasket acts as a seal to prevent gas leak. Occasionally, petroleum gauze can be wrapped around the bottom of the cannula to form a better seal. There are also disposable analogs that permit cannula-height adjustment without retying the stay sutures (Fig. 7–11). Another product uses expandable arms that secure the cannula from the inside the peritoneum and enables the surgeon to tent the peritoneum, allowing better exposure.

Although the use of the Hasson cannula was initially suggested for use in the patient with adhesions,

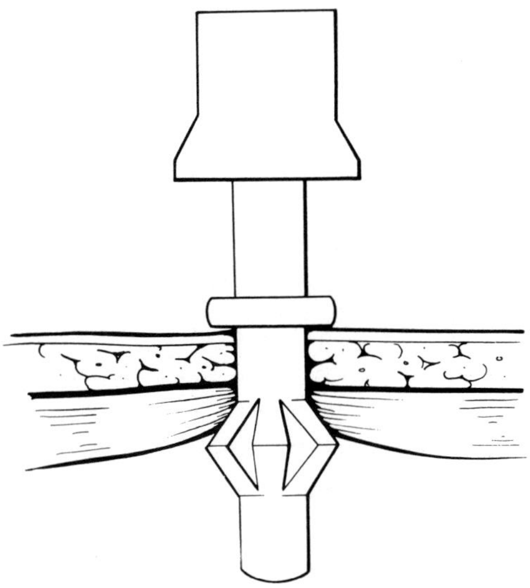

Figure 7–7. Expandable arms.

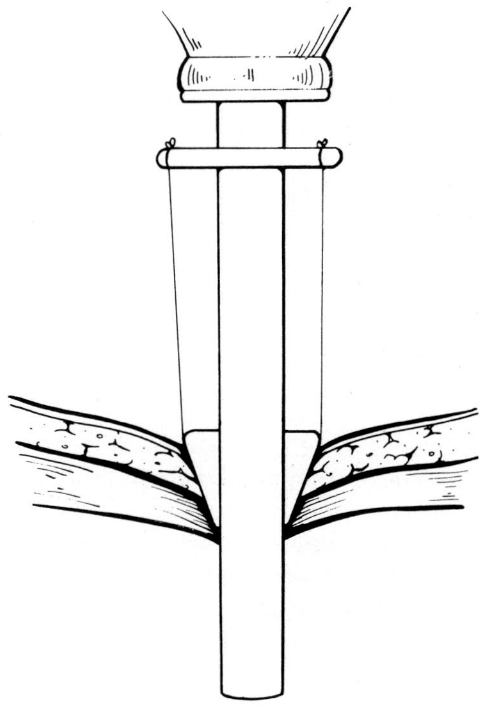

Figure 7–9. The Hasson cannula.

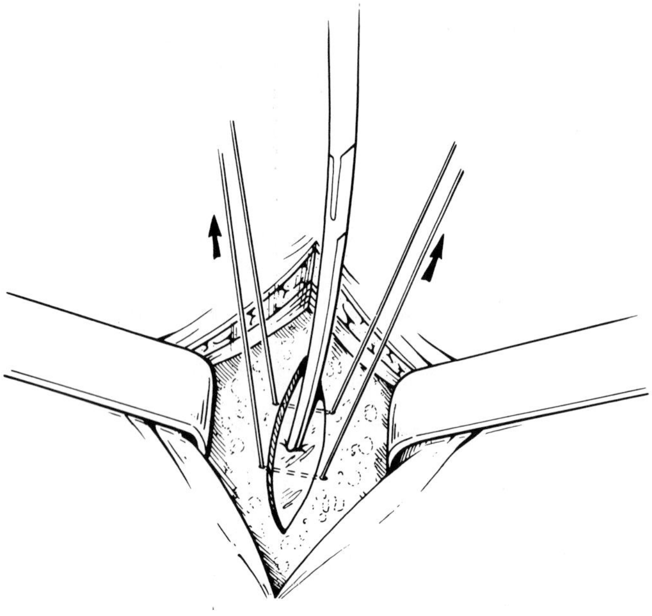

Figure 7–10. Technique for open laparoscopy.

it is invaluable when proper entry of the Verres needle and insufflation is complicated. The open method allows for greater patient safety and should be considered an essential part of the armamentarium for the laparoscopic surgeon.

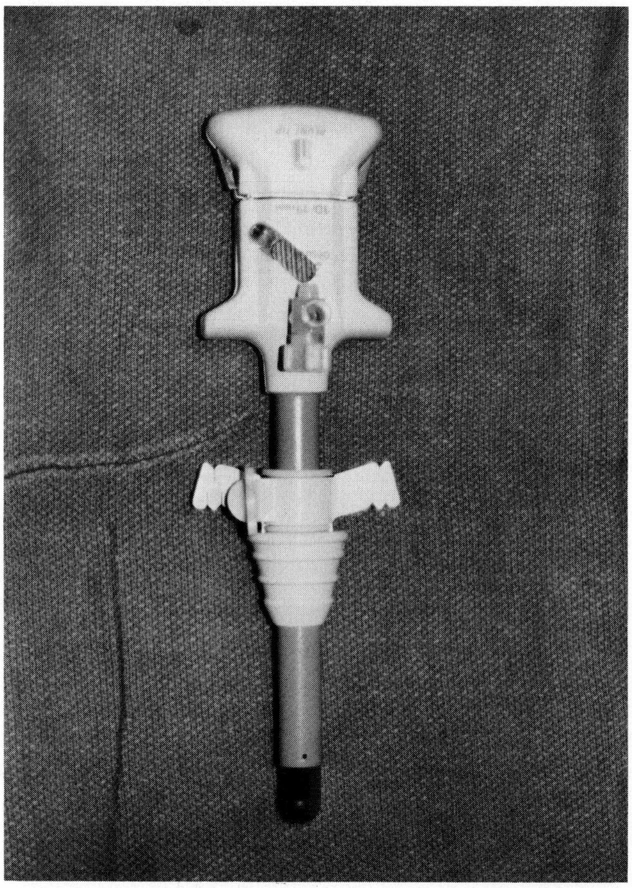

Figure 7–11. Disposable cannula for open laparoscopy.

Another area of debate is that of disposable versus reusable trocars. A recent study found that the disposable devices require half the force for entry as that of the reusable device.[9] It is uncertain if this reduction in force is associated with a decreased incidence of trocar-related injuries. However, it is conceivable that it may lessen the approximation of the abdominal wall to the spine and that the intervening bowel and vessels are therefore less vulnerable to injuries.

A major advance in laparoscopy is the safety shield feature available on several disposable trocars. As the trocar is depressed into the abdomen, a spring-loaded plastic shield is retracted into the cannula. This exposes the sharp trocar tip for penetrating the abdominal parieties. Once inside the peritoneal cavity, the plastic shield protrudes, automatically preventing the sharp end of the trocar from injuring the abdominal contents.

A potential criticism of the shielded products stems from the time interval between entry of the peritoneum and the shielding of the trocar tip. Under normal circumstances, with an adequately insufflated abdomen, this time interval is sufficient for the mechanism to work properly. However, with excessive entering force or an inadequate pneumoperitoneum there is increased risk of injury.

In summary, a shielded trocar can still cause injury to the bowel or major blood vessels, but when used carefully, it may indeed prove to be the standard for entry trocars. We currently recommend a shielded trocar for initial entry.

Insertion of Trocar

The ease of insertion of the trocar depends on the diameter of the cannula and the size of the skin incision. The umbilical incision can be elongated if necessary and can be deepened to the level of the rectus fascia, a small opening being made in the fascia. An 11-mm trocar is firmly grasped in the dominant hand with the index or middle finger placed along the length of the cannula to act as a brake against a sudden forceful movement through the abdominal wall (Fig. 7–12). Alternatively, the opposite hand may be placed around the cannula while resting the ulnar hand surface on the anterior abdominal wall. Elevation of the abdominal wall with towel clips can also increase the margin of safety. The trocar should be angled downward toward the hollow of the sacrum. A slight twisting movement is employed to facilitate passage of the trocar.

The penetration of the peritoneum is often appreciated by a sudden drop in resistance and an audible pop. With successful entry, a rush of gas may be heard escaping through the cannula when the trocar is removed or through the stopcock if it is left in the open position. The insufflating line should now be con-

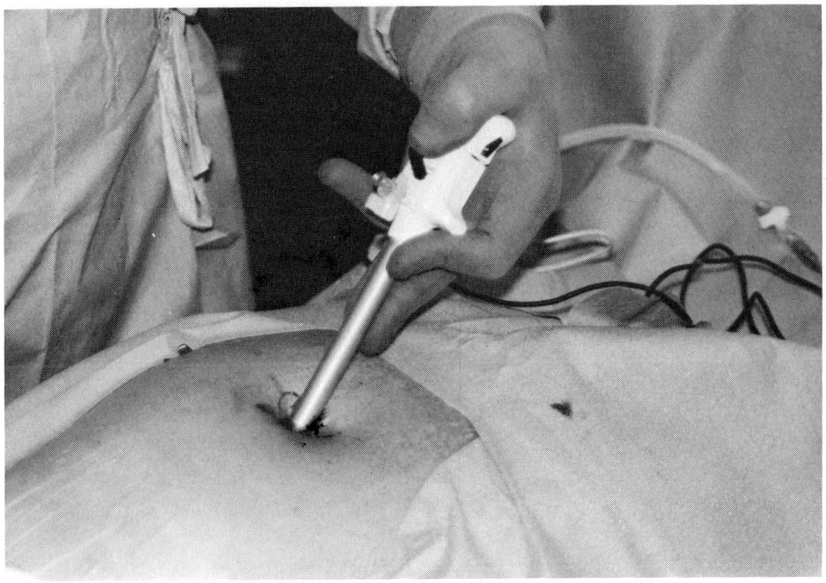

Figure 7–12. Proper bracing of the trocar.

nected to the cannula and placed on automatic flow to maintain intraperitoneal pressure at 12 to 15 mm Hg.

The laparoscope is now introduced (10 mm in diameter, at 0° or 30°), and inspection of the peritoneal cavity is commenced. The area that should be examined first is the region traversed by the Verres needle and the trocar. This is a 360° excursion, and injury to the intestine and the retroperitoneum surrounding the large vessels must be ruled out. Retroperitoneal injuries may not be heralded by free peritoneal blood; rather, they may be associated only with a fullness noted in the retroperitoneum.

It must be stressed that any hypotension mandates thorough examination of the peritoneal cavity. This must not be attributed to anesthesia-related events since a catastrophic large-vessel injury may go unnoticed. If laparotomy is warranted, one can torque the trocar or laparoscope and cut down on it with a scalpel. The retroperitoneal hematoma is evacuated and control of the injured vessel is accomplished.

After major vessel or visceral injury has been ruled out, a thorough survey of the entire abdomen should be undertaken and evidence of metastatic disease or other pathology that was unsuspected should be noted. Obviously, a metastatic deposit in the liver or gross peritoneal seeding precludes laparoscopic lymph node dissection, although biopsy of the metastasis can be performed to confirm the diagnosis.

PLACEMENT OF ACCESSORY PORTS

Depending on the nature of the laparoscopic procedure, additional ports will be required (Fig. 7–13). The cannula widths will vary from 5 mm to 12 mm, depending on the width of the instruments necessary for the procedure. All these can be placed under video monitoring. The lower abdomen should be transilluminated so that larger subcutaneous vessels, especially the superficial epigastric, can be avoided. In a thin patient, even the deep epigastric vessels may be transilluminated. It is imperative to observe the pointing of the peritoneum at the site where the trocar will enter and then to visualize the trocar penetrating the peritoneum. If the trocar appears to overshoot and strike the viscera or posterior peritoneum, one should examine carefully for possible injuries. It is our preference to connect the gas tubing to a port not holding the laparoscope as we believe this will reduce fogging of the camera lens. Only when all accessory ports have been placed and injury has been ruled out can the surgeon commence the operative phase of the laparoscopic procedure.

COMPLETION OF PROCEDURE

Once the operative phase of the laparoscopic procedure is completed there is a tendency to become less vigilant, since the more challenging phase of the procedure has passed. However, it is extremely important to remain focused and to be meticulous regarding the exiting procedure; failure to do so can result in serious complications.

The abdominal pressure should be decreased to 5 mm to allow better identification of potential sources of hemorrhage. A careful survey of the operative field for hemostasis and a thorough examination of the entire abdomen is essential. One may spot areas of bleeding that were not adequately controlled initially or sources of bleeding at sites remote from the operative field that were caused inadvertently. Additionally, there should be inspection for more lymphatic tissue that may have separated from the nodal packet during

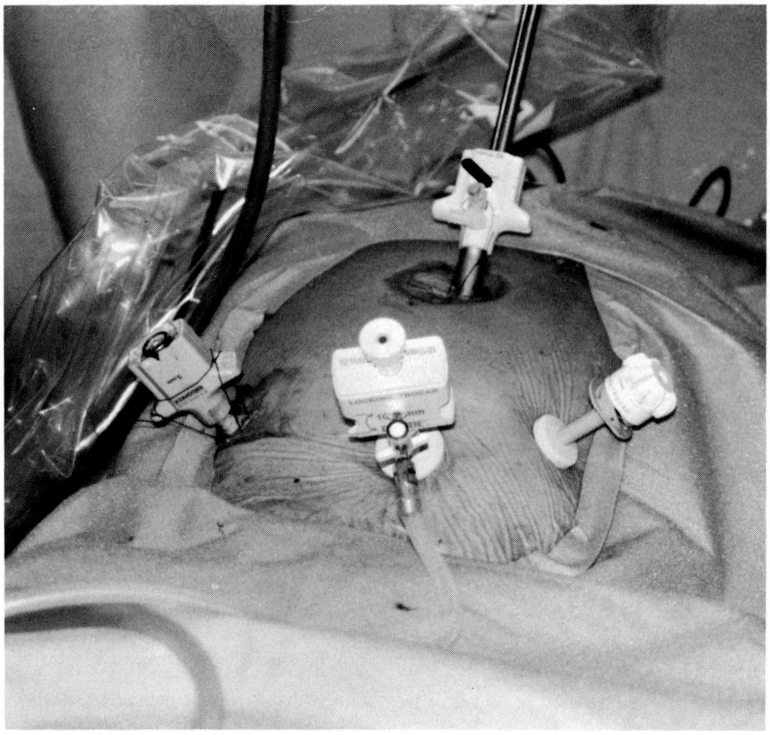

Figure 7–13. Configuration of ports for laparoscopic lymphadenectomy.

its removal. The entry sites of the cannulas should be inspected serially for any bleeding, especially from the deep epigastric vessels.

While removing the cannulas, one must remember that the subumbilical cannula was placed blindly and therefore its entry site into the peritoneum must be observed for bleeding; if this site is not inspected, even a through and through bowel injury may go unnoticed. Therefore the laparoscope is placed through the suprapubic or one of the lateral cannulas, and the entry site of the subumbilical cannula is inspected as the latter is removed from the abdomen. The CO_2 is then removed from the peritoneal cavity with the patient in a more horizontal position to facilitate full evacuation, especially from the subphrenic space. Failure to do this can frequently result in diaphragmatic irritation and postoperative shoulder pain. The anesthesiologist should be asked to hyperventilate the patient and provide deep inspirations. The remaining cannulas are then removed. When the last cannula is to be removed, the laparoscope should be placed within it; the cannula is then removed over the laparoscope. This ensures that omentum or viscera is not pulled out by the tip of the cannula. As an additional measure of safety, the laparoscope can be removed under vision to ensure that any omentum or viscera is not protruding through the defect in the fascia or peritoneum. All trocar sites greater than 10 mm in diameter should be closed with a single 2-0 polydioxanone suture through the anterior fascia to prevent dehiscence or herniation.[10] Any smaller sites do not warrant fascial sutures. The skin can be closed with subcuticular sutures or simply reapproximated with sterile adhesive strips.

CONTROL OF HEMORRHAGE

Hemorrhage requiring further intervention occurs in about 0.64% instances.[11] As a general rule, the large-diameter trocars tend to cause greater vascular injury than the Verres needle, but Verres needles have also been implicated in major vascular injuries. Minor bleeding can occur at the puncture site and is usually well controlled with the use of a suture or a pressure dressing. Small abdominal wall hematomas from the superficial epigastric vessels may require suture ligation and rarely require a subsequent evacuation. Bleeding from the parietal peritoneum can be controlled by electrocautery through the working port and may be lessened by the tamponade effect of the cannula, especially those with internal retaining mechanisms. Injury to the inferior epigastric vessels is often detected by the dripping of blood around the cannula or the observation of a properitoneal or rectus sheath hematoma. Although simple external pressure is often recommended to control hemorrhage, in practice it is often relatively ineffective. If the bleeding is moderate, it can be controlled by electrocautery of the vessels at their origin or by applying the electrocautery to the parietal peritoneum both above and below the cannula entry site.

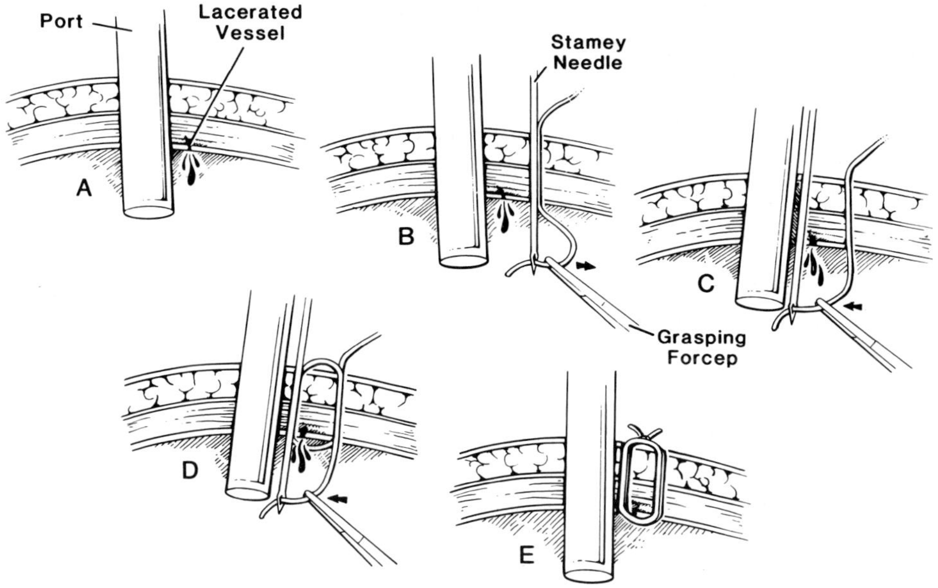

Figure 7–14. Management of epigastric vessel injury; technique of repair. *A*, Lacerated vessel medial to port. *B*, Stamey needle with Prolene ligature has been percutaneously introduced 1 cm medial to the port; the ligature is grasped with grasping forceps and the needle is withdrawn. *C*, The empty needle has been reintroduced, this time alongside the port; grasping forceps are used to thread ligature through the eye of the needle. *D*, The needle has been withdrawn and the entire procedure repeated. *E*, Figure-of-eight suture, ensuring hemostasis. (Courtesy of L. Green, MD.)

With severe bleeding, full-thickness sutures can be placed above and below the bleeding site to control hemorrhage. Intracorporeal suturing can also be attempted, but brisk hemorrhage may obscure the view through the laparoscope. It may be possible to pass percutaneously a Stamey urethropexy needle with a suture attached, and after the suture is grasped with laparoscopic forceps, the Stamey needle can be withdrawn and reintroduced. By repeating such technique, hemostatic sutures can be placed under direct vision (Fig. 7–14).[12]

A Foley catheter can be passed through the incision into the peritoneal cavity and with use of a hemostat can be placed on traction for several hours. If any of these measures are unsuccessful, the abdomen should be opened to obtain direct control of the bleeding vessel.

Perhaps the most serious complication associated with laparoscopy is the injury of a major blood vessel. The incidence of this type of injury is unknown, but the result can be catastrophic with a reported mortality rate of 15%.[11] The distal aorta and common iliac vessels are most often involved, and injuries to the inferior vena cava, iliac veins, and mesenteric vessels are also reported. In one study, the Verres needle was responsible for the majority of the injuries, whereas in another study, the Verres needle and the trocar were equally implicated. Recognition usually occurs because of sudden hypotension. However, with venous injury, the pneumoperitoneum can exert a tamponading effect on the vein, progressive hemorrhage occurring after the pneumoperitoneum is removed. Regardless of the source, upon laparotomy nearly all patients have minimal blood in the peritoneum with large retroperitoneal hematomas. Almost all these hemorrhages can be repaired with a vascular suture.

Several factors are common among the cases of major vascular injuries.[13] Inexperience of the surgeon, dull trocars, improper positioning, lack of elevation of the abdominal wall, perpendicular insertion of the needle or trocar, off-center insertion of the needle or trocar, inadequate pneumoperitoneum, and failure to note important anatomic landmarks have been implicated.

REFERENCES

1. Winfield, HN; Donovan, JF; See, WE; et al: Urological laparoscopic surgery. J Urol 146:941–947, 1991.
2. Saleh, J: Laparoscopy. Philadelphia, WB Saunders, 1988, pp. 253–260.
3. Hulka, J: Textbook of Laparoscopy. Orlando, FL: Grune & Stratton, 1985, pp. 52–71.
4. Phillips, JM: Laparoscopy. Baltimore, Williams & Wilkins, 1977, pp. 220–246.
5. Clayman, RV; Griffith, DP; Kavoussi, LR: Laparoscopy: Tips on technique. Contemp Urol 3:23, 1991.
6. Semm, K: Operative Manual for Endoscopic Abdominal Surgery. Chicago, Year Book Medical Publishers, 1987, pp. 130–151.
7. Reddick, EJ; Olsen, DO: Laparoscopy for the General Surgeon. Tuttlingen, W Ger: Braun-Druck, 1989, pp. 2–18.
8. Reich, H; McGlynn, F: Short self-retaining trocar sleeves for laparoscopic surgery. Am J Obstet Gynecol 162:453–454, 1990.
9. Corson, SL; Batzer, FR; Gocial, G; Maislin, G: Measurement of the force necessary for laparoscopic trocar entry. J Reprod Med 34:282–284, 1989.
10. Kavoussi, LR; Sosa, RE; Capelouto, C: Complications of laparoscopic surgery. J Endourol 6:95–98, 1992.
11. Baadsgaard, SE; Sille, S; Egeblad, K: Major vascular injury during gynecologic laparoscopy. Acta Obstet Scand 68:283–285, 1989.
12. Green, LS; Loughlin, KR; Kavoussi, LR: Management of epigastric vessel injury during laparoscopy. J Endourol 6:99–101, 1992.
13. Penfield, AJ: How to prevent complications of open laparoscopy. J Reprod Meld 30:660–663, 1985.

SECTION IV

LAPAROSCOPIC UROLOGIC PROCEDURES

CHAPTER 8

Laparoscopic Procedures in Pediatric Urology

Sakti Das, MD, FACS

In this era of minimally invasive surgery, laparoscopy probably constitutes the most epochal event. All areas of the abdominothoracic anatomy are now subject to the diagnostic and therapeutic intrusion of laparoscopy. In urology, laparoscopy continues to progress in quantum leaps through the tenacity and scientific pursuit of the pioneers. It is a historical paradox, however, that although the primitive experiments with laparoscopy involved the versatility of the urologic cystoscope, for more than half a century the art and practice of laparoscopy blossomed mostly in the hands of gynecologists. Subsequently, the urologic use of the laparoscope was initiated and for a long time was limited to the field of pediatric urology. In 1973 Gans and Berci were the first to include laparoscopic evaluation of a patient with genitourinary pathology, namely intersex, in their report on 16 pediatric patients.[1] Cortesi and colleagues in 1976 pioneered the more common urologic expediency of laparoscopy in the localization of bilateral interabdominal testes and commended this diagnostic approach as a prelude to surgical exploration in the management of nonpalpable testes.[2] During the same period, Paramo, in Spain, had utilized laparoscopy in six males with cryptorchidism, although this was belatedly communicated by Eason in a letter to the *Journal of Urology*.[3] Thereafter until the recent blitz of urologic laparoscopy, the only serious involvement of the urologists with the laparoscope has been for the localization and evaluation of nonpalpable testes.

Human ingenuity and perseverance, aided by technologic advancements, has prompted us to extend the use of endoscopy beyond the realm of diagnostic exploration. Developments in laparoscopic dissection, initially from gynecologists, have led to more complex urologic surgeries through the laparoscope. As techniques and expertise mature, the indications are prudently extended to the extremes of ages. In the pediatric arena, the current indications of laparoscopy fall into three nonexclusive categories—diagnostic, extirpative, and reparative. Diagnostic categories include visual evaluation with necessary biopsy of intersex states, nonpalpable testes, and pelvic malignancies. Extirpative surgeries imply laparoscopic removal of genitourinary organs for benign and malignant pathologies. Reparative surgeries through the laparoscope are in a state of evolution and include a spectrum of indications from varicocelectomy to more complex and challenging urologic reconstructions. Laparoscopic urology carries special significance in our pediatric population because the reduced trauma of access with minute scars and rapid recovery lead to less psychologic trauma and easier acceptance of surgery by this select group of patients. The following sections elaborate the general techniques of pediatric laparoscopy and the existing indications and techniques for specific laparoscopic procedures in pediatric urology with special emphasis on cryptorchidism.

PEDIATRIC LAPAROSCOPY

In older children and adolescents we utilize the same technique and instruments as in adults (see Chap. 7). Special caution and considerations are imperative during laparoscopy in younger children. Depending upon the indications, laparoscopy has been reported even in a 1-day[1] and a 1-week-old[4] neonate. The smaller accesses, accommodating smaller instruments and optics, often reduce illumination and clarity of the video image. Direct visual examination may be necessary in these circumstances. The surgeon and the assistant should be vigilant about the ports and instruments because the small abdominal girth of young children effectively reduces the critical working distance. General endotracheal anesthesia is supplemented by a caudal block for pelviscopic procedures. For more prolonged surgeries such as nephrectomy and the like, nitrous oxide is avoided to minimize intestinal distension.

The patient is placed supine and the bladder is drained with a no. 8 French feeding tube. A small semilunar incision is made just inside the infraumbilical fold. The Veress needle is introduced after lifting the lower abdominal wall either manually or with Kocher clamps applied to the fascia. In neonates, because the umbilical cord is prominent and the umbilical ring is distensible, the Veress needle and camera port is established at the lateral margin of the rectus abdominis, below the umbilical line. Proper intraperitoneal placement of the Veress needle is ascertained with the aspiration, saline injection, and saline drop test. Carbon dioxide insufflation is begun after setting the maximum intraperitoneal pressure to 14 mm Hg. Low initial pressure of less than 4 mm Hg indicates proper placement of the needle. Undue initial rise of pressure may occur because of the needle's position in the properitoneal space or lying against a loop of bowel, in which case the needle has to be carefully repositioned. Adequate abdominal distention for trocar insertion is usually achieved with instillation of 1.5 to 2.0 L of CO_2 in young children.

The Veress needle is withdrawn and the laparoscopic trocar is introduced. For diagnostic laparoscopy, a 5-mm trocar that accommodates 0° or 30° pediatric laparoscopic lens is usually used. The first objective of visual assessment is to ensure proper intra-abdominal placement of the laparoscope and to check for any intra-abdominal injury or bleeding. Establishment of accessory working ports, patient positioning, and so forth is dictated by the indications and procedure to be undertaken.

CRYPTORCHIDISM

During the last 17 years since the original reports of Cortessi and Paramo, a large body of experience has accumulated substantiating the merits of laparoscopy in the diagnostic localization as well as for definitive surgical procedures for nonpalpable testes.[2–22] In a patient with nonpalpable testes, laparoscopy may be useful for the purposes of (1) localization and evaluation of the missing testis, (2) two-step orchiopexy, (3) laparoendoscopic orchiopexy, and (4) orchiectomy.

Localization and Evaluation

About 20% of patients in most series of undescended testes have nonpalpable testes. Traditionally, nonpalpable testes are approached through a groin incision, and if the inguinal canal is found to be void of any gonadal structures, the incision is extended for intraperitoneal and retroperitoneal exploration. Proper localization and anatomic assessment of the status of the nonpalpable gonad before exploratory surgery should allow rational planning for the more suitable orchiopexy, and such planned surgery may yield better testicular salvage. Other localization procedures for the cryptorchid testes include spermatic venography,[23] spermatic arteriography,[24] herniography,[25] radionuclide scanning, abdominal ultrasound,[26] computed tomography (CT),[27] and magnetic resonance imaging (MRI).[28] Arteriography and venography are invasive procedures requiring separate general anesthesia. Abdominal ultrasound, radionuclide scanning, and CT yield inconsistent results. The hazards of imaging radiation exposure to the younger boys with some of these procedures is of added concern. MRI is poorly tolerated by younger children because of the claustrophobia aggravated by prolonged scanning time. It is not cost effective, and often imaging of the smaller intra-abdominal testes is obscure. Laparoscopy immediately prior to exploration, on the other hand, has proved successful in up to 100% of instances in correctly localizing or identifying the cryptorchid testes.

There are three potential laparoscopic findings in patients with nonpalpable testes: (1) Intra-abdominal testes are visible inside the abdomen proximal to the deep inguinal ring (Figure 8–1). The degree of testicular atrophy and associated epidiymal anomalies are visually assessed. (2) In canalicular testes the vas deferens and spermatic vessels are seen to converge and exit at the deep inguinal ring (Fig. 8–2). Milking the inguinal canal, often associated with an indirect inguinal hernia, may cause the testis to emerge into the neck of the hernia at the deep inguinal ring (Fig. 8–3). It is often possible to negotiate the laparoscope into the inguinal hernia through the deep ring and visualize more distal canalicular testes. Presence of an inguinal hernia does not automatically imply that the

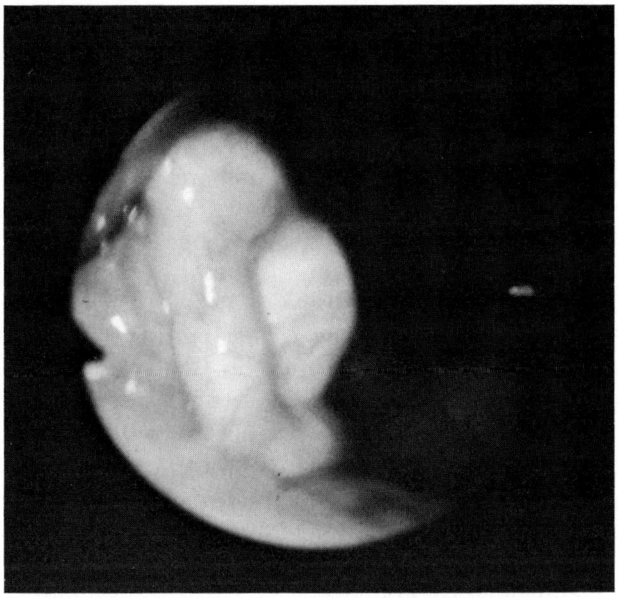

Figure 8–1. Intra-abdominal testis. See also Color Plate 1.

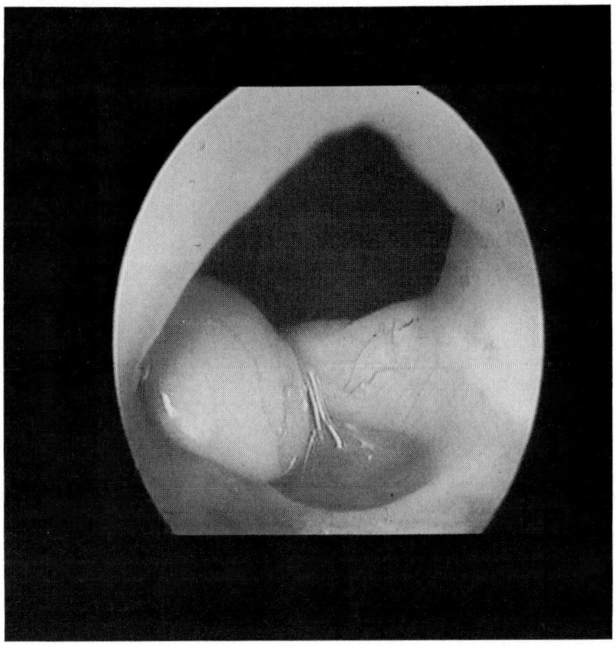

Figure 8–3. Inguinal hernia with canalicular testis. See also Color Plate 2.

testicular structures are distal to the deep ring. We have treated a child who underwent an inguinal hernia repair and on subsequent laparoscopy two years later was proved to have a high-lying intra-abdominal testis. (3) In anorchia, or vanishing testes, blind termination of the vas deferens and spermatic vessels is found (Fig. 8–4). Laparoscopic observation of the vas deferens and gonadal vessels with blind endings proximal to the deep inguinal ring is convincing enough evidence of vanishing testes so that no further surgical exploration is necessary. In recent series 45% to 64% of unilateral nonpalpable testes were found to have blind-ending cord structures. Of these, in 14% to 27% of cases the cord structures ended proximal to the deep ring and therefore laparoscopy was beneficial in obviating an extended groin exploration.[22,29]

One must however observe the blind-ending gonadal vessels before a diagnosis of anorchia can be entertained. In the literature, there has never been a report of a testis located geographically away from the termination of its vessels. On rare occasions when the vas deferens is seen to end blindly with no testis or spermatic vessels in the vicinity, one should explore for the latter structures, because they may be lying high and disjunct from the vas deferens. But whenever a testes is present, it cannot be disjunct from the

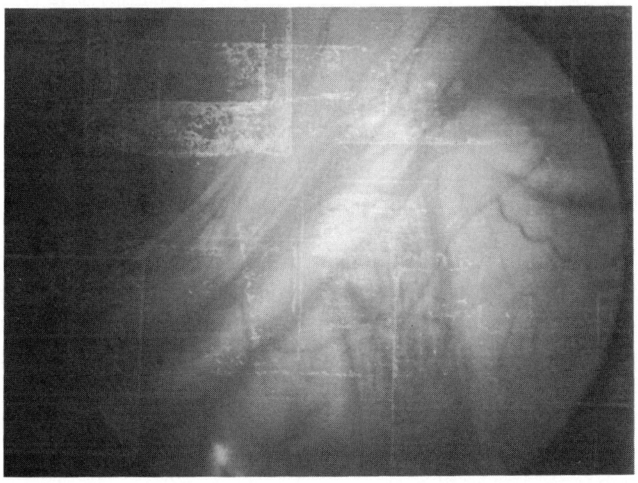

Figure 8–2. Right canalicular testis. Vas deferens and spermatic vessels can be seen exiting at the deep inguinal ring. See also Color Plate 2.

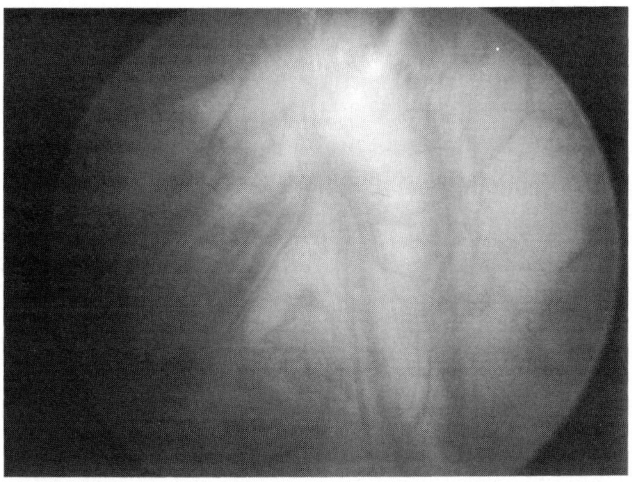

Figure 8–4. Anorchia. Blind termination of vas deferens and spermatic vessels. See also Color Plate 2.

termination of its vessels. One of our patients and another in the series of Weiss and Seashore[12] affirm the therapeutic axiom that whether by laparoscopic or by open exploration, if the termination of the gonadal vessels is not identified, a meticulous transperitoneal search should be undertaken to locate or exclude the possibility of a proximal high-lying testes.

Our laparoscopic experience dictates that inguinal exploration alone for nonpalpable testes often is deceptively inadequate, especially when evidences of gonadal elements and cord structures are not unequivocally established. Boddy and associates[11] reported on 13 boys declared to have no testes after extensive inguinal exploration and found five salvageable intra-abdominal testes on subsequent laparoscopy. The perils of subsequent malignancies in missed supracanalicular testes cannot be overemphasized. Brothers and co-workers[30] reviewed 13 instances of testicular tumors arising in patients believed to be missing a testis that later became malignant, including four who had undergone previous explorations without results.

Compared with other localization procedures, laparoscopy is an extremely specific and sensitive test that provides direct visual evidence of the location and anatomic status of the nonpalpable testes. It has only rare false-negative and no false-positive interpretations.

Two-Step Orchiopexy

Following laparoscopic localization of a salvageable abdominal testis in younger children or in older boys with a compromised contralateral gonad, it may be worthwhile to preserve and relocate the testis toward the scrotum. Testicular autotransplantation[5,31] and staged orchiopexy[32] are difficult although feasible surgical options in the management of a high-lying testis, but the preferred approach has been the Fowler-Stephens orchiopexy[33] whereby the spermatic vessels are divided and the testis is mobilized on the vas deferens with the hope that the vasal blood supply will sustain the vascular needs of the testis. Stephens stated that the anatomic criteria for a successful Fowler-Stephens orchiopexy include a long-loop vas deferens, short spermatic vessels and prune-belly syndrome.[34] Unfortunately, these criteria are rarely fulfilled, and specifically a long-loop vas, which is the most important criteria, is not a common form of vasal anatomy. Even in highly selected patients, the success rate of Fowler-Stephens orchiopexy ranged from 50% to 86%. In 1982 Duckett proposed preliminary in situ ligation of the spermatic vessels with the intent that vasal collaterals to the testis would be enhanced and that subsequent later division of the spermatic vessels and vas-based orchiopexy would have improved potential for success. In laboratory animal study, Pascual and colleagues[35] observed that following spermatic vascular interruption, blood flow to the testes was reduced by 80% at 1 hour but returned to normal by 30 days. Ransley and associates[36] in 1984 reported favorable results in their series of boys subjected to this staged Fowler-Stephens procedure.

With the advent of laparoscopy, Bloom[37] utilized the concept of in situ ligation by applying hemostatic clips to interrupt the spermatic vessels from the testes. A second trocar of 10 mm diameter is necessary for passage of the clip applicator. About 6 months after clipping, the patient is explored for the stage 2 of two-step orchiopexy. The spermatic vessels are ligated and divided cephalad to the clip. After inscribing a wide peritoneal cuff around the testis and vas deferens, the latter structures are carefully mobilized to gain length for placement in the scrotum. Early results of two-step orchiopexy in the albeit small series reported by Bloom are encouraging. Six of seven testes showed normal size and growth compared with that of the contralateral gonad at 6 to 39 months follow-up. The only failure was in a boy who already had testicular atrophy following two prior inguinal explorations. Waldschmidt and Schier[4] advocated spermatic vessel ablation by laser with the obvious advantage of using a smaller trocar for the laser probe. They successfully accomplished the second stage 4 weeks following the laparoscopic vascular interruption. Based on the laboratory data of Pasqual and co-workers, it should be feasible and may be advisable to carry out the second stage at an earlier date after waiting 4 weeks.

There are several distinct advantages of laparoscopic two-step orchiopexy for high-lying testis over the orthodox single-stage Fowler-Stephens procedure. It is applicable for any salvageable abdominal testis whether or not associated with a long-loop vas deferens. Proximal clip ligation or laser ablation interrupts the spermatic vessels with virtually no dissection or disturbance of the testis or the vasal arcades of circulation. Although the two-step procedure requires two separate anesthesias and operative interventions, the laparoscopic first step is rapid and minimally invasive. The second stage is of known quantity and is executed with no uncertainty of exploration, and a precisely contrived dissection optimizes the success of vasal pedicle orchiopexy.

Orchiectomy

Removal of an intra-abdominal testis becomes imperative in situations such as postpubertal patients and obviously atrophic nonsalvageable testes. A unilateral high-lying testis with a normal contralateral gonad constitutes a relative indication for orchiectomy. Carcinoma in situ and obvious malignancies have been reported in as many as 8% of these abnormally descended testes.[38]

With the available instrumentation for laparoscopic dissection, orchiectomy can be carried out expeditiously at the time of laparoscopy by clipping and dividing the spermatic vessels and vas deferens in sequence and then dissecting the distal peritoneal and gubernacular attachments. The freed testis is contained in a laparoscopic pouch and removed through a port.[39]

Laparoendoscopic Orchiopexy

A new technique of laparoscopic orchiopexy was reported by Jordan and associates[40] whereby a high-lying intra-abdominal testis was first mobilized by laparoscopic dissection of the spermatic vessels, vas deferens, and the associated inguinal hernia. A 10-mm trocar was then introduced through the scrotal Dartos pouch into the peritoneal cavity. The mobilized testis was grasped through the scrotal trocar, brought down into the Dartos pouch, and anchored there. The authors claim that the delayed second stage orchiopexy following laparoscopic in situ clipping of the spermatic vessels also should be feasible by their laparoendoscopic technique thereby obviating an open laparotomy incision.

INTERSEX STATES

In suspected intersex patients with ambiguous genitalia, laparoscopy constitutes the most definitive and minimally invasive procedure for the inspection and necessary biopsy or removal or intra-abdominal gonadal structures (see Chap. 9).

Even during laparoscopy for cryptorchidism, one should entertain the possibility of finding muellerian structures. Lowe and co-workers[7] reported one patient with gonadal dysgenesis in their laparoscopy series of 33 patients with nonpalpable testes. Wolfman and Kreutner[41] reported their laparoscopic experience with 13 adolescents having gonadal dysgenesis, three with vaginal agenesis and two with gonadal agenesis. Waldschmidt and Schier[4] recently reported a large series of laparoscopy in neonates and infants that included diagnostic laparoscopy of six patients with ambiguous genitalia, five of which also underwent laparoscopic gonadectomy. The spectrum of laparoscopic findings in intersex states in the several reports included absent gonads, streak gonads, and normal-appearing gonads with various abnormal muellerian derivatives. With the available laparoscopic expertise, a diagnostic open laparotomy in these children can no longer be condoned.

ADOLESCENT VARICOCELES

Varicoceles in the adolescent are unique abnormalities of unknown etiology and natural history. Consequently there is no consensus regarding their management. Varicoceles are not observed in childhood, but their prevalence is between 14.7% and 16.2% in 10- to 14-year-old adolescent males.[42,43] More than one third of these varicoceles are pronounced—25% are grade II and 11% are grade III. The effects of various factors, such as increased scrotal temperature and altered hormonal milieu, can lead to progressive testicular atrophy. Okuyama and associates[44] carefully followed 40 adolescents with varicoceles, including 24 who were subjected to varicocelectomy and 16 who were only observed. Significant improvement of pre-existing testicular atrophy and normalization of seminal patterns were observed more commonly in the males subjected to varicocelectomy. The adolescents followed up with no surgical venous interruption continued to have deterioration of testicular size and seminal patterns. Internal spermatic vein ligation is therefore recommended in adolescents with varicoceles whenever there is 20% or more discrepancy in testicular size secondary to testicular atrophy.

Laparoscopic internal spermatic vein ligation has several distinct advantages over open vein ligation in this age group. The relatively smaller incisions for access are more cosmetically appealing. Significantly less pain allows quicker recovery and early resumption of activities such as sports and education. Open internal spermatic vein ligation has been associated with a 5% to 16% recurrence rate.[45] The majority of these recurrences are attributable to missed accessory internal spermatic veins or aberrant tributaries communicating with cremasteric, vasal, and presacral veins.[46] The retroperitoneal anatomy at and above the internal inguinal ring is clearly depicted during laparoscopy and should allow better identification of all the venous channels, leading to a more thorough venous interruption and, it is to be hoped, less incidence of recurrence.[47]

The cardinal reason for internal spermatic vein interruption in adolescents with varicoceles is to prevent and often reverse testicular atrophy. Therefore every effort must be made to identify and preserve the integrity of the testicular artery during the dissection and clipping of the venous channels. It is advisable not to use electrocautery during laparoscopic varicocelectomy to prevent inadvertent arterial injury or spasm. Identification of a testicular artery in spasm is often aided by laparoscopic Doppler probes and facilitated by sprinkling papaverine solution in the area of dissection. On the whole, the magnification and more focused surgical dissection allows sparing of the artery and lymphatics with a higher degree of precision than does open surgery.

MISCELLANEOUS SURGERIES

Nephrectomy, Nephroureterectomy, and Partial Nephrectomy. As a logical extension of our adult experience, laparoscopic nephrectomy, partial nephrectomy, and nephroureterectomy becomes more technically feasible in the pediatric population because most commonly the indications involve small, minimally functioning or atrophic kidneys. We have successfully accomplished nephroureterectomy in an 11-year-old girl to remove an end-stage shrunken kidney secondary to vesicoureteric reflux.[48] The child went home on the second postoperative day and did not require parenteral analgesics. Laparoscopic removal of a multicystic dysplastic kidney has been carried out on a 6-month-old child, although such pathologies do not require extirpation unless the diagnosis is equivocal or associated conditions mandate exploration (LR Kavoussi, MD, personal communication). Similarly, removal of congenital hypoplastic kidneys causing hypertension and partial nephrectomy in duplex kidneys with obstruction, ectopia, or reflux can be accomplished by laparoscopic dissection.

Renal Biopsy. Laparoscopic renal biopsy offers the advantage of direct visual hemostasis, especially when percutaneous biopsy is contraindicated. We prefer to perform this by retroperitoneal laparoscopic technique (see Chap. 14).[49] Bleeding from the biopsy site is usually controlled by direct pressure application of microfibrillar collagen with a special laparoscopic applicator, and laparoscopic suturing of the renal capsule is rarely necessary.

Pyeloplasty. Early experience with laparoscopic dismembered pyeloplasty for ureteropelvic junction obstruction proves the feasibility of such a low-morbidity approach.[50] With increasing experience, technical advancements, and improvement in our surgical finesse, especially in endoscopic suturing, laparoscopic pyeloplasty can be expected to establish itself as the prudent surgical choice. Similarly, anastomotic procedures such as pyeloureterostomy and ureteroureterostomy for pathologies associated with duplicated ureters should become feasible laparoscopically in the near future.

Antireflux Surgery. Experimental works are in progress in attempting laparoscopic antireflux surgery in the form of extravescial ureterovesicoplasty.[51] Whether such techniques will prove clinically feasible with results comparable to the well-established open techniques of ureteral reimplantation remains a challenging question.

Bladder Surgeries. Simple cystectomy, partial cystectomy, removal of urachal cysts, and bladder diverticulectomy have been reported in adults and can be employed for specific indications in the pediatric population. Waldschmidt and Schier[4] reported on laser ablation of urachal fistula in a child. Augmentation as well as reduction cystoplasties should be feasible with improvement of endosuturing techniques and development of absorbable stapling devices. Ehrlich has mentioned carrying out laparoscopic seromyotomy for bladder autoaugmentation.[52]

Pediatric Hernia Repair. Although endoscopic hernia repair has become an established procedure in adults, the morbidity and potential complications of such procedure through multiple ports does not make it less invasive than the conventional hernia surgery in children. Pediatric laparoscopic hernia repair may be carried out only in conjunction with another primary endoscopic procedure.

Laparoscopic Exploration and Biopsy of Pelvic Malignancies. Laparoscopy provides a minimally invasive tool for inspection and biopsy for initial diagnosis as well as for monitoring chemotherapeutic responses in pelvic sarcomas.

CONCLUSIONS

Laparoscopic procedures in urology were initiated in the domain of pediatric urology with evaluation of nonpalpable testes. Expanding on the diagnostic experience and aided by advancements in laparoscopic dissection techniques, laparoscopy has now extended to surgical management of high-lying intra-abdominal testes with staged orchiopexy, laparoscopic orchiopexy, or orchiectomy. In addition, the various adult urologic laparoscopic procedures are now applicable for similar indications in the pediatric population. The unavoidable challenge of transformation to laparoscopic urology is perceptible in pediatrics as much as in other spheres of urology. It is essential, however, to exercise extra precaution during laparoscopy in children because of their small size and certain anatomic characteristics that are liable to result in injuries to the bladder, intestines, and stomach. Administration of anesthetics with care and vigilance toward respiratory compromise and complications of hypercarbia should be emphasized from the onset. Caution and prudence assume extraordinary significance when pragmatic decision is poised between the extremes of safety and therapeutic excellence.

"If you can meet with triumph and disaster and treat those two imposters just the same. . . ."

RUDYARD KIPLING

REFERENCES

1. Gans, SL; Berci, G: Peritoneoscopy in infants and children. J Pediatr Surg 8:399, 1973.
2. Cortesi, N; Ferrari, P; Zambarda, E; et al: Diagnosis of bilateral abdominal cryptorchidism by laparoscopy. Endoscopy 8:33, 1976.
3. Eason, AC: Laparoscopy for cryptorchidism. (Letter) J Urol 128:829, 1982.
4. Waldschmidt, J; Schier, F: Laparoscopical surgery in neonates and infants. Eur J Pediatr Surg 1:145, 1991.
5. Silber, SJ; Cohen, R: Laparoscopy for cryptorchidism. J Urol 124:928, 1980.
6. Scott, JES: Laparoscopy as an aid in the diagnosis and management of the impalpable testis. J Pediatr Surg 17:14, 1982.
7. Lone, DH; Brock, WA; Kaplan, GW: Laparoscopy for localization of nonpalpable testes. J Urol 131:728, 1984.

8. Malone, PS; Guiney, EJ: The value of laparoscopy in localizing the impalpable undescended testes. Brit J Urol 56:429, 1984.
9. Manson, AL; Terhune, D; Jordan, G; et al: Preoperative laparoscopic localization of the nonpalpable testes. J Urol 134:919, 1985.
10. Paramo, PG; Gutierrez del Olmo, A; Paramo, PS Jr; et al: Estudio comparativo entre los metodos diagnosticos preoperatonos del testiculo intra-abdominal III: precesion de la laparoscopia. Actas Urol Esp 9:331, 1985.
11. Boddy, S; Corkery, JJ; Gornall, P: The place of laparoscopy in the management of the impalpable testes. Br J Surg 72:918, 1985.
12. Weiss, RM; Seashore, JH: Laparoscopy in the management of nonpalpable testes. J Urol 138:382, 1987.
13. Bloom, DA; Ayers, JWT; McGuire, EJ: The role of laparoscopy in the management of nonpalpable testes. J Urol (Paris) 94:465, 1988.
14. Das, S; Amar, AD: The impact of laparoscopy on modern urologic practice. Urol Clin North Am 15:537, 1988.
15. Naslund, MJ; Gearhart, JP; Jeffs, RD: Laparoscopy: Its selected use in patients with unilateral nonpalpable testes after human chorionic gonadotrophin stimulation. J Urol 142:108, 1989.
16. Guiney, EJ; Corbally, M; Maline, PS: Laparoscopy and the management of the impalpable testis. Br J Urol 63:313, 1989.
17. Doig, CM: Use of laparoscopy in children with impalpable testis. Int J Androl 12:420, 1989.
18. Elder, JS: Laparoscopy and Fowler-Stephens orchiopexy in the management of the impalpable testes. Urol Clin North Am 16:399, 1989.
19. Castilho, LN: Laparoscopy for the nonpalpable testis: How to interpret the endoscopic findings. J Urol 144:1215, 1990.
20. Das, S: Laparoscopic evaluation of nonpalpable testes. Urology 37:460, 1991.
21. Peloquin, F; Kiruluta, G; Quiros, E: Management of an impalpable testis: The role of laparoscopy. Can J Surg 34:587, 1991.
22. Heiss, KF; Shandling, B: Laparoscopy for the impalpable testes: Experience with 53 testes. J Pediatr Surg 27:175, 1992.
23. Diamond, AB; Meng, CH; Kodroff, M; et al: Testicular venography in the nonpalpable testis. Am J Roent 129:71, 1977.
24. Ben-Menachem, Y; DeBerardinis, MC; Salinas, R: Localization of intra-abdominal testes by selective testicular arteriography: A case report. J Urol 112:493, 1974.
25. White, JJ; Shaker, IJ; Oh, KS; et al: Herniography: A diagnostic refinement in the management of cryptorchidism. Am Surg 39:624, 1973.
26. Weiss, RM; Carter, AR; Rosenfield, AT: High resolution real-time ultrasonography in the localization of the undescended testis. J Urol 135:936, 1986.
27. Wolverson, MK; Jagannapharao, B; Sundram, M; et al: CT in localization of impalpable cryptorchid testes. Am J Radiol 134:725, 1980.
28. Kogan, BA; Hricak, H; Tanagho, EA: Magnetic resonance imaging in genital anomalies. J Urol 138:1028, 1987.
29. Caldamone, AA: Laparoscopy for the impalpable testis. Dialog Pediatr Urol 15:5, 1992.
30. Brothers, LR; Weber, CH Jr; Ball, TP Jr: Anorchism versus cryptorchidism: The importance of a diligent search for intra-abdominal testes. J Urol 119:707, 1978.
31. Upton, J; Schuster, SR; Colodny, AH; et al: Testicular autotransplantation in children. Am J Surg 145:514, 1983.
32. Corkery, JJ: Staged orchiopexy—a new technique. J Pediatr Surg 10:515, 1975.
33. Fowler, R Jr; Stephens, FD: The role of testicular vascular anatomy in the salvage of high undescended testes. Aust NZ J Surg 29:92, 1959.
34. Stephens, FD: Fowler-Stephens orchiopexy. Semin Urol 6:103, 1988.
35. Pascual, JA; Villanueva-Meyer, J; Salido, E; et al: Recovery of testicular blood flow following ligation of testicular vessels. J Urol 142:549, 1989.
36. Ransley, PG; Vordermark, JS; Caldamone, AA; et al: Preliminary ligation of the gonadal vessels prior to orchiopexy for the intra-abdominal testicle: A staged Fowler-Stephens procedure. World J Urol 2:266, 1984.
37. Bloom, DA: Two-step orchiopexy with pelviscopic clip ligation of the spermatic vessels. J Urol 145:1030, 1991.
38. Krabbe, S; Skakkebaek, NE; Berthelsen, JG; et al: High incidence of undetected neoplasia in maldescended testes. Lancet 1:999, 1979.
39. Castilho, LN; Ferreeira, U; Esteves, SC; et al: Laparoscopic orchiectomy. J Urol 145:206A, 1991.
40. Jordan, GH; Robey, EL; Winslow, BH: Laparoendoscopic surgical management of the abdominal/transinguinal undescended testis. J Endourol 6:159, 1992.
41. Wolfman, WL; Kreutner, K: Laparoscopy in children and adolescents. J Adolesc Health Care 5:261, 1984.
42. Oster, J: Varicocele in children and adolescents: An investigation of the incidence among Danish school children. Scand J Urol Nephrol 5:27, 1971.
43. Steeno, O; Knops, J; Declerck, L; et al: Prevention of fertility disorders by detection and treatment of varicocele at school and college age. Andrologie 8:47, 1976.
44. Okuyama, A; Nakamura, M; Namiki, M; et al: Surgical repair of varicocele at puberty: Preventive treatment for fertility improvement. J Urol 139:562, 1988.
45. Zaontz, MR; Firlit, CF: Use of venography as an aid in varicocelectomy. J Urol 138:1041, 1987.
46. Kogan, SJ: Prevention of persistent varicocele. Soc Pediatr Urol Newsletter, p. 6, Feb 22, 1984.
47. Hagood, PG; Mehan, DJ; Parra, R: Laparoscopic varicocelectomy: Preliminary report of a new technique. J Urol 147:73, 1992.
48. Das, S; Keizur, JJ; Tashima, MK: Laparoscopic nephroureterectomy for end-stage reflux nephropathy in a child. Surg Lap Endosc 3:462, 1993.
49. Keizur, JJ; Tashima, M; Das, S: Retroperitoneal laparoscopic renal biopsy. Surg Lap Endosc 3:60, 1993.
50. Vancaillie, TG; Schuessler, WW; Preminger, GM: Laparoscopic dismembered pyeloplasty. J Urol 149:958A, 1993.
51. Atala, A; Goldstein, DS; Kavoussi, LR; et al: Laparoscopic correction of vesicoureteral reflux. J Urol 149:960A, 1993.
52. Ehrlich, R; Gershman, A; Fuchs, G; et al: Expanding horizons in pediatric laparoscopy. J Urol 149:190A, 1993.

CHAPTER 9

Laparoscopy in the Management of Intersex States

Ubirajara Ferreira, MD
Nelson Rodrigues Netto, Jr, MD
Sandro Cassiano Esteves, MD

The normal development of the reproductive systems requires that a series of interrelated and organized steps occur in an orderly and sequential manner (Fig. 9–1). The first step in this process is the establishment of the genetic sex; this determines the gonadal sex, which determines the phenotypic sex. Any disturbance along this sequence may be reflected clinically as disorder of sexual differentiation.

It is imperative for the physician to recognize such a disorder as soon as possible following birth. The most obvious phenotypic clue is the presence of ambiguous genitalia.

In three of four diseases that result in ambiguous external genitalia, disorders of androgen synthesis or action are usually present, and cryptorchidism is frequently detected. However, clinical and laboratory assessment may not diagnose all intersex disorders. In such cases, gonadal biopsy and exploratory laparotomy are indicated to detect testicular, ovarian, or gonadal streak tissue.

In order to avoid the surgical procedure, laparoscopy can be indicated to localize müllerian duct remnants and gonadal tissue in intersex states and even to perform gonadal biopsy or gonadectomy.

AMBIGUOUS EXTERNAL GENITALIA

Ambiguous external genitalia is observed in four different sex disorders (Table 9–1): (1) female pseudohermaphroditism, (2) male pseudohermaphroditism, (3) mixed gonadal dysgenesis, and (4) true hermaphroditism (Fig. 9–2).

Female Pseudohermaphroditism

Female pseudohermaphroditism is the most common cause of ambiguous external genitalia in the newborn period. The patient has 46 XX karyotype, bilateral ovaries, internal müllerian ducts, and varying degrees of virilization of the external genitalia.[1] This virilization may be caused by (1) excessive androgen secretion by the adrenal glands (adrenogenital syndrome in which 21-hydroxylase and 11β-hydroxylase deficiencies are the most common),[2] (2) an androgen-secreting adrenal tumor in a pregnant woman, or (3) ingestion of virilizing drug during pregnancy.[3]

The degree of virilization of the external genitalia is determined by the stage of sexual differentiation at the time of exposure to this extragonadal source of androgens.

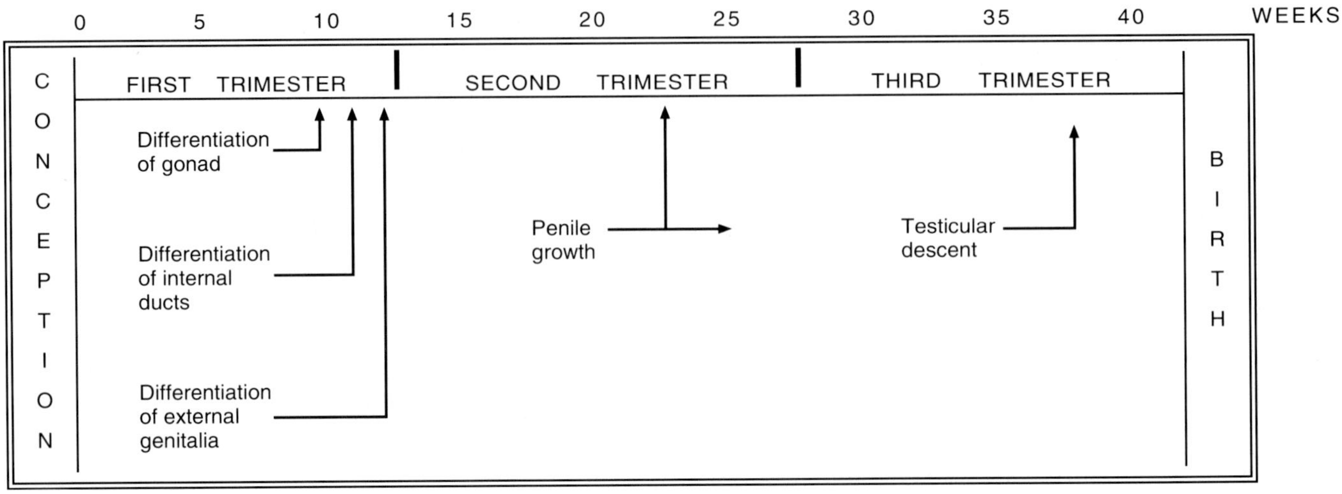

Figure 9–1. Normal sexual differentiation. (From Rajfer, J: Disorders of sexual differentiation. In: Rajfer, J: Urologic Endocrinology. Philadelphia, WB Saunders, 1986.)

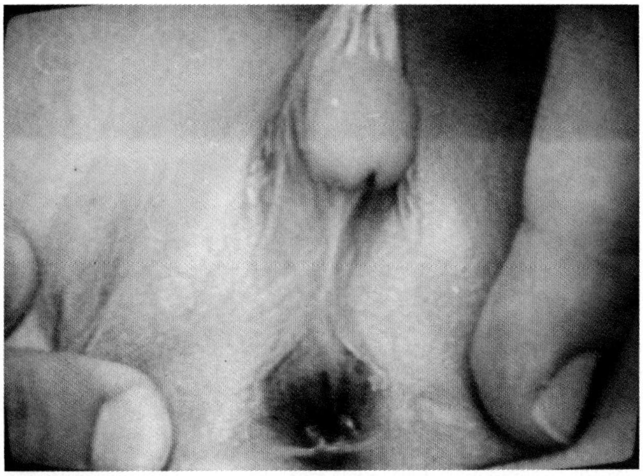

Figure 9–2. Six-year-old male patient with ambiguous external genitalia.

Male Pseudohermaphroditism

Male pseudohermaphroditism is a disorder in which a 46 XY karyotype patient with bilateral testes differentiates completely or partly as a phenotypic female as a result of a defect in either testosterone synthesis or action.[4,5]

Defects in Testosterone Synthesis

Clinical presentation of these patients may vary from those with hypospadias or cryptorchidism or both to those who are normal phenotypic women. Because the fetal testes secrete testosterone that acts locally to establish the wolffian ducts, a total or partial deficiency of testosterone secretion may result in incomplete wolffian duct development.[1]

Defects in Androgen Action

Testosterone is metabolized by 5α-reductase to dihydrotestosterone (DHT), which has greater affinity than testosterone itself for the intracellular androgen receptor protein. Any defect of testosterone or DHT intracellularly may result in incomplete virilization of the external genitalia. This may be due to either a defect in the 5α-reductase enzyme or absence of the androgen receptor itself.

In 5α-reductase deficiency, the clinical features can

Table 9–1. DISORDERS RESULTING IN AMBIGUOUS EXTERNAL GENITALIA

	Genetic Sex			Internal Müllerian Ducts	Gonads
	Baar Body	H-Y Antigen	Karyotype		
Female pseudohermaphroditism	+	–	46 XX	+	O + O
Male pseudohermaphroditism	–	+	46 XY	–	T + T
Mixed Gonadal dysgenesis	–	+	45 XO/46 XY 46 XY	+	T + S
True hermaphroditism	+	+	46 XX; 46 XY	+	T + O

O, ovary; T, testis; S, streak.

be summarized as showing male internal genital structures and female external genitalia.

Abnormalities of the androgen receptor can be expressed clinically as four main phenotypes, two predominantly female and two male. The female forms are complete and incomplete testicular feminization, and the male forms are Reifenstein's syndrome and the infertile male syndrome.[6,7]

Mixed Gonadal Dysgenesis

Mixed gonadal dysgenesis is characterized by the presence of a testis on one side and a streak gonad on the contralateral side.[8] This disorder probably represents the second most common cause of ambiguous external genitalia in the newborn period and appears to be the result of a testicular differentiation fault during embryogenesis. The most common karyotype is 45 XO/46 XY.

All patients have a uterus and at least one fallopian tube, cryptorchidism, and/or hypospadias. Approximately 25% of the gonads, including streak gonads, will undergo malignant degeneration if followed into adulthood.[9]

True Hermaphroditism

True hermaphroditism is the rarest of the intersex disorders. Its feature is the presence of ovarian and testicular tissue in the same patient. The ovarian and testicular tissue may be found in separated gonads either on the same side or on opposite sides, or they may be found within the same gonad (ovotestis), either unilaterally or bilaterally.

Usually, there is a suggestion of virilization in the external genitalia, and, indeed, the majority of patients with true hermaphroditism have been reared as males. Hypospadias, cryptorchidism, and labioscrotal fusion are present in such cases. In addition, almost all patients have a urogenital sinus.[10] Internally, a uterus is usually present, whereas the ductal system usually corresponds to the adjacent gonad. When an ovotestis is detected, a fallopian tube and vas deferens may be seen on the same side. The testis or ovotestis may be found anywhere between the abdominal cavity and the scrotum along the line of normal testicular descent. The ovary, however, is usually intra-abdominal, although it has occasionally been found in the hemiscrotum.[11]

LAPAROSCOPY

Many series have shown that laparoscopy is an accurate means to localize nonpalpable testes, identifying preoperatively almost 100% of the abdominal testes.[12–15] On the other hand, when the testes are not present, laparoscopy allows the visualization of spermatic vessels, accompanied or not by a vas deferens.[16,17] This procedure may establish the diagnosis of vanishing testis,[18] when the spermatic vessels and vas deferens end blindly above the internal inguinal ring, precluding a confirmatory open exploration.

A confirmatory open exploration is also not necessary if no vascular, ductal, or testicular structures are found under laparoscopic examination (testicular absence).[17]

In the management of intersex states, laparoscopy is a useful investigative instrument in selected cases. The procedure allows the exploration of the pelvis to localize müllerian and wolffian duct remnants. Gonadal biopsy and gonadectomy may be indicated to confirm the diagnosis of selected disorders of sexual differentiation. Laparoscopy can avoid the exploratory laparotomy in such cases and may constitute the last step in the management of intersex states (Fig. 9–3).[19,20]

Management of Intersex Disorders

Gonadal biopsy is valuable in the diagnosis of true hermaphroditism, particularly in patients with ovotestes from whom either the ovarian or the testicular component must be removed in keeping with the sex of rearing. Biopsy is also useful in establishing the diagnosis of gonadal dysgenesis, particularly in patients with normal or XO/XY mosaic karyotypes. Gonadal biopsy can confirm the presence of testicular tissue in an intra-abdominal gonad in cases of male pseudohermaphroditism.[5]

The testes or dysgenetic gonads must be removed in early childhood in all XY patients assigned to the female gender. There is a risk of malignancy if such gonads are left in situ.[21] In patients with dysgenetic testes, these should preferably be removed before puberty, unless they are located well within the scrotum and are regularly examined.

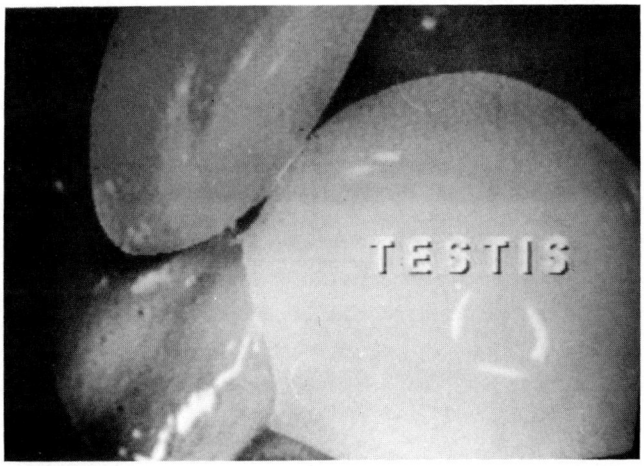

Figure 9–3. Laparoscopic view of an abdominal testis from the same patient.

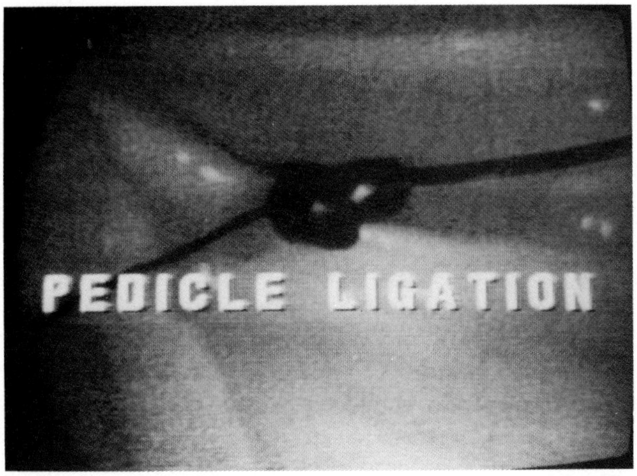

Figure 9–4. Pedicle ligation of the abdominal testis with 2–0 chromic catgut sutures.

In patients with complete androgen insensitivity, the testes should also be removed because of the increased incidence of malignancy, but this is best deferred until late teens when spontaneous feminization is complete. In contrast, in order to avoid virilization at puberty, early gonadectomy is usually indicated in patients with incomplete androgen insensitivity or deficient testosterone production who have been brought up as girls.[5]

Laparoscopic gonadectomy can be performed in small gonads. Under general anesthesia, a pneumoperitoneum with ambient air is created by means of a subumbilical needle and hand-held syringe. The telescopic system is inserted in the abdominal cavity immediately below the umbilicus. The patient is examined in the Trendelenburg position. After observation of the abdominal cavity, two 5-mm incisions are made, one in the left and one in the right inguinal area, and trocars are inserted into the abdominal cavity.[19] A prehensile forceps is used to grasp the gonad. With endoscopic scissors, a biopsy can be performed. The gonadectomy can also be performed after the placement of two endoloops in the pedicle of the gonad (Fig. 9–4).[19]

After gonadectomy appropriate sex hormone replacement should be given.[19]

Fig. 9–5 shows a diagnostic scheme that should be followed in the management of disorders of sexual differentiation. Physical examination is the first step to be evaluated. Sex assignment is best made in the newborn period to define the best sex in which to rear the child. Laparoscopy is an important tool in achieving this final decision.

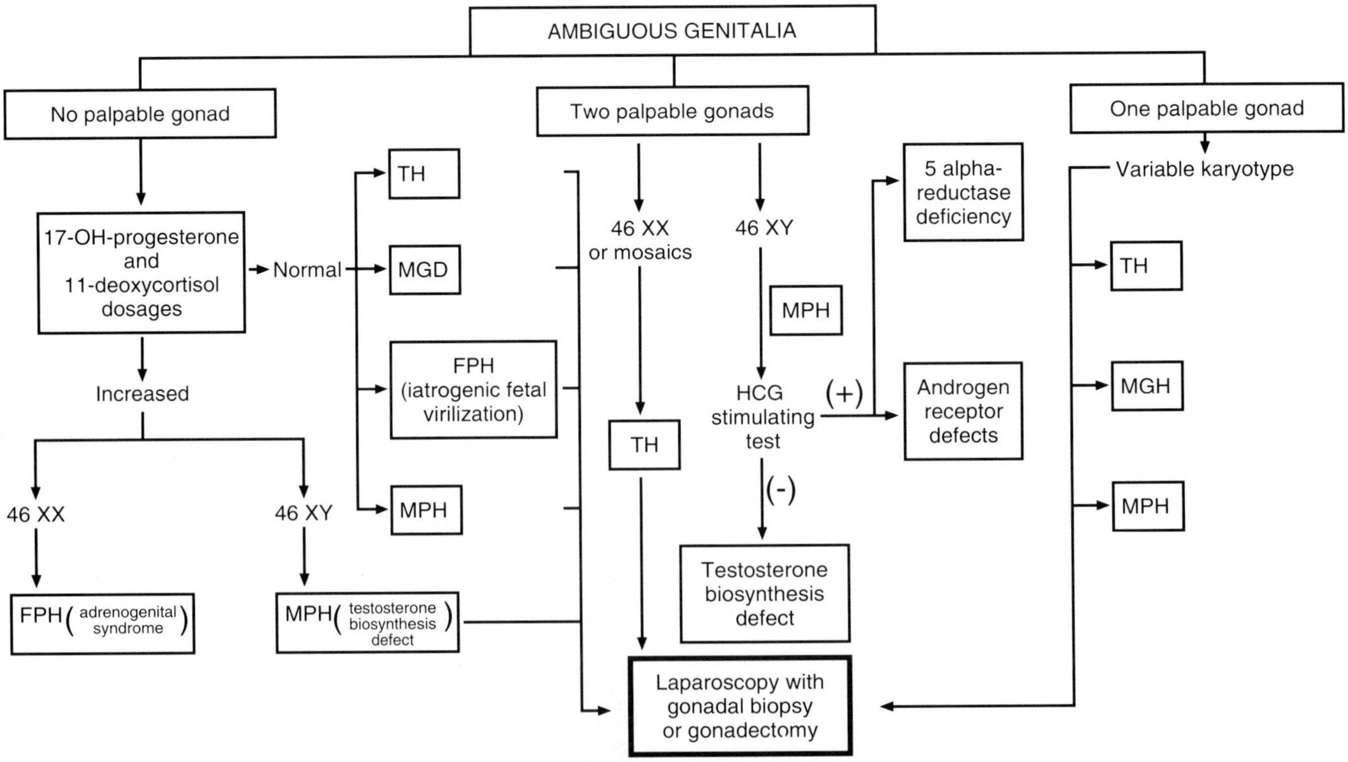

Figure 9–5. Diagnostic scheme for the management of genital ambiguity based on physical examination. FPH, female pseudohermaphroditism; MGD, mixed gonadal dysgenesis; MPH, male pseudohermaphroditism; TH, true hermaphroditism.

REFERENCES

1. Grumbach, MM; Conte, FA: Disorders of sex differentation. In: Williams, RH, ed: Textbook of Endocrinology, 6th ed. Philadelphia, WB Saunders, 1981.
2. Childs, B; Grumbach, MM; Vanwyck, GG: Virilizing adrenal hyperplasia: A genetic and hormonal study. J Clin Invest 35:213, 1956.
3. Bongiovanni, AM; DiGeorge, AM; Grumbach, MM: Masculinization of the female infant associated with estrogen therapy alone during gestation. J Clin Endocrinol Metab 19:1004, 1959.
4. Rajfer, J: Disorders of sexual differentation. In: Rajfer, J, ed: Urologic Endocrinology. Philadelphia, WB Saunders, 1986.
5. Savage, MO: Clinical aspects of intersex. In: Brook, CGD, ed: Clinical Paediatric Endocrinology, 2nd ed. London. Blackwell Scientific Publications, 1989.
6. Givens, JR; Wiser, WL; Summitt, RL; et al: Familial male pseudohermaphroditism without gynecomastia due to deficient testicular 17-ketosteroid reductase activity. N Engl J Med 291:938, 1974.
7. Wilson, JD; Harrod, MJ; Goldstein, JL; et al: Familial incomplete male pseudohermaphroditism. Type 1: Evidence for androgen resistance and variable clinical manifestations in a family with Reifenstein syndrome. N Engl J Med 290:1097, 1974.
8. Pollack, M; Levine, LS; Duchon, M: Prenatal diagnosis of CAH due to 21-hydroxylase deficiency by HLA typing of amniotic fluid cells. (Abstract) Pediatr Res 13:384, 1979.
9. Aarskog, D: Intersex conditions masquerading as hypospadias. Birth Defects 7:122, 1971.
10. Federman, DD: Abnormal sexual development. Philadelphia, WB Saunders, 1967.
11. Jones, HW, Jr; Scott, WW: True hermaphroditism. In: Jones, HW, Jr; Scott, WW, eds: Hermaphroditism, Genital Anomalies, and Related Endocrine Disorders. 2nd ed. Baltimore, Williams & Wilkins, 1971, pp. 290–317.
12. Guinoy, EJ; Corbally, M; Malone, PS: Laparoscopy and the management of the impalpable testis. Br J Urol 63:313, 1989.
13. Lowe, DH; Brock, WA; Kaplan, GW: Laparoscopy for localization of nonpalpable testes. J Urol 31:728, 1984.
14. Silber, SJ; Cohen, R: Laparoscopy for cryptorchidism. J Urol 124:928, 1980.
15. Weiss, RM; Seashore, JH: Laparoscopy in the management of the nonpalpable testis. J Urol 138:382, 1987.
16. Bloom, DA; Ayers, JWT; MacGuire, EJ: The role of laparoscopy in management of nonpalpable testis. J Urol 94:465, 1988.
17. Castilho, LN: Laparoscopy for the nonpalpable testis: How to interpret the endoscopic findings. J Urol 144:1215, 1990.
18. Abeyaratne, MR: The vanishing testis. Lancet 2:822, 1969.
19. Castilho, LN; Ferreira, U; Rodrigues Netto, H, Jr; et al: Laparoscopic pediatric orchiectomy. J Endourol 6:155, 1992.
20. Scott, JES: Laparoscopy as an aid in the diagnosis and management of the impalpable testis. J Pediatr Surg 17:14, 1982.
21. Savage, MO; Chaussain, JL; Evain, D; et al: Endocrine studies in male pseudohermaphroditism in childhood and adolescence. Clin Endocrinol 8:219, 1978.

CHAPTER 10

Laparoscopic Varicocelectomy

Paul G. Hagood, MD
Raul O. Parra, MD, FACS

The utility of varicocelectomy for the treatment of infertility seems incontrovertible. The beneficial effects have been well documented by many authors.[1-3] A review by Pryor and Howards found that between 50% and 80% of the patients improve their semen parameters and 30% to 40% can expect to initiate pregnancy after varicocelectomy.[4] Increase in size and improvement of the histology of the testicle often follows surgery.[5,6] Varicoceles therefore represent the most common surgically treatable disorder in patients presenting for infertility and when found, are a source of encouragement to the patient and physician.

There has arisen, however, a significant difference of opinion as to the proper surgical method of varicocele ablation. The inguinal and high retroperitoneal approaches (with or without magnification) are the most commonly performed procedures at this time.[7,8] Recently, Sanchez-de Badejos[9] in Spain and a number of independent investigators in the United States published reports of laparoscopic varicocelectomies.[10-12] Laparoscopic varicocelectomy is essentially a high retroperitoneal ligation. These reports indicated that this procedure may offer significant advantages to the patient by decreasing the morbidity of standard incisions and increasing the efficacy of the operation.

HISTORICAL BACKGROUND

Varicoceles are an ancient pathologic process, described as early as the first century A.D. The association with infertility was guessed at early in the nineteenth century, and treatment of varicoceles was recommended by Barwell in 1855.[13] Unfortunately, the varicocele was generally neglected until in 1954 Tulloch reported on a series of varicocelectomies and the subsequent improvement in male fertility.[1] The bulk of the surgical series since Tulloch has demonstrated a significant advantage to the patient.

Few modifications in techniques have been presented over the years. In 1960 Ivanissevich described his experience of more than 40 years with an inguinal approach to the pampiniform plexus.[7] In 1969 Palomo proposed a high retroperitoneal approach to the internal spermatic veins, citing ease of vein identification as the major advantage.[8] The application of optical magnification to assist in the isolation of all offending veins was suggested by Wosnitzer and Roth in 1983.[14] There are three reasons for the proliferation of techniques. First, the pathologic anatomy and physiology is controversial. Second, many consider present surgical methods to be excessively morbid for an elective procedure. Third, there is a significant surgical and physiologic failure rate. The laparoscopic variation is an attempt to address all of the persistent questions.

ANATOMIC CONSIDERATIONS

Venous Anatomy

In its most basic form, a varicocele represents an inappropriate increase in pressure in the spermatic vein that causes engorgement of the pampiniform plexus. The dilation encompasses the entire spermatic vein system but is seen clinically in the scrotum. The major vein is the *internal spermatic*,[15] arising from the renal vein on the left and the inferior vena cava on the right. Other veins cited as possible contributors include the cremasteric or external pudendal (for our purposes, the *external spermatic*), draining into the external iliac system; the *deferential*, feeding into superior or inferior vesical; and the *scrotal* veins (including the gubernacular veins).[16,17]

The clinical interest in the external spermatic system was initiated by Coolsaet's description of a nutcracker effect on the renal and the iliac vein. He found venographic compression of the left renal vein in 56% of patients with varicocele. In this same study, he proposed a distal nutcracker effect with partial obstruction of the left common iliac vein causing dilation of the external spermatic.[18]

In Beck and associates' series of 115 surgical dissections, dilated external spermatic veins larger than 2 mm were identified 74% of the time.[17] Hill and Green found incompetent cremasteric veins in 25 of 48 patients by venography. They believed that 15 of these patients had no other identifiable cause of a varicocele.[19] Sayfan and colleagues found a 12% incidence of dilated cremasteric veins.[20]

In contrast to this, a venographic study by Kaufman and associates found that collateral channels from the internal iliac veins were not present in 70 patients studied, nor was there a pressure gradient across the left iliac vein detected in any of the seven patients who underwent spermatic venography in follow-up for failed varicocele ligation. All five patients who had recurrent varicoceles following surgical ligation were found to have collateral internal spermatic veins that were not ligated primarily.[21]

To complicate the anatomy, many have described a network of fine veins surrounding the testicular artery.[14] Beck and associates saw this in 30% of their dissections. They also found veins exiting the tunica vaginalis and transversing the gubernaculum in 79% of the patients. Sixty percent of these veins were larger than 2 mm in diameter. As stated, however, the role of any of these vessels in the pathogenesis of the varicocele is uncertain.[17]

Circuit Flow

In a study by Dennison and Tibbs, in which four patients underwent internal spermatic venography, it was noted that the venous flow passed through the varicose pampiniform plexus, out through the ductus deferens, obturator, circumflex, and superficial epigastric veins. In all patients, it was possible to see outflow via pelvic veins to the common iliac vein at some stage, and in one patient there was a clear communication with the long saphenous. The researchers concluded that the varicocele is an example of a venous retrograde circuit that represents a dynamic phenomenon, not merely static distention.[22] Such a retrograde circuit must have a substantial outlet, as in these cases, through the cremasteric and other veins. To accommodate this view of the pathology, venous shunt procedures have been described.[23,24] Experimental models have shown that acute venous occlusion produces the same degree of testicular ischemia as arterial occlusion.[25] Certainly, ligation of all outflow veins would therefore be inappropriate. To some this implies that the appropriate level of transection of the vein should be above the internal inguinal ring. Hart and colleagues described the resolution of dilation of external veins in 100% (5/5) of patients after simple ligation of the internal spermatic vein above the internal ring.[26] Gill and associates described identical results in all 16 patients with dilated external veins.[27] In numerous series, the recurrence rate following high ligation is less than 10%.[4] This must be contrasted with the reported 74% incidence of dilated external spermatic veins.[17] Obviously, few of these veins can reasonably be considered contributors to the varix pathology.

Bilaterality

Traditionally, a varicocele is considered to be a left-sided abnormality. Classic studies have reported that 75% to 90% of all varicoceles occurred in the left hemiscrotum, most often as solitary entities.[28,29] Recently, however, anatomic and radiographic studies have demonstrated a greater incidence of right-sided and bilateral varicoceles.[30–32] The importance of the right varicocele is emphasized by the Amelar and Dubin series of 41 patients who had undergone a left varicocelectomy without improvement and were later found to have a small right varicocele. Subsequent right varicocelectomy produced semen improvement in 23 (56%), and pregnancy in 21 (43%).[33] In modern surgical series, bilateral varicocelectomies are performed in up to 70% of patients.[34,35]

Even when only a clinically obvious left varix is identified, the defect in spermatogenesis is bilateral. No satisfactory explanation for this is universally accepted. Some believe this is secondary to generalized increase in scrotal temperature from the left varix.[36] On the other hand, some anatomic studies have shown that there are numerous vessels crossing from left to right. Perhaps more important may be the so-called subclinical varicocele.

Subclinical or ultrasound-diagnosed right-sided varicoceles are obviously more common than those clinically diagnosed.[37,38] Dubin and Amelar found no correlation between size of the varix found on physician examination and the degree of impairment of spermatogenesis.[39] Dhabuwala and co-workers demonstrated equivalent improvement in semen parameters in men with clinical and subclinical varicoceles undergoing varix ligation.[40] Many investigators have since come to believe that ultrasound-diagnosed varicoceles are as significant as larger ones.[37,38]

The importance of crossing vessels is debatable. In Wishahi's study of cadavers, the single trunk of the spermatic vein divided into medial and lateral divisions at L4 in all male cadavers studied. Twenty-two of 40 men (55%) had cross-communications between the left and right spermatic veins arising from the medial division of the spermatic vein.[41] A year later he published the results of a venographic study of 17 men but could not identify any crossing vessels below the inguinal ring. Unfortunately, he did not compare the two studies, and in an editorial, discounted the cross-communication theory.[42] Cross-communication was not seen in venographic studies by Narayan.[31] It is not clear from the literature that either high or low cross-communication exists.[43,44] It is clear that in a significant number of infertile men, bilateral retrograde flow is more common than expected from physical examination.

PATHOLOGY

Numerous studies have been conducted to elucidate the pathology of the impaired spermatogenesis. At this time, the most proximal etiology is still in question. However, a few facts are unique and impact on treatment.

In 1941 MacLeod and Hotchkiss proposed that elevated temperature of the scrotum diminished sperm production.[45] In 1973, Zorgniotti and MacLeod accurately measured the scrotal temperature in 50 patients with varicoceles and in 35 controls.[36] They found that the varix subjects had a higher scrotal temperature by 0.6° to 0.8°C. Agger found in a select group that surgery resulted in a decrease of 0.5°C in the scrotal temperature.[46] It is routinely suggested that elevated testicular temperature is the most reasonable explanation for the diminished spermatogenesis in patients with varicoceles.[47]

Second, in multiple animal studies, researchers have found increased perfusion of both testes with partial occlusion of the left renal vein.[47,48] Although the effect is uniformly seen, the cause of the increased blood flow is uncertain. In Turner and Lopez's study, reflux of the spermatic vein could not be identified and is an unlikely cause of this increased blood flow.[49]

Finally, the pathologic effect of the varicocele is probably progressive. Chehval and Purcell point out that an untreated varicocele can serially decrease a patient's sperm count.[50] Nagoa found impaired spermatogenesis in fertile men with varicoceles as compared with men having none.[51] Weese and associates have investigated the generation of oxygen radicals in sperm and found increased reactivity to chemotactins in both fertile and infertile men with varicoceles. Oxygen radical formation is destructive to lipid components of sperm and was significantly increased in men with varices compared with matched controls.[52] The bottom line is that the varix pathology is progressive and is dependent on increased blood flow and temperature. Any procedure that can decrease the blood flow should be helpful.

INDICATIONS FOR THERAPY

By far the most common reason for varicocelectomy is infertility. In patients presenting because of infertility, a complete history with attention to the past fertility, the partners' fertility, and the possibility of associated anomalies or syndromes is taken. Obviously, the discussion of a complete evaluation of male infertility goes beyond this chapter, but when contemplating a varix operation, it should be remembered that a varicocele is a common finding in the general population, and may not be the most significant factor in the couple's infertility problem.

The physical examination should focus on the size of both testicles. Bilaterally small testicles even with a large varicocele should alert the clinician to the possibility of other syndromes. The varicocele is typically graded by size I to III. We also give special attention to the exclusion of any right-sided varix. If the diagnosis of a varicocele is uncertain, a scrotal ultrasound with Doppler effect can be useful. Veins larger than 2 mm with Valsalva maneuver are considered varicose. There is no reason to request venography unless simultaneous embolization is contemplated.

A minimum of two seminograms are required. MacLeod described the stressed sperm pattern (increased tapered forms) in 1965.[53] This is not pathognomonic of a varicocele but rather is a finding associated with any abnormal spermatogenesis.[28] The sperm should be examined for motility, viability, and density. All patients with a sperm density less than 10×10^6 microns/ml are required to have serum follicle-stimulating hormone, luteinizing hormone, and testosterone assays. Generally, the sperm counts are quite diminished, commonly to less than 20 million/ml. Asthenospermia is generally recognized as a critical indicator of sperm dysfunction.[54] We also perform a cervical mucus–penetration test, using the automated Penetrak system.*

Another reason for surgery is pain from a large or cumbersome varicocele. The pain is usually dull, aggravated by long period of standing, and often relieved by lying down. Overall, this is unusual, and other causes of inguinal, scrotal, and perineal pain need to be investigated before resorting to varicocelectomy. In our experience, patients with pain need to be advised that if surgery is contemplated, it does not ensure the resolution of their symptoms.

Studies of adolescents (as well as adults) with varicoceles have demonstrated testicular atrophy to be a relatively common association. Unfortunately, adolescent fertility studies have not been undertaken, and predicting a patient's future fertility is not possible. After varicocelectomy in adolescents, Kass and Belman demonstrated a significant increase in testicular volume, which they refer to as "catch up growth."[5] Also, as previously noted the pathology of the varix is probably progressive. Some authors seem to recommend the prophylactic ligation of all large varicoceles.[52] Testicular atrophy associated with varicoceles is generally considered an appropriate indication.[55,56] Without atrophy or impaired sperm production, however, the question of who should undergo operation is not settled at this time.

SURGICAL APPROACHES

Surgical treatment can basically be divided into only two types: a high versus a low approach, dependent on the location of the incision in relation to the internal ring. This dichotomy is based on the fact that the confluence of the internal spermatic tributaries is usually above the inguinal ring. Below the inguinal ring and certainly in the pampiniform plexus, it is quite common to find multiple spermatic veins.[8,17] Obviously, the true disadvantage of the high technique, aside from its muscle-splitting morbidity is that it does not allow identification and ligation of the cremasteric veins.[17]

Furthermore, careful consideration must be given to the need for preservation of the spermatic artery and the ligation of the accompanying venae spermatica comitans. In his original surgery, Palomo did not heed the artery and divided it without any reported atrophy.[8]

*Serono-Baker Diagnostics, Inc., Allentown, PA.

Kass and Marcol found that the Palomo technique of mass high retroperitoneal ligation had a lower incidence of varicocele recurrence compared either with a high retroperitoneal artery sparing or a modified inguinal technique. In this study, 102 varicocele ligations were performed using 4.5 power optical magnification. In 53 cases, an inguinal incision was made at the internal ring and all dilated internal and external veins were ligated. In 17 patients, a modified Palomo retroperitoneal technique with sparing of the internal spermatic artery was used. Finally, in 32 patients, a standard Palomo technique without spermatic artery sparing was performed. No postoperation varicoceles were noted in the 32 patients who had a mass high retroperitoneal ligation, although 9/53 (16%) recurred in the inguinal and 2/17 (12%) recurred in the artery-sparing high ligation. Postoperative testicular atrophy did not occur in any patient.[57]

Experience of others with the Palomo technique parallels this. Hosli[58] and Okuyama and co-workers[59] have also reported excellent results without testicular atrophy using a traditional mass ligation technique. In our laparoscopic Palomo technique, we emphasize arterial sparing but having performed more than 90 laparoscopic procedures, we have yet to see a recurrence. In their laparoscopic experience, Donovan and Winfield have seen one recurrence in 47 men.[60] We and others who have performed laparoscopy believe that the exposure of the veins is far superior compared with a muscle-splitting approach. Conversely, Beck and associates reported a low recurrence rate of 0.5% with microsurgical inguinal varicocelectomies.[17] Obviously, a microsurgical technique is not accessible to the majority of practitioners. Taken together, it would appear that total vein ablation by mass ligation or efficient microscopic surgery is equally effective either above or below the internal ring. Therefore although the anatomy is well described, the significance of the individual scrotal veins is a matter of considerable controversy. Until the pathophysiology is clearly defined, no blanket statement regarding the appropriate level or extent of venous ligation is warranted.

LAPAROSCOPIC VARICOCELECTOMY

Preoperative Evaluation

In preparation for general anesthesia, the condition of the patient should always be assessed. Contraindications to laparoscopy include a history of extensive abdominal scarring, herniations, bowel adhesions with peritonitis or intestinal obstruction, or uncorrectable coagulopathy. The patient's respiratory function must be adequate to handle the increase in arterial Pco_2 from the pneumoperitoneum. Informed consent should emphasize the unique possible complications of laparoscopy. It should also include a discussion of the nonsurgical options, the experimental nature of laparoscopy, and the possibility of conversion to an open procedure. No bowel preparation is required, nor is blood typing and banking done. We do empirically give a broad spectrum antibiotic 1 to 2 hours before surgery.

Operative Technique

The procedures performed at our institution are all done with general endotracheal anesthesia. Matsuda has performed the operation using local anesthesia.[61] A Foley catheter is used to decrease the potential for bladder perforation. Rarely, we have used a nasogastric tube. We place the patient in modest Trendelenburg position to displace the bowels away from the pelvis. The arms are tucked at the side to allow for maximum movement by the surgical team. As the operation proceeds, the table can be tilted from side to side to further displace the bowels away from the inguinal ring. A full abdominal scrub is performed should a laparotomy become necessary. The perineum and scrotum are also scrubbed for two reasons. First, traction on the testicle may be helpful in identifying the cord structures during dissection, and, second, decompression of the pneumoscrotum is most easily accomplished at the termination of the case, before removal of the trocars.

A 1-cm subumbilical curvilinear incision is made, and the fascia identified. The skin is grasped with towel clips, and the bowel is allowed to fall away from the abdominal wall. A Verres needle is then inserted into the peritoneum through this incision and directed into the pelvis. The saline drip technique is used to ensure proper placement. In these patients, we have been compelled to use a Hasson cannula at times, and the surgeon should be comfortable with this mini-laparotomy technique.[62] Perforation of bowel or the aorta with a trocar has been reported, and the risk can be decreased with the use of the Hasson cannula.

CO_2 insufflation is accomplished via the cannula. Intra-abdominal pressure is maintained at less than 15mm Hg by automatic monitoring. With adequate pneumoperitoneum, three trocars are placed—a midline laparoscopic trocar of at least 10 mm and then bilateral 5- and 10-mm working ports. The bilateral ports are lateral to the epigastric vessels, approximately 5 to 10 cm below the umbilicus. Donovan and Winfield recommend a fourth midline suprapubic trocar.[11] This may be useful if the chief surgeon is the only operator and uses one port for retraction and the other for dissection. In our University practice, both the chief and assistant perform the dissection in concert. The use of two instruments in mirror image placement may necessitate occasional crossing of instruments or, preferably, exchange of duties as retraction needs dictate. The operating surgeon should be opposite the varix being ligated, the first assistant ipsilateral to the dissection, and the laparoscope operator cephalic to the surgeon or assistant. In most instances, it is preferable to have the operating surgeon work in line with the laparoscope to eliminate the reversed image effect seen when the scope is facing the surgeon.

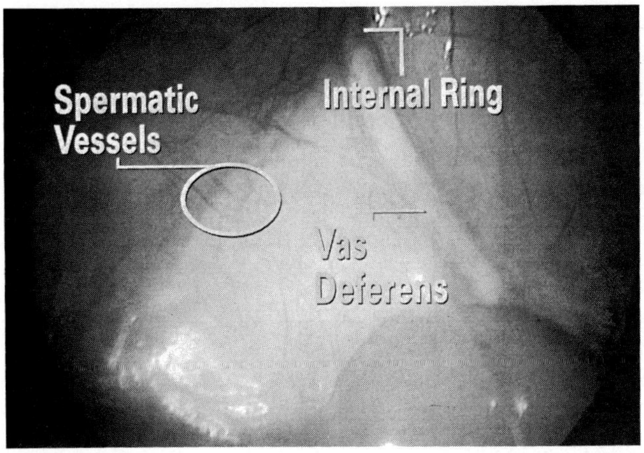

Figure 10–1. View at left internal ring. See also Color Plate 2.

In most cases, the inguinal ring is easily identified with the vas deferens looping medial and inferior and the spermatic vein and artery running in a cephalic direction (Fig. 10–1). On the left, it may be necessary to mobilize the sigmoid colon, and lateral adhesions are actually common, even in this young group of patients. The peritoneum is opened with electrocautery scissors immediately superior to the spermatic veins, approximately 2 to 3 cm above the internal ring (Fig. 10–2). Dissection too close to the ring can lead to injury of the vas deferens or epigastric vessels. Extending the dissection too far cephalad may result in the surgeon's missing important collaterals or crossing veins. A "T" incision in the peritoneum is described, although simple traction on the peritoneum is usually

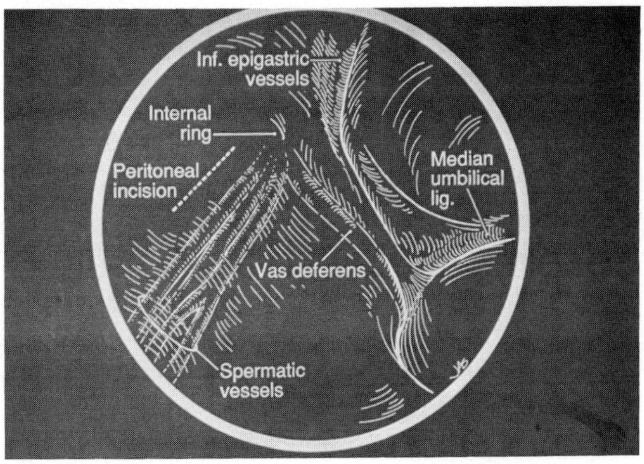

Figure 10–2. Anatomy at left internal ring and position of peritoneal incision. See also Color Plate 2.

sufficient to completely expose the vascular bundle. If an incision is made over the vessel, to avoid arterial damage or spasm, electrocautery should not be used.[60]

Before significant dissection is undertaken, an initial inspection is made in an attempt to identify the artery. If the vascular bundle is not evident, traction on the scrotum may be useful. When the vascular bundle is fully and carefully exposed, a blunt probe is passed under it (Fig. 10–3), and an edge is grasped and retracted to thin out the complex as much as possible. The artery can often be identified immediately, and the artery and the bulk of the vein complex are separated from each other by blunt dissection. This is the most efficient method of separating out the artery. Transmitted pulses from the external iliac can be mistaken for spermatic artery activity. Papaverine (30 mg/ml) or lidocaine (2% without epinephrine) may unmask an artery in spasm. Scrotal[12] or translaparoscopic Doppler probe[63] has been used to assist in arterial identification, although Donovan is less than enthusiastic about it.[60] With the artery isolated, the rest of the spermatic veins then can be clip-ligated and divided (Fig. 10–4). Careful attention should be given to the spermatic artery, because small veins are usually closely adherent. Although they may appear to be noncontributary to the varix process, it has been well documented that these residual veins can dilate and cause a recurrence of the varicocele. An Nd:YAG laser or fine-tipped, right-angled hook electrocautery probe can be used to obliterate these.[64,65] Obviously, the laser adds considerable cost to the operation. On occasion veins are seen through the peritoneum, lateral or medial to the bulk of the cord vessels. These may be colonic or renal collaterals and should be obliterated. It should be remembered that the epigastric vessels are anteromedial and the genitofemoral nerve is posterolateral. Winfield and Donovan reported transient sensory loss in the anterior thigh in one patient.[66] We have seen one patient who developed transient nerve damage 5 days after surgery, presumably from late nerve compression from a hematoma. When it has been ensured that all veins have been divided, the artery is examined for persistent pulsations. Finally, as noted in the discussion above, complete sacrifice of the vascular bundle (artery included) eliminates all veins and by most reports does not increase the risk of testicular atrophy. Although this method is decidedly simpler and faster, it needs further study before it can be recommended.

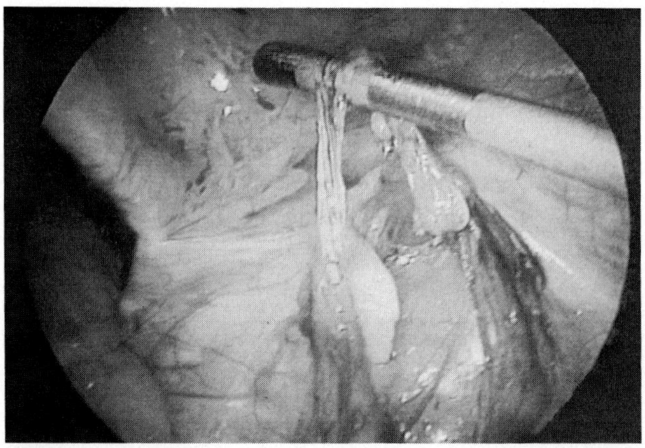

Figure 10–3. Blunt probe under the vascular bundle. See also Color Plate 2.

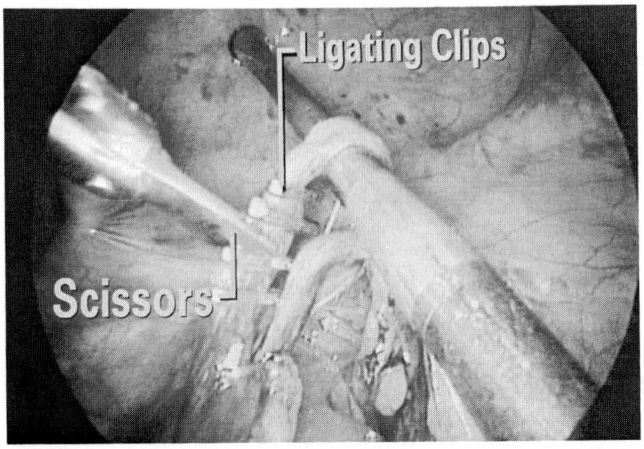

Figure 10–4. Ligating clips on vein bundle. The spermatic artery is below the blunt probe. See also Color Plate 3.

Quite often bilateral varicocelectomy is performed. The dissection is identical right to left, although the need for bowel mobilization and adhesiolysis is usually minimal on the right. We have on occasion, in examining a right-sided internal spermatic system, been impressed by the size of the veins and have ligated them without a clinically evident varicocele.

On both sides, the number of veins ligated is variable, but we have rarely seen fewer than two veins and, occasionally, four or five. When all veins have been ligated and hemostasis has been assured, any pneumoscrotum is decompressed and pneumoperitoneum is vented. All trocars are removed, and the fascia is closed with No. 1 polyglycolic acid sutures. It may be advisable in larger men to close the lateral wounds with laparoscopic visualization of suture placement before the pneumoperitoneum is released. At the very least, visual and manual inspections with an index finger is necessary to ensure that no bowel or omentum is incarcerated. We have seen one bowel herniation in our series of over 200 general laparoscopic cases. We infiltrate the fascia and subcutaneous tissue with a long-acting anesthetic (bupivacaine) and give a nonsteroidal anti-inflamatory drug at the close of the operation. The skin is then closed in a subcuticular fashion. If a nasogastric tube has been placed, it is removed. The urethral catheter is removed before the patient leaves the recovery room. A moderate-strength oral analgesic (acetaminophen with codeine) is prescribed, and the patient is advised to limit his activity for the first 48 hours and then to increase it as he judges best.

Laparoscopic Results

More than 90 laparoscopic varicocelectomies have been performed at our institution. Only two patients have failed to return to normal activity within 3 days, and all but two patients have been discharged from the hospital within 24 hours, most on the same day. No major complication has been seen. One persistent hydrocele developed. Minimal testicular aching was reported by approximately one third of the patients but did not require analgesics and resolved within 7 to 10 days. Three patients had shoulder pain, and three minor wound infections have been seen. No recurrent varicoceles have occurred. The operative time ranged from 35 to 140 minutes with an average 63 minutes for bilateral operations. There is no significant difference when comparing unilateral and bilateral operations. Most of the unilateral operations were performed early in our experience.

Mehan and colleagues have reviewed the fertility results from the St. Louis University program.[67] Thirty-eight patients were available for more than 6 months' follow-up. Pregnancy was achieved in 16 of 38 cases (42%). Five patients reporting pregnancies refused postoperative semen analysis. Postoperative seminograms are available in 11 of the successful cases, and 10 of these showed improvement of greater than 50% in the sperm density. Viability improved in 77% to some degree and in the two cases achieving pregnancy who failed to improve in density, there was a significant increase in the viability. All cases but one had increased motility.

Of the 22 cases not achieving pregnancy, 9, or 41%, had a 50% rise in the sperm density and 8, or 36%, demonstrated an increase in viability and motility. Thirteen men showed no improvement in any parameter. In total, 17 of 33 (51%) cases suitable for evaluation, had a statistically significant improvement in sperm density. In 15 of 33 (45%) cases, there was improved viability and motility.

At the University of Iowa in a series of 26 patients, pregnancies occurred in 24%. An overall operative time of 105 minutes and 167 minutes for a bilateral procedure was reported. One recurrence has been seen (2%). The average time of return to full activity was 3.7 days.[60] Similar results have also been published by Aaberg and associates[12] and Matsuda and coworkers.[61]

CONCLUSIONS

These results compare quite favorably with all other surgical and radiologic techniques. Morbidity is low, and this technique has proven advantages in terms of simplicity of spermatic vein dissection, preservation of the spermatic arteries, and access to bilateral veins. As the competing technologies are examined, it is reasonable to conclude that the laparoscopic varicocelectomy is a legitimate alternative approach to the surgical correction of the varicocele.

REFERENCES

1. Tulloch, WS: Consideration of sterility factors in the light of subsequent pregnancies: Subfertility in the male. Trans Edinburgh Obstet Soc Edinburgh Med J 59:29, 1952.
2. Dubin, L; Amelar, RD: Nine hundred eighty-six cases of varicocelectomy: A 12-year study. Urology 10:446, 1977.
3. Mehan, DJ: Results of ligation of internal spermatic vein in the treatment of infertility in azoospermic patients. Fertil Steril 27:110, 1976.
4. Pryor, J; Howards, SS: Varicocele. Urol Clin North Am 14:499, 1987.
5. Kass, EJ; Belman, BA: Reversal of testicular growth failure by varicocele ligation. J Urol 137:475, 1987.
6. Johnson, SG; Agger, P: Quantitative evaluation of testicular biopsies before and after operation for varicocele. Fertil Steril 29:58, 1978.
7. Ivanissevich, O: Left varicocele due to reflux; experience with 4470 cases in 42 years. J Int Coll Surg 34:742, 1960.
8. Palomo, A: Radical cure of varicocele by a new technique: Preliminary report. J Urol 61:604, 1969.
9. Sanchez-de Badajoz, E; Diaz-Ramirez, F; Vara-Thorbeck, C: Endoscopic varicocelectomy. J Endourology 4:317, 1990.
10. Hagood, PG; Mehan, DJ; Worischeck, JH; et al: Laparoscopic varicocelectomy: Preliminary report of a new technique. J Urol 147:73, 1992.
11. Donovan, JF, Jr; Winfield, HN: Laparoscopic varix ligation. J Urol 147:77, 1992.
12. Aaberg, RA; Vancaillie, TG; Schuessler, WW: Laparoscopic varicocele ligation: A new technique. Fertil Steril 56:776, 1991.
13. Barwell, R: One hundred cases of varicocele treated by the subcutaneous wire loop. Lancet 1:978, 1885.
14. Wosnitzer, M; Roth, JA: Optical magnification and Doppler ultrasound probe for varicocelectomy. Urology 22:24, 1983.
15. Williams, PL; Warwick, R; Dyson, M; Bannister, LH; eds: Gray's Anatomy, 37th ed. New York, Churchhill Livingstone, 1989, p. 818.
16. Hanley, HG; Harrison, RG: The nature and surgical treatment of varicocele. Br J Surg 50:64, 1962.
17. Beck, EM; Schlegel, PN; Goldstein, M: Intraoperative varicocele anatomy: A macroscopic and microscopic study. J Urol 148:1190, 1992.
18. Coolsaet, BLRA: The varicocele syndrome: Venography determining the optimal level for surgical management. J Urol 124:833, 1980.
19. Hill, JT; Green, NA: Varicocele: A review of radiological and anatomical features in relation to surgical treatment. Br J Surg 64:747, 1977.
20. Sayfan, J; Halevy, A; Oland, J; Nathan, H: Varicocele and left renal vein compression. Fertil Steril 41:411, 1984.
21. Kaufman, SL; Kadir, S; Barth, KH; et al: Mechanisms of recurrent varicocele after balloon occlusion or surgical ligation of the internal spermatic vein. Radiology 147:435, 1983.

22. Dennison, AR; Tibbs, DJ: Varicocele and varicose veins compared: A basis for logical surgery. Urology 28:211, 1986.
23. Flati, G; Porowska, B; Flati, D; Carboni, M: Microsurgical treatment of varicocele: Selecting most appropriate shunt. Urology 35:121, 1990.
24. Fox, U; Romagnoli, G; Colombo, F: The microsurgical drainage of the varicocele. Fertil Steril 41:475, 1984.
25. Huang, EJ; Kelly, RE; Masuda, H; et al: Deleterious effects of testicular venous occlusion in young rats. Surg Gynecol Obstet 171:382, 1990.
26. Hart, RR; Rushton, GH; Belman, BA: Intraoperative spermatic venography during varicocele surgery in adolescents. J Urol 148:1514, 1992.
27. Gill, B; Kogan, SJ; Maldonado, J; et al: Significance of intraoperative venographic patterns on the postoperative recurrence and surgical incision placement of pediatric varicoceles. J Urol 144(Part 2):502, 1990.
28. Saypol, DC; Lipshultz, LI; Howards, SS: Varicocele. In: Lipshultz, LL; Howards, SS; eds: Infertility in the Male. New York, Churchill Livingstone, 1983.
29. Dubin, L; Amelar, RD: Varicocelectomy: Twenty-five years of experience. Int J Fertil 33:226, 1988.
30. Bigot, JM; Barret, F; Henelon, C: Phlebography of the right spermatic vein in varicoceles. In: Jecht, EW; Zeitler, E; eds: Varicocele and Male Infertility. New York, Springer-Verlag, 1982, p.59.
31. Narayan, P; Amplatz, K; Gonzalez, R: Varicocele and male subfertility. Fertil Steril 36:92, 1981.
32. Gonzales, R; Reddy, P; Kaye, KW; Narayan, P: Comparison of Doppler examination and retrograde venography in the diagnosis of varicocele. Fertil Steril 40:96, 1983.
33. Amelar, RD; Dubin, L: Right varicocelectomy in selected infertile patients who have failed to improve after previous left varicocelectomy. Fertil Steril 47:833, 1987.
34. Amelar, RD; Dubin, L: Therapeutic implications of left, right, and bilateral varicocelectomy. Fertil Steril 30:53, 1987.
35. Cockett, ATK; Takihara, H; Cosentino, JM: The varicocele. Fertil Steril 41:5, 1984.
36. Zorgniotti, AW; MacLeod, J: Studies in temperature, human semen quality, and varicocele. Fertil Steril 24:40, 1973.
37. McClure, DR; Hricak, H: Scrotal ultrasound in the infertile man: Detection of subclinical unilateral and bilateral varicoceles. J Urol 135:711, 1986.
38. Greenburg, SH; Lipshultz, LI; Wei, AJ: A preliminary report of "subclinical varicocele": Diagnosis by Doppler ultrasonic stethoscope. Examination and initial results of surgical therapy. J Reprod Med 22:77, 1979.
39. Dubin, L; Amelar, RD: Etiologic factors in 1294 consecutive cases of male infertility. Fertil Steril 22:469, 1971.
40. Dhabuwala, CB; Hamid, S; Moghissi, KS: Clinical versus subclinical varicocele: Improvement in fertility after varicocelectomy. Fertil Steril 57:854, 1992.
41. Wishahi, MM: Detailed anatomy of the internal spermatic vein and the ovarian vein. Human cadaver study and operative spermatic venography: Clinical aspects. J Urol 145:780, 1991.
42. Wishahi, MM: Anatomy of the spermatic venous plexus (pampiniform plexus) in men with and without varicocele: Intraoperative venographic study. J Urol 147:1285, 1992.
43. Walsh, PC; White, RI: Balloon occlusion of the internal spermatic vein for the treatment of varicoceles. JAMA 246:1701, 1981.
44. Morag, B; Rubinstein, ZJ; Goldwasser, B; et al: Percutaneous venography and occlusion in the management of spermatic varicoceles. Am J Roetgenol 143:635, 1984.
45. MacLeod, J; Hotchkiss, RS: The effect of hyperperexia on spermatozoa counts in men. Endocrinology 28:780, 1941.
46. Agger, P: Scrotal and testicular temperature: Its relation to sperm counts before and after operation for varicocele. Fertil Steril 22:286, 1971.
47. Nagler, HM; Zippe, CD: Varicocele: Current concepts and treatment. In: Lipshultz, LI; Howards, SS; eds: Infertility in the Male. Chicago, Mosby Year Book, 1991, p. 313.
48. Turner, TT: Varicocele: Still an enigma. J Urol 129:695, 1983.
49. Turner, TT; Lopez, TJ: Effects of experimental varicocele require neither adrenal contribution nor venous reflux. J Urol 142:1372, 1989.
50. Chehval, MJ; Purcell, MH: Deterioration of semen parameters over time in men with untreated varicoceles: Evidence of progressive testicular damage. Fertil Steril 57:174, 1992.
51. Nagoa, RR; Plymate, SR; Berger, RE; et al: Comparison of gonadal function between fertile and infertile men with varicoceles. Fertil Steril 46:930, 1986.
52. Weese, DL; Peaster, ML; Himsl, KK; et al: Stimulated reactive oxygen species generation in spermatazoa of infertile men. J Urol 149:64, 1993.
53. MacLeod, J: Seminal cytology in the presence of varicoceles. Fertil Steril 16:735, 1965.
54. McConnell, JD: Abnormalities in sperm motility: Technics of evaluation and treatment. In: Lipshultz, LI; Howards, SS: Infertility in the Male. Chicago, Mosby Year Book, 1991, p. 313.
55. Lipshultz, LI; Corriere, JN, Jr: Progressive testicular atrophy in the varicocele patients. J Urol 117:175, 1977.
56. Lyon, RP; Marshall, S; Scott, MP: Varicocele in childhood and adolescence: Implication in adulthood infertility? Urology 19:641, 1982.
57. Kass, EJ; Marcol, B: Results of varicocele surgery in adolescents: A comparison of techniques. J Urol 148:694, 1992.
58. Hosli, PO: Varicocele—results after early treatment in children and adolescents. Z Kinderchir 43:213, 1988.
59. Okuyama, A; Nakamura, M; Namiki, M; et al: Surgical repair of varicocele at puberty: Preventive treatment for fertility improvement. J Urol 139:562, 1988.
60. Donovan, JF, Jr: Laparoscopic varix ligation. In Clayman, RV; McDougall, EM; eds: Laparoscopic Urology. St. Louis, Quality Medical Publishing, 1993.
61. Matsuda, T; Horii, Y; Higashi, S; et al: Laparoscopic varicocelectomy: A simple technique for clip ligation of the spermatic vessels. J Urol 147:636, 1992.
62. Hasson, HM: Open laparoscopy: A report of 150 cases. J Reprod Med 12:234, 1974.
63. Loughlin, KR; Brooks, DC: The use of a Doppler probe to facilitate laparoscopic varicocele ligation. Surg Gynecol Obstet 174:326, 1992.
64. Donovan, JF, Jr; Winfield, HN: Laparoscopic varix ligation with Nd:YAG laser. J Endourol 6:165, 1992.
65. Clayman, RV: Laparoscopic varix ligation (editorial). In: Clayman, RV; McDougall, EM; eds: Laparoscopic Urology. St. Louis, Quality Medical Publishing, 1993.
66. Winfield, HN; Donovan, JF, Jr: Laparoscopic varicocelectomy. Semin Urol 10:143, 1992.
67. Mehan, DJ; Andrus, CH; Parra, RO: Laparoscopic internal spermatic vein ligation: Report of a new technique. Fertil Steril 58:1263, 1992.

CHAPTER 11

Laparoscopic Nephrectomy, Nephroureterectomy, and Partial Nephrectomy

E. M. McDougall, MD, FRCSC
R. V. Clayman, MD, FACS

The first nephrectomy was performed in 1869 by Simon for ureterovaginal fistula.[1] During the more than 100 years since that first nephrectomy, dramatic changes in anesthesia, antibiotics, and surgical technique have improved access to the kidney and its vasculature, facilitated removal of the diseased kidney, and hastened patients' recovery from the operative procedure.

Laparoscopy was first reported in 1901 by Kelling of Dresden after he used a Nitze cystoscope to examine the abdominal cavity of a dog.[2] In that report he described the instrumentation required and speculated on the future possibilities for the technique. In 1910 Jacobeus of Sweden described and reported on laparoscopy in a series of human patients.[3] The initial diagnostic laparoscopy in the United States was performed by Bernheim in 1911, using a cystoscope and room light to examine the abdominal cavity.[4] Following these reports, investigators struggled to develop new instrumentation to improve the access and diagnostic yield of the laparoscope. Verres of Hungary developed a new needle for the atraumatic induction of pneumothorax in 1938.[5] This new needle was subsequently found to be ideal for establishing a pneumoperitoneum. An automatic insufflation device to monitor intra-abdominal pressure and gas flow was developed in the 1960s by Semm, a gynecologist and engineer from Kiel, Germany.[6] However, for many subsequent decades laparoscopy was considered to be a less than optimal procedure and was therefore not accepted by many surgeons. Nevertheless, many pioneering individuals continued in the 1960s and 1970s to report with enthusiasm the value of laparoscopy as a diagnostic and therapeutic modality.[7–11]

The laparoscope was first used for urologic purposes in 1976 when Cortesi and associates utilized the technique to localize a cryptorchid testicle.[12] However, the development of computed tomography (CT) and ultrasonographically directed biopsies further limited the pursuit of laparoscopy in urology.[13] Indeed, in adult urology, the use of the laparoscope was limited to case reports in which the instrument was used to help monitor the establishment of a percutaneous nephrostomy tract in a stone-laden pelvic kidney.[14]

Similarly, Wickham and subsequently Clayman and associates reported single cases of retroperitoneoscopy for the removal of ureteral calculi.[15,16] It wasn't until the pioneering work of Scheussler and colleagues that laparoscopy was finally introduced into general adult urology. Their report in 1989 of laparoscopic pelvic lymphadenectomy in a patient with prostatic carcinoma initiated a new era in urologic surgery.[17]

Laparoscopists in all the surgical disciplines were not content with using laparoscopy for diagnostic purposes alone and began to investigate its use for operative procedures.[18,19] A variety of urologic surgical problems previously approached by a flank or abdominal incision have since been managed laparoscopically: varicocele,[20] pelvic lymphocele,[21] retroperitoneal fibrosis,[22] stress incontinence,[23] renal cysts,[24] and most recently, end-stage renal disease[25] and renal malignancy.

The development of a surgical entrapment sack and a 10-mm high-speed tissue morcellator has facilitated the removal of the kidney through an entirely laparoscopic approach. The first laparoscopic nephrectomy was performed in June 1990.[26] Since then there have been more than 50 laparoscopic nephrectomies performed worldwide.[27] In addition, the technique has been used to successfully complete laparoscopic nephroureterectomy with concomitant excision of a cuff of bladder and to manage other renal disease processes such as renal cysts, nephroptosis, calyceal diverticulum, and lobar renal disease.

INDICATIONS

At present laparoscopic nephrectomy is indicated for all patients in whom the kidney requires removal for benign disease. This would include the poorly functioning or nonfunctioning kidney associated with flank pain, chronic obstruction and infection, persistent renovascular hypertension, and occasionally the multicystic kidney.

Laparoscopic nephrectomy and nephroureterectomy have been used in selected patients for low-grade or small malignant tumors of the kidney or upper collecting system or both. There remains considerable controversy as to the appropriateness of the generalized use of laparoscopic removal of malignant renal tissues. The process of tissue morcellation allows for accurate identification and grading of the tumor cells. However, the ability to accurately stage the local disease by its depth of invasion is not possible with this technique. Although the degree of invasiveness may have implications for the patient's prognosis in respect to survival or renal cell carcinoma or transitional cell carcinoma, the status of perirenal lymph nodes appears to have the most significant impact on this issue. Hilar lymph nodes can be sampled as separate specimens at the time of laparoscopic surgery, thereby limiting this concern. In addition, the degree of local invasion does not alter the subsequent therapeutic management of patients with these urologic malignancies.

The fragmentation of the entire tissue specimen for removal by the morcellator raises a concern for macroscopic or microscopic seeding of tumor cells within the abdominal cavity or at the incision site. There have been three reports in the literature in which patients with known intra-abdominal malignancy underwent laparoscopic biopsy and subsequently developed incisional tumor. Two of these cases involved patients with malignant ascites.[28–30] All the principles of surgery for renal cell carcinoma are maintained during laparoscopic nephrectomy. The dissection is performed while retaining the Gerota fascial containment of the cancer-bearing kidney and securing first the renal artery and then the renal vein before transection. The entrapment sack into which the surgical specimen is placed is completely impermeable. Studies in our laboratory have shown the Lapsack (Cook Urologic) to maintain its impermeability to indigo carmine, albumin, and tumor cells for up to 24 hours after renal morcellation. The blunt tip of the morcellator requires that the renal tissue be cored out before the recessed blades can fragment the tissue for aspiration. To date, in 23 nephrectomies performed laparoscopically, no entrapment sack perforations have occurred.

Alternatively, the risk of seeding and proper tumor grade and stage can accurately be determined if the kidney is removed intact. To do this, the sack can be withdrawn from the abdomen by making a 2 to 3 cm extension of the trocar insertion site. The tumor is at no time exposed or biopsied.

Another concern in approaching upper urinary tract malignancy by the laparoscope is the ability to successfully remove all of the disease. The entrapment sacks have a maximum size of 5.5 × 8.0 inches (volume, 700 ml). Large tumors (i.e., >5 cm) affecting a normal-sized kidney are therefore not amenable to laparoscopic removal. Another problem is the need to remove the adrenal gland for renal malignancy. However, Robey and Schellhammer showed that the adrenal gland does not need to be removed for lower-pole or midsection cancers of the kidney.[31] In these cases, Gerota's fascia is entered at the upper pole of the kidney, and the adrenal gland is not removed. For upper-pole renal tumors, additional time is spent to perform an adrenalectomy and thereby keep the Gerota fascia intact.

At Washington University School of Medicine, we have completed 25 laparoscopic nephrectomies since June 1990. Seventeen patients underwent a simple transabdominal laparoscopic nephrectomy for benign disease (Table 11–1). The average age in this group of

Table 11–1. TRANSABDOMINAL LAPAROSCOPIC NEPHRECTOMY: DEMOGRAPHICS

		Upper Tract Mass	
	Benign Disease	***Renal Tumor***	***Transitional Cell CA***
Patients	17	2	6
Male/female	4/13	0/2	5/1
Age (average): (years)	42	87.5	60.8
Range (years)	(16-72)	(85-90)	(58-83)
Prior abdominal surgery	6	1	1
Renal disease			
Obstruction/pain	6		
Obstruction/infection	10		
Hypertension	1		
Oncocytoma		1	
Renal cell CA		1	

CA, Carcinoma

patients was 42 years (range 16 to 72 years), and the average rating of the American Society of Anesthesiologists was 1.7 (range 1 to 3) (Table 11–2). The initial 6 patients had renal artery embolization just before arriving in the operating suite. In all subsequent patients, arterial embolization was not done. The average operating time was 5.2 hours (range, 2.5 to 7.75 hours) with an average estimated blood loss of 223 ml (range, 50 to 500 ml). The majority of the 17 patients had chronic inflammation or nephrosclerosis or both as the final pathologic diagnosis (Table 11–3). This group of patients had a quick recovery and a short hospital stay (Table 11–4).

The complication rate in the group of 17 patients with benign disease was 11% (Table 11–5). One patient failed a laparoscopic approach because of marked obesity and operator inability to safely secure the renal artery; an open laparotomy was performed to complete the nephrectomy. This patient also sustained a postoperative right brachial nerve palsy, which was managed conservatively. Two initial patients received blood transfusions (1 and 2 units, respectively) for immediate postoperative declines in the hematocrit. Both of these patients developed congestive heart failure that resolved with medical management; there was no evidence of myocardial injury in either patient. One patient developed an angiographically confirmed pulmonary embolus and received 6 months' therapy with anticoagulant.

Eight patients with malignant disease were treated with laparoscopic surgical excision (see Tables 11–1 to 11–5). Two patients had renal cell carcinoma. One patient had a midpole left renal cell carcinoma and underwent a laparoscopic radical nephrectomy with preservation of the adrenal gland. This patient was 90 years of age with an ASA rating of 3; the procedure required 9 hours of operating time; 600 ml of blood loss occurred, necessitating transfusion of one unit of packed red blood cells. This patient also had a prolonged ileus and atrial fibrillation postoperatively and was discharged from the hospital on the tenth postoperative day. A second patient underwent a left radical nephrectomy and adrenalectomy for a 3-cm upper-pole renal tumor. Despite a lymphocele, this 72-year-old man had an uneventful recovery and was discharged from the hospital on the fourth postoperative day. One patient had an oncocytoma that was diagnosed preoperatively.

Six of the eight patients had transitional cell carcinoma of the upper tract (see Tables 11–1 to 11–4). The average age in this group was 60.8 years (range, 58 to 83 years), and the average ASA rating was 2.6 (range, 2 to 4). All of these patients had cystoscopic unroofing of the ureter immediately preceding the

Table 11–2. TRANSABDOMINAL LAPAROSCOPIC NEPHRECTOMY—OPERATIVE DETAILS

		Upper Tract Mass	
	Benign Disease	***Renal Tumor***	***Transitional Cell CA***
ASA rating: average	1.7	2.5	2.6
Preoperative renal artery embolization	1st 6 of 17	0	0
Operating room time (h)			
Average	5.2*	7.8*	8.7†
Range	2.5–7.75	6.75–9.0	6.67–10.6

*Includes stent placement.
†Includes cystoscopy and ureteral unroofing.
CA, carcinoma; h, hours.

Table 11–3. TRANSABDOMINAL NEPHRECTOMY: PATHOLOGY

		Upper Tract Mass	
	Benign Disease	***Renal Tumor***	***Transitional Cell CA***
Weight of specimen (g)			
Average	134.2	235	362
Range	31–410	190–280	229–550
Pathologic diagnosis			6
Nephrosclerosis	5		
Chronic inflammation	5		
Acute and chronic inflammation + calculus	7		
Oncocytoma		1	
Renal cell CA		1	

CA, carcinoma.

laparoscopic procedure. Laparoscopically, the ureter was completely dissected, and a cuff of bladder was excised intact with the nephrectomy specimen. Of the six patients undergoing laparoscopic nephroureterectomy for transitional cell carcinoma, three had the specimen removed intact in the entrapment sack for pathologic staging and grading. The operative time was longer than for simple nephrectomy and averaged 8.7 hours (range, 6.67 to 10.6 hours), including the time required to unroof the ureter. Among five of these patients the average hospital stay was 6.3 days. First oral intake averaged 1.5 days, and the amount of postoperative parenteral analgesia averaged 24.3 mg of morphine sulfate. One patient with preoperative cardiac disease and chronic obstructive pulmonary disease (COPD) underwent nephroureterectomy for transitional cell carcinoma. He developed postoperative bleeding, necessitating emergency laparotomy. Bleeding from a venous branch at the inferior edge of the adrenal was noted and controlled, but the patient received transfusion of 8 units of blood. He subsequently developed adult respiratory distress syndrome and expired.

In conclusion, laparoscopic nephrectomy in comparison with open surgical nephrectomy requires longer operative time. However, in general, patients undergoing laparoscopic nephrectomy resume oral alimentation more quickly, require less postoperative analgesia, and return to their normal activity level more quickly. Laparoscopic nephrectomy does have associated significant complications of which the surgeon and patient should be aware. Attention to surgical detail will minimize the risk of these complications. Meticulous postoperative care alerts the surgeon regarding any developing problems, thereby permitting prompt intervention to reduce risks of long-term sequelae.

Table 11–5. COMPLICATIONS IN TRANSABDOMINAL LAPAROSCOPIC NEPHRECTOMY

Complication	No. of Patients
Benign Disease (17 Patients)	
Intraoperative	
Failed laparoscopic approach, open nephrectomy*	1
Postoperative	
Congestive heart failure†	1
Pulmonary embolus	1
Right brachial plexus injury*	1
Transfusions (2 units)	1
Renal Tumor Disease (8 Patients)	
Postoperative (0 Intraoperative)	
Postoperative bleeding (laparotomy)‡	1
Respiratory failure and death‡	1
Atrial fibrillation and prolonged ileus	1
Transfusions	
8 units‡	1
1 unit	2

*In same patient.
†In same patient.
‡In same patient.

Table 11–4. TRANSABDOMINAL LAPAROSCOPIC NEPHRECTOMY—POSTOPERATIVE COURSE

		Upper Tract Mass	
	Benign Disease	***Renal Tumor***	***Transitional Cell CA***
First oral intake (days)	1.4	2	1.1
Parenteral analgesics (mg of morphine sulfate)	41	14	24
Hospital stay (days)	3.6	8.5	5.4
Return to regular activity (weeks)	1.75		3.0*

*Follow-up on three of six patients.
CA, carcinoma.

PATIENT PREPARATION

The patient considered an appropriate candidate for laparoscopic nephrectomy because of the disease process or concomitant medical status is fully informed of the surgical options. The patient is told that all of the inherent risks of open surgical nephrectomy are similarly associated with laparoscopic nephrectomy. These risks can include injuries to vascular structures, the bowel, the bladder, and other intra-abdominal structures (spleen, liver, or pancreas). These injuries may be life-threatening or may necessitate opening the abdomen in a traditional manner for appropriate management or both. Similar risks of postoperative infection, bleeding, and venous thromboembolic abnormalities can occur with laparoscopic nephrectomy, but the risk of these complications should be low. Also, technical problems with tissue dissection and renal entrapment or removal may require an open incision to complete the procedure. The patient is informed that the laparoscopic procedure will require five 0.25- to 0.5-inch abdominal wall incisions. The abdominal wall incisions are small yet just as with the traditional open abdominal incision, bowel adhesions, herniation, or both can occur. In addition, there usually is some degree of postoperative discomfort associated with the trocar sites. The patient is also told that laparoscopy poses some unique life-threatening, as well as other minor, risks, such as gas embolus, arrhythmias, and subcutaneous emphysema.

All patients undergo routine preoperative evaluation with serum electrolytes, complete blood cell counts, urinalysis, and urine culture. Those patients with malignancy have preoperative staging that may include CT of the abdomen, pelvis, and chest and any or all of the following: bone scan, chest radiograph, liver function tests, and Doppler ultrasound imaging of the renal vein. Depending on the patients' medical status, they may also require ECG, chest radiograph, and pulmonary function tests or cardiac stress testing or both.

The patient is routinely typed and crossmatched for two units of packed red blood cells. Alternatively, the patient is allowed the opportunity to provide two units of autologous whole blood for an electively planned procedure.

A complete mechanical and antibiotic bowel preparation is administered on an outpatient basis. This consists of 4 L of GoLYTELY the day before surgery and nothing by mouth after midnight preoperatively. The patient is also given neomycin 2 g and metronidazole 2 g by mouth at 1900 hours and 2300 hours on the day before the surgery.

On call to the operating room, the patient receives an intravenous dosage of a broad-spectrum antibiotic (cephalosporin or ampicillin and gentamicin).

Although our first seven laparoscopic nephrectomy patients underwent renal artery embolization just before their planned procedure, we have subsequently found that this additional step is not necessary. The last 13 patients have not had renal artery embolization, and no significant problem with intraoperative bleeding has occurred. In one patient, the renal vascular pedicle could not be properly secured, necessitating open exploration and nephrectomy. Preoperative embolization may be of benefit in the surgeon's early experience with laparoscopic nephrectomy or when difficulty with the renal hilar dissection is anticipated.

For patients undergoing laparoscopic nephrectomy or nephroureterectomy, an indwelling ureteral catheter is placed immediately before the planned operative procedure. Placement can usually be performed in the cystoscopy suite, using intravenous sedation or local anesthesia with 2% xylocaine gel per urethra or both. A flexible cystoscope is used to access the ureteral orifice, and a 0.035-inch Bentson guide wire is inserted into the involved ureter under fluoroscopic control. After satisfactory positioning of the guide wire in the upper collecting system, the cystoscope is removed. A no. 7 Fr, 11.5-mm occlusion balloon catheter is passed over the guide wire until the tip of the catheter is in the renal pelvis. The guide wire is removed, and a retrograde pyelogram is performed, using 5 to 10 ml of dilute contrast (50% normal saline and 50% Conray 60). Under fluoroscopic control, the catheter balloon is inflated with one ml of contrast through a one-way stopcock. After inflating the balloon in the renal pelvis, the Bentson guide wire is exchanged for an 0.035-inch Amplatz Super Stiff guide wire. A side-arm adapter is passed over the Super Stiff guide wire and fixed to the distal end of the occlusion balloon catheter. The side-arm adapter is then tightly screwed down to secure it to the guide wire. A Foley catheter is placed alongside the occlusion balloon catheter to drain the bladder. Both catheters are placed in a sterile plastic bag for transport to the main operating room.

Before leaving the cystoscopy suite while under fluoroscopic control, the balloon in the renal pelvis is localized on the abdominal skin, using the tip of a metal clamp. A 25-gauge needle is used to inject 0.1 ml of indigo carmine subcutaneously. This subcutaneous "blue dot" helps to localize the area of the renal pelvis in order to facilitate trocar port placement directed towards the renal pelvis.

The patient is transported to the main operating room where general anesthesia is induced with cuffed endotracheal intubation. Throughout the procedure, the patient is monitored with a central venous pressure line (CVP), capnometry, arterial line for blood gas calculations, Foley urethral catheter, and a nasogastric tube. In patients with a history of coronary artery disease or cardiac arrhythmias, Swan-Ganz catheter monitoring is preferable to a CVP line.

After induction of anesthesia and initial supine positioning, a full skin preparation is carried out from xiphoid to symphysis pubis and from the lateral aspect of the contralateral rectus muscle to the posterior axillary line on the ipsilateral side. Under sterile conditions, the catheters are removed from the plastic bag. For access throughout the operative procedure, the perineum and shaft of the urethral catheter and an equal length of the ureteral catheter are prepared and draped separately.

PATIENT POSITIONING

The patient is initially positioned supine on a deflatable bean bag with both arms extended on arm boards. To avoid brachial plexus injury, care should be taken to ensure that the shoulders are not hyperabducted. The kidney region of the flank should be positioned over the kidney rest and the break in the table. Pneumatic compression stockings are applied to both legs and thighs. In the supine position, the first three ports are inserted: a 12-mm umbilical port, a 5-mm midclavicular subumbilical port, and a 12-mm midclavicular subcostal port.

The patient is then placed in the lateral decubitus position to expose the appropriate flank. The two 5-mm axillary line ports are then placed: one subcostally and one at the umbilical line. To maintain a sterile operative field, redraping is often necessary following this. In the lateral decubitus position, the lower leg is flexed 30° at the knee and hip, and the top leg is left extended with one or two pillows placed between the legs. The upper arm is supported over the patient by securing it to an ether screen or an elevated arm board. The axilla should be padded to protect the brachial plexus of the lower arm. All bony prominences should be inspected and padded as necessary. The pulse oximeter is placed on the dependent arm. The Foley catheter and ureteral catheter are maintained in a sterile field. The table is flexed. The bean bag is molded and deflated to support the patient's position. Additional sandbags may be required at the shoulders and hips to maintain the lateral decubitus position. Two straps are affixed, one at the shoulders and one at the knees, to help maintain the patient's position.

REQUIRED INSTRUMENTS

1 No. 12 hook blade and scalpel handle
2 sharp towel clips
2 toothed forceps
1 10-ml syringe
1 Verres needle (14-gauge)
1 Kelly clamp
1 ring forceps
2 12-mm trocars
1 10-mm laparoscope
3 5-mm trocars
1 5-mm laparoscope
6 trocar reducers 10.5-mm (2); 5.5-mm (2); 4.5-mm (2)
1 5-mm electrosurgical monopolar scissors
3 5-mm atraumatic grasping forceps (2 spoon-shaped, 1 dolphin)
4 5-mm traumatic, locking, grasping forceps
1 5-mm or 10-mm curved or right-angle dissector or both
1 5-mm Babcock locking forceps
1 9-mm clip applier
1 11-mm Endoclip applier
1 surgical entrapment sack (5.5 × 8.5 inches)
1 5-mm irrigator/aspirator
1 10-mm tissue morcellator
2 Kocher clamps
2 Sinn retractors
1 11-mm retractor (fan-type)
1 needle holder
1 5-mm retractor (fan-type)
4 2–0 nonabsorbable sutures or LR cutting needles
2 4–0 absorbable sutures
1 umbilical tape: 4 inches
Steri-Strips

OPTIONAL INSTRUMENTS

2 Army-Navy retractors
1 12-mm GIA vascular stapler (3 cm length)
1 12-mm GIA tissue stapler (3 cm length)
1 5-mm or 10-mm Babcock forceps

OPERATING ROOM SETUP (Fig. 11–1)

The surgeon and camera operator (second assistant) stand on the side of the table opposite (i.e., contralateral to) the side of dissection. The first surgical assistant stands opposite the surgeon on the side of the table ipsilateral to the operative site. The cart holding the primary video monitor, CO_2 insufflator, light source, and recorder are positioned on the ipsilateral side of the table just above the shoulder of the first assistant. The secondary video monitor is positioned above the surgeon's shoulder on the contralateral side of the table. The electrosurgical generator and its cord are placed behind the surgeon. The irrigator/aspirator tubing enters from the ipsilateral side of the table.

The scrub nurse is positioned next to the first assistant with the sterile setup table behind him or her and a Mayo stand crossing the bottom of the operative

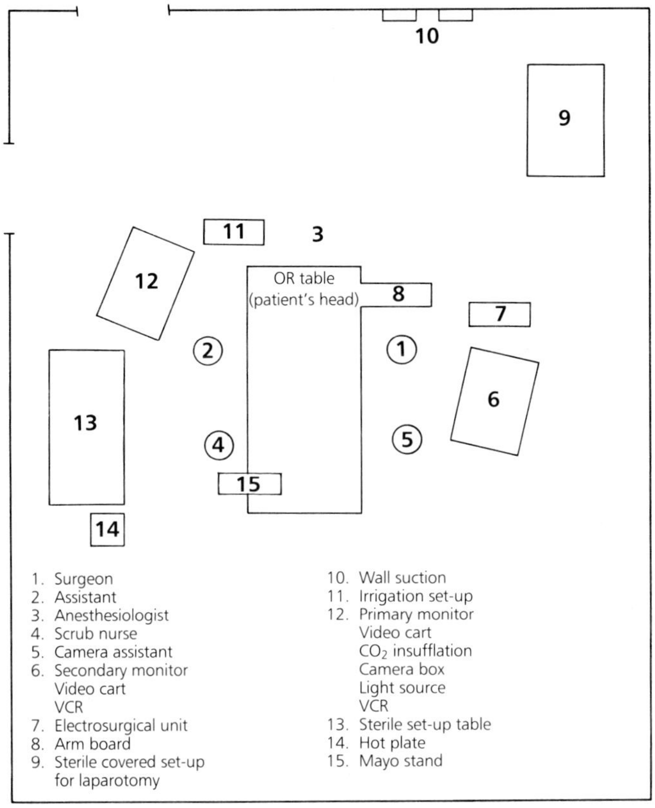

Figure 11–1. Operating room setup for laparoscopic nephrectomy. (From Clayman, RV, McDougall, EM: Laparoscopic Urology. St. Louis, Quality Medical Publishing, 1993.)

table. The anesthesiologist is at the head of the table behind a horizontal sterile barrier drape.

PNEUMOPERITONEUM

The No. 12 hook scalpel blade is used to make a 12-mm incision in the supra-umbilical line. A 14-gauge Verres needle is inserted perpendicular to the skin while the skin edge is stabilized by the assistant with sharp towel clips on either side. The Verres needle is held like a dart between the thumb and index finger; the hypothenar eminance rests against the abdominal wall for stabilization. As the Verres needle passes through the anterior fascia and peritoneum, two distinct "pops" will be felt and the red indicator marker will spring down each time. A 10-ml syringe with 5 to 7 ml of normal saline is connected to the Verres needle, and the stopcock on the needle is opened. Aspiration on the syringe should return a few bubbles of gas. If blood or green or brown fluid is obtained, the needle is incorrectly positioned and should be removed. After gas has been obtained, a few ml of saline should be injected; this should flow into the abdomen without any resistance. Re-aspiration of the syringe should again obtain bubbles of gas and no fluid. The syringe is disconnected from the needle and with the abdomen slightly raised by the towel clips, the saline remaining in the hub of the needle should rapidly flow down the needle into the peritoneal cavity. This procedure confirms accurate placement of the needle in the peritoneal cavity.

The CO_2 insufflation tubing is connected to the Verres needle, and flow is commenced at one L/minute. The immediately recorded abdominal pressure as flow commences should be less than 10 mm Hg and should remain below 10 mm Hg for the first 500 ml of CO_2 insufflated. If pressures are greater than 10 mm Hg, the needle can be rotated 180°. If pressures are still greater than 10 mm Hg, the needle should be pulled from the abdomen and reinserted.

After 0.5 L of CO_2 has been insufflated and the abdominal pressure has remained below 10 mm Hg, the flow rate can be increased. The maximum flow rate that can be achieved through the Verres needle is approximately 2.3 to 2.5 L/minute. CO_2 insufflation is continued until the intra-abdominal pressure is 20 to 25 mm Hg; in the adult, this pressure is usually reached after approximately 4.5 to 5.0 L of CO_2 have been insufflated. At this maximum pressure, the insufflation is discontinued, and the Verres needle is removed.

PORT PLACEMENT (Fig. 11–2)

The incision in the umbilical crease in enlarged to 12 mm. Kelly forceps are used to spread the subcutaneous tissues and anterior fascia of the supraumbilical incision. The sharp towel clips at the edges of the incision are replaced to stabilize the abdominal wall. The 12-mm trocar is held in the dominant hand with the middle finger extended along the shaft of the trocar to act as a brake during insertion. The trocar tip is inserted through the skin. A twisting motion using constant pressure is used to advance the trocar through the abdominal wall, directing it toward the renal pelvis. There is a "give" as the trocar passes into the peritoneal cavity, and the rush of gas through the open sidearm of the trocar confirms its proper position in the peritoneal cavity. The trocar's obturator is removed, and the CO_2 insufflation tubing is connected to the stopcock. A 10.5-mm reducer is placed on the trocar and the 10-mm laparoscope is inserted. This will confirm satisfactory positioning of the trocar's sheath in the peritoneal cavity, since loops of bowel should readily be identifiable. The abdominal cavity should be examined for bowel adhesions to the anterior abdominal wall that might affect positioning of additional trocars. Also, the abdomen should be scanned as part of a routine examination before beginning the nephrectomy.

By palpating on the abdominal wall, the proposed trocar site can be observed with the laparoscope to

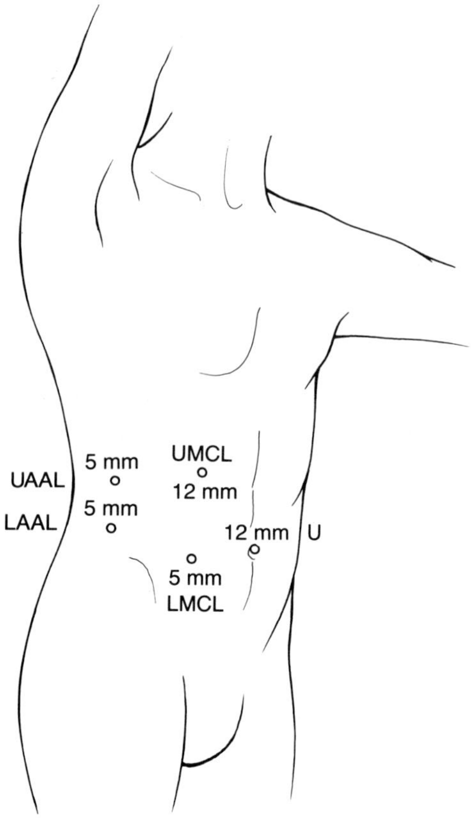

Figure 11–2. Port placement for laparoscopic nephrectomy. LAAL, lower anterior axillary line; LMCL, lower midclavicular line; U, umbilicus; UAAL, upper anterior axillary line; UMCL, upper midclavicular line. (From Clayman, RV, McDougall, EM: Laparoscopic Urology. St. Louis, Quality Medical Publishing, 1993.)

ensure that adhesions, bowel, or other viscera will not interfere with port placement. The proposed site is transilluminated to identify any large abdominal wall vessels, which can thereby be avoided. The site below the costal margin in the midclavicular line (MCL) is examined, and a skin incision is made with the no. 12 hook scalpel blade to admit another 12-mm trocar. The trocar is held in the same manner as the initial trocar and is inserted with a constant, twisting pressure directed towards the renal pelvis. This maneuver is monitored with the laparoscope to avoid injury to any intra-abdominal structure. The trocar is advanced until 1 to 2 cm of the sheath is below the level of the peritoneum; the obturator is removed, and the stopcock is closed. A no. 2 Proline suture is passed through to the skin at the base of the trocar and then tied to the stopcock sheathing, thereby securing the port to the skin. This maneuver precludes inadvertent removal of the sheath during the procedure.

In a similar manner, with transillumination, the site for the 5-mm trocar is identified in the MCL, 3 to 4 cm below the umbilicus. The tip of the no. 12 hook blade is used to just puncture the skin and anterior fascia. A Kelly clamp is used to spread the skin incision to accept the 5-mm trocar. Holding the trocar in the same manner as the 12-mm trocar, under laparoscopic visualization, the 5-mm trocar is inserted and is directed toward the area of the renal pelvis. The 5-mm sheath is advanced 1 to 2 cm into the peritoneal cavity, the puncture site in the peritoneum is examined for hemostasis, and the sheath is then sutured to the skin with a no. 2 Proline suture.

A 10.5-mm reducer is placed on the 12-mm midclavicular trocar, and the laparoscope is removed from the umbilical port and inserted through the midclavicular 12-mm trocar. The peritoneal side of the umbilical sheath is examined for hemostasis and 1 to 2 cm of sheath is positioned in the abdominal cavity; no. 2 Proline is used to also secure this sheath to the skin.

As previously described, the patient is in the lateral decubitus position. The laparoscope is inserted through the umbilical port and is used to transilluminate the anterior axillary line (AAL) just below the costal margin. The no. 12 hook scalpel blade is used to create a puncture incision at the tip of the 12th rib, and this site is dilated with the Kelly forceps. A 5-mm trocar is directed toward the renal pelvis and is inserted under direct laparoscopic visualization. In the same fashion as the previous sheath, it is secured to the skin with no. 2 Proline suture.

The skin site for the last 5-mm trocar is identified in the anterior axillary line, opposite the umbilicus. This trocar is also inserted with laparoscopic visualization, directed toward the renal pelvis, and secured to the skin with no. 2 Proline suture.

INCISION OF THE LINE OF TOLDT (Fig. 11–3)

The laparoscope remains in the umbilical port. The surgeon works with an atraumatic grasping forceps through the 5-mm MCL port and the electrosurgical scissors through the 12-mm MCL port. The first assistant uses grasping forceps through the two 5-mm anterior axillary ports to provide countertraction superior and lateral to the surgeon's grasping forceps, thereby allowing the surgeon to incise the peritoneum between the grasping forceps. The peritoneum is incised along the line of Toldt from its inferior aspect up to and including the hepatic (on the right side) or the splenic (on the left side) flexure. A sweeping motion with the grasping forceps mobilizes the colon medially to expose the retroperitoneum overlying the kidney and ureter. It is important to fully mobilize the respective flexure of the colon in order to completely expose the upper pole of the kidney. Care must be taken to avoid laceration of the liver or spleen or injury to the bowel during this dissection. Small vessels are controlled with electrocautery. By further developing the plane between the bowel and the Gerota

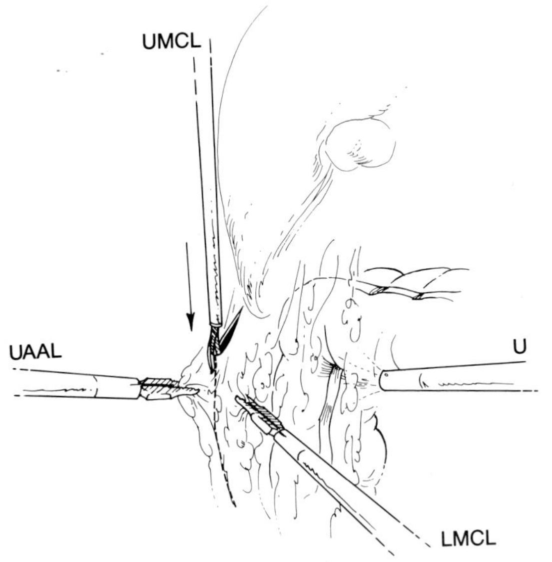

Figure 11–3. Incision of the line of Toldt. (From Clayman, RV, McDougall, EM: Laparoscopic Urology. St. Louis, Quality Medical Publishing, 1993.)

fascia, the bowel can be mobilized far medially. On the right side, the duodenum is also moved medially, while on the left side, the aorta is uncovered.

SECURING THE URETER (Fig. 11–4)

Once the bowel is completely mobilized, attention is directed to the retroperitoneum below the kidney in order to localize the ureter. Manipulation of the ureteral catheter where it exits the urethral meatus produces movement of the ureter in the retroperitoneum that aids in ureteral localization. Also the ureteral catheter and Amplatz Super Stiff guide wire provide rigidity to the ureter, which can be felt as an overriding ridge as the forceps is passed across the retroperitoneum. If this fails to identify the ureter, then attention is directed to the region of the pulsation of the common iliac vessels. Careful, blunt, and anteriorly directed sharp dissection in this area will usually delineate the ureter as it passes over the iliac vessels.

After identifying the ureter, it is sharply and bluntly dissected to create a "window" free of periureteral connective tissue around the ureter. A Babcock forceps can then be inserted through the lower 5-mm AAL port and can be used to secure the ureter and retract it superiorly and laterally. Alternatively, the 4-inch piece of umbilical tape can be inserted through the lower AAL port. This is placed around the ureter and is grasped with a 5-mm locking forceps. This maneuver allows dissection of the ureter to proceed up to the renal pelvis and hilar region.

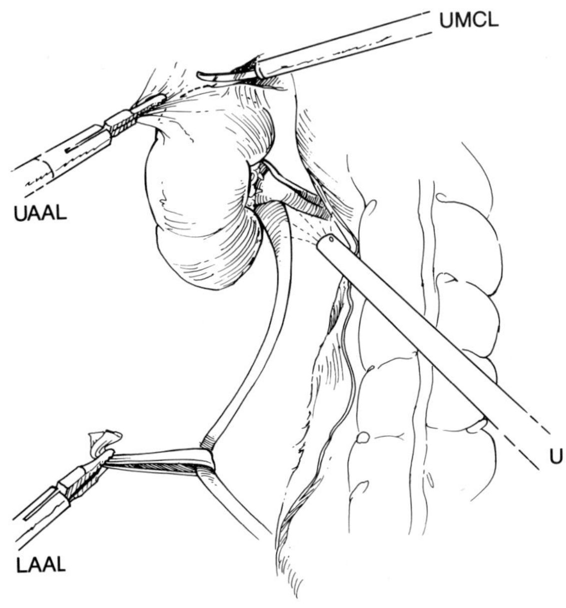

Figure 11–4. Securing the ureter and dissecting the upper pole of the kidney. U, umbilicus; UAAL, upper anterior axillary line. (From Clayman, RV, McDougall, EM: Laparoscopic Urology. St. Louis, Quality Medical Publishing, 1993.)

DISSECTING THE UPPER AND LOWER POLES OF THE KIDNEY (see Fig. 11–4)

The camera remains at the umbilical port, and the surgeon works through the two MCL ports with countertraction provided by the first assistant's graspers through one or both AAL ports.

Having dissected the ureter up to the renal hilum, Gerota's fascia overlying the lower pole of the kidney can be incised. To perform this, the assistant uses the lower AAL port grasper to retract laterally, and the surgeon uses the lower MCL port grasper to countertract medially; the electrocautery scissors are used through the upper MCL port to incise and dissect Gerota's fascia. This dissection is continued along the lateral border of the kidney proceeding superiorly. The assistant can then position the lower AAL port grasper medial to the lower pole of the kidney to bluntly retract the lower pole laterally. The upper AAL port grasper then retracts Gerota's fascia of the upper pole laterally while the surgeon's lower MCL grasper provides medial traction, and the scissors through the upper MCL port are used to incise and dissect the upper pole of the kidney free from Gerota's fascia. The upper AAL port grasper is then placed just medial to the upper pole of the kidney, and the upper pole is bluntly retracted laterally.

SECURING THE HILAR VESSELS (Fig. 11–5)

By retracting the upper and lower poles of the kidney with the grasping forceps through the two AAL ports, the first assistant places the hilar vessels on slight

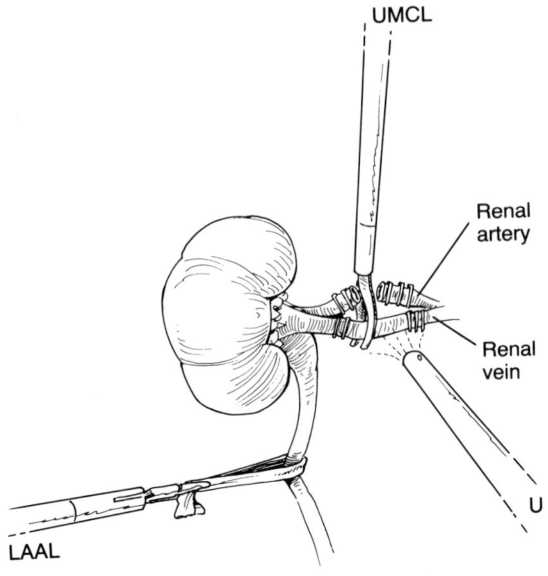

Figure 11–5. Securing the hilar vessels. LAAL, lower anterior axillary line; U, umbilicus; UMCL, upper midclavicular line. (From Clayman, RV, McDougall, EM: Laparoscopic Urology. St. Louis, Quality Medical Publishing, 1993.)

stretch, which facilitates their dissection. The surgeon continues to work through the two MCL ports using an atraumatic straight or curved dissector through the lower MCL port and the electrosurgical scissors from the upper MCL port. Blunt dissection along the line of the vessels strands out the fatty connective tissue and lymphatic vessels, which can be coagulated and incised. This exposes the anterior surface of the renal vein. On the left side, care must be taken to identify the gonadal vein, posterior lumbar vein, and adrenal vein. These are individually dissected free and are secured with four 9-mm clips before being transected between the second and third clip. To apply the vessel clips, the instrument in the upper 12-mm trocar is removed, and the 5.5-mm reducer is exchanged for a 10.5-mm reducer. The clip applier is inserted through this port as the grasper in the lower MCL port exposes the vessel. After the clips are applied, the clip applier is removed. A 5.5-mm reducer is reapplied to the 12-mm MCL sheath, and the scissors are introduced through the port to transect the vessel. On the right side, the gonadal vein can be identified and requires securing with clips before transection in a similar manner.

Having secured these smaller veins, the main renal vein is identified and dissected. The posterior aspect of the vein is then mobilized, and the renal artery can usually be seen pulsating just posterior to the renal vein. The periarterial connective tissue is dissected to expose the renal artery; the artery is circumferentially freed for a length of 1 to 1.5 cm. After a complete "window" has been created around the artery, the 9-mm clip applier is inserted through the 12-mm MCL port while an atraumatic grasper through the lower MCL port maintains exposure of the artery. A clip is fired into the jaws of the clip applier. The clip applier is passed across the artery until both tips traverse the body of the artery. The engaged clip is partially closed, approximating the tips of the clip as the handle is closed to its halfway position. The clip can then be slid along the vessel and can be positioned proximally as far as possible. Once in a satisfactory position on the vessel, the handle is completely closed, causing the clip to tightly approximate the vessel wall. Distal to the first clip, this procedure is repeated four more times. The clip applier is removed, and the scissors are inserted through the upper MCL port; the renal artery is transected between clips 3 and 4, thereby leaving 3 clips on the stump of the renal artery. If there is only one artery, the renal vein will decrease significantly in size after ligation of the artery.

A complete "window" around the renal vein is confirmed, and then the 9-mm or 11-mm clip applier (depending on the size of the renal vein) is inserted through the upper MCL port. Again, five clips are applied, and the vein is transected between clips 3 and 4, thereby leaving 3 clips on the stump of the renal vein. It is important to visualize the tips of the clip as it is being applied to ensure that the vessel is *completely* contained within the clip.

Occasionally, the main renal vein may be too wide for even the 11-mm clips to completely secure it. In this instance, the renal vein can be dissected distally to where it branches and each branch can be individually dissected and clipped with 9-mm or 11-mm clips. Alternatively, a 12-mm GIA vascular stapler can be used to secure the renal vein. This instrument can place six 3-cm long rows of staples and simultaneously incise the renal vein between the third and fourth row of staples.

Once the hilar vessels are secured and transected, the medial dissection of the kidney is next completed with caution to ensure that no small renal vessels remain in these tissues. The posterior aspect of the kidney can then be freed, using sharp and blunt dissection. With this process completed, the kidney remains attached only by the ureter.

DIVIDING THE URETER (Fig. 11–6)

The circulating nurse deflates the balloon on the occlusion balloon catheter. The ureteral catheter and guide wire are then completely removed. The 9-mm clip applier is inserted through the 12-mm MCL sheath, and an atraumatic grasper is passed through the 5-mm MCL sheath. Two clips are placed on the ureter above and below the Babcock clamp or tape, approximately 5 cm from the ureteropelvic junction.

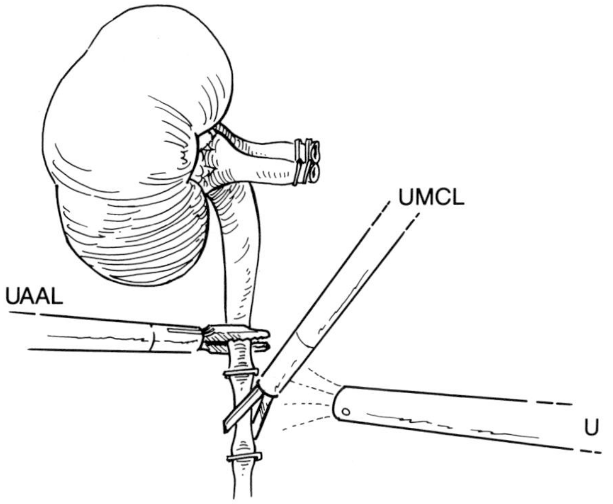

Figure 11–6. Incising the ureter. U, umbilicus; UAAL, upper anterior axillary line; UMCL, upper midclavicular line. (From Clayman, RV, McDougall, EM: Laparoscopic Urology. St. Louis, Quality Medical Publishing, 1993.)

The clip applier is removed and replaced by scissors, which are used to transect the ureter. If present, the umbilical tape is cut and is removed from the abdomen. A traumatic locking grasper is inserted through the upper 5-mm AAL port and is used to secure the freed ureter. The grasper on the ureter is used to displace the kidney into the ipsilateral upper quadrant, to overlie the liver or the spleen (Fig. 11–7).

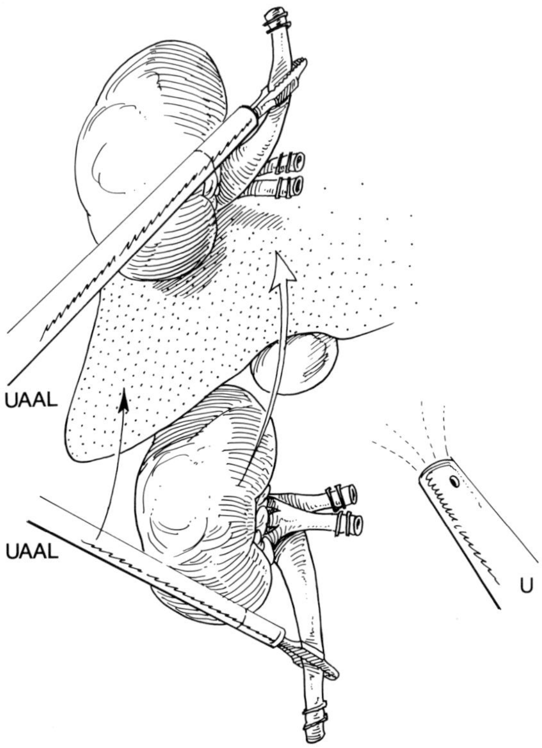

Figure 11–7. Displacing the kidney into the ipsilateral upper quadrant. U, umbilicus; UAAL, upper anterior axillary line. (From Clayman, RV, McDougall, EM: Laparoscopic Urology. St. Louis, Quality Medical Publishing, 1993.)

INSERTION OF THE ENTRAPMENT SACK
(Fig. 11–8)

The 5-inch × 8-inch organ entrapment sack is then carefully rolled in its introducer. It is important that the drawstrings of the bag be laid along the body of the bag and that they be incorporated well within the rolls of the bag so that they do not become caught in the flap valve of the trocar during sack insertion.

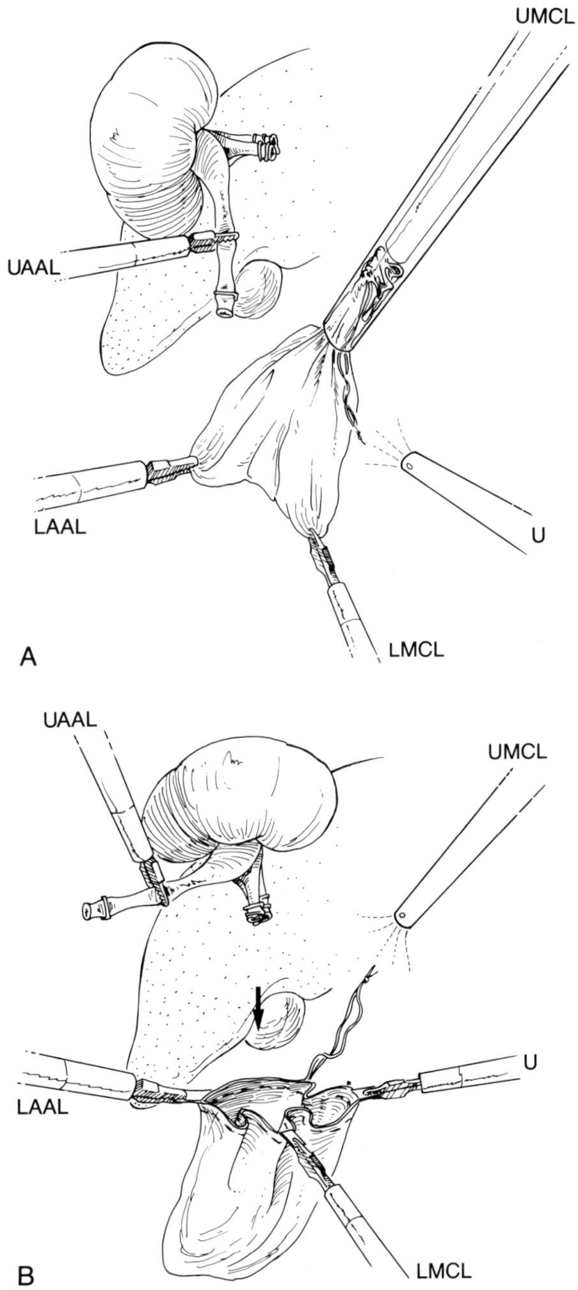

Figure 11–8. *A*, inserting the entrapment sack. *B*, Opening the entrapment sack. LAAL, lower anterior axillary line; LMCL, lower midclavicular line; U, umbilicus; UAAL, upper anterior axillary line; UMCL, upper midclavicular line. (From Clayman, RV, McDougall, EM: Laparoscopic Urology. St. Louis, Quality Medical Publishing, 1993.)

The 12-mm MCL port is used for insertion of the entrapment sack. The sack introducer is inserted under constant laparoscopic visualization to avoid intra-abdominal injuries. Atraumatic graspers are used through the lower 5-mm AAL port and the 5-mm MCL port to assist in pulling the bag well down into the pelvis (Fig. 11–8*A*). They are used to unfurl the sack within the abdomen, and the introducer is then removed.

Once the sack is positioned satisfactorily, the laparoscope is moved from the umbilical port to the 12-mm MCL port. Traumatic locking graspers are inserted through the lower 5-mm AAL sheath, the 5-mm MCL sheath, and the 12-mm umbilical sheath. These graspers are then secured on the lateral, middle, and medial tabs of the bag opening, respectively (Fig. 11–8*B*). By using traction and countertraction, the graspers triangulate open the entrapment sack. The laparoscope is moved forward into the open bag, and by use of a circular motion, the bottom of sack is also spread open. The laparoscope is then withdrawn from the sack. The ureter, still secured with the locking grasper through the upper 5-mm anterior axillary port is moved into the entrapment sack, thereby dragging the kidney into the sack (Fig. 11–9*A*). The grasper is then released from the ureter and is withdrawn leaving the kidney within the sack. The grasper, passed through the umbilical sheath, is then used to locate and grasp the end of the sack's drawstrings. The drawstrings are removed from the abdominal cavity and are drawn into the sheath of the umbilical port, but not through the port, thereby closing the sack on the kidney (Fig. 11–9*B*). The other two traumatic graspers on the tabs of the bag edge are then released and removed from the abdominal cavity. The abdominal pressure is reduced to 5 mm Hg, and the abdomen, surgical site, and trocars are re-examined to ensure that no active bleeding is present. Any bleeding should be thoroughly controlled at this point. Electively the abdomen can be irrigated with 250 to 500 ml of Ringer lactate, containing 5000 units of heparin/L and 500 mg of cefazolin/L. The irrigant is aspirated from the abdomen using the suction irrigator.

The patient is now returned to the supine position, and the laparoscope is maintained through the 12-mm MCL port. The grasper with the drawstring is drawn up through the umbilical trocar. This draws the edge of the sack up against the sheath's tip. The grasper is removed, and the 12-mm sheath is then also removed, allowing the drawstring to be manually grasped by the surgeon as it exits the abdomen. An assistant's finger over the port site helps to maintain pneumoperitoneum. Under laparoscopic visualization, the drawstrings are further pulled up through the 12-mm port site, delivering the neck of the sack onto the abdominal wall. This maneuver is monitored endoscopically

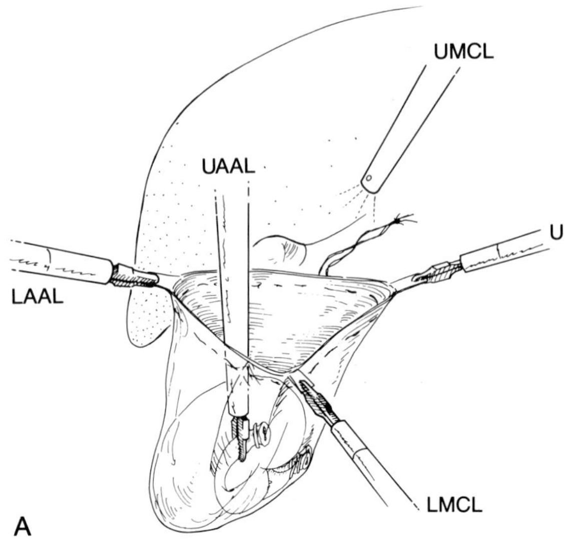

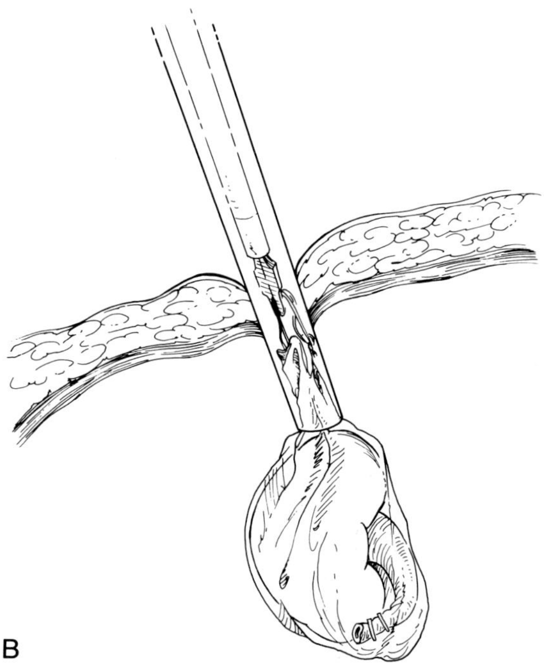

Figure 11–9. *A*, Placing the kidney in the entrapment sack. *B*, Drawing the drawstrings of the entrapment sack into the umbilical port sheath. LAAL, lower anterior axillary line; LMCL, lower midclavicular line; U, umbilicus; UAAL, upper anterior axillary line; UMCL, upper midclavicular line. (From Clayman, RV, McDougall, EM: Laparoscopic Urology. St. Louis, Quality Medical Publishing, 1993.)

to be certain that no bowel or omentum is entrapped alongside the sack or is pulled into the port site.

TISSUE MORCELLATION VS. WHOLE TISSUE DELIVERY

The surgeon and assistant use their nondominant hands to grasp the edge of the sack and pull it up firmly. Laparoscopically, the bag should be seen to hold the kidney tightly against the abdominal wall with no redundancy in the bag. The laparoscope should remain in the 12-mm MCL port for constant visual monitoring of the morcellation process.

The morcellator is plugged into the electrical outlet and the activating foot pedal is placed opposite the surgeon's foot. The handle of the morcellator is connected to wall suction. The neck of the sack is pulled taut by the assistant and the surgeon; the surgeon inserts the 10-mm barrel of the morcellator with his dominant hand until it firmly contacts the kidney. The valve on the handle of the morcellator is turned to the aspiration position. The morcellator is activated by depressing the foot pedal. The tip of the morcellator barrel must be cored into the renal tissue in order to deliver the tissue to the recessed rotating cutting blade. Therefore, it is best to use a firm downward motion to push the tip of the morcellator deeply into the kidney (Fig. 11–10*A*). Also, the morcellator should be moved backward and forward, and its direction should be changed so that it does not rest in one position within the bag, because this can result in a build-up of heat at the tip of the morcellator and can potentially damage the bag. In this respect, the tip of the morcellator can be moved around an imaginary clock face within the sack. The bag must at all times be pulled tightly upward against the abdominal wall to provide countertraction for effective coring of the tissue and to prevent any folds from developing in the sack, which could be damaged by the morcellator (Fig. 11–10*B*).

The mesh trap in the handle of the morcellator should be cleaned out every 3 to 5 minutes to ensure maximum suction and thus facilitate tissue morcellation. Each time the morcellator is removed from the sack, the sack should be again firmly drawn up against the abdominal wall to keep the renal tissue tautly applied to the underside of the abdominal wall. Constant laparoscopic monitoring is essential to preclude entrapment of omentum or bowel in the folds of the sack.

It is also crucial to be alert for any perforation of the sack during morcellation. This is very unlikely to happen if the preceding suggestions are followed. However, if the sack develops folds because it is not being drawn up firmly, then the fold may be sucked into the morcellator tip and perforated by the morcellating blades. This will result in a sudden loss of pneumoperitoneum; the bowel will immediately surround the sack. If this problem is not immediately recognized by the surgeon, the bowel may be injured by the morcellator, thereby necessitating open surgical repair. Quite simply, the morcellation process should be stopped whenever the surgeon notes any contact between the sack and the bowel.

If the kidney is fibrotic then there may be some residual renal tissue that cannot completely be morcellated. In this instance, the tip of a Kelly clamp can be gently inserted and used to grasp the tissue and pull it from the sack with a twisting motion. This part of the procedure should also be laparoscopically monitored.

Following extraction of the renal tissue, the empty sack can easily be withdrawn from the abdominal cavity (Fig. 11–10*C*). The assistant places a finger over the port site to maintain the pneumoperitoneum. All the tissue retrieved from the wire mesh trap is submitted to the pathologist for histologic evaluation.

For kidneys being removed for renal cell carcinoma it may be desirable to remove the tissue intact for more accurate staging of the tumor. In this instance, the technique is the same as just described until the

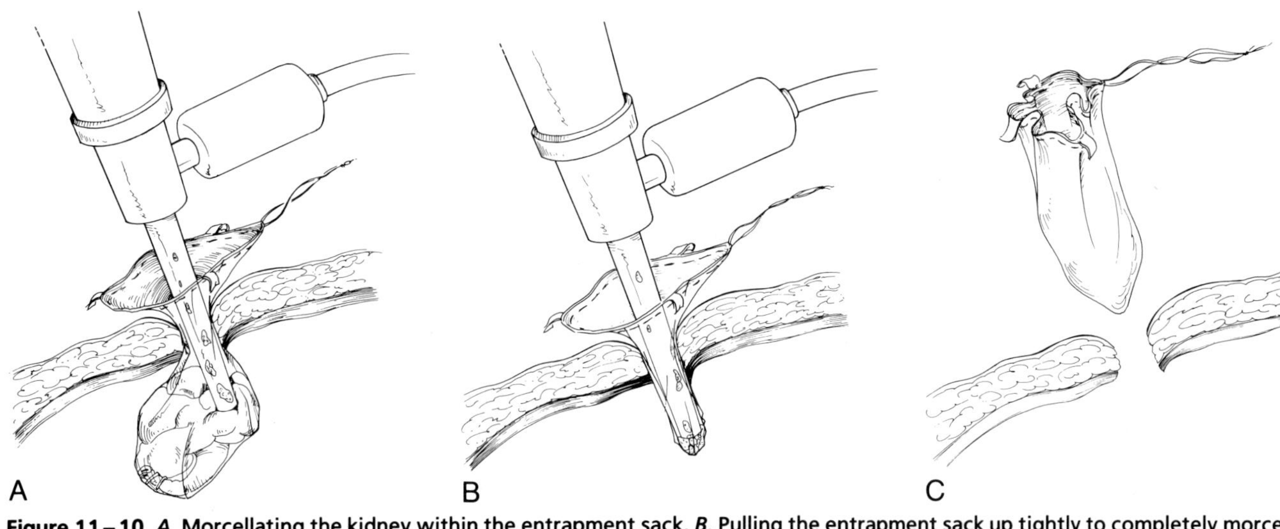

Figure 11–10. *A*, Morcellating the kidney within the entrapment sack. *B*, Pulling the entrapment sack up tightly to completely morcellate the kidney. *C*, Withdrawing the empty entrapment sack from the abdominal cavity. (From Clayman, RV, McDougall, EM: Laparoscopic Urology. St. Louis, Quality Medical Publishing, 1993.)

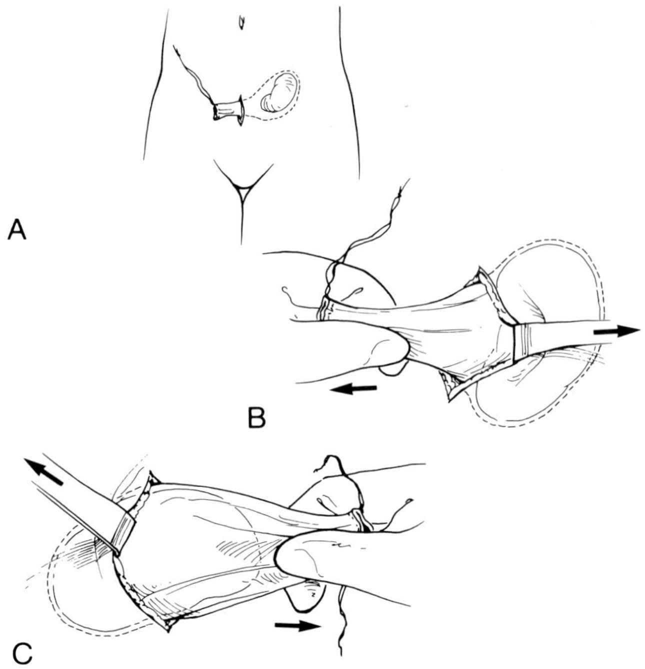

Figure 11–11. *A* to *C*, Removing the surgical specimen intact in the entrapment sack. (From Clayman RV, McDougall EM: Laparoscopic Urology. St. Louis, Quality Medical Publishing, 1993.)

entrapment sack edge has been delivered to the abdominal surface. Then the umbilical skin incision or a suprapubic incision is extended vertically and inferiorly, for a total length of 3 to 4 cm (Fig. 11–11*A*). Army-Navy retractors are used to retract the skin edge and the rectus fascia is similarly incised. The Army-Navy retractor is then placed on the skin and fascial edges of the incision to work as a wedge (Fig. 11–11*B*). Using a side-to-side winching motion, the entrapment sack with the intact kidney is worked out of the abdomen (Fig. 11–11*B* and *C*).

EXITING THE ABDOMEN

After the kidney and the entrapment sack have been removed from the abdomen, the assistant either places a finger over the 12-mm port site (i.e., after morcellation) or proceeds to close the 3- to 4-cm abdominal incision (i.e., after intact removal) with interrupted no. 1-0 absorbable sutures placed in a figure-eight configuration. The pneumoperitoneum is then reestablished.

The 10-mm laparoscope is removed, and a 5-mm laparoscope is inserted through the 5-mm MCL sheath. The second, and if present third, 12-mm trocar is then removed, and the fascia is approximated, under laparoscopic control, with a single figure-eight, 2-0 absorbable suture. The two AAL 5-mm sheaths are removed, under laparoscopic control, and an assistant places a finger over each skin site to maintain the pneumoperitoneum. The 5-mm laparoscope is then withdrawn until it extends just past the end of the last 5-mm sheath. The laparoscope and 5-mm sheath together are withdrawn slowly from the abdomen so that the sheath's tract through the abdominal wall can carefully be examined for bleeding. When all the trocars have been removed, the pneumoperitoneum is allowed to escape from the 5-mm port sites. The skin edges of the 12-mm trocar sites are approximated, using a 4-0 absorbable subcuticular suture. All wounds are cleansed and dried, and adhesive skin strips are applied.

POSTOPERATIVE MANAGEMENT

Following laparoscopic nephrectomy, the nasogastric tube is removed, and the patient is returned to the postoperative recovery area. The CVP monitor is usually discontinued before the patient returns to his or her hospital room. The urethral catheter is removed the morning following the operative procedure, and ambulation commences. Alimentation is begun with clear liquids on the evening the patient returns from the operating room. This diet is advanced to regular meals usually by the end of the first postoperative day.

Initially, postoperative analgesia is provided by parenteral morphine sulfate through a patient-controlled analgesic device. However, by the end of the first or second postoperative day, this is replaced by oral analgesia as requested. Oral analgesia is rarely required postoperatively for more than 4 to 5 days. Parenteral antibiotics are continued postoperatively fro 24 hours and then discontinued. The patient is discharged usually by the third or fourth postoperative day with non-narcotic analgesia and no activity restriction.

NEPHROURETERECTOMY

For patients with transitional cell carcinoma, historically there is a 30% to 60% chance of recurrent tumor in the remaining ureteral stump following nephrectomy.[32] For this reason, the accepted management of upper-tract transitional cell carcinoma is nephroureterectomy. This can also be done laparoscopically by using the endoscopic GI stapler to resect a bladder cuff to complete the ureterectomy portion of the procedure.

The laparoscopic procedure in these patients consists of unroofing the affected distal ureter. Under anesthesia in the cystoscopy suite, the bladder is examined and a 7 Fr, 5-mm × 5-cm dilating balloon ureteral catheter is inserted into the distal affected ureter over a preplaced Bentson (0.035-inch) guide wire under fluoroscopic guidance. The balloon is inflated to less than 1 atmosphere of pressure and is left in posi-

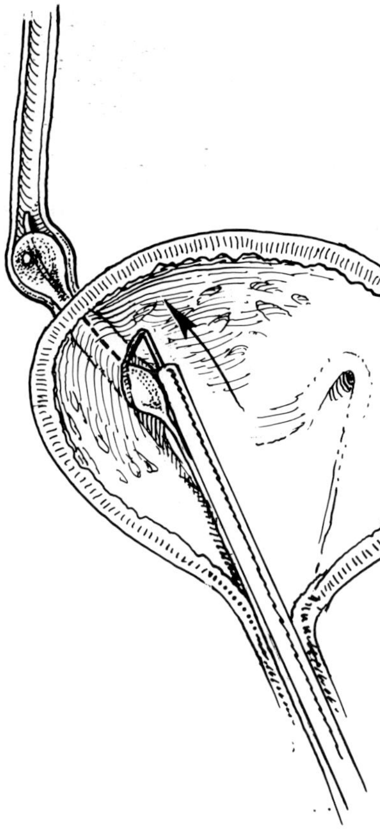

Figure 11–12. Incising the ureteral tunnel over a ureteral dilating balloon catheter with the Orandi knife. (From Clayman, RV, McDougall EM: Laparoscopic Urology. St. Louis, Quality Medical Publishing, 1993.)

tion. The cystoscope is removed, leaving the catheter in position. A 24 Fr resectoscope equipped with an Orandi knife is then inserted. The ureteral orifice and ureteral tunnel is incised anteriorly over the balloon with the Orandi knife electrode (Fig. 11–12). It is important to completely incise through the ureter to expose the balloon; however, the incision in the ureter should end at the intramural ureter near the uretero-vesical junction (UVJ). When the incision is complete, the 24 Fr resectoscope is removed from the bladder, and the dilating balloon catheter is deflated and removed; only the 0.035-inch guide wire remains in position in the upper tract. A 7 Fr, 11.5-mm occlusion balloon catheter is inserted fluoroscopically over the guide wire and is advanced to the renal pelvis. The balloon is inflated with one cc of dilute contrast. The Bentson guide wire is replaced with a 0.035-inch Amplatz Super Stiff guide wire. A side-arm adapter is passed over the Super Stiff guide wire and fixed to the distal end of the occlusion balloon catheter. The side-arm adapter is then tightly screwed onto the guide wire. A 16 Fr Foley urethral catheter is inserted alongside the occlusion balloon and is secured to it with a 2-0 silk suture. Both catheters are placed in a sterile bag, and the patient is transferred to the main operating room.

The patient preparation, room setup, and port placement are essentially the same as for the laparoscopic nephrectomy. However, an additional 12-mm trocar is inserted in the midline, approximately 2 to 3 cm above the symphysis pubis for passage of the 12-mm GIA tissue stapler. The initial dissection is also essentially the same as for the nephrectomy, although the dissection of the ureter is extended distally into the pelvis. The course of the ureter is followed over the iliac vessels and down to the crossing of the vas deferens or round ligament. The same technique as described for the nephrectomy is followed to dissect the proximal ureter and the upper and lower poles of the kidney, to secure the renal vessels, and finally to completely free the kidney.

Instead of clipping and incising the ureter, the dissection is again directed to the pelvic ureter. The superior vesical artery is dissected as it crosses the ureter. It is secured with four 9-mm clips and is transected between the second and third clips. Next, the vas deferens or round ligament is electrocoagulated and transected (Fig. 11–13). The ureter is dissected until the detrusor muscle fibers of the UVJ are identified. At this point, by placing a grasping forceps through the lower AAL, the ureter can be firmly retracted

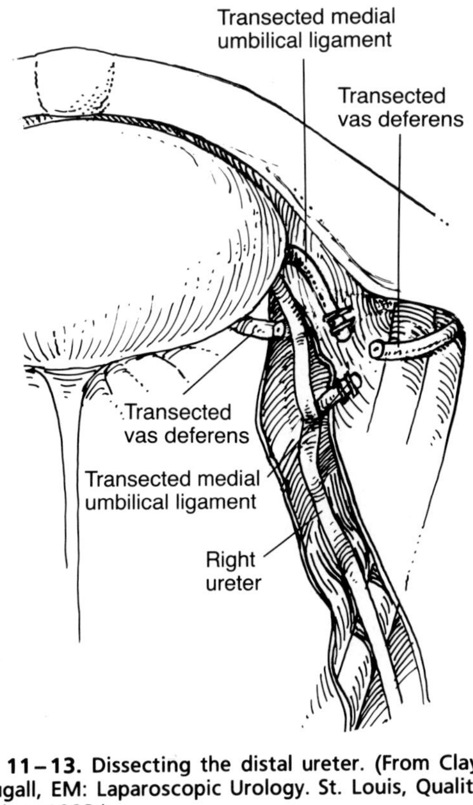

Figure 11–13. Dissecting the distal ureter. (From Clayman, RV, McDougall, EM: Laparoscopic Urology. St. Louis, Quality Medical Publishing, 1993.)

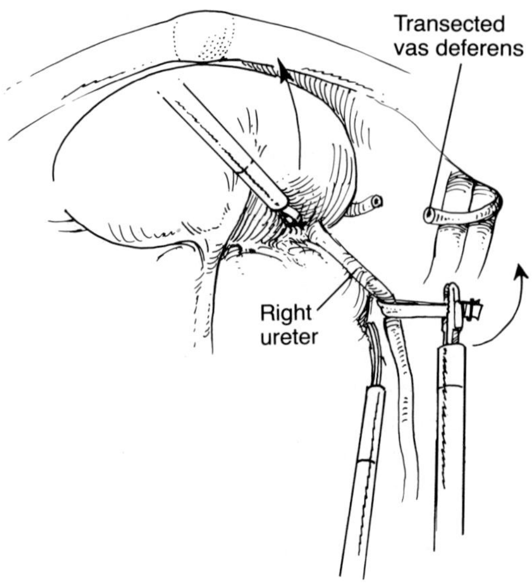

Figure 11–14. Retracting the ureter superiorly and laterally, thereby tenting up the wall of the bladder. (From Clayman, RV, McDougall, EM: Laparoscopic Urology. St. Louis, Quality Medical Publishing, 1993.)

superiorly and laterally, thereby tenting up the wall of the bladder (Fig. 11–14). Once there is a satisfactory circumferential dissection of the UVJ, the 12-mm GIA tissue stapler is inserted through the lower midline 12-mm port. The occlusion balloon is deflated, and the 7 Fr ureteral catheter is removed. The opened jaws of the GIA stapler are placed across the cuff of bladder. The stapler jaws are then closed, thereby opposing the bladder wall beneath the UVJ (Fig. 11–15*A*). Before firing the stapler, it is important to be sure that the cuff of bladder is completely contained within the jaws of the instrument. By rotating the closed stapler 90°, the designated "cut" line on both jaws should be visualized; this line should lie well beyond the edge of bladder to ensure complete stapling and transection (Fig. 11–15*B*). Once positioning is satisfactory, the lock on the handle is released, and the handle is squeezed. Six 3-cm rows of titanium staples are laid down, and an instrument-contained knife blade cuts between the third and fourth rows of staples. The lever release is then opened and the jaws are allowed to open, thereby exposing the two stapled and now incised edges of the bladder cuff (Fig. 11–15*C*). The nephroureterectomy specimen should now lie completely free in the abdomen. By using the locking traumatic grasping forceps passed through the upper AAL port, the proximal ureter is secured, and the specimen is dragged up and laid over the liver or the spleen, according to the side of dissection.

The retrieval of the kidney and ureter specimen is the same as described for laparoscopic nephrectomy. Morcellation is completed as previously described. However, these specimens can also be removed intact to facilitate staging and grading of a renal pelvic malignancy. In this instance, the string of the entrapment sack is drawn through the 12-mm midline suprapubic port site. The port site is extended inferiorly in the midline for 2 inches. After incising the fascia, the entrapment sack and intact specimen are removed with the aid of the Army-Navy retractors as previously described.

Exiting the Abdomen

If the intact kidney has been removed through an incision in the midline suprapubic site, then the fascia is closed under direct vision, using interrupted no. 1-0 absorbable sutures placed in a figure-eight pattern. After this closure is complete, the pneumoperitoneum is re-established, the remaining sheaths are removed, and the incision site is closed as previously described for the laparoscopic nephrectomy.

Postoperative Management

The postoperative care of the nephroureterectomy patient is essentially the same as for that of the nephrectomy patient. However, the Foley catheter is left in

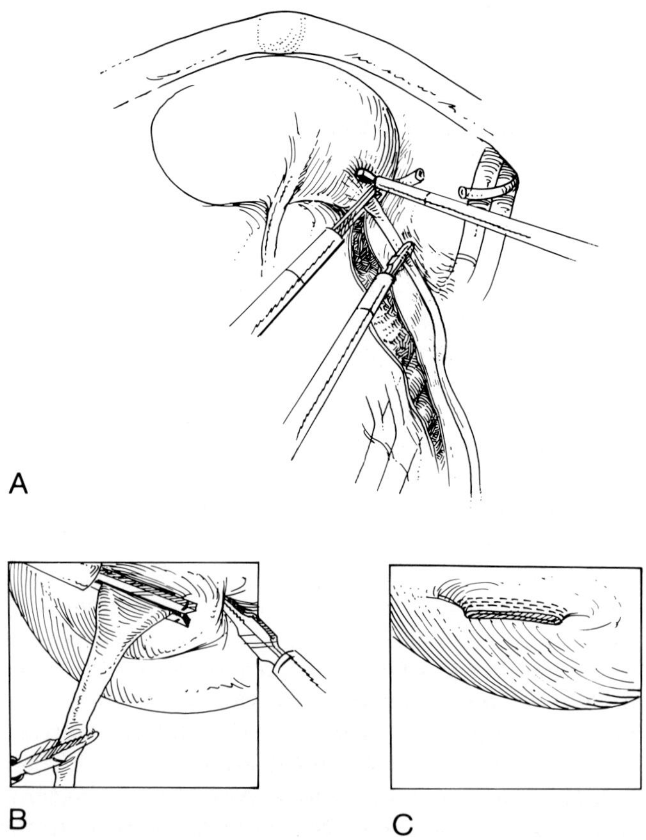

Figure 11–15. *A*, Placing the GIA stapler across the bladder wall beneath the ureterovesical junction. *B*, The "cut" line of the stapler should lie well beyond the edge of the bladder. *C*, The incised and stapled edge of the bladder cuff. (From Clayman, RV, McDougall, EM: Laparoscopic Urology. St. Louis, Quality Medical Publishing, 1993.)

place for 2 to 3 days; then a cystogram is performed to confirm that the bladder closure is satisfactory.

RETROPERITONEOSCOPY

For renal surgery, a more direct retroperitoneal approach to the kidney has several surgical advantages. There is less chance of injury to intra-abdominal organs such as bowel, liver, or spleen by avoiding the peritoneal cavity. Less dissection and retraction is necessary for exposure of the kidney, thereby decreasing the operative time. A posterior approach to the kidney facilitates early control and ligation of the renal artery. Also, other retroperitoneal stuctures, such as the adrenal gland on the right side, can more easily be exposed by a retroperitoneal approach. The extraperitoneal approach avoids CO_2 contact with the peritoneal membrane and reduces hypothermia and postoperative pain secondary to diaphragmatic irritation. Initially, we described our laboratory and clinical experience using CO_2 insufflation to perform laparoscopic retroperitoneal nephrectomy.[33] This technique appeared unsatisfactory due to a longer operative time and more difficulty in performing organ entrapment as a result of the restricting smaller retroperitoneal space.

Of late we have modified the technique described by Gaur, using a home-made dilating balloon to obtain access to the retroperitoneum.[34] We are creating a Verres needle pneumoretroperitoneum and are inserting a 12-mm port at Petit's triangle (posterior lumbar triangle). Next, the middle finger of a size 8 sterile surgeon's glove is tied with 2-0 silk ties on the tip of a 16 Fr red rubber catheter; the end of the catheter is back-loaded through a 28 Fr or 30 Fr Amplatz sheath. The Amplatz sheath is passed through the 12-mm laparoscopic sheath, and the balloon-tipped catheter is pushed forward into the retroperitoneal space. The balloon is distended with 1 L of normal saline. The balloon is then aspirated, withdrawn into the Amplatz sheath, and the sheath and balloon are removed from the 12-mm port. The laparoscope is inserted through the 12-mm sheath, and CO_2 insufflation is commenced with pressure limit set at 15 mm Hg. Under direct laparoscopic visualization, additional ports are inserted into the retroperitoneal space. On examination of the retroperitoneum after balloon dilation, the psoas muscle, ureter, and often the gonadal vein are clearly exposed. The area of the kidney surrounded by Gerota's fascia and fat is also evident. We have not been successful, as described by Gaur, in directly dilating with the balloon within Gerota's fascia. However, sharp dissection of these tissues will expose the kidney.

The limitation of retroperitoneal space for organ entrapment remains somewhat challenging and results in operative times that are essentially the same for retroperitoneoscopy compared with the transperitoneal approach for laparoscopic nephrectomy.

LAPAROSCOPIC PARTIAL NEPHRECTOMY

As an extension of our work to evaluate the potential application of laparoscopy to urologic surgery, we explored the feasibility of using this minimally invasive approach for performing a partial nephrectomy in the animal model.[35] Laparoscopic partial nephrectomy (LPN) was performed on nine female pigs using a plastic cable tie (15 mm × 4 mm × 1 mm) to achieve renal ischemia and an argon-beam coagulator (ABC) probe to fulgurate the transected surface. These studies showed that LPN is a feasible procedure in the pig and that there is excellent function of the renal remnant, no arteriovenous fistula formation and no evidence of renovascular hypertension.

All laparoscopic procedures were performed on the right renal unit. Initially, cystoscopy was performed, and a 7.1 Fr pigtail external ureteral stent was inserted on the right side.

After CO_2 pneumoperitoneum was established, and five laparoscopy ports were placed: (1) an 11-mm port was inserted in the midline at the umbilicus, (2) a 12-mm port was placed in the MCL at the costal margin, (3) a 5-mm port was inserted at the MCL approximately 3 to 5 cm below the umbilicus, and (4) two 5-mm ports were inserted along the AAL at the costal margin and at the level of the umbilicus after the animal was placed in the left lateral decubitus position.

The right line of Toldt was incised, and the peritoneum was retracted medially. The renal hilar vessels were dissected en masse, and a vascular loop was placed around the vessel bundle. The upper pole of the right kidney was completely dissected. A preformed plastic cable tie was inserted through the 11-mm umbilical port. The loop was positioned around the upper pole of the kidney and was tightly cinched down against the parenchyma. The ABC probe was inserted through the 11-mm umbilical port and was used to fulgurate the proposed line of renal incision. The vascular loop was tightened to occlude the vessels, and the cable tie was further tightened to compress the parenchyma. Electrocautery scissors were then used to excise the kidney lying superior to the cable tie. The ABC probe was reinserted through the 12-mm MCL port and was used to fulgurate the entire cut surface of the kidney (140 watts at 4 L/minute/hour). The hilar vascular loop and cable tie were then removed.

The excised renal tissue was removed from the abdomen using an organ entrapment sack and a 10-mm high-speed electrical tissue morcellator.

The plastic cable tie allowed the kidney to be easily

manipulated during excision of the renal tissue and ABC fulguration of the transected surface. The ABC produces effective closure of the transected vascular structures and collecting system at the surgical site. No extravasation or delayed bleeding occurred in any of the pigs.

The same basic principle and technique have been used to successfully perform laparoscopic partial nephrectomy in the clinical setting. Winfield and coworkers performed a left partial nephrectomy on a woman with a lower-pole calyceal stone and diverticulum unresponsive to endoscopic management.[36]

REFERENCES

1. Simon, G: Extirpation ciner miere am Menschen. Deutsch Klin 22:137, 1870.
2. Kelling, G: Uber Oesophagoskopie, gastroskopie und koelioskopie. Munch Med Wochenschr 49:21, 1901.
3. Jacobeus, HC: Uber die moglichkeit die zystoskopie be: Untersuchung seroser Hchlungen anzuwenden. Munch Med Wochenschr 57:2090, 1910.
4. Bernheim, BM: Organoscopy: Cystoscopy of the abdominal cavity. Ann Surg 53:764, 1911.
5. Verres, J: Neues Instrument zur Ausfuhrung von brustoder Bachpunktionen und Pneumothorax-behundlung. Deutsch Med Wochenschr 64:1480, 1938.
6. Semm, K: Operative Manual for Endoscopic Abdominal Surgery. Chicago, Year Book Medical Publishers, 1987, pp. 175–216.
7. Steptoe, PC: Laparoscopy in Gynecology. New York, Churchill Livingstone, 1967, pp. 12–18.
8. Gomel, V: Laparoscopy. Can Med Assoc J 111:167, 1974.
9. Hulka, JF; Mercer, JP; Fishburne, JI; et al: Spring clip sterilization: One year follow-up of 1,079 cases. Am J Obstet Gynecol 125:1039, 1976.
10. Hasson, HM: Open laparoscopy: A report of 150 cases. J Reprod Med 12:234, 1974.
11. Daginni, G: Incidenti della laparscopia: Rapporto su 7870 casi. G Gastroenterol Endosc 3:914, 1980.
12. Cortesi, N; Ferrari, P; Zumbarda, E; et al: Diagnosis of bilateral abdominal cryptorchidism by laparoscopy. Endoscopy 8:33, 1976.
13. Gandofi, L; Rossi, A; Leo, P; et al: Indications for laparoscopy before and after the introduction of ultrasonography. Gastrointest Endosc 31:1–3, 1985.
14. Eshghi, AM; Roth, JS; Smith, AS: Percutaneous transperitoneal approach to a pelvic kidney for endourological removal of staghorn calculus. J Urol 134:525, 1985.
15. Wickham, JEA: The surgical treatment of renal lithiasis. In: Wickham, JEA ed: Urinary Calculus Disease. New York, Churchill Livingstone, 1979, pp. 145–198.
16. Clayman, RV; Preminger, GM; Franklin, JR; et al: Percutaneous ureterolithotomy. J Urol 133:671, 1985.
17. Schuessler, WW; Vancaillie, TG; Reich, H; Griffith, DP: Transperitoneal endosurgical lymphadenectomy in patients with localized prostate cancer. J Urol 145:988, 1991.
18. Gomel, V: Operative laparoscopy: Time for acceptance. Fertil Steril 51:1–11, 1989.
19. Reddick, EJ; Olson, DO; Daniel, JF; et al: Laparoscopic laser cholecystectomy. Laser Med Surg News 7:38–40, 1989.
20. Donovan, JF; Winfield, HN: Laparoscopic varix ligation. J Urol 145:325A, 1991.
21. McCullough, CS; Soper, NJ; Clayman, RV; et al: Laparoscopic drainage of a post-transplant lymphocele. Transplantation 51:725, 1991.
22. Kavoussi, LR; Clayman, RV; Brunt, LM; Soper, NJ: Laparoscopic ureterolysis. J Urol 147:426, 1992.
23. Vancaillie, TG; Schuessler, WW: Laparoscopic bladderneck suspension. J Laparoendosc Surg 1:169, 1991.
24. Stoller, ML; Irby, PB; Carroll, PR; Osman, M: Laparoscopic renal cyst resection. J Endourol 6:556, 1992.
25. Clayman, RV; Kavoussi, LR; Soper, NJ; et al: Laparoscopic nephrectomy. (Letter) N Engl J Med 324:1370, 1991.
26. Clayman, RV; Kavoussi, LR; McDougall, EM; et al: Laparoscopic nephrectomy: A review of 16 cases. Surg Laparosc Endosc 2:1, 1992.
27. Rassweiler, J; Potempa, DM; Henkel, TO; et al: The technique of transperitoneal laparoscopic nephrectomy. J Endourol 6:S153, 1992.
28. Stockdale, AD; Pocock, TJ: Abdominal wall metastasis following laparoscopy: A case report. Eur J Surg Oncol 11:373, 1985.
29. Cava, A; Roman, J; Quintela, AG; et al: Subcutaneous metastasis following laparoscopy in gastric adenocarcinoma. Eur J Surg Oncol 16:63, 1990.
30. Dobrento, Z; Wittmann, T; Kracsony, G: Rapid development of malignant metastases in the abdominal wall after laparoscopy. Endoscopy 10:127, 1978.
31. Robey, EL; Schellhammer, PF: The adrenal gland and renal cell carcinoma: Is ipsilateral adrenalectomy a necessary component of radical nephrectomy? J Urol 135:453, 1986.
32. Cummings, KB: Nephroureterectomy: Rationale in the management of transitional cell carcinoma of the upper urinary tract. Urol Clin North Am 7:569, 1980.
33. Kerbl, K; Figenshau, RS; Clayman, RV; et al: Retroperitoneal laparoscopic nephrectomy: Laboratory and clinical experience. J Endourol 7:23, 1993.
34. Gaur, DD: Laparoscopic operative retroperitoneoscopy: Use of a new device. J Urol 148:1137, 1992.
35. McDougall, EM; Clayman, RV; Chandhoke, PS; et al: Laparoscopic partial nephrectomy in the pig model. J Urol (in press).
36. Winfield, HH; Donovan, JF; Godet, AS; Clayman, RV: Human laparoscopic partial nephrectomy—case report. Minim Invas Ther 1 (supplement):66, 1992.

CHAPTER 12

Extraperitoneal Endoscopic Surgery for Benign Renal Cysts

Adley Raboy, MD
Lawrence S. Hakim, MD
George Ferzli, MD, FACS
Peter S. Albert, MD, FACS

Simple renal cysts occur in 39% to 50% of the population.[1,2] Despite their high prevalence, these cysts infrequently require treatment. Conservative intervention by needle aspiration and percutaneous drainage, with or without injection of sclerosing agents, although initially effective, can cause recurrence of the symptomatic cyst.[3,4] Various surgical approaches have been described for the treatment of symptomatic renal cysts. These include open surgical resection and less invasive means such as ureteronephroscopic marsupialization and laparoscopic unroofing. However, these interventions may be associated with significant morbidity.[5–8] In order to avoid the potential complications associated with transperitoneal laparoscopic surgery, the extraperitoneal endoscopic approach can be used for various urologic procedures, including pelvic lymph node dissection for the staging of prostatic and bladder carcinomas and vesicourethral suspensions for the treatment of stress urinary incontinence.[9–12] We have applied the extraperitoneal endoscopic approach for the unroofing of symptomatic benign renal cysts as a minimally invasive alternative to open surgical or transperitoneal laparoscopic resection of benign renal cysts when conservative measures fail.

In this chapter, we discuss the various diagnostic and therapeutic methods available for the treatment of symptomatic renal cysts, with emphasis on the newer, "minimally invasive" techniques. Indications for treatment, radiologic studies, and associated complications are also discussed. An algorithm for the approach to renal cysts, including a detailed description of the extraperitoneal endoscopic technique, is presented.

DIAGNOSIS

Most renal cysts are asymptomatic, especially when they are small. When large, cysts may manifest with pain or discomfort in the flank, as palpable flank masses, or infrequently, with hematuria. Cysts may also occur with hypertension, proteinuria, or even with jaundice. In general, renal function is preserved, even with large cysts. The diagnosis of a simple, uncomplicated renal cyst is often made incidentally by renal ultrasound, excretory urogram, abdominal computed tomography, or magnetic resonance imaging for an unrelated cause. Renal cysts are easily recognized sonographically because of their intrinsic characteristics. Simple cysts are spherical and echo-free; have a smooth, sharply defined back wall with distinct margins; and can be acoustically enhanced with good through-transmission.[13]

INDICATIONS FOR TREATMENT

Although renal cysts can be found in as much as 50% of the adult population, the majority never manifest clinically, nor do they require any treatment throughout the patient's lifetime.[1,2] However, renal cysts can become symptomatic, requiring treatment. Patients may present with flank pain due to enlargement of the cyst with encroachment on surrounding structures or with spontaneous hemorrhage. Renal cysts can also cause problems by impinging on the renal parenchyma, leading to hypertension, ischemia, urinary obstruction, and ultimate loss of renal function. In these circumstances, urologic intervention becomes necessary. The optimal treatment should be minimally invasive yet provide definitive resolution of the cyst with a low probability of morbidity or recurrence.

THERAPEUTIC MODALITIES

Initial treatment of symptomatic renal cysts should include percutaneous aspiration, possibly with sclerotherapy. Simple cyst aspiration allows immediate decompression and is useful in demonstrating that the origin of symptoms is indeed from the cyst. Unfortunately, it has been shown that the cyst usually reaccumulates, and symptoms return following aspiration alone.[3] Following cyst aspiration, the injection of various sclerosing agents, including tetracycline, 95% ethanol, phenol, polidocanol, and bismuth-phosphate has been reported. However, aspiration and sclerotherapy are associated with a significant risk of recurrence ranging from 4% to 35% in various series.[5–8,14,15] Complications of this technique include extravasation of the sclerosing agent into the peripelvic tissue with resultant fibrosis and ureteropelvic junction obstruction.[16] In addition, the occurrence of a severe inflammatory reaction requiring nephrectomy following sclerotherapy with lipiodol has been reported.[12]

In cases of *recurrent* symptomatic renal cysts, various alternative therapies have been used. Open surgical unroofing, although effective, is associated with a significant morbidity, especially postoperative pain and patient discomfort. Percutaneous resection and ureteroscopic intrarenal marsupialization, requiring fluoroscopic control, provides minimally invasive treatment of cysts but requires violation of the renal parenchyma and collecting system to achieve its results.[17–19] This procedure can result in significant bleeding and possible extravasation into the retroperitoneal space with resultant electrolyte and fluid abnormalities. In addition, with progression of the percutaneous procedure, collapse of the cyst cavity leads to diminished visibility with increased risk of bleeding and iatrogenic injury. Patient discomfort from a large percutaneous nephrostomy tube must also be considered. Gelet and associates reported their experience with percutaneous resection and sclerotherapy and found a 25% recurrence rate and a 20% rate of secondary infection of the cysts following treatment.[20] Using percutaneous resection of renal cysts, Hubner and associates reported complete resolution of the cysts in only 57% of patients. Cyst size was reduced in 6 of the 14 patients; however, one patient remained symptomatic.[21]

The transperitoneal laparoscopic treatment of symptomatic renal cysts has lately been described in the urologic literature.[22,23] However, since this is a "transperitoneal" procedure, several serious risks may be associated with it. These include the possibility of viscous injury, ileus, peritonitis, adhesions, hernia, uncontrolled bleeding, hypercapnia, and hypothermia.[24,25] The use of a sterile "balloon-glove" for retroperitoneoscopy has also been proposed.[26] However, the risks of injury from the blind inflation of the balloon and balloon rupture, such as bleeding; tearing of the peritoneum; tension pneumoperitoneum (from high insufflation pressures); and surgical emphysema of the chest, scrotum, abdomen, and face must be considered. In our experience, the use of CO_2 insufflation at low pressures in patients with no prior open retroperitoneal surgery is more than adequate for the development of the extraperitoneal cavity.

We have shown that extraperitoneal endoscopic unroofing of renal cysts can easily be done as a minimally invasive operative technique.[27] The procedure is performed through a dorsal lumbar approach, and the anatomical considerations are similar to those encountered during a dorsal lumbotomy.[28] In addition, no muscle-splitting is required, since the incision is carried down to and through the lumbodorsal fascia. Despite early less successful attempts at direct retroperitoneal renal endoscopy, we have found that insufflation of the retroperitoneum with low CO_2 pressures is well tolerated and provides excellent access to the kidney under video guidance.[29] More important, as opposed to laparoscopy, there is no need to enter the peritoneal cavity; hence intraperitoneal complications can be avoided. Additionally, the need for fluoroscopy with its associated radiation exposure is completely avoided with the extraperitoneal endscopic technique. This endoscopic approach is also ideal for other urologic procedures that have been performed laparoscopically, including renoscopy and renal biopsy, ureterolithotomy, para-aortic lymph node biopsy, ligation of the internal spermatic vein, and nephrectomy.[30,31]

EXTRAPERITONEAL ENDOSCOPIC UNROOFING OF RENAL CYSTS: OPERATIVE TECHNIQUE

After induction of general anesthesia with endotracheal intubation, the patient is placed in the lateral decubitus position with the table flexed and the kidney rest raised and is prepped and draped in a sterile fashion. A 1.5-cm incision is made in the skin just lateral to the sacrospinalis muscle, midway between the 12th rib and iliac crest, and is carried down to the lumbodorsal fascia. Retractors are placed in the operative site to retract the sacrospinalis and quadratus lumborum muscles medially, exposing the lumbodorsal fascia. Two stay sutures are placed in the lumbodorsal fascia, which is then incised. Blunt finger-dissection is used to pierce the transversalis fascia and to enter the pararenal space. A 10-mm Hasson trocar is placed in the space and is secured with the previously placed stay sutures. Insufflation tubing is attached to the cannula and an insufflation pressure of 8 mm Hg maintained. A 10-mm zero-degree operating laparoscope is introduced through the Hasson trocar, and the pararenal space is dissected under video guidance using a blunt probe through the 5-mm working channel. This is illustrated in Figure 12–1 (see also reproduction in color). Dissection is first carried out posteriorly, using the psoas muscle as a landmark. Dissection is then directed medially, and Gerota's fascia is entered, as shown in Figure 12–2 (see also reproduction in color). Blunt dissection is continued down to the kidney, clearly exposing the renal cyst (Fig. 12–3; see also reproduction in color). A 5-mm

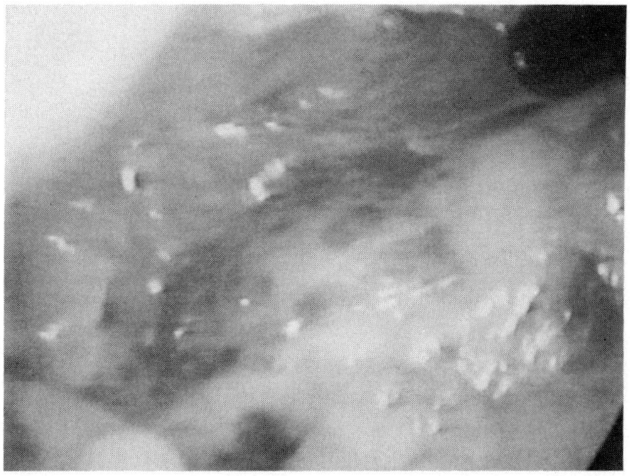

Figure 12–2. Dissection of the renal cyst is illustrated. See also Color Plate 3.

trocar is placed superior to the Hasson trocar, through which grasping forceps can be introduced, to allow countertraction in unroofing the cyst. Endoscopic hook electrocautery or an endoscissors may be placed through the operating laparoscope to excise the cyst wall, which is then removed through the 5-mm port and sent for pathologic examinations (Fig. 12–4; see also reproduction in color). The cyst fluid is removed by suction aspiration and is sent for cytology. The cauterized edges are inspected for bleeding, and inspection of the cyst base is performed for the presence of tumor (Fig. 12–5). If a suspicious area is seen, a biopsy can be taken at this time. At the conclusion of the procedure, the retroperitoneum is desufflated, the trocars are removed under vision, the stay sutures are tied together, and the skin edges are reapproximated.

The endoscopic extraperitoneal procedure is well tolerated by the patient with minimal postoperative discomfort. The operative time is less than 1 hour with minimal blood loss. The patient can be fed a regular diet the evening of surgery and is discharged home on the following day.

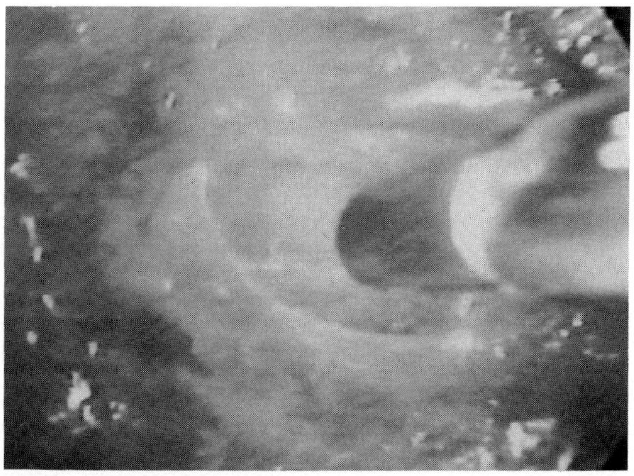

Figure 12–1. This intraoperative photograph illustrates the initial incision into the Gerota fascia. See also Color Plate 3.

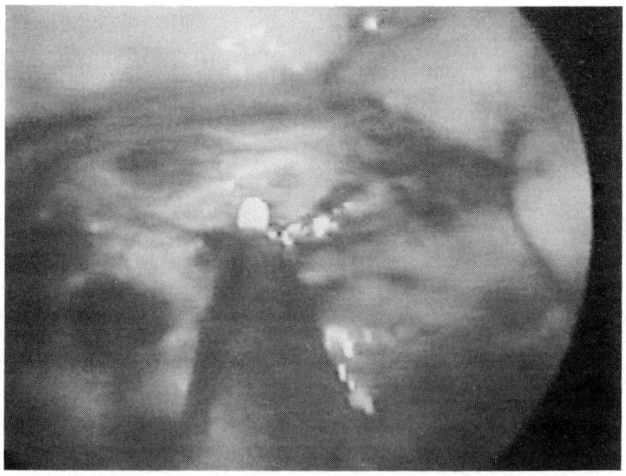

Figure 12–3. The endoscopic hook cautery device is used to incise the cyst wall and achieve hemostasis. See also Color Plate 3.

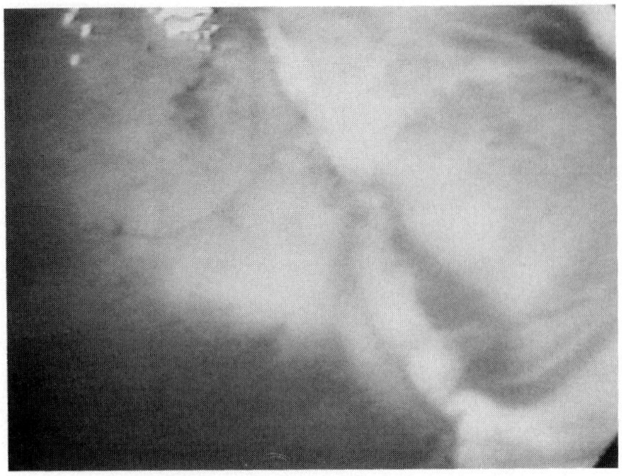

Figure 12–4. Careful visual inspection of the inside of the cyst is performed; cyst fluid is seen at the base (aspirated and sent for cytology). See also Color Plate 3.

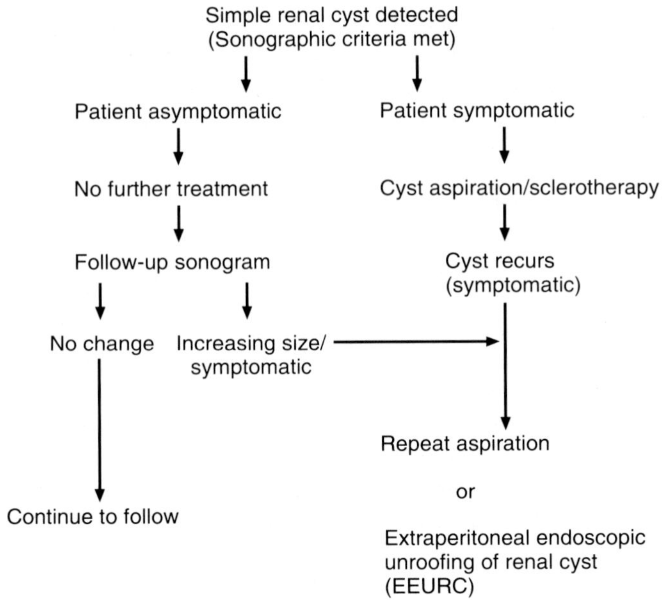

Figure 12–5. Algorithm for the management of benign renal cysts.

CONCLUSIONS

Although simple renal cysts have a relatively high prevalence in adults, most remain asymptomatic and undetected, never requiring urologic intervention. However, when treatment is deemed appropriate, based on specific clinical findings and defined indications, various treatment options are available. For the initial treatment of these symptomatic, simple renal cysts, the least invasive therapy is ultrasound-guided percutaneous aspiration, with or without sclerotherapy. However, for recurrent cysts, a more aggressive therapy may be necessary for resolution. An algorithm for the management of benign renal cysts is illustrated in Figure 12–6.

Extraperitoneal endoscopic unroofing of renal cysts is a minimally invasive procedure that is well tolerated and provides excellent access to the kidney under video guidance.[29] Extraperitoneal endoscopic surgery avoids the potential complications of transperitoneal laparoscopy and open surgical resection, including those associated with CO_2 insufflation and those associated with Verres needle and trocar placement. We believe that in principle the extraperitoneal approach

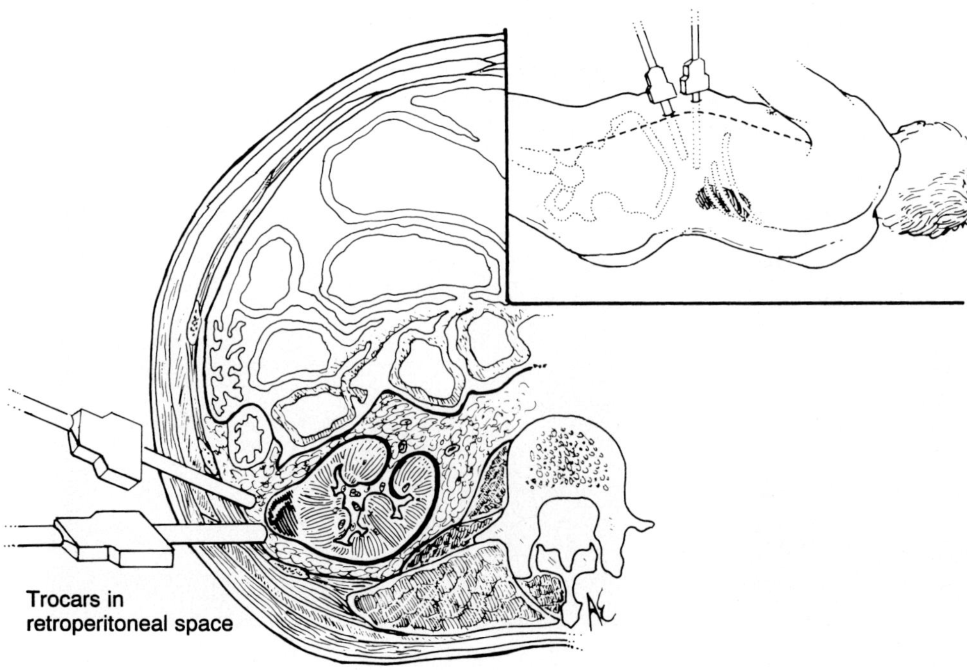

Figure 12–6. Cross-sectional view of the abdomen is illustrated, demonstrating trocar placement within the retroperitoneum. A 10-mm trocar is anchored to the lumbodorsal fascia; a 5-mm working port is superiorly placed. *Inset:* Patient is shown in lateral decubitus position with placement of trocars at the posterior axillary line.

to endoscopic surgery is advantageous whenever the analogous open surgical procedure is performed extraperitoneally. In this exciting era of minimally invasive surgery for urologic diseases, this promising new operative technique will soon become an integral component of our clinical resources for treatment.

REFERENCES

1. Kissane, JM: The morphology of renal cystic disease. In: Gardner, KD, Jr, ed: Cystic Diseases of the Kidney. New York, John Wiley & Sons, 1976, p. 31.
2. Reis M; Faria, V; Lindoro, J; Adolfo, A: The small cystic and noncystic, noninflammatory renal nodules: A postmortem study. J Urol 140:721, 1988.
3. Bartholomew, TH; Sloves, TL; Kroovand, RL; Corbett, DP: The sonographic evaluation and management of simple renal cysts in children. J Urol 123:732, 1980.
4. Hobarth, K; Kratzik, C: Percutaneous sclerosing of kidney cysts with alcohol. Urologe [A] 30:189, 1991.
5. Garcia Novio, F; Rey Rego, R; Mateo Cambon, L; Perez Mendana, P: Symptomatic simple cyst of the kidney. Treatment using puncture-aspiration and sclerosis with 95% ethanol. Arch Esp Urol 43:269, 1990.
6. Forster, P; Wieland, W; Rossler, W: Percutaneous kidney cysts sclerosing. Fortschr Med 110:354, 1992.
7. Zhang, XZ: CT-guided puncture aspiration with sclerosing treatment of renal cyst. Chung Hua Fang She Hsueh Tsa Chih 23:337, 1989.
8. Zellweger, U; Meyenberger, C; Buhler, H; Ammann, R: Ultrasonically guided sclerosing of kidney and liver cysts using polidocanol. Schweiz Rundsch Med Prax 79:1412, 1990.
9. Ferzli, G; Trapasso, J; Raboy, A; Albert, PS: Extraperitoneal endoscopic pelvic lymph node dissection. J Laparoendosc Surg 2:39, 1992.
10. Ferzli, G; Raboy, A; Kleinerman, D; Albert, PS: Extraperitoneal endoscopic pelvic lymph node dissection versus laparoscopic lymph node dissection in the staging of prostatic and bladder carcinoma. J Laparoendosc Surg 2:219, 1992.
11. Albert, PS; Raboy, A: Extraperitoneal endoscopic pelvic lymph node dissection (EEPLND). Cur Surg Techniques Urol 5:1, 1992.
12. Raboy, A; Hakim, LS; Ferzli, G; Albert, PS: Extraperitoneal endoscopic vesicourethral suspension (EEVUS). J Laparoendosc Surg (in press).
13. Goldman, SM; Hartman, DS: The simple renal cyst. In: Pollack, HM, ed: Clinical Urography. Philadelphia, WB Saunders, 1990, p. 1063.
14. Reiner, I; Donnell, S; Jones, M; et al: Percutaneous sclerotherapy for simple renal cysts in children. Br J Radio 65:281, 1992.
15. Holmberg, G; Hietala, SO: Treatment of simple renal cysts by percutaneous puncture and instillation of bismuth-phosphate. Scand J Urol Nephrol 23:207, 1989.
16. Camacho, MF; Bondhus, MJ; Carrion, HM; et al: Ureteropelvic junction obstruction resulting from percutaneous cyst puncture and intracystic isophendylate injection: An unusual complication. J Urol 124:713, 1979.
17. Beyer, D; Fiedler, V: Is renal cyst puncture an available diagnostic procedure for differentiation of avascular, space-occupying renal lesions? Urologe [A] 16:339, 1977.
18. Hulbert, JC; Hunter, D: Percutaneous techniques for intrarenal marsupialization of difficult symptomatic renal cysts by stereotactic methods. Presented at the 85th AUA meeting, New Orleans, 1990.
19. Kavoussi, LR; Clayman, RV; Mikkelsen, DJ; and Mertyk, KS: Ureteronephroscopic marsupialization of obstructing peripelvic renal cyst. J Urol 146:411, 1991.
20. Gelet, A; Sanseverino, R; Martin, X; et al: Percutaneous treatment of benign renal cysts. Eur Urol 18:248, 1990.
21. Hubner, WA; Floth, A; Pfab, R; et al: Treatment of renal cysts by percutaneous resection. Presented at the 85th AUA meeting, New Orleans, 1990.
22. Morgan, C, Jr; Rader, D: Laparoscopic unroofing of a renal cyst. J Urol 148:1835, 1992.
23. Nieh, PT; Bihrle, W III: Laparoscopic marsupialization of massive renal cyst. J Urol 150:171, 1993.
24. Winfield, HN; Donovan, JF; See, WA; et al: Urologic laparoscopic surgery. J Urol 146:942, 1991.
25. Zucker, K: Surgical Laparoscopy. St Louis, Quality Medical Publishing, 1991, pp. 258–260.
26. Gaur, DD: Laparoscopic operative retroperitoneoscopy: Use of a new device. J Urol 148:1137, 1992.
27. Raboy, A; Hakim, LS; Ferzli, G; Albert, PS: Extraperitoneal endoscopic unroofing of renal cysts (EEURC): A new minimally-invasive technique. J Laparoendosc Surg (in press).
28. Freed, SZ: The present status of bilateral nephrectomy in transplant recipients. J Urol 115:8, 1976.
29. Wickham, JEA; Miller, RA: Percutaneous renal access. In: Percutaneous Renal Surgery. New York, Churchill Livingstone, 1983, pp. 33–39.
30. Clayman, RV; Kavoussi, LR; Soper, NJ; et al: Laparoscopic nephrectomy: Initial case report. J Urol 146:278, 1991.
31. Raboy, A; Ferzli, G; Ioffreda, R; Albert, PS: Laparoscopic ureterolithotomy. Urology, 39:223, 1992.

CHAPTER 13

Laparoscopic Ureteral Surgery

David M. Albala, MD
Louis R. Kavoussi, MD

Historically, retroperitoneal ureteral pathology has been accessible only through an open surgical approach. Over the past 15 years, the development of therapeutic endoscopes and miniaturized instrumentation has allowed minimally invasive treatment of disease affecting the interior of the upper collecting system (e.g., stones, strictures, and neoplasms). The ureter, renal pelvis, and calyces have been reached by natural channels or keyhole incisions, markedly reducing the morbidity previously seen with an open incision. Unfortunately, a number of diseases affecting the ureter have still required incisional surgery for cure.

Investigators have made attempts to minimize the morbidity of accessing ureteral pathologies not amenable to standard endoscopic techniques. The first percutaneous approach directly to the retroperitoneum was by Wickham in 1979.[1] Using a laparoscope, he reported a case of retroperitoneoscopy for the purpose of removing a ureteral calculus. A similar report was given by Clayman in 1985 in which a percutaneous tract was placed to the level of a ureteral stone.[2] Both these cases demonstrated that the ureter could be approached in a minimally invasive fashion. However, lack of a systematic technique of access, risk of fluid absorption, and limited instrumentation hindered this approach from becoming widely applicable.

Now, transabdominal laparoscopic techniques have been developed to treat a variety of ureteral pathologies. Laparoscopic techniques for ureterolysis, ureterectomy, ureterolithotomy, and ureteral reanastomosis (ureteroureterostomy) have all been described. This chapter discusses current indications, surgical considerations, techniques, postoperative management and preliminary results for patients undergoing laparoscopic ureteral surgery.

ANATOMIC CONSIDERATIONS

When approaching any organ laparoscopically, a clear understanding of anatomic relationships is critical. The ureter lies entirely in the retroperitoneal space, and its length ranges from 20 to 30 cm. The upper ureter lies loosely within Gerota's fascia. After crossing the iliac vessels in the pelvis, the ureter adheres to the underside of the parietal peritoneum, where it is relatively fixed.

For surgical purposes, the ureter is divided into two portions; the abdominal (upper) ureter and pelvic (lower) ureter. The abdominal ureter runs from the ureteropelvic junction at the level of the transverse process of the first lumbar vertebra to the iliac vessels. It passes over the body of the psoas muscle, and enters the pelvis after being crossed anteriorly by the gonadal vessels. The genitofemoral nerve passes behind the ureter at the level of the fourth lumbar vertebra.

The pelvic ureter begins at the level of the iliac vessels and continues to the ureterovesical junction.

On the right, the lower ureter usually crosses the right external iliac artery; and on the left, it crosses the left common iliac artery. The lower ureter courses anterior and medial to the hypogastric artery, obturator nerve, and vessels. It passes posterior and medial to the medial umbilical ligament, also known as the obliterated umbilical artery at this level. The pelvic ureter enters the bladder obliquely, passing through a submucosal tunnel.

When the distal ureter is surgically approached, the superior vesical artery needs to be transected to obtain adequate working space. In the male, the vas deferens, crossing anteriorly, can inhibit access and should be retracted or divided. In female patients, the uterine artery and occasionally the broad ligament of the uterus may need to be transected to obtain adequate visualization.

SURGICAL CONSIDERATIONS

As with all laparoscopic surgical procedures, patient selection and preparation are critical to obtain an optimal surgical result. Patients must be candidates for laparoscopic intervention as outlined elsewhere in this textbook. The presence of vascular aneurysms, prior transabdominal or retroperitoneal surgery, retroperitoneal fibrosis, and variation in body habitus may markedly alter anatomic relationships. Preoperative x-ray studies outlining the exact course of the ureter and its position relative to the surrounding structures are mandatory.

Before undertaking ureteral surgery, one needs to master laparoscopic suturing techniques. The ureter is a fragile organ, and great care must be taken during its handling. Extracorporeal knotting can put excessive strain on delicate ureteral tissue. Unless the trocar through which the knot is being passed directly overlies the surgical field, intracorporeal knots should be used for ureteral repair when necessary.

Patients undergoing laparoscopic ureteral surgery should have a full mechanical and antibiotic bowel preparation. This decompresses the intestine to increase exposure during dissection and allows for conservative repair if any inadvertent bowel injury occurs during the procedure.

Preoperatively, patients are given an intravenous dose of a broad spectrum antibiotic just before surgery. All patients are typed and screened for possible blood transfusion.

In general, when treating pathologies of the upper ureter, the patient should be placed in a lateral position. For laparoscopic approach to the lower ureter, the patient should be positioned supine in the Trendelenburg position with the ipsilateral side of pathology elevated. When possible, it is helpful to have an external ureteral stent to aid in localization of the ureter during laparoscopy.

Access to the upper ureter can be by a transperitoneal or complete retroperitoneal approach, depending on the pathology being treated.[3,4] A transperitoneal procedure allows easier orientation and a larger working space than the retroperitoneal route. However, transperitoneal access carries with it the potential for injury to intra-abdominal organs and postoperative small-bowel obstruction.

SURGICAL PROCEDURES

Ureterolysis

The indications for laparoscopic ureterolysis are similar to those for open repair.[5–7] The objectives of treatment are to relieve ureteral obstruction, to prevent recurrence, and to preserve renal function. Ureteral entrapment by retroperitoneal fibrosis may occur secondary to a number of pathologic processes, including inflammatory bowel disease, pelvic inflammatory disease, endometriosis, neoplasms, previous radiation therapy, surgery, or use of drugs such as methysergide (Sansert).[5–7] It is important preoperatively to make every attempt to rule out malignancy as a cause of retroperitoneal fibrosis since ureterolysis alone without treatment of the underlying neoplasm would be unsuccessful in such patients.

Surgical Technique

With the patient under general anesthesia, a nasogastric tube is passed to decompress the stomach and a Foley catheter is inserted to drain the bladder during the surgery. At the beginning of the procedure, a no. 7.1 Fr occlusion balloon catheter is positioned under fluoroscopic guidance at the level of the ureteropelvic junction. A super stiff guide wire is passed through the lumen of the catheter into the renal pelvis. This will help identify and aid in the dissection of the ureter.

The patient is placed in a left lateral position to allow gravity to retract the bowel away from the operative field. After the pneumoperitoneum is established, four laparoscopic ports are placed. A 10-mm trocar is placed at the umbilicus for the camera. A 12-mm trocar is placed in the midclavicular line below the level of the costal arch. The 12-mm size of the trocar is necessary for the hernia stapler, which is used to reapproximate the peritoneum. A 5-mm trocar is placed at the level of the umbilicus in the anterior axillary line, and a second, 5-mm trocar is placed in the midline, 5 cm below the umbilicus (Fig. 13–1). When necessary, a fifth trocar may be utilized to aid in the dissection.

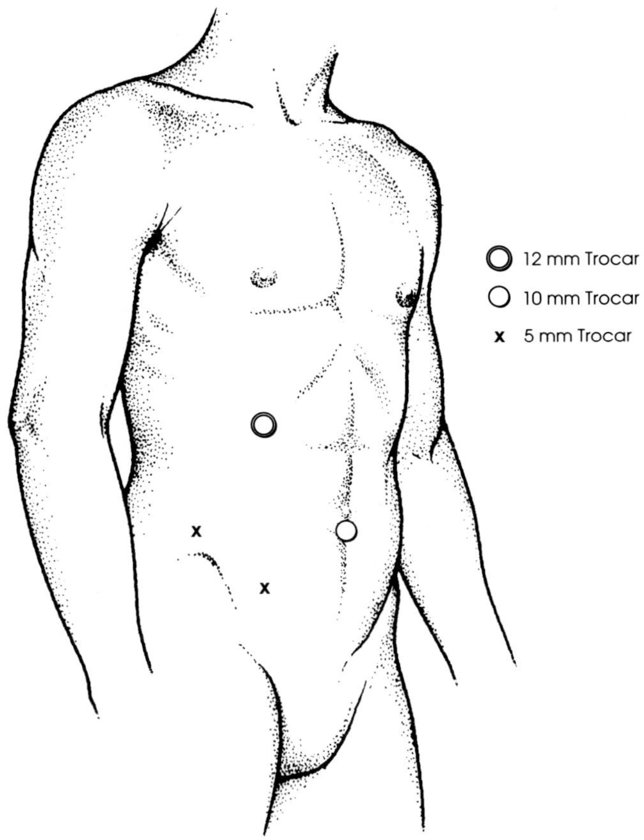

Figure 13–1. Trocar placement for laparoscopic ureterolysis. Four trocars are usually used: a 10-mm trocar in the umbilicus, a 12-mm trocar below the ribs in the midclavicular line, a 5-mm trocar below the umbilicus in the midclavicular line and a 5-mm trocar in the anterior axillary line at the level of the umbilicus. A fifth dissecting trocar may be used when necessary.

The line of Toldt is incised with electrocautery scissors, and the colon is reflected medially. Adequate mobilization is necessary to identify the entire course of the ureter (Fig. 13–2). The incision should be carried inferiorly over the iliac vessels and medial to the medial umbilical ligament. Proximally, the incision should free the hepatic flexure on the right side and splenic flexure on the left side.

Once the colon is adequately mobilized, the ureter should be identified where it is uninvolved by the fibrotic process. This is usually near the ureteropelvic junction or in the pelvis below the iliac vessels. Manipulation of the external ureteral stent is helpful in locating the ureter. Once the ureter is identified, several biopsies of the periureteral retroperitoneal tissue are taken, using the laparoscopic biopsy forceps, and are sent for immediate frozen-section examination to rule out the presence of malignancy.

After isolating a segment of ureter, an umbilical tape can be introduced into the abdominal cavity and looped around the ureter to act as a tractor (Fig. 13–3). Gentle traction is applied to aid in the ureteral dissection, avoiding excessive force that might tear or avulse the ureter.

The ureter is dissected free from the surrounding fibrous tissue with both blunt and sharp dissection. Use of electrocautery should be minimized to avoid ureteral injury. When dissecting the proximal ureter, the gonadal vessels are usually encountered and need to be ligated and transected for adequate mobilization. The dissection must be carried out until normal ureter is identified both proximally and distally.

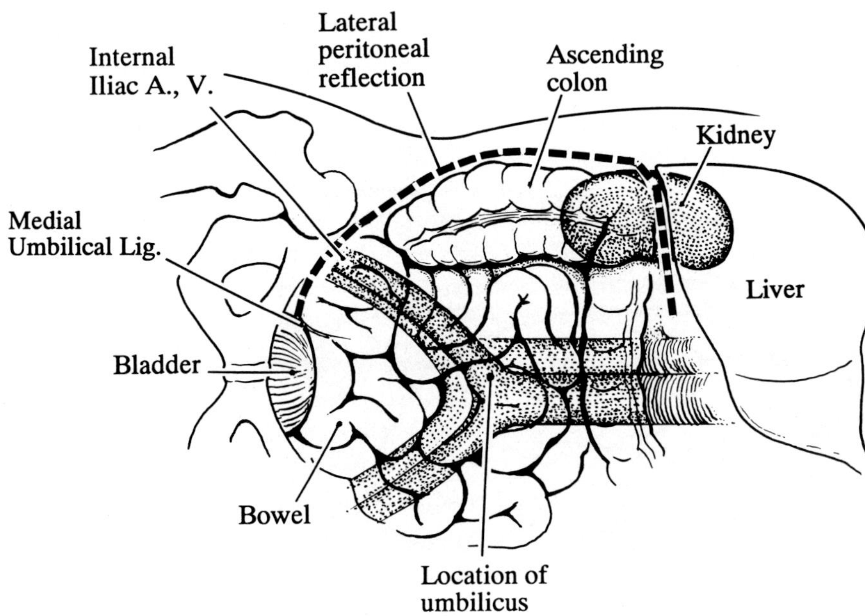

Figure 13–2. This diagram demonstrates where the incision should be carried to reflect the colon in order to access the ureter by a transperitoneal approach. A, artery; Lig, ligament; V, vein.

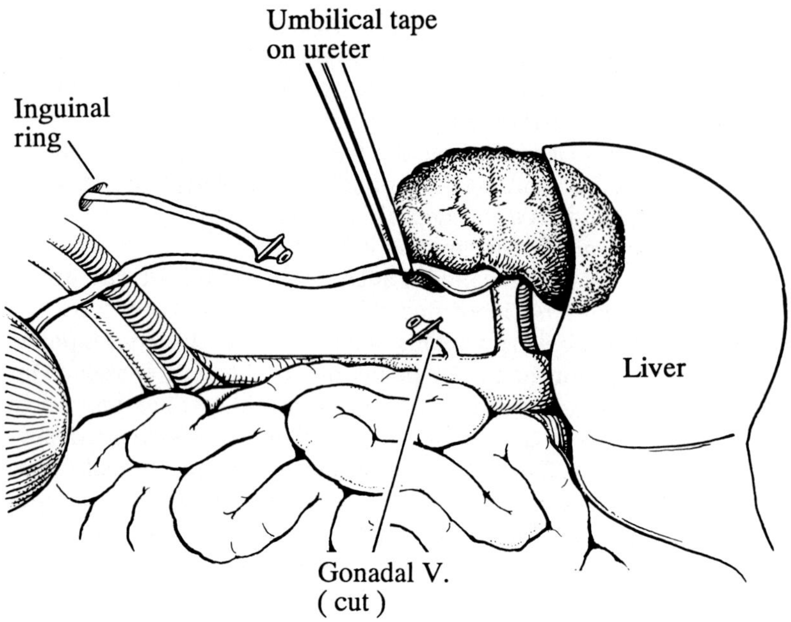

Figure 13–3. Umbilical tape passed alongside a trocar can act as a tractor to facilitate dissection. Note: while working on the upper ureter, the gonadal vessels may need to be transected. V, vein.

Once freed from the fibrous tissue, the ureter is then retracted into the peritoneal cavity. Grasping forceps are used to draw the cut peritoneal edges together behind the ureter (Fig. 13–4). These edges are carefully clipped together with a hernia stapler. In order to prevent obstruction, care is taken not to close the peritoneum too tightly where the ureter enters and exits the peritoneal cavity. Alternatively, omentum may be used to wrap around the ureter. Again, this is held in place with clips and staples. When using omentum for bilateral ureterolysis, it can be split with the GIA stapler. This will provide sufficient length to wrap both the ureters.

At the conclusion of the procedure, the pneumoperitoneum is deflated, and the trocars are removed. The external ureteral catheter is exchanged for an indwelling stent (Fig. 13–5).

Postoperative Care

The nasogastric tube and Foley catheter are removed at the conclusion of the operation, and the patient's diet is advanced as tolerated. The ureteral stent remains in place for 2 weeks, and afterwards patients are permitted to resume activities as tolerated. Radiographic imaging is obtained at 3, 6, and 12 months after the procedure in order to rule out recurrent ureteral obstruction (Fig. 13–6).

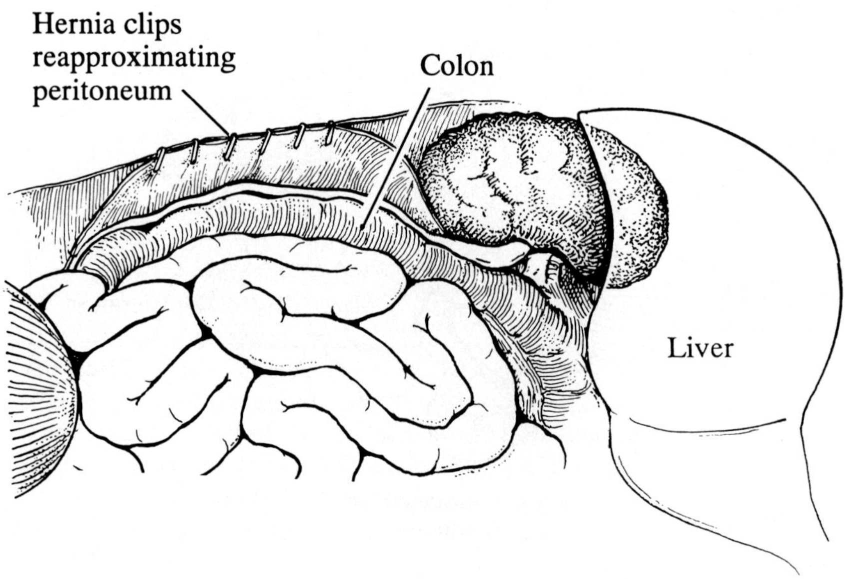

Figure 13–4. Diagram illustrating the peritoneum closed behind the ureter. Hernia staples are used to reapproximate edges. An omental wrap may be performed.

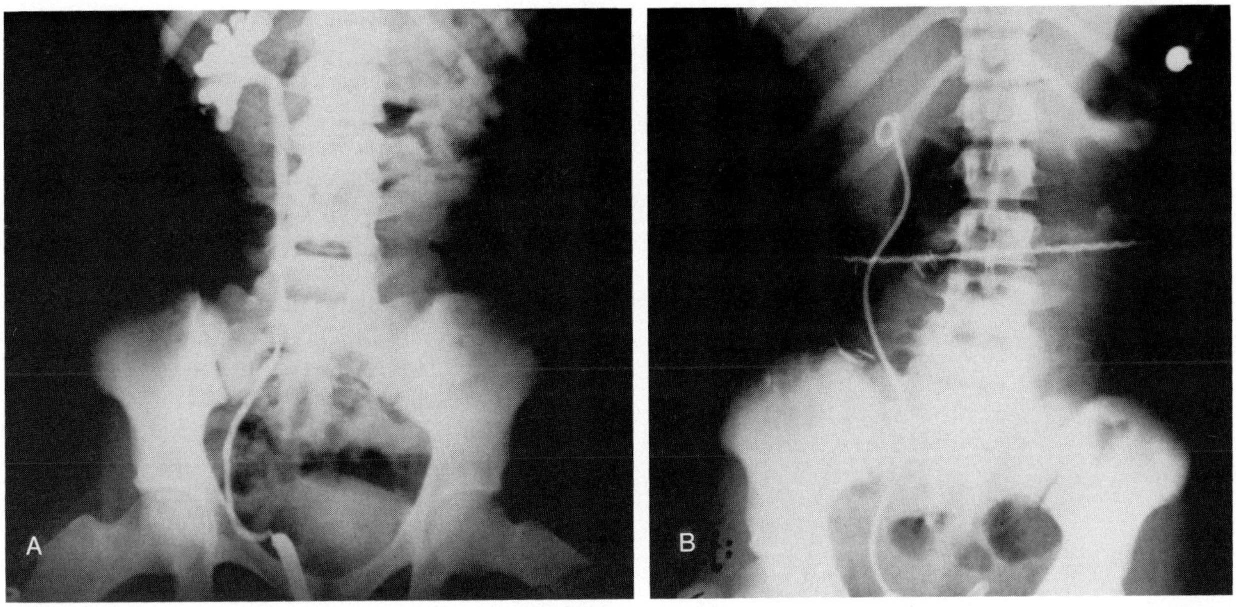

Figure 13–5. *A*, A retrograde pyelogram demonstrates medial displacement of the ureter in a patient with retroperitoneal fibrosis. There is no evidence of intrinsic obstruction. *B*, An indwelling ureteral stent has been placed after laparoscopic ureterolysis. Note that the medial clips have been placed on the gonadal vessels, whereas the lateral clip was used to reapproximate the peritoneal edge.

Results

To date a limited number of laparoscopic ureterolysis procedures have been reported.[8,9] We have performed this procedure successfully in three patients. All patients were discharged on the third postoperative day, utilized minimal narcotic analgesia, and returned to full unrestricted activity once the ureteral stents were removed. With follow-up, two patients remain unobstructed for more than 1 year. The third patient was found to have unsuspected carcinoma in the retroperitoneum and developed recurrent obstruction.

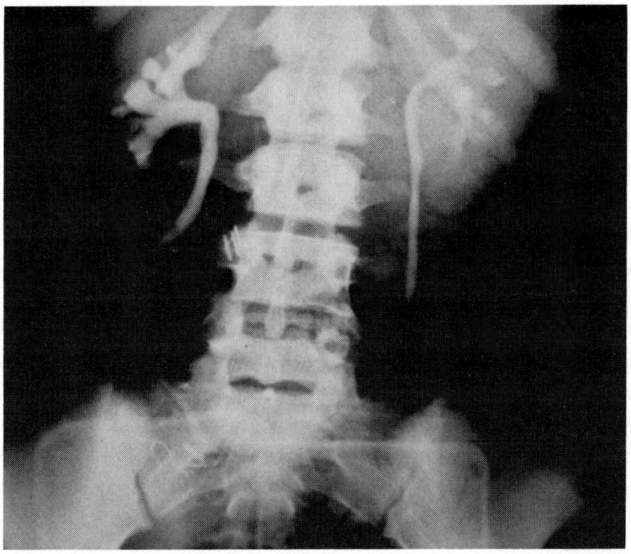

Figure 13–6. Postoperative intravenous urography showing ureteral drainage and maintenance of surgically achieved lateral placement of the right ureter.

Puppo recently reported on bilateral ureterolysis for idiopathic retroperitoneal fibrosis.[9] Although the operation took 10 hours, the patient was discharged on the second postoperative day and fully recovered in 2 weeks. Three months' follow-up demonstrated no evidence of recurrent obstruction.

Ureterectomy

Ureterectomy is most frequently carried out in conjunction with a nephrectomy in patients with primary neoplasms of the renal pelvis or ureter. Other conditions that may require ureterectomy include persistent infections in a refluxing system with end-stage nephropathy. Segmental ureterectomy may be necessary for stricture, tuberculosis, ectopic ureteroceles, ureteral valves, primary mega-ureter, benign neoplasms, or localized malignant neoplasm in a solitary ureter.

Surgical Technique

The patient's genitalia are prepped into the operative field. A no. 7 Fr occlusion balloon catheter is placed up to the renal pelvis. Using the Collin knife and a resectoscope, the ureteral orifice is excised circumferentially, and a tunnel is opened into the bladder. The periureteral area within the bladder is fulgurated for approximately 1 cm on either side of the incised tunnel. The fulguration mark will help identify if an adequate cuff of bladder has been obtained at the conclusion of the procedure. A Foley catheter is then placed alongside the external ureteral stent.

If the ureterectomy is performed in conjunction with a nephrectomy, five trocars are placed (Fig. 13–

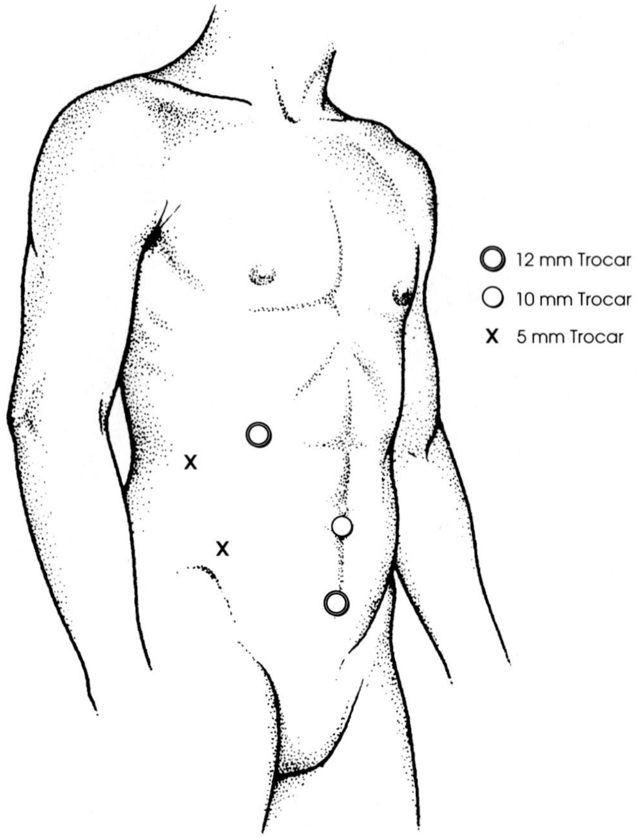

Figure 13–7. Five trocars are placed for ureterectomy. Placement is similar to that for a laparoscopic nephrectomy except that the lower trocar is placed in the midline and is 12-mm in size to allow for passage of the GIA stapling device.

7). A 10-mm trocar is placed at the umbilicus for the laparoscope. A 12-mm trocar is placed in the midclavicular line just below the level of the costal arch with a second 12-mm trocar in the midline between the umbilicus and the symphysis pubis. The 12-mm trocars are necessary for the endoscopic GIA stapler, which is used to control and transect the renal vein and bladder cuff. Two 5-mm trocars are placed: one subcostally in the anterior axillary line and one above the iliac crest in the anterior axillary line. If ureterectomy alone is being performed, one of the two 5-mm anterior axillary line ports can be omitted, and a 10-mm port can be substituted for the 12 mm midclavicular port.

The kidney is dissected as described in Chapter 11. The ureter is then carefully freed from the kidney to the level of the pelvic inlet. At this point, the patient is placed in the Trendelenburg position with the ipsilateral side elevated to mobilize the distal ureter. As in ureterolysis, the peritoneal incision needs to be extended distally, *medial* to the medial umbilical ligament, to above the pubic symphysis. To avoid injuring the bladder, care must be taken not to incise too far medially.

As the ureter is dissected distally into the pelvis, the superior vesical vessels are encountered crossing anteriorly. These need to be secured with clips and divided.

In the male, for adequate exposure, the vas deferens needs to be transected. In the female, the uterine artery is divided between hemostatic clips, and in some cases, the broad ligament may also need to be opened to gain adequate exposure.

The ureter is freed caudally to the level of the ureterovesical junction. The dissection is then continued around the bladder over sufficient area to obtain an adequate bladder cuff. The ureteral catheter is removed, and the ureter is transected with a cuff of bladder, by use of a laparoscopic GIA stapler. Cystoscopy is then performed to assure that the entire distal ureter with a cuff of bladder has been removed. Usually, no staples are visible in the bladder lumen, and no extravasation is noted.

As described for nephrectomy, the entire surgical specimen is maneuvered into a sack that has been introduced into the abdomen. The neck of the sac is delivered through the sheath of the 12-mm lower midline trocar. Care is taken so that the distal ureter is delivered last within the neck of the sack. In this manner, the distal ureter can be pulled from the bag, clipped, cut, and examined as a separate specimen. The remaining specimen can then be morcellated or removed intact by slightly extending the trocar incision.

Postoperative Care

The nasogastric tube is removed at the end of the procedure; however, the Foley catheter is left in to drain the bladder for 7 days. A cystogram is obtained before removal of the catheter to rule out extravasation. The patient's diet and activity can be advanced as tolerated. Surveillance cystoscopy is performed as indicated by the primary pathology.

Results

Clayman and associates have reported performing six laparoscopic nephroureterectomies.[10,11] The average patient age was 69 years (range, 52 to 83 years), and average length of surgery was 9.1 hours (range, 8 to 11 hours). Patients remained in the hospital an average of 5 days and required a combined average of 19 mg of morphine sulfate for analgesia. Patients returned to their preoperative level of activity within 4 weeks of surgery. Clayman also reported a successful ureterectomy in a patient who had undergone a prior open nephrectomy and was subsequently found to have a transitional cell carcinoma on final pathologic analysis.[11]

Some concerns exist regarding use of staples to close the bladder. Although a suture closure can be accomplished, this procedure is slower and more arduous than using the GIA stapler. Studies have demonstrated that the GIA stapler allows for a secure, water-tight closure of the bladder.[12] Concerns regarding possibility of stone formation on the staple line also exist. Experiments in a porcine model with the use of stapler for bladder closure have not demonstrated exposed clips or stones at 6-months' follow-up.[12] To date, these concerns have not been demonstrated to be a clinical problem; however, long-term evaluation is necessary.

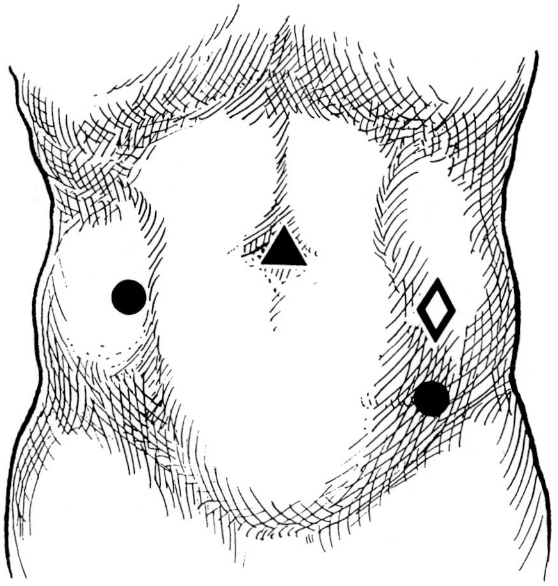

Figure 13–8. Trocar placement for distal ureteral surgery: a 10-mm trocar in the umbilicus, a 12-mm trocar at the level of the umbilicus, lateral to the contralateral side being treated, and a 5-mm trocar in each lower quadrant.

Ureterolithotomy

The need for open ureterolithotomy has markedly decreased owing to the recent advances in endourologic techniques and shock-wave lithotripsy. In rare instances, however, shock-wave lithotripsy and endoscopic approaches are unsuccessful, and an open ureterolithotomy is necessary. In selected patients, the laparoscopic removal of a calculus from the ureter may reduce the morbidity of an open procedure.

Surgical Technique

Preoperative and intraoperative x-ray imaging is crucial in locating the calculus. The genitalia are prepped for endoscopic access to the ureter during the procedure. A 5 Fr open-ended external ureteral stent is placed in the ureter under fluoroscopic guidance. In many instances, the catheter can be passed only up to the level of the stone. A Foley catheter is placed adjacent to the stent.

The number and location of trocars vary, depending on the position of the stone. For upper ureteral calculi, the trocars are placed as shown for ureterolysis. When treating lower ureteral stones, four trocars are used (Fig. 13–8). A 10-mm port is placed at the level of the umbilicus for the camera. A 10-mm trocar is placed at the level of the umbilicus lateral to the ipsilateral rectus muscle. A 5-mm trocar is placed in each lower quadrant lateral to the rectus muscle.

As with ureterolysis, the colon is reflected to expose the ureter over the level of the stone. The ureter is usually dilated to just above the level of the calculus and in most instances the stone can be found by gentle palpation with graspers. Alternatively, intraoperative fluoroscopy or ureteroscopy can aid in localization.

The ureter is incised in a longitudinal fashion directly over the stone. Care must be taken to extract and adequately grasp the stone intact. The stone should be kept in the visual field during removal through the 10-mm port. This will facilitate locating the stone if it is accidently knocked out of the grasper's jaws. A larger port may be necessary for removal, depending upon the size of the stone. Alternatively, the stone may be placed in an organ entrapment sac and removed through a port site after removing the trocar.

Once the calculus is removed, the ureteral stent can be manipulated past the point of obstruction into the renal pelvis. The ureter may be allowed to heal over the stent or loosely reapproximated, using interrupted absorbable 4-0 polydioxanone suture. A retroperitoneal drain should be left exiting through the ipsilateral lateral trocar site and the peritoneum should be reapproximated over the repair.

At the conclusion of the procedure, the pneumoperitoneum is deflated, and the trocars are removed. The external ureteral stent is exchanged for an indwelling double-pigtail stent.

Postoperative Care

The Foley catheter is removed at the end of the procedure, and the patient's diet and activity are advanced as tolerated. The retroperitoneal drain is removed when no drainage is noted, and the stent is left indwelling for 6 weeks. Follow-up radiographic imaging should be performed postoperatively to ensure adequate healing without obstruction.

Results

Several authors have reported on laparoscopic ureterolithotomy.[3,13,14] Harewood has removed ureteral calculi in five patients using this surgical technique.[14] In all these patients, previous endoscopic attempts at stone removal had failed. Following laparoscopic removal, all patients were discharged from the hospital within 2 postoperative days and required only minor analgesia for discomfort. Mean follow-up of 3 months revealed no evidence of obstruction.

Gaur has reported on completing retroperitoneal laparoscopic ureterolithotomies in two patients.[3] Blunt dissection allowed access into the retroperitoneal space through a 2-cm skin incision just above the iliac crest. A balloon introduced into the retroperitoneum lifted the peritoneum atraumatically and created sufficient working space for stone removal.

Ureteral Reconstruction

Ureteral reconstruction may be indicated in patients with iatrogenic or congenital ureteral obstruction. Ureteroureterostomy may be performed for short postoperative fibrotic strictures, congenital strictures, intraoperative laparoscopic ureteral injury, or endometriosis involving the ureter.

Ureteropelvic junction obstruction can be repaired by a Y-V plasty or dismembered pyeloplasty. The primary contraindication to any ureteroureterostomy is inadequate ureteral length, preventing a tension-free anastomosis.

Surgical Technique

Patient preparation and port placement are similar to that described for ureterolithotomy. When possible, a double-pigtail indwelling catheter is placed. After adequate localization of the diseased segment, the ureter is dissected from the surrounding tissue. It is helpful to place a stay stitch to align and manipulate the anastomosis during suture placement. The ureter is then transected with minimal mobilization so as not to disrupt the blood supply, and the diseased segment is removed. Care is taken not to cut the stent or to make spiral the incision in the ureter. Articulating scissors are useful in precisely incising the ureter. The most important factor influencing the success of the repair is the creation of a watertight anastomosis free of tension. Mobilization of the kidney and lower-pole fixation to the psoas fascia may reduce anastomotic tension and provide additional ureteral length.

The proximal and distal ends of the anastomosis are spatulated, using atraumatic grasping forceps and scissors. If earlier the stent could not be passed above the area of stricture, it is now advanced into the proximal ureter and renal pelvis. The ureteral anastomosis is performed, using four absorbable 4-0 sutures in an interrupted fashion. For ureteroureterostomy, sutures are placed at the 6, 12, 9, and 3 o'clock positions to approximate the proximal and distal ureteral edges. For pyeloplasty, six sutures are usually needed to complete the ureteropyelostomy, and a running suture may be helpful to close the incision in the renal pelvis. A retroperitoneal drain is left exiting through the lateral trocar site. The peritoneum is then reapproximated over the repair, using a hernia stapler or clips.

Postoperative Care

The Foley catheter is left in overnight. The retroperitoneal drain is removed once urinary drainage has decreased. The ureteral stent is left indwelling for a minimum of 2 weeks. Again, follow-up imaging studies are required to assess long-term effectiveness and to rule out complications.

Results

As with other areas of laparoscopic ureteral surgery, only isolated clinical reports are currently available to assess results. Nezhat and associates have accomplished a partial ureteral resection and ureteroureterostomy in a 36-year-old woman with a long-standing history of endometriosis and left ureteral obstruction.[15] In their report, the estimated blood loss was less than 100 ml, and the duration of the procedure was 117 minutes. The patient was discharged from the hospital on the first postoperative day and on follow-up has no evidence of obstruction.

Schuessler and associates have performed laparoscopic pyeloplasties in five patients.[16] The operative times have ranged from 3 to 10 hours, and both primary and secondary obstruction have been repaired. No intraoperative or postoperative complications were noted; however, one case had to be aborted secondary to difficulty with dissection.

Kavoussi and Peters have performed pyeloplasty in a patient in whom a crossing lower-pole vessel was responsible for obstruction.[17] This patient required only two doses of postoperative parenteral narcotic analgesia and was back to full unrestricted activity 10 days following surgery. Initial results of these laparoscopic ureteral reconstruction procedures are promising; however, long-term efficacy data are not yet available.

Other Applications

In laboratory models, several centers have evaluated the effectiveness of treating vesicoureteral reflux by extravesicular ureteral reimplantation.[18,19] Trials are currently under way in a refluxing porcine model to test the effectiveness of a laparoscopically performed Lich-Gregoire procedure, using both absorbable and nonabsorbable staples to create the extravesical tunnel for the ureter. At 6 months' follow-up, neither recurrent reflux nor clip erosion into the ureteral lumen has been noted.

Urinary diversion techniques are being investigated as an alternative to chronic percutaneous drainage to treat patients with malignant ureteral obstruction. Goldstein and associates have been able to develop a laparoscopic technique for cutaneous ureterostomy in the porcine model.[20] This procedure has been performed successfully with minimal morbidity and long-term effectiveness. Kozminski and co-workers have reported on successful laparoscopic ileal conduit urinary diversion.[21] Long-term efficacy with these procedures awaits confirmation by further clinical trials.

Research is currently under way to facilitate ureteral reconstructive techniques. Poppas and colleagues have combined low-power laser energy with a protein solder and light-absorbing chromophore to perform ureteral and ureteroenteric anastomosis.[22] This technology may prove to be an easier alternative to current suturing techniques. Another area being investigated is the use of fibrin glue (a mixture of fibrinogen and thrombin) to seal ureteroureteral anastomosis.[22] Although the glue does not provide tensile strength to an anastomosis, its role in reinforcing and "waterproofing" sutured or stapled anastomosis may improve healing. With improved instrumentation and techniques, laparoscopic reconstructive surgery, including pyeloplasty, ureteral reimplantation, and ureteroenteric anastomosis can be routinely performed and may supplant current open operative alternatives.

CONCLUSIONS

Recent developments in laparoscopic techniques and technology have the promise to revolutionize modern urologic surgery. The potential advantages of decreased postoperative pain with a shorter hospital stay and convalescence clearly offer significant advantages over traditional open surgery in properly selected patients.

Although laparoscopic ureteral surgery has been successfully performed in a number of clinical centers, limited data are available, and several shortcomings still remain. These procedures are technically difficult and require expertise in laparoscopic surgical techniques, especially in intracorporeal suturing. In order for a laparoscopic approach to urologic pathologies to become standard practice, simplification in these techniques must occur. Moreover, laparoscopic procedures are lengthy and expose patients to the risk of prolonged anesthesia. Finally, as with any new surgical procedure, long-term efficacy and outcomes need to be carefully assessed. Since a limited number of procedures have been performed to date in a highly select group of patients, very little information regarding complications is available.

The future role of laparoscopic surgery in approaching ureteral pathology is still evolving. As techniques and instrumentation mature, laparoscopy may assume a prominent role in the treatment of diseases affecting the upper urinary tract.

REFERENCES

1. Wickham, JEA: The surgical treatment of renal lithiasis. In: Wickham, JE, ed: Urinary Calculus Disease, New York, Churchill Livingstone, 1979, pp. 145–148.
2. Clayman, RV, Preminger, GM; Franklin, JR; et al: Percutaneous ureterolithotomy. J Urol 133:671, 1985.
3. Gaur, DD: Laparoscopic operative retroperitoneoscopy: Use of a new device. J Urol 148:1137, 1992.
4. Rubinstein, S; Hulbert, J; Pharand, D; et al: Laparoscopic ablation of symptomatic renal cysts. (Unpublished.)
5. Sosa, RE; Vaughan, ED, Jr; Gibbons, RT: Retroperitoneal fibrosis. AUA Update Series, Vol. 6, Lesson 21, 1987.
6. Sufrin, G; Hubrin, R: Postsurgical ureteral stenosis. In: Resnick, M; Kursh, E, eds: Current Therapy in Genitourinary Surgery. Philadelphia, B.C. Decker, 1987, pp. 183–186.
7. Lepor H; Walsh, PC: Idiopathic retroperitoneal fibrosis. J Urol 122:1, 1979.
8. Kavoussi, LR; Clayman, RV; Brunt, LM; Soper, NJ: Laparoscopic ureterolysis. J Urol 147:425, 1992.
9. Puppo, P: Bilateral laparoscopic ureterolysis. (Unpublished.)
10. Clayman, RV; Kavoussi, LR; Figenshau, RS; et al: Laparoscopic nephroureterectomy: Initial clinical case report. J Laparoendosc Surg 1:343, 1991.
11. Clayman, RV: Personal communication, 1993.
12. Figenshau, RS; Albala, DM; Clayman, RV; et al: Laparoscopic nephroureterectomy: Initial laboratory experience. Minim Invas Ther 1:93, 1991.
13. Raboy, A; Ferzli, GS; Ioffreda, R; Albert, PS: Laparoscopic ureterolithotomy. Urol 29:223, 1992.
14. Harewood, L: Personal communication, 1993.
15. Nezhat, C; Nezhat, F; Green, B; Gonzalez, G: Laparoscopic ureteroureterostomy. J Endourol 6:143, 1992.
16. Schuessler, WW: Grune, MT; Tecuanhuey, LV; Preminger, GM: Laparoscopic dismembered pyeloplasty. J Urol 150:1795, 1993.
17. Kavoussi, LR; Peters, CA: Laparoscopic pyeloplasty. J Urol 150:1891, 1993.
18. Clayman, RV; McDougall, EM; Chandhoke, PS; et al: Laparoscopic ureteral reimplantation: Initial laboratory studies. J Endourol 6:5144, 1992.
19. Atala, A; Kavoussi, L; Goldstein, D; et al: Laparoscopic correction of vesicoureteral reflux in an animal model. J Endourol 6:S168, 1992.
20. Goldstein, DS; Ho, GT; Scott, JA; et al: Laparoscopic cutaneous ureterostomy: Porcine model. J Endourol 6:S167, 1992.
21. Kozminski, M; Partamian, KO: Case report of laparoscopic ileal loop conduit. J Endourol 6:147, 1992.
22. Poppas, DP; Sutaria, P; Sosa, E; et al: Re-establishing continuity of the ureter using laser tissue-welding technique: Evaluation of new laser tissue-welding solders for laparoscopic surgery. J Urol 147:1244A, 1992.

CHAPTER 14

Retroperitoneoscopy

John J. Keizur, MD
Sakti Das, MD, FACS

Embryologically, the urogenital system is mostly developed from the derivatives of primitive mesoderm behind the coelomic cavity. In their fully developed state, the genitourinary organs are therefore sequestrated in the depths of retroperitoneum. Consequently, our open surgical approaches to the kidneys, ureters, and pelvic organs are extraperitoneal whenever feasible, unless special surgical circumstances warrant a transperitoneal approach.

Traditionally, laparoscopic surgeries are performed by transperitoneal approach following establishment of pneumoperitoneum by closed technique using the Verres needle or by the open mini laparotomy. The parietal peritoneum is then secondarily incised and dissected to obtain access to the retroperitoneal target organs like kidneys, ureters, adrenals, and lymph nodes. This orthodox transperitoneal laparoscopy, although seemingly expeditious, invites the potential calamities of possible vascular and visceral injuries and morbidities of intraperitoneal surgeries, and increased time and dissection is necessary to reach the retroperitoneal organs. On the other hand, after a few sporadic endeavors, retroperitoneal laparoscopy has undergone a premature obsolescence because of the perceived difficulties in working in a contained limited space.[1] However, with technical refinements, several recent reports of successful retroperitoneoscopic surgeries have proved the feasibility and distinct advantages of this approach.[2,3]

HISTORICAL PERSPECTIVE

Retroperitoneoscopy has experienced a delayed development and acceptance compared with peritoneoscopy. Difficulties in providing adequate visualization and room for surgical maneuvering as well as concerns about deleterious effects of insufflating the retroperitoneal space account for this retarded progression. Although pneumoretroperitoneum has been used safely for more than 70 years to aid in radiographic visualization of the kidneys and adrenals,[4] the conjunctive use of endoscopes has only recently been attempted.

Early animal experiments confirmed the technical feasibility and safety of insufflating gas directly into the retroperitoneum. Using a fetoscope, Roberts[5] injected carbon dioxide within the Gerota fascia in rhesus monkeys and was able to visualize the posterior surface of the kidneys. Kaplan and associates[6] established a true pneumoretroperitoneum in canines by insufflating nitrous oxide through a presacrally placed spinal needle. A separate approach through the flank with the laparoscope reliably identified the kidneys, renal vessels, ureters and adrenals. No animals suffered ill effects from the pneumoretroperitoneum.

Retroperitoneoscopy through the flank in a human was pioneered by Wickham, who performed an extraperitoneal laparoscopic ureterolithotomy in 1978.[7] From subsequent investigations in cadavers, Wickham noted that although the posterior aspects of the kidneys can be explored with the laparoscope, the overall quality of pneumoretroperitoneum was poor. Clayman and associates[8] also reported similar experience of removing a ureteral stone in one patient using retroperitoneal endoscopy with fluid irrigation in the retroperitoneum.

Extraperitoneal endoscopy in the pelvis has focused on lymph nodal staging procedures. Earliest techniques, termed pelviscopy, utilized a mediastinoscope to bluntly dissect within the pelvic retroperitoneum to sample pelvic lymph nodes.[9–13] The obvious disadvantage of such technique has been the difficulty in exposing the obturator nodes, precluding the performance of an adequate staging lymphadenectomy. In the initial series reported by Hald and Rasmussen,[9] 4 of 12 patients had no lymph nodes found in their surgical specimen. With refinements of surgical techniques, subsequently more complete pelviscopic node dissections have been reported.[10]

SURGICAL TECHNIQUE

Probably the most important initial step in retroperitoneoscopy is the expansion and distention of the retroperitoneal space by an expanding device. We have successfully utilized a balloon device modified after that of Gaur.[14] The fingers of a latex rubber glove are tied off, and the glove is secured over the distal end of the catheter (Chap. 16, Fig. 16–1). The device is placed in the retroperitoneum and expanded by injecting saline through the catheter. Special trocars are available with transparent balloons at their inner end that can be inflated with air or fluid to allow laparoscopic visibility of retroperitoneum through the clear distended balloon (Fig. 14–1).

Retroperitoneoscopy Through the Flank

This approach is applicable to surgery on adrenals, kidneys, and upper ureters. The patient is placed in a lateral decubitus position with slight forward tilt. A small incision is made about 2 cm below the twelfth rib, just lateral to the sacrospinalis. The incision is deepened through the fused lamellae of lumbar fascia to enter the perinephric space. The latter is further dissected by blunt digital exploration. The expanding device is introduced into the retroperitoneal space, and about 800 to 1000 ml saline are injected to inflate the balloon. The balloon is then deflated and removed. Laparoscope lens in an 11-mm trocar is introduced into the retroperitoneal space and high-flow carbon dioxide insufflation is continued to maintain a pressure of about 14 mm Hg. With the posterior parietal peritoneum pushed away by the expanding device, the retroperitoneal space is widely opened by continued insufflation, and subsequent working ports are established under camera vision. The number and location of accessory ports are determined by the surgical procedure to be undertaken. However, it is usually advisable to keep the ports posterior to the anterior axillary line to avoid transgressing the lateral peritoneal reflection. During laparoscopic dissection it is often helpful to move the laparoscope to the anterior ports for better visibility as the situation may dictate.

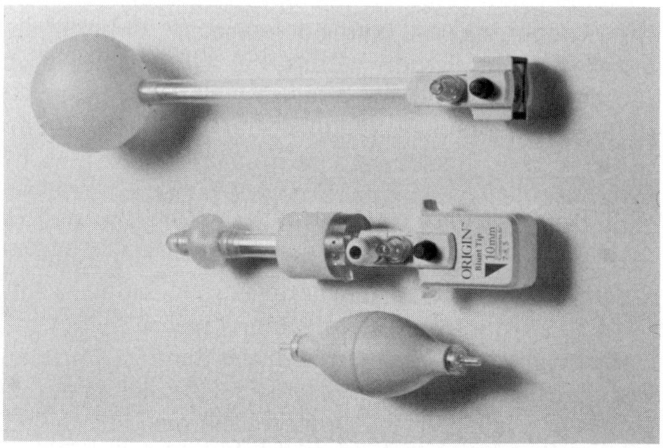

Figure 14–1. Trocar balloon for extraperitoneal distention.

Retroperitoneoscopy: Anterolateral

For surgery on mid and lower ureters and for internal spermatic vein ligation, the retroperitoneum is reached by a small incision at McBurney's point. The external oblique aponeurosis is incised, and underlying fibers of the internal oblique and transverse muscles of the abdomen are split to reach the extraperitoneal space. Following careful digital dissection, the expanding device is introduced and inflated in the retroperitoneum. The remainder of the procedure is the same as that previously discussed.

Retroperitoneoscopy: Pelvic

We have found the pelvic retroperitoneoscopy ideal for bilateral staging pelvic lymph node dissection and bladder-neck suspension procedures. A small midline incision is made about 2 cm below the umbilicus. The linea alba is opened, and underlying extraperitoneal space is developed by digital dissection behind the rectus muscle of the abdomen. The expanding device is introduced and expanded by injecting about 1200 ml saline solution. The balloon is decompressed and removed. The laparoscope is introduced with high-flow carbon dioxide insufflation. Anatomic landmarks of the symphysis pubis, superior pubic rami, bladder neck, and external iliac vein pulsations in the pelvis are easily identified. Complete bilateral staging lymphadenectomy is accomplished by en bloc dissection of the fibrofatty lymphatic tissue from the triangular area bounded laterally by the external iliac vein, proximally by the hypogastric artery, and inferiorly by the endopelvic fascia (see Chapter 16).

CONCLUSIONS

The pioneering concept of retroperitoneal expansion by Gaur and co-workers[14] has led to the resurgence of retroperitoneoscopy. Artificial balloon expansion creates the necessary space and retraction of neighboring viscera, so that subsequent insufflation can maintain the open space for surgical maneuvering. In a way, this technique simulates the steps of dissection and retraction traditionally used during open surgery.

Aside from obviating the potential hazards of transperitoneal access and intraperitoneal dissection, there are certain distinct advantages of retroperitoneoscopy in patient positioning, intestinal retraction, anatomic approach to the renal hilum, and postoperative wound drainage. For retroperitoneal approaches to the adrenals, kidneys, and ureters the patient is placed in the lateral decubitus, as opposed to the initial supine position for pneumoperitoneum; then lateral tilting or turning maneuvers necessary in transperitoneal laparoscopy. The intestines contained within the intact peritoneal envelope remain displaced during retroperitoneal dissection, thereby avoiding extensive colonic mobilization and constant retraction of bowel. During nephrectomy, the renal hilum is approached from the posterior aspect, allowing easier initial control of the renal arteries. Similar exposure of other retroperitoneal structures such as the adrenal gland in the right side is relatively easier than with the anterior approach. The closed extraperitoneal space allows more effective postoperative drainage, especially following reconstructive and reparative surgery such as pyeloplasty, partial nephrectomy, pyelolithotomy, and ureterolithotomy. The perceived difficulties of surgical dissection of kidneys and adrenal glands in a restricted environment during retroperitoneoscopy has not proved true with the present technique of initial balloon expansion. However, organ entrapment, especially of large specimens, in the limited space is difficult.

The anterolateral extraperitoneal approach allows access for ureterolithotomy on the lower ureter at and above the pelvic inlet (Fig. 14–2). We have performed internal spermatic vein ligation extraperitoneally for treatment of varicocele. The extraperitoneal dissection appears however to be more extensive, and such an approach will not be suitable for bilateral varicocele surgery.

In the pelvis, the excellent anatomic appearance of the bladder, bladder neck, and symphysial structures makes the extraperitoneal approach ideally suited for procedures such as laparoscopic bladder-neck suspension (see Chap. 21) and surgery for urachal pathologies. The majority of bladder diverticula are located posterolaterally and are therefore not often amenable to extraperitoneal excision. Although our experience with laparoscopic antireflux surgery has so far been limited to animal experimentations, an extravesical ureterovesicoplasty by extraperitoneal approach should be feasible in humans simulating the standard open procedures of Lich-Gregoire for correction of vesicoureteric reflux.

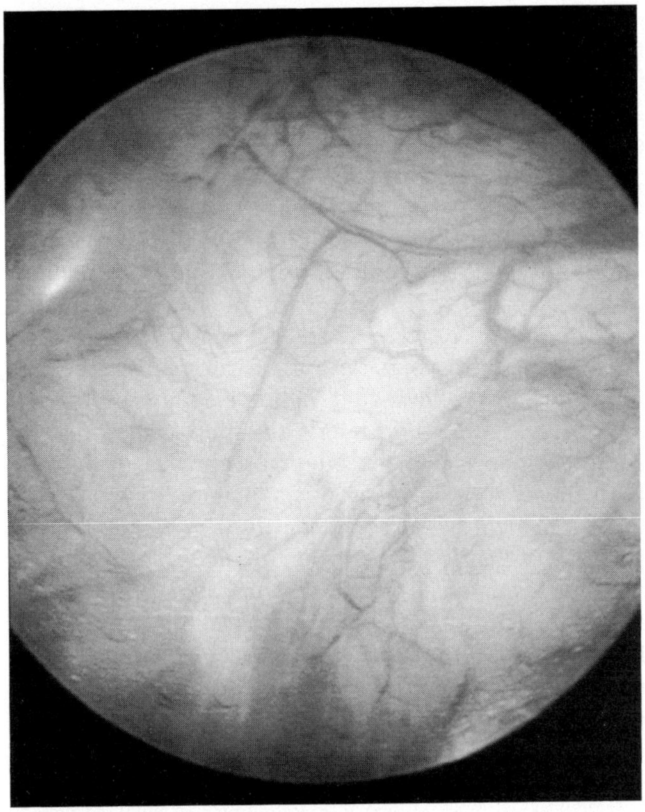

Figure 14–2. Ureter at the pelvic brim viewed through the distending balloon. See also Color Plate 3.

For the purpose of bilateral staging pelvic lymphadenectomy we have consistently used the extraperitoneal approach, proving its safety and feasibility (see Chapter 16). The lymph node dissection is anatomically precise, simulating the standards of open pelvic lymphadenectomy.

Although it has been conjectured that CO_2 insufflation during retroperitoneoscopy may lead to a greater degree of hypercapnia, we have not encountered a single instance of clinically significant hypercapnia in our patients. On careful monitoring of the end-tidal CO_2, the highest level registered was 48.5 mm Hg Pco_2 with no untoward cardiopulmonary effect. In comparison, the end-tidal CO_2 levels during our transperitoneal laparoscopies have been higher. We believe that the preliminary balloon expansion allows easier distention of the retroperitoneal space at lower inflow pressure of CO_2 during laparoscopic dissection. The overall absorptive surface of retroperitoneal space is much less than the extensive peritoneal surface area. Last, the relatively avascular extraperitoneal fat is probably less capable of CO_2 absorption than the well-perfused peritoneal surface. The other advantage of retroperitoneal CO_2 insufflation is that by avoiding CO_2 contact with the peritoneal membrane, there is less hypothermia and reduced postoperative pain from diaphragmatic irritation.

In conclusion, retroperitoneoscopy offers another viable option in the developing field of laparoscopy. Other workers have used blind or fluoroscopically monitored Verres needle placement for CO_2 insufflation before trocar insertion in the retroperitoneum. Hakim and colleagues (Chap. 17) advocate the use of operative laparoscopy for retroperitoneal dissection. However, we believe that balloon expansion of the retroperitoneum as a prelude to laparoscope and trocar placement is an excellent atraumatic procedure that allows superior anatomic exposure for laparoscopic surgical procedures in the flank and pelvis. The surgical indications that warrant an extraperitoneal approach in open surgery hold true for retroperitoneoscopy as well. As a minimally invasive technique, retroperitoneoscopy emulates the established standards and principles of open urologic procedures without compromising surgical efficiency and patient safety.

REFERENCES

1. Wickham, JEA; Miller, RA: Percutaneous renal access. In: Wickham, JEA, ed: Percutaneous Renal Surgery. New York, Churchill Livingstone, 1983, pp. 33–39.
2. Villers, A; Baron, JC; Anidjar, M; et al: Extraperitoneal endosurgical lymphadenectomy with insufflation for staging of pelvic malignancies. J Urol 147:407A, 1992.
3. Ferzli, G; Raboy, A; Kleinerman, D; Albert, P: Extraperitoneal endoscopic pelvic lymph node dissection vs laparoscopic lymph node dissection in the staging of prostate and bladder carcinoma. J Laparoendosc Surg 2:219–222, 1992.
4. Robertson, LH; Anderson, EE; Glenn, JF: Retroperitoneal contrast studies: Simplified bilateral perirenal carbon dioxide insufflation. J Urol 93:414–416, 1965.
5. Roberts, JA: Retroperitoneal endoscopy. J Med Primatol 5: 124–127, 1976.
6. Kaplan, LR; Johnston, GR; Hardy, RM: Retroperitoneoscopy in dogs. Gastrointest Endosc 25:13–15, 1979.
7. Wickham, JEA: The surgical treatment of renal lithiasis. In: Wickham, JEA, ed: Urinary Calculus Disease. New York, Churchill Livingstone, 1979, pp. 145–198.
8. Clayman, RV; Preminger, GM; Franklin, JR; Peters, PC: Percutaneous ureterolithotomy. J Urol 133:671, 1985.
9. Hald, T; Rasmussen, F: Extraperitoneal pelvioscopy: A new aid in staging of lower urinary tract tumors. A preliminary report. J Urol 124:245–248, 1980.
10. Mazeman, E; Wurtz, A; Gilliot, P; Biserte, J: Extraperitoneal pelvioscopy in lymph node staging of bladder and prostate cancer. J Urol 147:366–370, 1992.
11. Wurtz, A: L'endoscopie de l'espace retroperitoneal techniques. Résultats et indications actuelles. Ann Chir 43:475–480, 1989.
12. Taillandier, J; Boiteux, JP; Giraud, B: Pelvic lymphadenoscopy. A simple reliable method for the staging of pelvic cancers. Int Surg 77:211–213, 1992.
13. Fantoni, PA; Mondina, P; Tognoli, S; et al. Retroperitoneoscopy for biopsy of pelvic and medium low para-aortic lymph nodes and tissues. Int Surg 68:157–160, 1983.
14. Gaur, DD; Agarwal, DK; Purohit, KC: Retroperitoneal laparoscopic nephrectomy: Initial case report. J Urol 149:103–105, 1993.

CHAPTER 15

Laparoscopic Pelvic Lymphadenectomy

Raju Thomas, MD, FACS

Although urologists have traditionally been endoscopic surgeons and thereby have been instrumental in the development of the cystoscope and endoscopic procedures, laparoscopy did not enter mainstream urology until recent years.[1–3] As a consequence of improved instrumentation and paraphernalia, there has been intensive interest in the use of laparoscopes in urologic surgery. Although laparoscopic urologic procedures have been developed for localization, orchiopexy, and orchiectomy of abdominal testes; varicocele ligation; occasional ureterolithotomy; renal biopsy; nephrectomy; bladder neck suspension; lymphocele drainage; and so forth, the main impetus in endoscopic laparoscopy has been pelvic lymphadenectomy for staging of adenocarcinoma of the prostate.

This use of laparoscopes within the ever-expanding and ever-improving technology has major implications for the practicing urologist. With the advent of minimally invasive surgery and the public awareness of such procedures, there has been a practical stimulus for further development of laparoscopic procedures.

RATIONALE FOR PELVIC LYMPHADENECTOMY

Before instituting definitive therapy for clinically localized adenocarcinoma of the prostate, accurate staging is essential. Pelvic lymph node dissection is currently accepted as the most accurate method for evaluating lymph nodal metastases from prostatic, vesical, penile, and cervical carcinoma. Such accurate evaluation of the pelvic lymph nodes is essential, since Gervasi and associates have shown that patients with a single microscopic node displaying metastasis had a pattern of progression and cancer-specific mortality rate that was similar to patients with more extensive nodal metastases and markedly worse than patients with negative nodes.[4] Although the significance of minimal nodal metastases has still not been definitely established, some authors argue that patients with minimal nodal metastases can sometimes be treated effectively with treatment modalities such as pelvic lymphadenectomy and radical prostatectomy or extended field radiotherapy.[5] Flocks reported that the presence of positive pelvic lymph nodes did not affect the incidence of local recurrence or the 5-year survival free of disease.[6] By quantitating the nodal metastases, Barzell and colleagues reported that patients with minimal nodal metastases (less than 3 ml) have the same probability of being free from distant metastases at 5 years (74%) compared with patients with negative nodes (71%).[7] Reports by Kramer and co-workers[8] and Smith and Middleton[9] attest to their finding that positive lymph nodes, despite the microscopic nature of the metastases, had an ominous prognosis regardless of the therapeutic modality used. Zincke and Utz analyzed and reported a series of patients who underwent radical prostatectomy even with a single positive node. They concluded that the higher relapse rate indicates systemic disease and recommended adjunctive hormonal therapy for such patients.[10,11]

Thus it is clear that adequate evaluation of the status of the lymph nodes, although controversial, is vital before a definitive and often invasive therapy for cancer control is instituted. Several imaging and surgical techniques have been studied and described for this purpose. The most accurate means to assess pelvic lymph nodes for metastases is through histologic examination. However, traditional open surgical pelvic lymphadenectomy is associated with a large abdominal incision and increased morbidity.[12]

Although noninvasive imaging techniques to evaluate the status of pelvic lymph nodes seem attractive, the accuracy of these techniques has been found to be clinically inadequate. Computed tomography (CT) gives a high false-negative result, since microscopic nodal metastases cannot be detected. The reported sensitivity is 50% to 75% with a specificity of 80% to 100% and an average accuracy of 83% to 92%.[13–15] Other invasive imaging techniques such as pedal lymphangiography cannot demonstrate the microscopic spread that accounts for the high false-negative rate of 20% to 40% and an overall accuracy of approximately 80%.[16] Percutaneous, fine-needle aspiration of lymph nodes is an invasive procedure, and only radiographically positive nodes can be biopsied. Transrectal ultrasound of the prostate, in widespread use today, is associated with a high incidence of upstaging ranging from 16% to 54% and as high as 62% incidence of understaging of prostatic cancer.[17]

Magnetic resonance imaging (MRI), although believed promising, has a reported accuracy rate of 83% to 89%.[18,19] Endorectal surface coil MRI has demonstrated an accuracy rate of 82% in differentiating those patients with stages B and C prostatic cancer.[20] Neither MRI nor transrectal ultrasound of the prostate is sufficiently reliable to significantly help accurate staging and thereby to impact patient management.[21]

Laparoscopic pelvic lymph node dissection (LPLND) is now considered a less invasive method of assessing the status of the pelvic lymph nodes.[2,3] Parra and co-workers have demonstrated the safety and accuracy of LPLND as compared with open pelvic lymphadenectomy.[22] Querleu and colleagues reported a 100% sensitivity and specificity of laparoscopic pelvic lymph node dissection in 39 women with cervical cancer.[23] The use of LPLND is indicated in patients with clinically localized adenocarcinoma of the prostate before radical surgery or radiation therapy, and in patients with a high probability of metastases. These patients can be characterized as those having an elevated prostate-specific antigen (PSA) and a high Gleason histopathology grade (7 and above). Also, patients with a large primary tumor (stage B_2 or C) fall into this category.

LAPAROSCOPIC PELVIC LYMPHADENECTOMY: TECHNIQUE

Pneumoperitoneum is created by CO_2 insufflation through a Verres needle at the umbilicus. The Verres needle is withdrawn, and in its place a 10-mm trocar is introduced for the laparoscope. Accessory ports are then placed under laparoscopic vision to reduce the risk of any injury. Usually, an 11-mm suprapubic port is established about 5 cm above the symphysis pubis in the midline. Two lateral 5-mm ports are placed approximately midway between the anterior superior iliac spine and the umbilicus, just lateral to the rectus abdominus muscle (Fig. 15–1*A*, *B*).

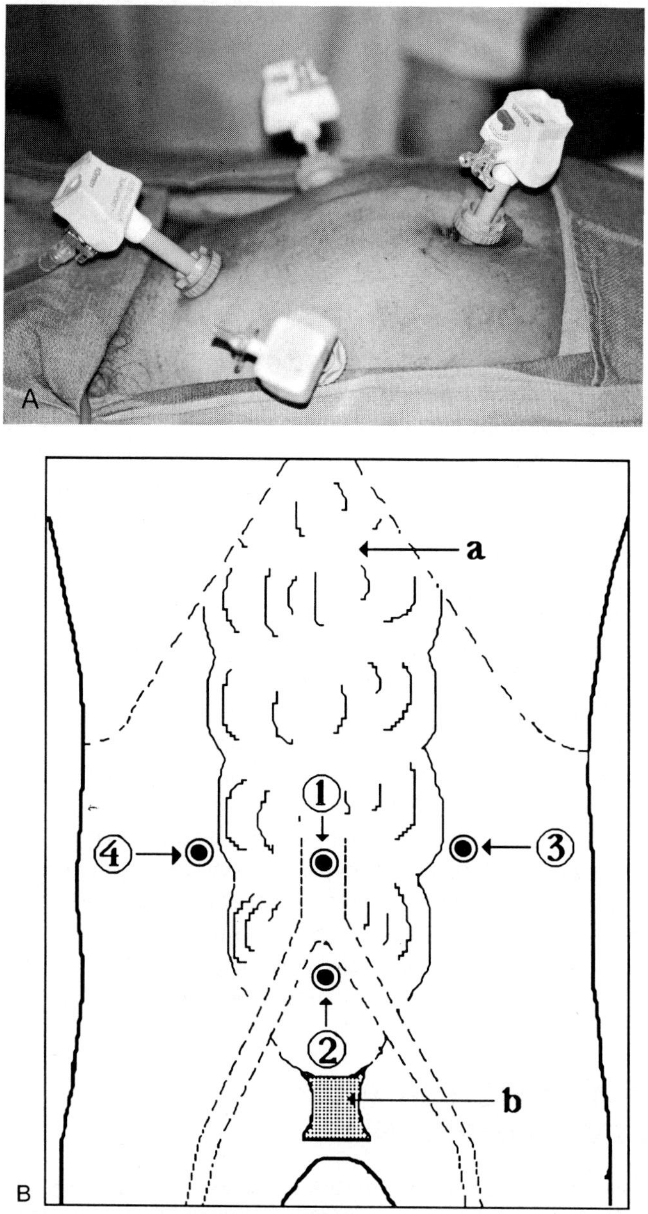

Figure 15–1. *A*, Trocar placement seen in a patient (Foley catheter denotes foot end). *B*, Usual sites for placement of trocars and introduction of video camera (1) and ancillary instrumentation (2, 3, and 4); a, rectus muscle; b, pubic symphises.

After successful placement of the abdominal trocars, the abdomen is laparoscopically examined for any trauma to the bowels or vasculature or any unexpected pelvic masses. LPLND is performed on the side ipsilateral to the prostatic nodule or with a positive histopathologic diagnosis. If the lymph nodes on this side show evidence of malignancy on frozen section, the contralateral pelvic node dissection is deemed unnecessary.

Before performing laparoscopic surgery in the pelvis, fundamental knowledge of the pelvic anatomy is essential (Fig. 15–2*A*, *B*). The median umbilical ligament (urachus) is seen in the midline. Moving laterally, the next major landmark is the medial umbilical ligament (obliterated umbilical artery), after which the next major landmark can be seen in the pulsations of the external iliac artery. In obese patients, this important landmark may not be clearly visualized. The internal inguinal ring with the spermatic vessels running laterally is also seen. The vas deferens takes a medial course over the iliac artery and the medial umbilical ligament. On the left pelvic wall, the sigmoid colon often has adhesions. The parietal peritoneal adhesions are released to dissect the sigmoid colon off the pelvic wall before left pelvic lymph node dissection.

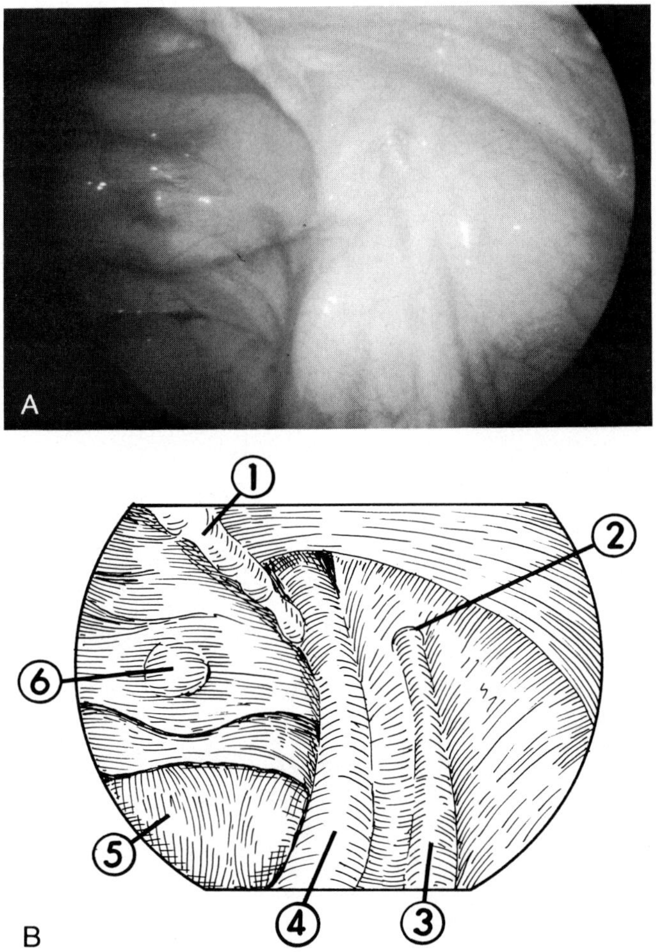

Figure 15–2. *A*, Photograph of important anatomic land marks for laparoscopic lymph node dissection. *B*, Drawing of *A*: (1) Medial umbilical ligament; (2) internal inguinal ring; (3) spermatic vessels; (4) iliac artery; (5) sigmoid colon; (6) tip of Foley catheter within bladder. See also Color Plate 4.

The initial parietal peritoneal incision is made just lateral to the medial umbilical ligament. This ligament is grasped and retracted medially to ensure that the incision is made just lateral to it. If the dissection is carried medially, then the ureter or bladder may be traumatized. This peritoneal incision is carried cephalad, and the vas deferens is encountered. The vas deferens can be either retracted (without transecting it) or transected at this time. The use of coagulating current at a lower power setting makes for an avascular dissection and prevents the nuisance of a bloody field. Although the bleeding is clinically insignificant, the magnification offered by the laparoscopic lens enhances even trivial bleeding. If the medial umbilical ligament is not readily visualized, the alternate site of incision should be that overlying the external iliac artery. Once again, traction and countertraction are obtained through the coordinated efforts of the surgeon and the assistant, and the incision, if made over the iliac artery, is carried distally toward the pelvic side wall and cephalad toward the bifurcation of the iliac vessels. The boundaries of the dissection are, medially, the medial umbilical ligament; laterally, the iliac vessels; distally, the pelvic side wall; inferiorly, the obturator nerve and vessels; and cephalad, the bifurcation of the iliac vessels. The fibrofatty lymphatic tissue between these landmarks is removed and submitted for histopathologic examination.

If the initial incision is made over the medial umbilical ligament, then the dissection is carried laterally, and tissue is swept laterally until the pulsatile external iliac artery is reached. At this point, the iliac vessels are stripped of the fibrofatty areolar tissue, and the external iliac vein should be encountered just beneath the artery. This vein is invariably collapsed because of the tension exerted by the pneumoperitoneum and by the Trendelenburg position of the patient. While approaching the lateral side walls, watch for the accessory obturator and circumflex iliac veins. A judicious use of graspers and curved scissors is recommended within the pelvis. The distal margin of resection should be the femoral canal, which contains the Cloquet node.

The nodal package is thus dissected, using blunt and sharp dissection between the boundaries mentioned above (Fig. 15–3*A*, *B*). As the package is developed, the incoming lymphatics and the attachment of this package to the pelvic side wall are transected. This can be done with the use of electrocautery, the contact-tip laser fiber, or endoscopic clips. The nodal package is then dissected around the obturator nerve, and this package is held at the bifurcation of the iliac

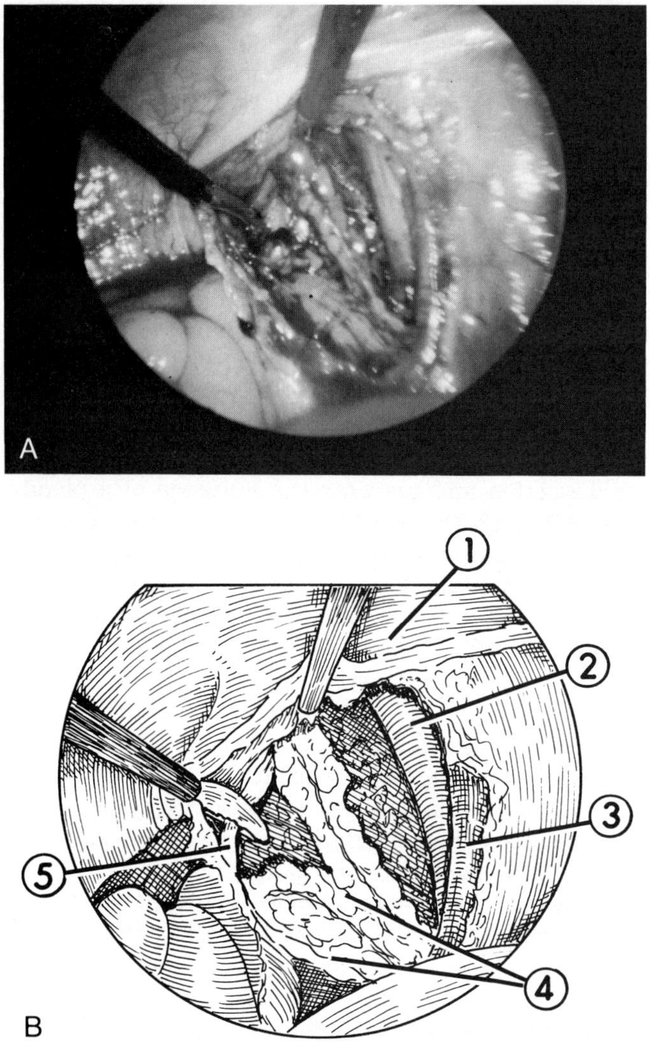

Figure 15–3. *A*, Nodal package being developed. *B*, Drawing showing (1) right pelvic side wall; (2) right external iliac vein; (3) right external iliac artery; (4) lymph node package; (5) forceps grasping right medial umbilical ligament. See also Color Plate 4.

vessels. The node-bearing package is dissected cephalad toward the bifurcation of the common iliac artery. Small vessels and lymphatics can be either cauterized or clipped.

Before dissecting the nodal package at the level of the bifurcation of the iliacs, it is essential to identify the ureter. Use of electrocautery in this area could cause thermal injury to the ureter unless it has been identified as being away from the cautery site. The nodal package is then clipped or cauterized, divided, and extracted through the 11-mm suprapubic port under laparoscopic vision. The flapper valve of the trocar sheath must be opened. A twisting motion facilitates extraction of the lymph node package. Alternatively, the lymph node package can be inserted into a disposable pouch, prior to its extraction through an 11-mm trocar sheath. The obturator fossa is then examined (Fig. 15–4*A*, *B*). Use of a suction irrigator is recommended. Remember to place the tip of the suction below fluid levels while suctioning in order to avoid aspirating the pneumoperitoneum.

Once the ipsilateral side pelvic node dissection has been completed, the contralateral pelvic lymph node dissection is performed. The table is rotated to the opposite side 30° to facilitate gravitational retraction of the bowel. After the bilateral pelvic lymphadenectomy has been completed, the abdomen is once again examined for any vascular injury or trauma to the bowels. Trocar removal and abdominal closure are then performed systematically.

POSTOPERATIVE CARE

The nasogastric tube is usually removed in the recovery room, and the Foley catheter is left in place until the patient has sufficiently recovered from the anesthetic to be able to void. Depending on the procedures

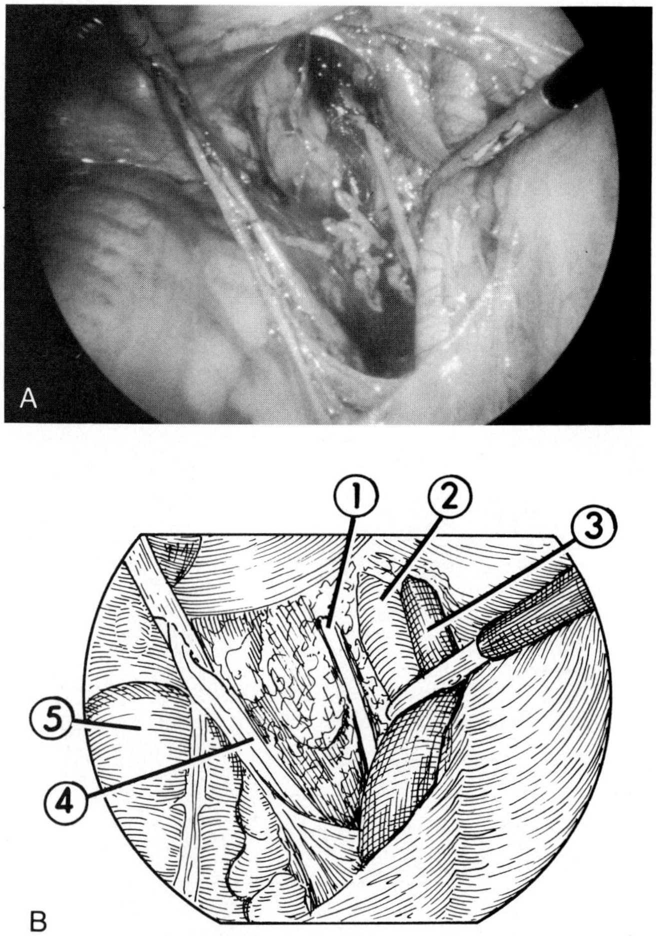

Figure 15–4. *A*, Completed laparoscopic right pelvic lymph node dissection. *B*, Drawing showing (1) obturator nerve; (2) right external iliac vein; (3) right external iliac artery; (4) medial umbilical ligament; (5) sigmoid colon. See also Color Plate 4.

performed (i.e., radical prostatectomy), diet is given as tolerated. Usually, patients who have just undergone an LPLND can be discharged the next morning or even in selected cases, the same evening.

COMPLICATIONS

In a cumulative multicenter retrospective analysis involving 372 patients, there was a significant learning curve associated with LPLND: during the first 8 cases performed in each institution, the majority of aborted procedures occurred.[24]

Vascular injuries, the most common complications reported, occurred during trocar placement or during dissection. Placement of the primary and secondary trocar using the technique mentioned earlier should prevent such injuries. If they do occur, laparoscopic-guided fulguration, cut-down to the injured vessel and suture ligation or placement of transcutaneous sutures guided by the laparoscope is recommended.[25] Intra-abdominal bleeding can often be managed with hemoclip application or safe use of electrocautery. If this does not suffice, the surgeon may have to resort to open laparotomy.

Ureteral injury, although it can be averted by identifying the ureter as it courses over the iliac vessels and by avoiding dissection medial to the obliterated umbilical artery (medial umbilical ligament), is usually repaired with open surgical techniques. However, laparoscopic ureteral reapproximation has been described and is recommended for the skilled laparoscopist.[26]

Bowel and bladder injury may occur during trocar insertion. Use of nasogastric tube and Foley bladder catheter should deter such occurrences. However, if significant trauma does occur during trocar placement or during LPLND, open repair may be necessary. Judicious use of monopolar electrocautery devices should prevent thermal injuries.

Other potential complications may be due to anesthesia (hypercapnia), obturator nerve injury, prolonged ileus, and so forth, and must be managed appropriately (see Chap. 4).

Thorough knowledge of laparoscopic instrumentation and its safe use and familiarity with anatomy as seen through the laparoscope should considerably reduce the risk of complications during LPLND. Appropriate patient selection and the importance of a laparoscopy team approach cannot be overemphasized.

Until the urologist is comfortable with this new surgical technique, the assistance of another laparoscopist familiar with the procedure is highly recommended. This will decrease the complication rate during the initial steep learning curve associated with performing LPLND.[24]

CONCLUSIONS

In summary, LPLND is a relatively newly introduced and rapidly developing alternative to open surgical lymphadenectomy. This procedure is indicated for patients with a high probability of metastases in these lymph nodes and before radiation therapy or radical perineal prostatectomy. The advantage of this minimally invasive surgery is the shortened hospital stay and a return to routine activities within 1 to 2 weeks. Since the results of LPLND compare favorably with open surgical lymph node dissection, LPLND and other laparoscopic procedures are revolutionizing urologic surgery.

REFERENCES

1. Das, S; Amar, A: Impact of laparoscopy on modern urologic practice. Urol Clin North Am 15:537, 1988.
2. Schuessler, WW; Vancaillie, TG; Reich, H; Griffith, DP: Transperitoneal endosurgical lymphadenectomy in patients with localized prostate cancer. J Urol 145:988, 1991.
3. Winfield, HN; Donovan, JF; See, WA; et al: Urologic laparoscopic surgery. J Urol 146:941, 1991.
4. Gervasi, LA; Marta, J; Easley, JD; et al: Prostatic significance of lymph node metastases in prostate cancer. J Urol 142:332, 1989.
5. Prout, GR, Jr; Heaney, JA; Griffin, PP; et al: Nodal involvement as a prognostic indicator in patients with prostatic cancer. J Urol 124:226, 1980.
6. Flocks, RH: The treatment of stage C prostatic cancer with special reference to combined surgical and radiation treatment. J Urol 109:461, 1973.
7. Barzell, W; Bean, NA; Hilaris, BS; Whitmore, WF, Jr: Prostatic adenocarcinoma: Relationship of grade and local extent to the pattern of metastases. J Urol 118:278, 1977.
8. Kramer, SA; Cline, WA, Jr; Farnham, R; et al: Prognosis of patients with stage D-1 adenocarcinoma. J Urol 125:817, 1981.
9. Smith, JA, Jr; Middleton, RG: Implications of volume of nodal metastasis in patients with adenocarcinoma of the prostate. J Urol 133:617, 1985.
10. Zincke, H; Utz, DC: Radical surgery for stage D-1 prostate cancer. Semin Urol 1:253, 1983.
11. Zincke, H; Utz, DC: Observations on surgical management of carcinoma of the prostate with limited nodal metastasis. Urology 24:137, 1984.
12. Donohue, RE; Mani, JH; Whitesel, JA; et al: Intraoperative and early complications of staging pelvic lymph node dissection in prostatic adenocarcinoma. Urology 35:223, 1990.
13. Morgan, CL; Calkins, RF; Cavalcanti, EJ: Computed tomography in the evolution, staging, and therapy of carcinoma of the bladder and prostate. Radiology 140:751, 1981.
14. Giri, PG; Walsh, JW; Hazra, TA; et al: Role of computed tomography in the evaluation and management of carcinoma of the prostate. Int J Radiol Oncol Biol Physiol 8:253, 1982.
15. Golimbu, M; Moralex, P; Al-Askari, S; Shulman, Y: CAT scanning in staging of prostatic cancer. Urology 18:305, 1981.
16. Koehler, PR: Current status of lyphography in patients with cancer. Cancer (Suppl 1) 37:503, 1976.
17. Andriole, GL; Coplen, DE; Mikkelsen, DJ; Catalona, WJ: Sonographic and pathological staging of patients with clinically localized prostate cancer. J Urol 142:1259, 1989.
18. Hricak, H; Dooms, GC; Jeffrey, RB; et al: Prostatic carcinoma: Staging by clinical assessment, CT and MR imaging. Radiology 162:331, 1987.

19. Biondetti, PR; Lee, JK; Ling, D; Catalona, WJ: Clinical stage B prostatic carcinoma: Staging with MR imaging. Radiology 162:325, 1987.

20. Schnall, MD; Imai, Y; Tomaszewski, J; et al: Prostate cancer: Local staging with endorectal surface coil MR imaging. Radiology 178:797, 1991.

21. Rifkin, MD; Zerhouni, EA; Gatsonis, CA; et al: Comparison of magnetic resonance imaging and ultrasonography in staging early prostate cancer. Results of a multiinstitutional cooperative trial. N Engl J Med 323:621, 1990.

22. Parra, RO; Andrus, C; Boullier, J: Staging laparoscopic pelvic lymph node dissection: Comparison of results with open pelvic lymphadenectomy. J Urol 147:875, 1992.

23. Querleu, D; Leblanc, E; Castelain, B: Laparoscopic pelvic lymphadenectomy in the staging of early carcinoma of the cervix. Am J Obstet Gynecol 164:579, 1991.

24. Kavoussi, LR; Sosa, E: Chandhoke, P; et al: Complications of laparoscopic pelvic lymph node dissection. J Urol 149:322, 1993.

25. Green, LS; Loughlin, KR; Kavoussi, LR: Management of epigastric vessel injury during laparoscopy. J Endourol 6:99, 1992.

26. Nezhat, C; Nezhat, F; Green, B: Laparoscopic treatment of obstructed ureter due to endometriosis by resection and ureteroureterostomy: A case report. J Urol 148:865, 1992.

CHAPTER 16

Laparoscopic Extraperitoneal Pelvic Lymphadenectomy

Miles Tashima, MD
Sakti Das, MD, FACS

Endoscopic lymphadenectomy was first reported by Hald and Rasmussen,[1] who used mediastinoscopic techniques for lymph node sampling. Querlue and associates[2] then performed an anatomic pelvic lymph node dissection on patients with cervical cancer. In the animal laboratory, Winfield and co-workers[3] further developed the technique of laparoscopic pelvic lymphadenectomy. Further clinical work by Schuessler and colleagues[4] has added to the acceptance of laparoscopic pelvic lymphadenectomy as an alternative to open pelvic lymphadenectomy. What most of these techniques have in common is the transperitoneal route of access to the pelvic lymph nodes. Although the peritoneal cavity affords an established window by which to view the pelvic contents, access through the abdominal wall into the peritoneal cavity has many potential inherent drawbacks. Kavoussi and associates[5] reported a 15% complication rate in the initial 372 cases of transperitoneal laparoscopic pelvic lymph node dissection. Understandably, many of those complications were related to the development of a new surgical technique. And yet the potential for injury to intraperitoneal organs exists whenever the Verres needle or trocar is being inserted.

Many advantages are gained when the peritoneal cavity is left intact during an extraperitoneal pelvic lymphadenectomy. One such advantage is that the intact peritoneal envelope keeps the bowel from entering the operative field and minimizes the need for Trendelenburg positioning. This improves visualization of the extraperitoneal pelvic anatomy and protects the bowel from iatrogenic trauma such as lacerations or cautery burns. Yet another advantage is that the hemodynamic compromise often occurring during peritoneal distention is reduced. A theoretical advantage is that the hypercapnia experienced in transperitoneal laparoscopy is reduced during extraperitoneal laparoscopy, since the exposed extraperitoneal surface (fat) is less well perfused than the bowel or peritoneum. Finally, by entering the space of Retzius, laparoscopic pelvic lymphadenectomy can be performed with the same landmarks that are used during open surgery.

SURGICAL TECHNIQUE

General anesthesia with endotracheal intubation is established with the patient in the supine position. After sterile preparation and draping of the anterior abdominal wall and genitalia, a Foley catheter is placed to empty the bladder. A 2-cm longitudinal midline incision is made approximately 4 cm below the umbilicus and is carried through the subcutaneous tissue and linea alba. Digital dissection is performed beneath the rectus abdominis muscle caudally and laterally so as to develop the extraperitoneal space of Retzius. A dissection balloon is created by tying off the fingers of a surgical glove, then securing the inverted glove over an 18 French urethral catheter (Fig. 16–1). The dissection balloon is then placed in the space of Retzius that was previously created. At this point approximately 1200 ml normal saline is instilled into the dissection balloon, thereby pushing the peritoneum cephalad and away from the pelvis. After the saline is drained out, the dissection balloon is removed. A 0° laparoscope is placed through a 12-mm sheath and passed through the incision under direct vision. High-flow CO_2 insufflation is used to maintain 12 to 14 mm Hg in the extraperitoneal space of Retzius. While viewing the inner surface of the anterior abdominal wall, three additional ports are established. A 10-mm trocar is passed about 3 cm above the symphysis pubis in the midline. Two 5-mm working ports are established lateral to the abdominal rectus muscle at a level midway between the umbilicus and symphysis pubis. The surgical landmarks seen during an open pelvic lymphadenectomy will now be evident. Laterally, the pulsations of the external iliac vessels can be seen, especially when temporarily lowering the CO_2 insufflation pressure (Fig. 16–2*A*).

The dissection is begun by first clearing the femoral canal of the node of Cloquet and continuing laterally to define the external iliac vein. If an accessory obturator vein is encountered, it may be preserved or divided between hemostatic clips. Additional clips are used throughout the dissection in order to obtain meticulous lymphostasis and hemostasis. As the dissection is extended inferiorly, the lateral wall of the true pelvis is viewed. Next, the obturator nerve is identified and dissected clean. The mobilized strip of lymph nodal tissue is held up with laparoscopic Babcock forceps so that proximal dissection can be continued to include the hypogastric lymph nodes (Fig. 16–2*B*). A useful maneuver at this point is to switch the laparoscope and Babcock forceps ports to better see the cephalad extent of the dissection. Once the lymph nodes are removed, the dissection is repeated on the opposite side (Fig. 16–2*C*). When the bilateral dissection is completed, the CO_2 insufflation pressure is lowered to 8 mm Hg so that the operative site can be checked for hemostasis (Fig. 16–2*D*). After hemostasis is confirmed, the CO_2 is vented, and the trocars are systematically removed under direct vision while the trocar sites are observed for any bleeding.

CONCLUSIONS

The distinct advantages of maintaining the integrity of the peritoneal cavity are well established from the experience reported on open pelvic lymphadenec-

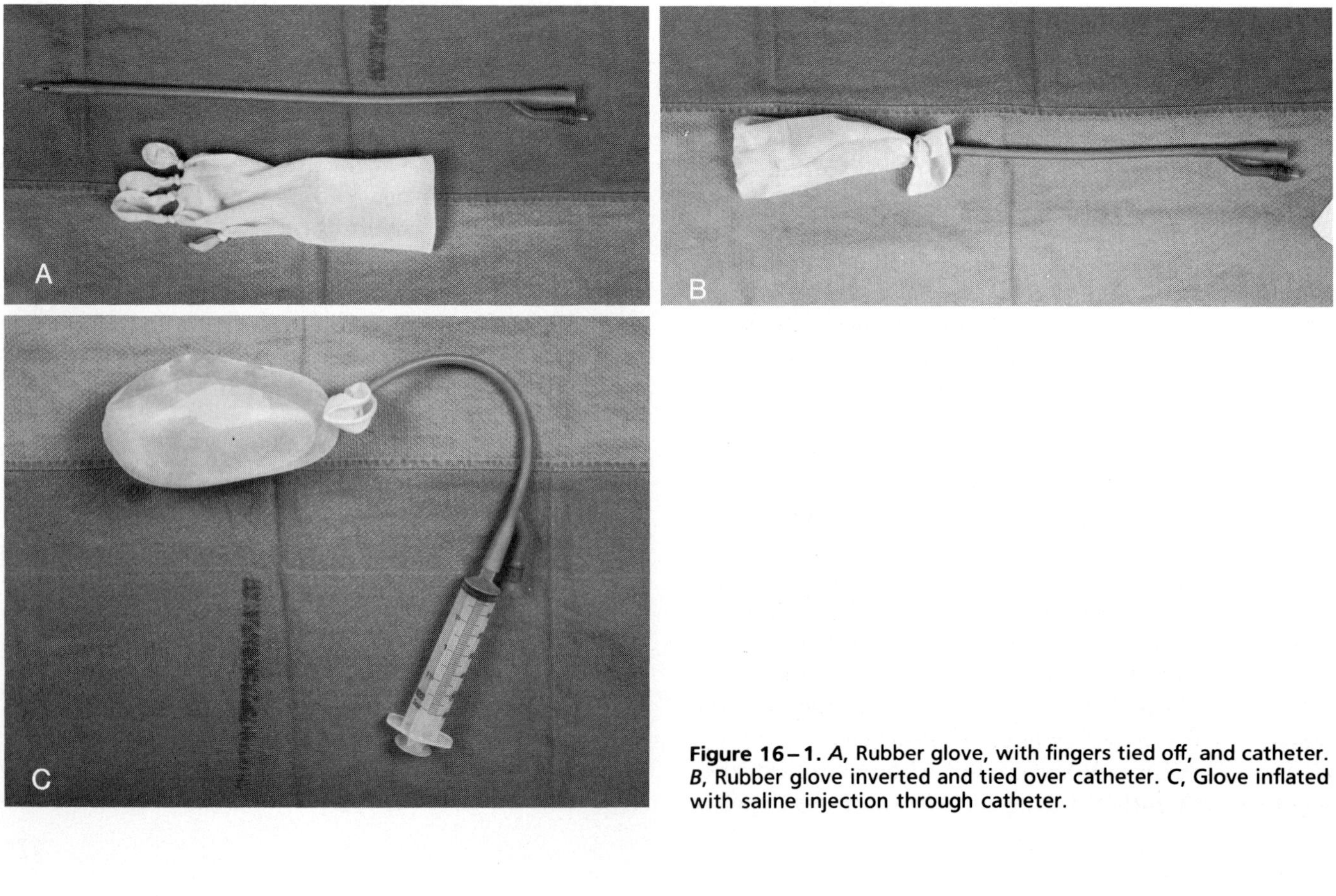

Figure 16–1. *A*, Rubber glove, with fingers tied off, and catheter. *B*, Rubber glove inverted and tied over catheter. *C*, Glove inflated with saline injection through catheter.

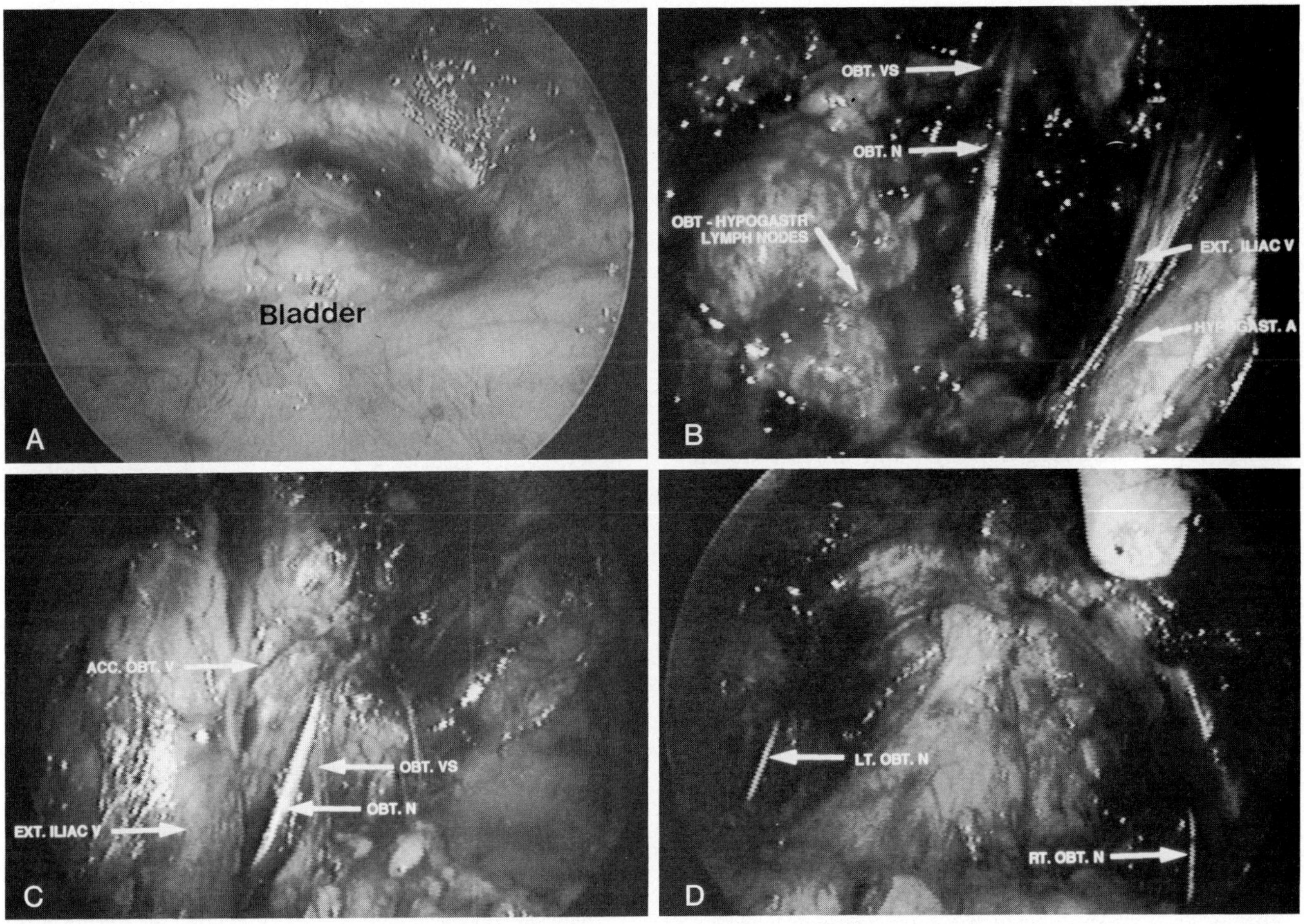

Figure 16–2. *A*, Initial laparoscopic view of extraperitoneal space. *B*, Dissection of right obturator-hypogastric lymph nodes. *C*, View after modified pelvic lymphadenectomy on left side. *D*, Laparoscopic view after bilateral modified pelvic lymphadenectomy. Acc obt v, accessory obturator vein; ext iliac v, external iliac vein; hypogast a, hypogastric artery; lt obt n, left obturator nerve; obt-hypogastr, obturator hypogastric; obt n, obturator nerve; obt vs, obturator vessels; rt obt n, right obturator nerve. See also Color Plate 5.

tomy.[6] Morbidities such as ileus, intestinal adhesions, intestinal obstruction, iatrogenic bowel injuries, and peritonitis can be obviated by avoiding entry into the peritoneal cavity. Morbidities unique to transperitoneal laparoscopic lymphadenectomy include subcutaneous emphysema and vascular and intestinal injuries. By following the techniques previously described, a Verres needle is not used, whereas the dissection balloon atraumatically develops the space of Retzius. This approach is especially useful in patients who have had prior abdominal surgery such as cholecystectomy, appendectomy, or inguinal herniorrhaphy in which the risk of intestinal trauma is higher because of intestinal adhesions to the anterior parietal wall.

Other concerns encountered during intraperitoneal laparoscopic surgery of the pelvis include bowel injuries and cautery burns of the intestines leading to missed or delayed perforation. The surgeon can employ steep Trendelenburg positioning in an effort to move the loops of intestine out of the surgical field, but this can lead to impaired cardiopulmonary function, increased cerebral and intraocular pressures, and brachial plexus injury.

While an intraperitoneal pelvic lymphadenectomy is being performed, a number of other anatomic structures encroach on the surgical field and need to be dealt with. Often the lateral peritoneal attachments of a redundant sigmoid colon have to be divided so that access to the left pelvic side wall can be attained. The medial umbilical ligament and its peritoneal investment may obscure the laparoscopic view if they are not properly retracted out of the way.[7] By using the described extraperitoneal route all of the aforementioned problems can be avoided.

Because of the use of CO_2 to establish the surgical field, the development and prevention of hypercapnia has been investigated. Villers and co-workers[8] have suggested limiting the surgery time to an hour in order to reduce the risk of hypercapnia. Sosa and associates[9] believed that significant hypercapnia developed only in patients with subcutaneous emphysema, which may be due to trocar dislodgement. As yet to be established is whether the absorption of CO_2 leading to hypercapnia is less during extraperitoneal laparoscopy when compared with intraperitoneal laparoscopy. The diffusion and absorptive capacity of the peritoneal cavity is well known and used for peritoneal dialysis. On the other hand, the less well-perfused fat in the extraperitoneal space along with its smaller surface area should present less potential for significant hypercapnia. Although Sosa and associates reported that during transperitoneal laparoscopy eight of their patients tolerated Pco_2 in the range of 60 to 75 mm Hg, in most cases of extraperitoneal pelvic lymphadenectomy, an end-tidal CO_2 can be consistently maintained below 40 mm Hg by increasing the ventilatory rate. With the development of mechanical body wall retractors, eliminating the need for pneumoperitoneum, concerns over the use of CO_2 leading to hypercapnia may be eliminated.

One reported advantage of the intraperitoneal approach to the pelvis has been the prevention of lymphoceles. In fact, it has been claimed that the creation of a large peritoneal window during intraperitoneal laparoscopic pelvic lymphadenectomy will obviate lymphocele formation by establishing peritoneal drainage. Despite this claim, lymphoceles have been known to occur following both intraperitoneal and extraperitoneal pelvic lymphadenectomy. What is important, as pointed out by Resnick and Kursh,[10] is adequate closure of the severed afferent lymphatic channels as a prophylactic measure against lymphocele formation. Rather than relying on postoperative drainage of leaking lymph into a peritoneal window, meticulous care should be taken to close the lymphatic channels with hemostatic clips to prevent lymphatic leakage.

Laparoscopic pelvic lymphadenectomy can be performed safely by the extraperitoneal route. The described technique reduces the complications associated with transperitoneal access and intraperitoneal laparoscopic dissection. The anatomic dissection during extraperitoneal pelvic lymphadenectomy adapts the new technology of laparoscopic surgery to established principles of open pelvic lymphadenectomy without compromising technical efficacy or patient care.

REFERENCES

1. Hald, T; Rasmussen, F: Extraperitoneal pelvioscopy: A new aid in staging of lower urinary tract tumors. A preliminary report. J Urol 124:245–248, 1980.
2. Querleu, D; Leblanc, E; Castelain, B: Laparoscopic pelvic lymphadenectomy in the staging of early carcinoma of the cervix. Am J Obstet Gynecol 164:579–581, 1991.
3. Winfield, HN; Donovan, JF; See, WA; et al. Urologic laparoscopic surgery. J Urol 146:941–948, 1991.
4. Schuessler, WW; Vancaillie, TG; Reich, H; Griffith, DP: Transperitoneal endosurgical lymphadenectomy in patients with localized prostate cancer. J Urol 145:988–991, 1991.
5. Kavoussi, LR; Sosa, E; Chandhoke, PJ; et al: Complications of laparoscopic pelvic lymph node dissection. J Urol 149:322–325, 1993.
6. Freiha, FS; Salzman, J: Surgical staging of prostatic cancer: Transperitoneal versus extraperitoneal lymphadenectomy. J Urol 118:616–617, 1977.
7. Griffith, DP; Schuessler, WW; Nickell, KG; Meaney, JT: Laparoscopic pelvic lymphadenectomy for prostatic adenocarcinoma. Urol Clin North Am 19:407–415, 1992.
8. Villers, A; Baron, JC; Anidjar, M; et al: Extraperitoneal endosurgical lymphadenectomy with insufflation for staging of pelvic malignancies. (Abstract) J Urol 147:407A, 1992.
9. Sosa, RE; Weingram, J; Stein, B; et al: Hypercarbia in laparoscopic pelvic lymph node dissection. (Abstract) J Urol 147: 246A, 1992.
10. Resnick, MI; Kursh, ED: Extrinsic obstruction of the ureter. In: Walsh, PC; Retik, AB; Stamey, TA; Vaugh, ED, eds: Campbell's Urology, 6th ed, Vol 1. Philadelphia, WB Saunders, pp. 562–566, 1992.

CHAPTER 17

Extraperitoneal Endoscopic Gasless Pelvic Lymph Node Dissection

Lawrence S. Hakim, MD
Adley Raboy, MD
George Ferzli, MD, FACS
Peter S. Albert, MD, FACS

Although it has been demonstrated to be efficacious for the staging of prostatic carcinoma, laparoscopic pelvic lymph node dissection is associated with a significant number of complications, including Verres needle injuries such as viscus perforation and vessel injury, hypothermia, hypercapnia, peritoneal adhesions, hernia formation, and peritonitis.[1] The extraperitoneal approach to endoscopic surgery was developed to help obviate these serious complications, while maintaining the efficacy of minimally invasive techniques, and it has been applied to various urologic procedures. These have included pelvic lymph node dissection for the staging of genitourinary malignancies, vesical neck suspension for the treatment of stress urinary incontinence, and unroofing of symptomatic benign renal cysts.[2–4] Although early experience with this technique has been encouraging, there are certain drawbacks that may be associated with this procedure. First, if the peritoneum is entered early in the dissection using CO_2 insufflation, it may be necessary to convert to an intraperitoneal laparoscopic procedure, with its inherent morbidities. In addition, a somewhat longer operative time is required because of dissection of the preperitoneal space and a significant initial learning curve, especially for those unfamiliar with laparoscopic instrumentation. Also, an associated higher hospital expense is necessitated by the cost of the newer laparoscopic instruments.

In order to obviate these potential disadvantages, the authors developed the extraperitoneal "gasless" approach to endoscopic surgery. The technique is easy to learn and requires shorter operative time compared with laparoscopy. The procedure is accomplished by using an anterior abdominal retractor, Laprolift, and a preperitoneal distention balloon dilator* to assist in the initial dissection of the extraperitoneal space. The Origin balloon has a 7.5-inch (19-cm) sheath that will accept a standard 10-mm laparoscope through its lumen. It has a capacity of 1200 ml, and its diameter when inflated is 4.5 inches (12.7 cm). When fully inflated, the balloon approximates a spherical shape but becomes more oblong under the pressure of the perito-

*Both from Origin Medsystems Company, Menlo Park, CA.

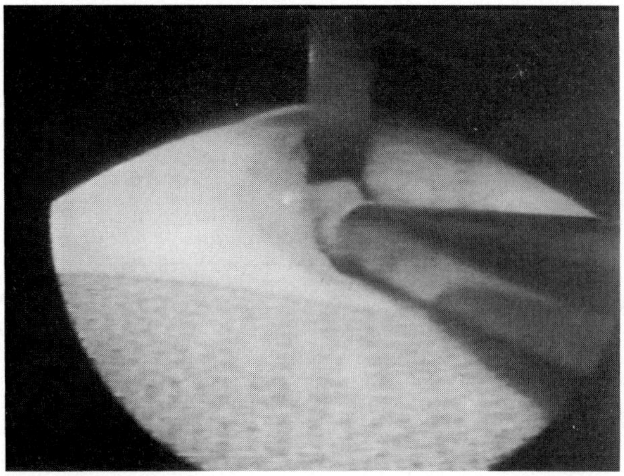

Figure 17–1. After blunt, finger dissection of the extraperitoneal space down to the pubic symphysis, the preperitoneal balloon dilator is shown being inserted to develop the extraperitoneal cavity. See also Color Plate 5.

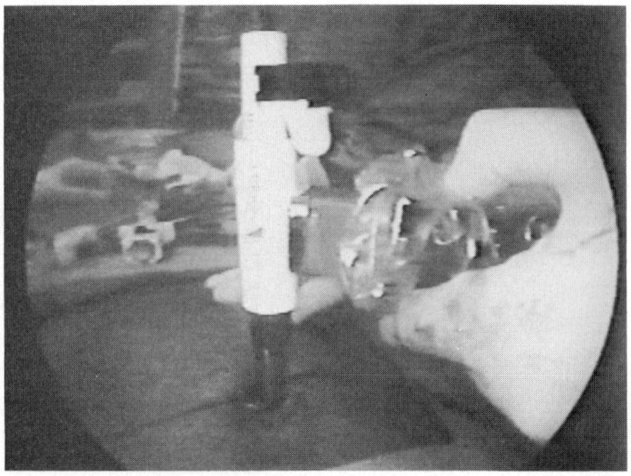

Figure 17–3. Attachment of the Laprolift to the Laprofan device positioned under each rectus muscle. See also Color Plate 6.

neal contents. Other significant advantages over conventional laparoscopy include the avoidance of any CO_2-related morbidities, use of standard surgical instruments, and performance of the procedure under spinal or epidural anesthesia.

OPERATIVE TECHNIQUE

After the induction of adequate regional or general anesthesia, the patient is placed in the supine position and prepared and draped in a sterile fashion. The bladder is decompressed with a urethral Foley catheter. An infraumbilical incision extending 1.5 cm is made and is deepened to the level of the rectus fascia. Two 0 Vicryl "stay" sutures are placed in the fascia on either side of the midline. After incision of the fascia, blunt finger dissection is used to develop the preperitoneal space, allowing insertion of the trocar Origin balloon dilator, shown in Figure 17–1. After placing a 25° endoscopic lens through the lumen of the Origin balloon for visual control, 1000 ml of air are manually injected to inflate the balloon. This enables initial dissection of the extraperitoneal space inferiorly toward the pubic symphysis and laterally toward the epigastric vessels, demonstrated in Figure 17–2. Under direct visual monitoring, a 1.5-cm incision is made midway between the umbilicus and pubic symphysis, and another incision is made just superior to the pubis. The Origin balloon is then deflated and removed, and a Laprofan* is inserted through the umbilical incision. The Laprofan is then spread open beneath the rectus muscles, and the Laprolift* is used to elevate the anterior abdominal wall (Fig. 17–3). Under video guidance, a 10-mm trocar sheath is inserted below the Laprolift to accommodate the 25° endoscopic lens (Fig. 17–4); and blunt dissection is performed laterally to the epigastric vessels (Fig. 17–

*Origin Medsystems, Menlo Park, CA.

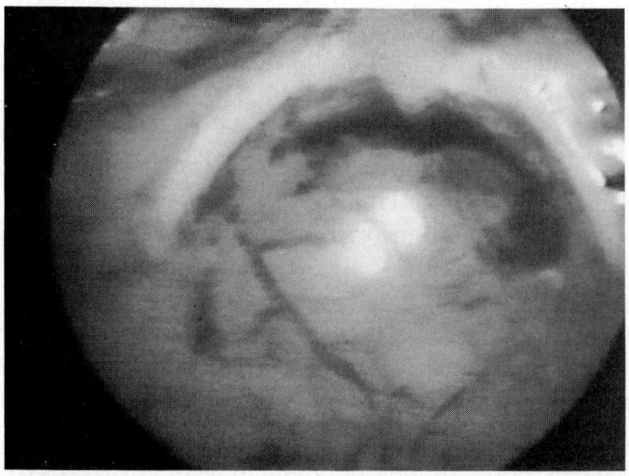

Figure 17–2. Preperitoneal dissection of the extraperitoneal space under visual control (as seen through the balloon trocar). See also Color Plate 5.

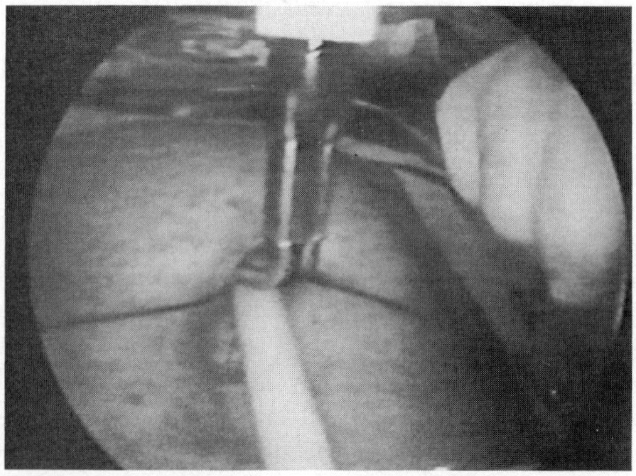

Figure 17–4. The 10-mm trocar is positioned under the Laprofan for placement of the endoscopic lens. See also Color Plate 6.

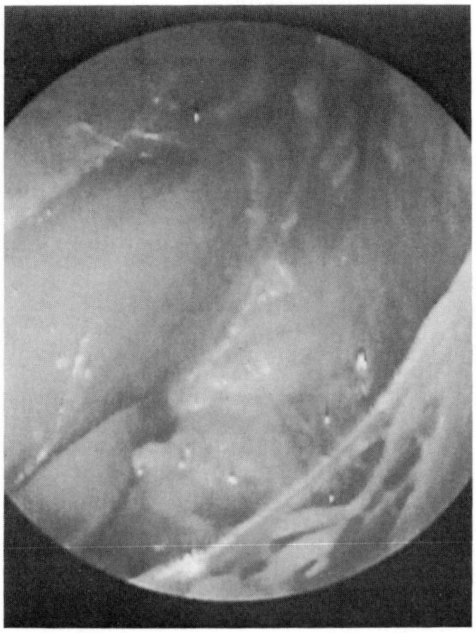

Figure 17–5. Position of Laprofan seen beneath the left rectus muscle. See also Color Plate 6.

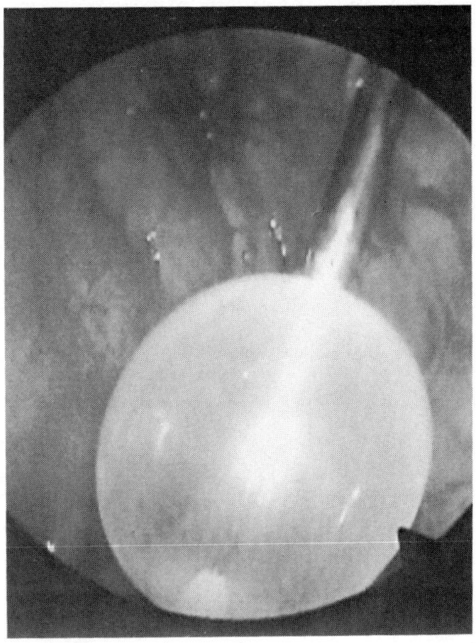

Figure 17–7. Either the Joystick balloon retractor or the endoscopic fan retractor can be used to retract the peritoneum superiorly and medially to provide exposure of the obturator fossa. See also Color Plate 7.

5). Two additional 0.5-cm incisions are then made lateral to the epigastric vessels to allow insertion of the standard surgical instruments under vision (Fig. 17–6). The peritoneum and its underlying contents can be deflected superiorly and medially using the balloon retractors, which affords exposure of the pelvic lymph nodes, as illustrated in Figures 17–7 and 17–8. Modified bilateral pelvic lymph node dissection requiring no special instrumentation or insufflation under direct visual video guidance is then performed (Figure 17–9). In addition, surgical clip applicators and electrocautery for maintaining hemostasis can be utilized with this technique. Once the nodal tissue is excised, the Laprofan and Laprolift are removed, and the camera is then removed. The rectus fascia is closed with interrupted 0 Vicryl sutures, the other incision sites are closed with 4-0 chromic sutures and the Foley catheter is removed.

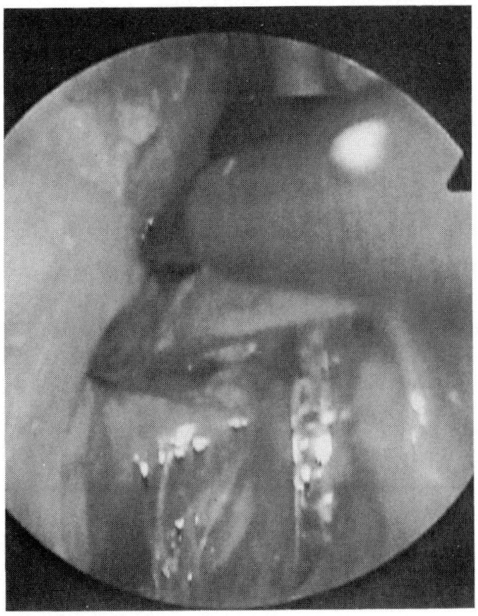

Figure 17–6. Endoscopic fan retractor. See also Color Plate 6.

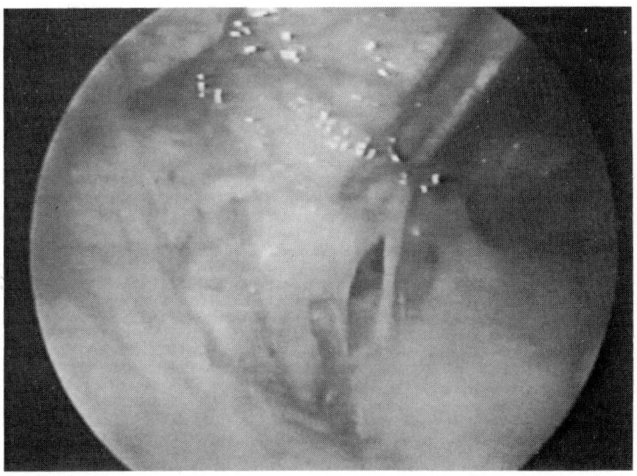

Figure 17–8. Initial dissection of the pelvic lymph node package from beneath the external iliac vein. See also Color Plate 7.

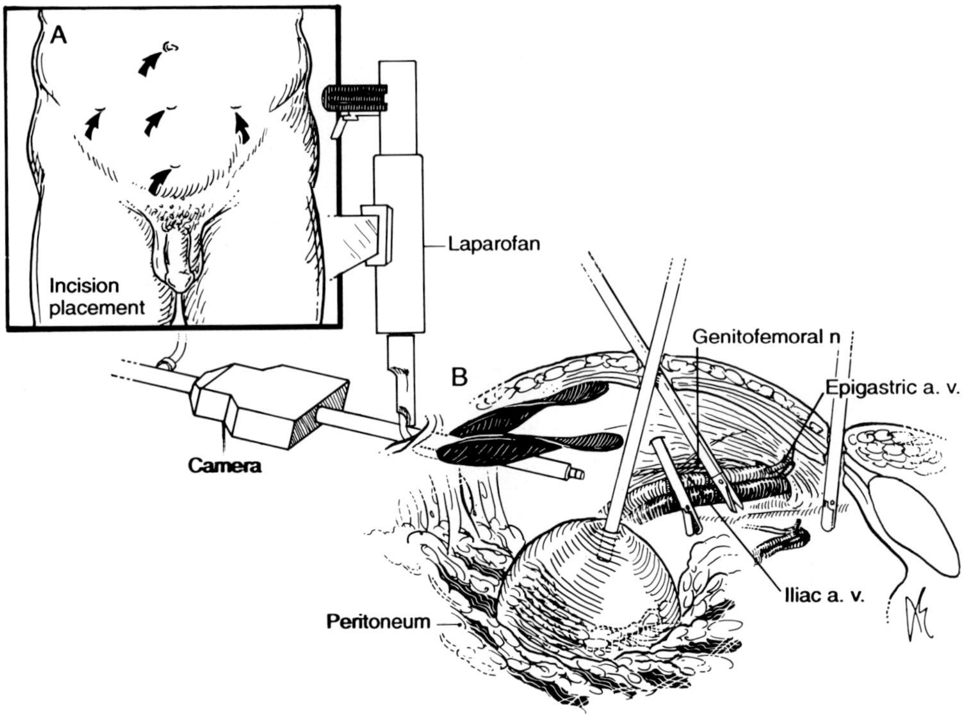

Figure 17–9. With the Laprolift in place, the extraperitoneal cavity is shown before pelvic lymph node dissection. The balloon retractor is shown aiding in exposure of the obturator fossa. *Inset*: Illustrated are the four small incisions in the extraperitoneal cavity through which standard surgical instruments can be placed to perform the pelvic lymph node dissection. The camera is placed at the level of the umbilicus.

Postoperative Care

Patients may resume their preoperative diet on the evening of surgery, and the majority of patients are discharged home from the hospital on the first postoperative day. Oral antibiotics are continued postoperatively for 48 hours.

CONCLUSIONS

There has recently been an explosion in the literature regarding minimally invasive approaches for surgical intervention in urologic diseases. Although laparoscopic pelvic lymph node dissection is effective in the staging of pelvic malignancies, it is associated with complications, including, but not limited to, viscus injuries, hemorrhage, and hypercapnia.[1] The extraperitoneal approach to endoscopic surgery, initially described as utilizing CO_2 insufflation and laparoscopic instrumentation, was developed as a minimally invasive alternative to laparoscopy, as a means of eliminating these potential morbidities. Although it is quite effective, we have been able to modify this extraperitoneal endoscopic technique by using state of the art technology, thus eliminating the need for CO_2 insufflation (hence gasless) or laparoscopic instruments, or both, indeed allowing for the use of standard surgical instruments. By using the preperitoneal balloon dilator the extraperitoneal space can be quickly and easily developed, facilitating the somewhat laborious dissection of the extraperitoneal space associated with standard laparoscopic instruments. In addition, epidural or spinal anesthesia can be used with this technique, obviating the need for general endotracheal anesthesia. With use of the Laprofan and Laprolift to elevate the anterior abdominal wall, there is no need for CO_2 insufflation of the extraperitoneal space. This eliminates the risk of CO_2-associated complications (e.g., hypercapnia, gas embolus) and also assures that the extraperitoneal approach can be maintained even if the peritoneum is inadvertently entered. There is also a significant cost benefit, since standard surgical instruments, instead of expensive laparoscopic instruments, are used. In summary, we believe that the extraperitoneal endoscopic gasless pelvic lymph node dissection is both a feasible and practical alternative to laparoscopy and a promising advancement in the field of endourology.

REFERENCES

1. Kavoussi, L; Sosa, E; Chandhoke, P; et al: Complications of laparoscopic pelvic lymph node dissection. J Urol 149:322, 1993.
2. Ferzli, G; Trapasso, J; Raboy, A; Albert, PS: Extraperitoneal endoscopic pelvic lymph node dissection. J Laparoendosc Surg 2:1, 1992.
3. Raboy, A; Hakim, LS; Albert, PS: Extraperitoneal endoscopic vesicourethral suspension (EEVUS). J Laparoendosc Surg (in press).
4. Hakim, LS; Raboy, A; Ferzli, G; Albert, PS: Extraperitoneal endoscopic unroofing of renal cysts (EEURC). J Urol (in press).

CHAPTER 18

Laparoscopic Retroperitoneal Lymph Node Dissection

Cliff Vestal, MD
E. David Crawford, MD, FACS

Laparoscopic urology is an everexpanding field; new procedures and indications continue to evolve. Procedures such as laparoscopic pelvic lymph node dissections for prostate, penile, and bladder cancers have become quite common. The evolution of laparoscopic technique has been driven by patient demand and improved postoperative outcome. The advancement of laparoscopic techniques and equipment has allowed the urologic surgeon to expand the number of procedures performed with less morbidity. Technically demanding surgeries such as laparoscopic nephrectomies and nephroureterectomies have become more common. Of the urologic procedures performed with laparoscopic techniques, the retroperitoneal lymph node dissection is perhaps the most challenging.

In patients with apparently low-stage nonseminomatous germ cell tumors (NSGCTs), open retroperitoneal node dissection is often required for accurate staging as well as for therapeutic purposes. However, the morbidities associated with the open surgery have stimulated research into more limited surgical dissection or surveillance protocols with no surgery. It is conceivable that laparoscopic retroperitoneal node dissection may offer a suitable alternative for reliable staging with minimal surgical morbidity.

ANATOMY

When dealing with NSGCT of the testes, several anatomic principles come into play. The skilled urologic surgeon must understand the anatomy of the retroperitoneum as it pertains to the vasculature, lymphatics, and nervous tissue. The lymphatics and sympathetic nerves play a key role in the current approach to testicular cancer.

Embryologically, the testes arise near the renal mesenchyme and migrate into the scrotum as the fetus develops. During this migration, the testes retain their original blood and lymphatic supply from near their origin. The left testis obtains its arterial supply from the anterior aorta, and its vein drains into the left renal vein. The right testis obtains its blood supply from the aorta near the right renal artery; its vein drains into the inferior vena cava. The lymphatics typically follow the vasculature.[1]

When performing a retroperitoneal lymph node dissection (RPLND), familiarity with the arterial supply to the intestines is important. The superior mesenteric artery supplies the entire midgut. It arises anteriorly from the aorta just posterior to the body of the pancreas. The inferior mesenteric artery arises from the anterior surface of the aorta, approximately 4 to 5 cm above the aortic bifurcation and opposite the third lumbar vertebra. The inferior mesenteric vein courses superiorly from its position above the rectum in a retroperitoneal position. When dissecting the aorta, these should be the only major vascular structures located on the anterior surface of the great vessels.[2]

Location of the kidneys and their anatomy are common knowledge for urologists. The renal veins are anteriorly placed, and the arteries are posterior to the veins. The ureters lie posterior to all vascular structures supplying the kidneys. The left renal vein crosses anterior to the aorta. The right renal artery lies posterior to the vena cava. The left testicular vein drains into the left renal vein, and the right testicular vein drains into the inferior vena cava just distal to the right renal vein. Quite commonly, an anomalous arterial supply to the kidneys is encountered, and during dissection, must be preserved, because they are end arteries, and any cessation of blood supply to the kidney from one of these accessory arteries leads to infarction of the area supplied.[2]

Ureteral location is important, since dissection around these structures is necessary. After arising from the renal pelvis, the ureters course inferiorly, where they cross the psoas major muscle. Once past the muscle they cross anterior to the iliac vessels.

Branches of the abdominal aorta and inferior vena cava are frequently encountered in this surgery. The renal and mesenteric arteries have already been mentioned. Both testicular arteries arise from the aorta on its anterior surface. Four pairs of lumbar arteries arise from the posterolateral aspect of the aorta. The lumbar veins take a course similar to their arterial counterparts and drain into the inferior vena cava. Difficulties in controlling the lumbar vessels by laparoscopic dissection often preclude posterior dissection of the retrocaval, retroaortic, or retrocrural lymphatics.

The sympathetic nervous system is a major concern during RPLND. The sympathetic nerves, which are involved in the act of emission and ejaculation, arise from the lumbar splanchnic nerves that form a profuse network of nerves on the anterior and lateral surfaces of the abdominal aorta. Damage to the sympathetic plexus that innervates the seminal vesicles, vas deferens, and bladder neck may cause ejaculatory impotence. The sympathetic nerves innervating these organs involved in emission and ejaculation arise from the T12 through L2 sympathetic chain.

The abdominal aorta is surrounded by a plexus of nerves that runs its entire length. A series of ganglia, including the celiac, superior mesenteric, aorticorenal, and inferior mesenteric ganglia, intercalate through a series of intertwining nerves. This plexus ceases at the inferior mesentery ganglia and leaves the aorta to reach the anterior surface of the sacrum as the hypogastric plexus.[2]

Lymphatic metastases from testicular neoplasms occur in a predictable manner. From the analysis of his 104 patients, Donahue elaborated the anatomic zones of lymphatic drainage of the testes.[4] For tumors on the right side, the primary metastatic sites are the interaortocaval zone and for tumors on the left side, these are the preaortic and left para-aortic zone. The observation of this zonal lymphatic drainage has led to the development of modified retroperitoneal lymph node dissection, allowing reliable staging information and at the same time minimizing ejaculatory dysfunction.

The anatomy of the retroperitoneum is complex. However, if addressed in a systematic manner and approached with good judgment and skill, few complications will be encountered, and emission and ejaculation can be preserved.

HISTORICAL BACKGROUND

The treatment of NSGCT has undergone remarkable changes over the past century. This disease entity was initially managed with aggressive bilateral retroperitoneal lymph node dissections. Dissection was done bilaterally above the renal hilum. The morbidity from this procedure was high and included complete ejaculatory impotence. However, using this approach with or without radiation therapy, survival statistics approaching 40% at 5 years were obtained in lower-stage tumors.[3]

Donahue and colleagues, using information from studies on the sites of metastases in NSGCT, envisioned less morbid surgery for this disease entity and indeed found the template method of RPLND to be an acceptable alternative to the standard bilateral RPLND.[4] In this modified procedure, the template dissection includes the area of ipsilateral primary lymphatic drainage. To minimize damage to the preaortic autonomic nerves supplying the ejaculatory system, the dissection of retroperitoneal lymph nodes below the inferior mesenteric artery is limited to the ipsilateral side.[5]

Management of NSGCT has become more controversial since the advent of surveillance protocols in the early 1980s.[6] The rationale was that platinum-based chemotherapy was so successful that surveillance of stage 1 tumors was acceptable. Caution should be used with this alternative to RPLND, since it appears from surveillance that an increased risk of mortality and morbidity to the patient and higher costs can occur.[7] Suffice it to say that surveillance is intense and should be limited to patients with appropriate pathologic and staging criteria in a center that can deal with potentially advanced disease. It therefore appears that for the patient with stage 1 NSGCT, the most prudent course is to perform a RPLND to establish the appropriate pathologic staging. In most instances, therapeutic benefit is derived in clinical stage 1 disease, which pathologically is found to be stage 2 following RPLND.[8]

The decision to proceed with either RPLND or observation should be based on available data and patient selection. Perhaps, if a technique that decreases the morbidity without compromising the benefits of the surgery could be performed, the controversy regarding treatment of stage 1 NSGCT could be avoided. The authors believe that in selected cases, laparoscopic RPLND accomplishing the template dissection may be such a procedure.

INDICATIONS

When evaluating a patient for RPLND, one must be cognizant of several factors that increase the chances of metastatic disease. Patients with embryonal tumors and involvement of the epididymis or tunica albuginea are at greater risk for metastatic disease. Vascular and lymphatic invasion likewise place the individual at risk of metastases. Failure of the serum markers alpha-fetoprotein and beta–human chorionic gonadotropin (beta-HCG) to normalize following radical inguinal orchiectomy usually indicates distant disease.[9] Any of these findings would argue against surveillance and for RPLND.

Appropriate staging studies should be undertaken before RPLND. A computed tomographic (CT) scan of the abdomen and pelvis determines if there is lymphadenopathy of the retroperitoneum. It must be cautioned that even with current accurate scanners, a 20% to 30% understaging occurs.[10] Chest radiographs indicate if there is pulmonary involvement. Serum markers are obtained to determine if they have normalized. If the CT scan shows no evidence of gross lymphadenopathy and the remaining tests are normal, it is considered appropriate to proceed with RPLND. Bulky disease should be managed with appropriate chemotherapy. This may be followed by a RPLND for residual masses, since these may harbor viable tumor or teratoma.

At this particular time, laparoscopic RPLND should be reserved for patients with clinical stage 1 disease. It has not been determined whether the laparoscopically performed RPLND can claim the same therapeutic benefits as the open procedure. Perhaps follow-up lymphangiograms, CT scans, or both will determine the completeness of the laparoscopic procedure. Until that time, it would be prudent to use the laparoscopic template dissection of retroperitoneal lymph nodes as a staging procedure alone.

PREPARATION

After appropriate staging studies are performed, the patients are informed about the risks involved in the standard RPLND. They are also informed of the risks with laparoscopy in general. They are advised that the procedure may be converted to an open RPLND as a result of technical difficulty or intraoperative complications, including hemorrhage and/or bowel, renal, or ureteral injury.

Steps are taken preoperatively to decrease the likelihood of morbidity or mortality. All patients undergo mechanical and antibiotic bowel preparations. A broad-spectrum antibiotic is also given before surgery. Blood products should be available in all cases. Preoperative laboratory studies should include serum tumor markers, complete blood count, and a full chemistry panel.

SURGICAL TECHNIQUE

Perhaps of greatest importance to this operation is the placement of the laparoscopic trocars. The anesthetized patient is positioned so that the ipsilateral abdomen is at a 30° angle from the table. The ipsilateral arm is draped over the chest. The positioning is comparable to a standard thoracoabdominal RPLND.

Pneumoperitoneum is then accomplished with either the Verres needle or an open technique. Once insufflation is complete, a 12-mm trocar is placed supraumbilically. Then with the camera in place, two 12-mm trocars are placed along the midclavicular line just below the costal margin and approximately 4 to 5 cm below the umbilicus. With this accomplished, two 5-mm trocars are placed along the ipsilateral anterior auxiliary line. One is placed just above the ileal crest approximately parallel to the umbilicus, the other just below the costal margin. Additional trocars may be placed on the contralateral side for retraction purposes (Fig. 18–1). Once the camera is in position, the abdomen should be inspected. With the endoscissors, an incision into the ipsilateral white line of Toldt is made. This allows mobilization of the bowel and mesentery and their retraction medially. The retroperitoneum is then inspected. Particular attention is directed to the lymphatic structures overlying the great vessels. If gross disease is noted, perhaps the most prudent step is to biopsy the mass, and if frozen section is positive for tumor, then to withdraw and proceed with an open RPLND. However, if there is no evidence of bulky disease, the operation should continue. Visualization and mobilization of the ipsilateral spermatic cord should be undertaken at this time. With the endoscissors, the peritoneum should be reflected away from the cord structures. Dissection of the cord to the internal inguinal ring is completed.

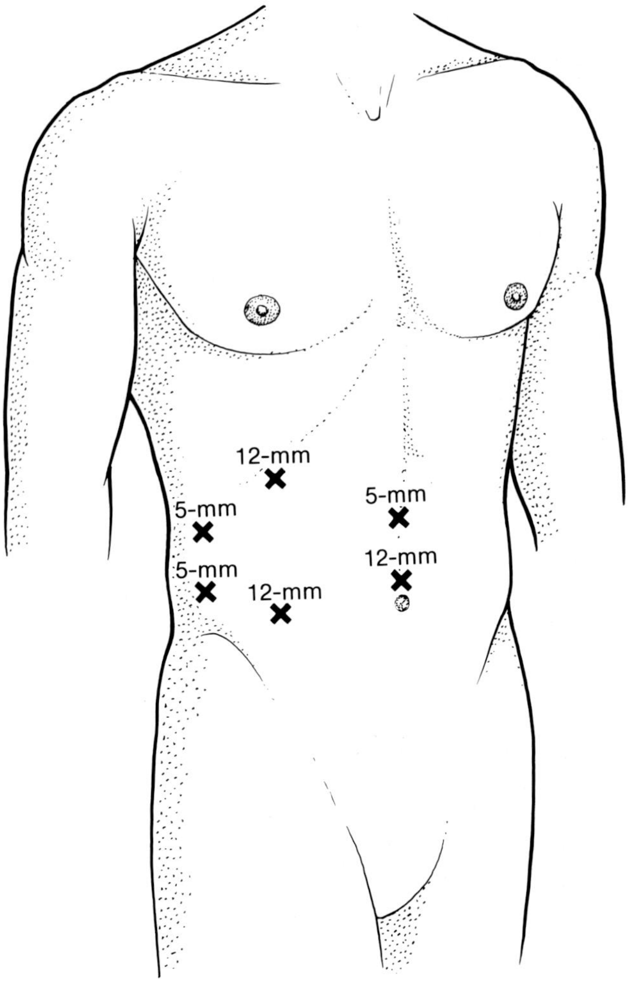

Figure 18–1. Trocar sites for retroperitoneal lymph node dissection on the right side.

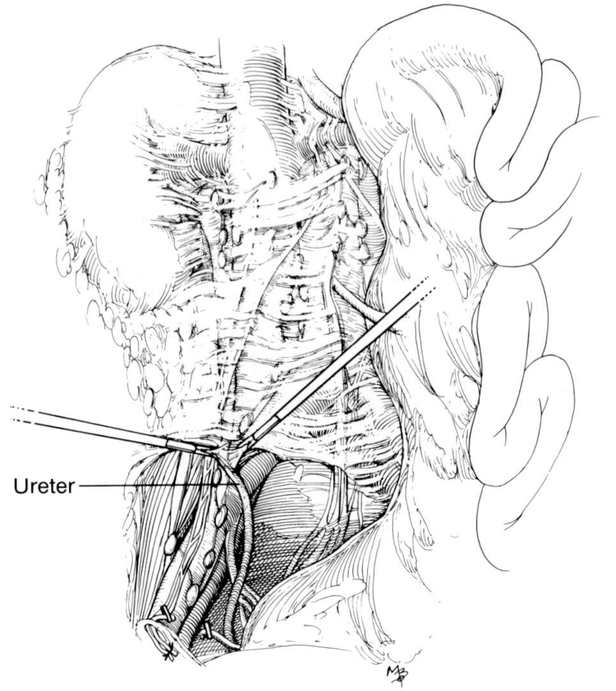

Figure 18–3. Beginning of ureteral dissection just above the iliac vessels.

Identification of the previously placed silk tie on the distal cord structures helps to limit the distal dissection (Fig. 18–2). The cord is dissected proximally to the aortic bifurcation. With use of the previously incised white line of Toldt to retract the mesentery con-

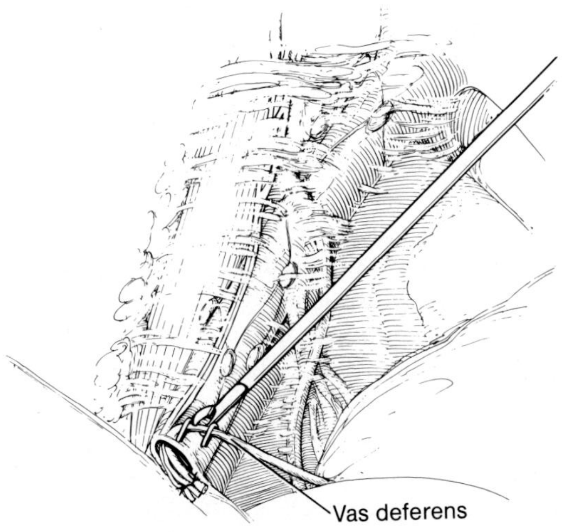

Figure 18–2. Laparoscopic dissection of the distal end of the spermatic cord.

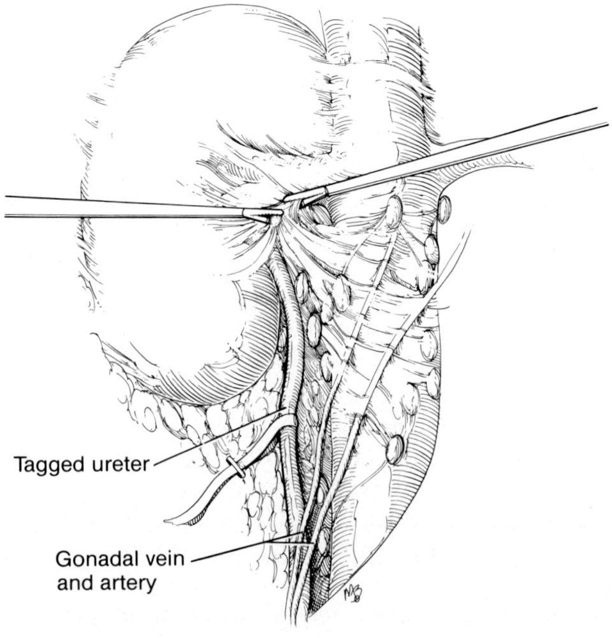

Figure 18–4. The ureter isolated and tagged for easier identification and retraction.

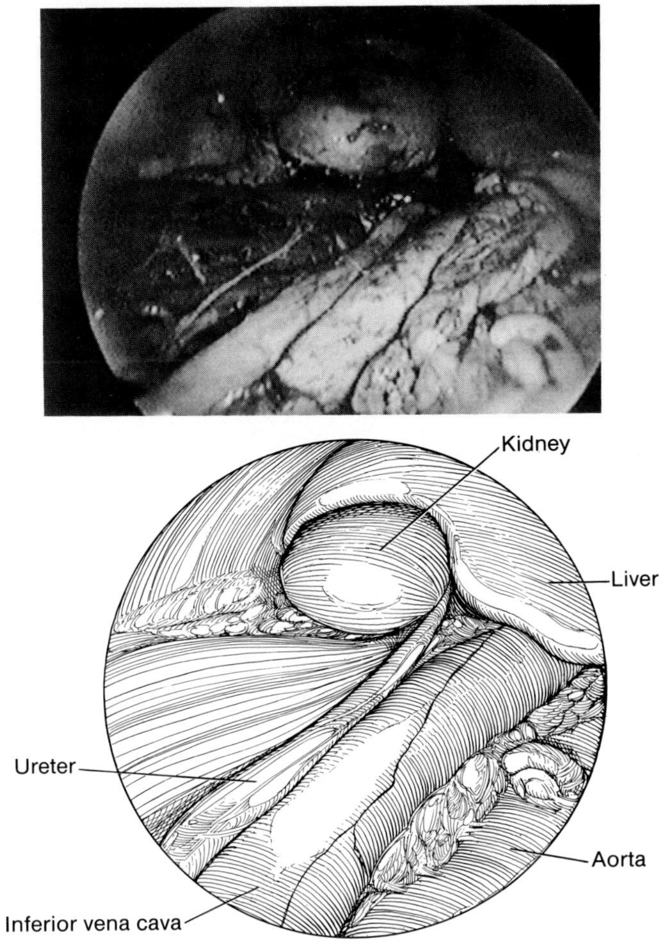

Figure 18–5. Dissection of Gerota's fascia, exposing the lower pole of the kidney.

tralaterally, the great vessels should again be seen. If the inferior mesenteric vein limits the dissection, it can be sacrificed by dividing it between laparoscopically applied clips. Dissection of the ureter away from surrounding areolar tissue begins above the iliac vessels (Fig. 18–3). Once isolated, the ureter can be dissected up to the kidney. A vessel loop or umbilical tape can be placed around the ureter to help in its retraction and identification (Fig. 18–4). After dissection of the ureter to the lower pole of the kidney, careful dissection to identify the renal vein should be undertaken. Dissection is then performed to remove Gerota's fascia from the renal capsule. This should allow easy identification of the renal hilum, which has been partially exposed with previous dissection (Fig. 18–5). Care must be taken when dissecting this area to avoid injury to any inferior polar artery. With the renal hilum exposed, the dissection can proceed to the contralateral great vessel. The nodal tissue is gently teased from around both the vena cava and aorta. This is done in a caudad direction. When dissecting the contralateral great vessel, care should be taken to identify the ureter and to avoid injury to the structure. Careful dissection along the aorta will expose the sympathetic nerve fibers, which can easily be seen with laparoscopic magnification (Fig. 18–6). The contralateral dissection is carried up to the inferior mesenteric artery. The ipsilateral dissection is carried to the ipsilateral iliac vessels. At this point, a previously dissected spermatic cord is incorporated into the specimen package (Fig. 18–7). When the package is free of surrounding tissues, it can be placed in a tissue bag or condom (Fig. 18–8). The abdomen is reexamined to assure the surgeon that there is no bleeding and that the kidney or ureter does not appear ischemic. The lymph node package is removed through a 12-mm port. The laparoscopic ports are withdrawn under direct camera view, and all port incisions are closed with absorbable sutures.

Patients undergoing this procedure are carefully observed with routine postoperative care. Once the patient has passed flatus and tolerated liquids, diet is advanced. Movement should begin soon after the surgery. Follow-up of these patients should be as diligent as that for an open RPLND. Monthly aquisition of serum markers and chest x-rays is a necessity because of a propensity for testicular tumors to recur quickly. CT scans can be used at the discretion of the surgeon. This type of follow-up should be undertaken for the first year and continue every other month for the second year.

CONCLUSIONS

Laparoscopic RPLND is a technically feasible but demanding operation that takes a much longer surgical time than the open procedure.[11] At present it can not compare with the open procedure in performance. Aside from limited exposure, the major difficulty entails controlling and dissecting the lumbar vessels. Although lymphatic tissue can often be teased from around these vessels, a thorough dissection posterior to the great vessels is not yet possible. Therefore, although it yields adequate staging information, laparoscopic RPLND cannot yet claim the same therapeutic benefit as the orthodox open RPLND. However, it seems that the patients tolerate the procedure well, and as a general rule, their hospitalization is shorter than that of patients undergoing open RPLND. With further refinements in instrumentation and technique, the procedure should become more widely accepted. Therefore, in certain individuals, the laparoscopic RPLND may be the procedure of choice.

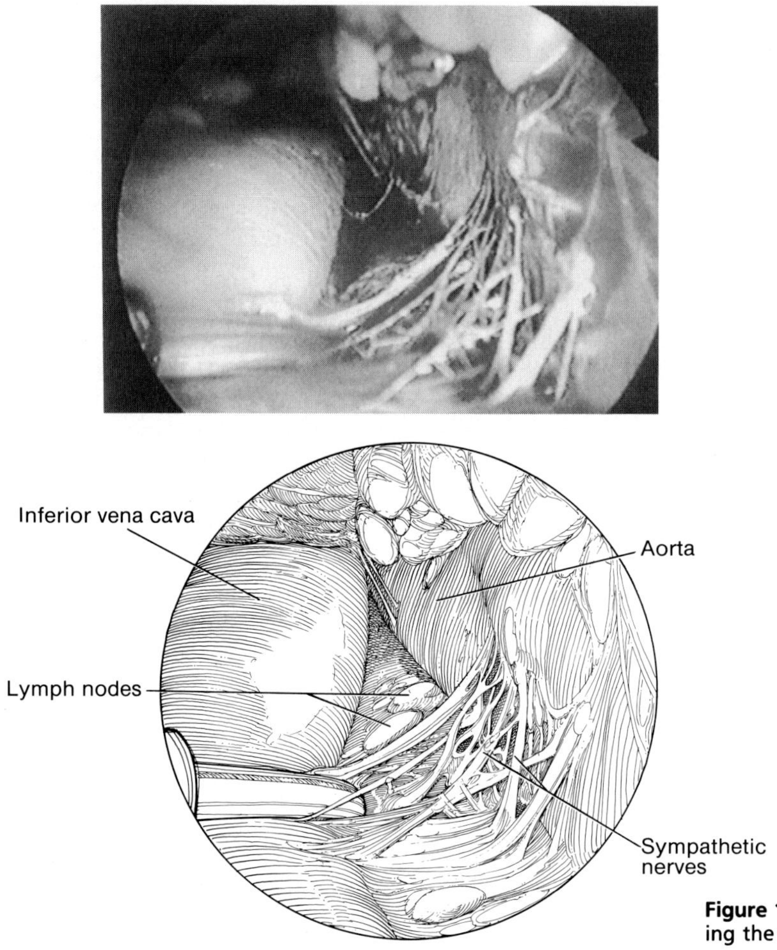

Figure 18–6. Dissection between the aorta and vena cava, exposing the sympathetic nerves and lymphatics.

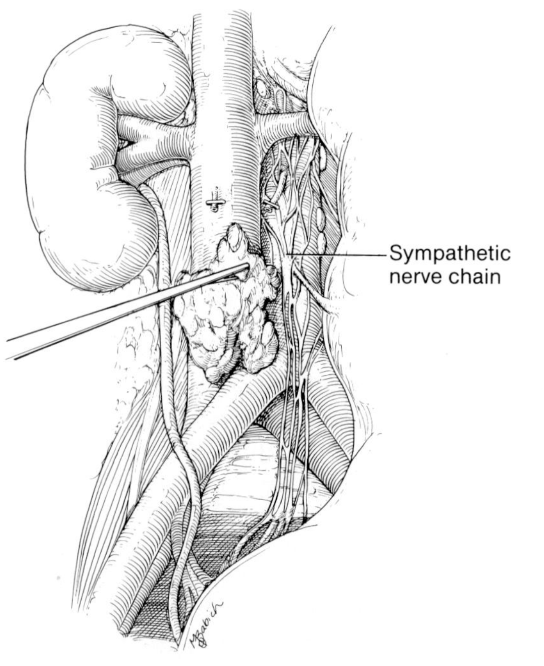

Figure 18–7. Lymph nodal package incorporated with the ipsilateral spermatic cord.

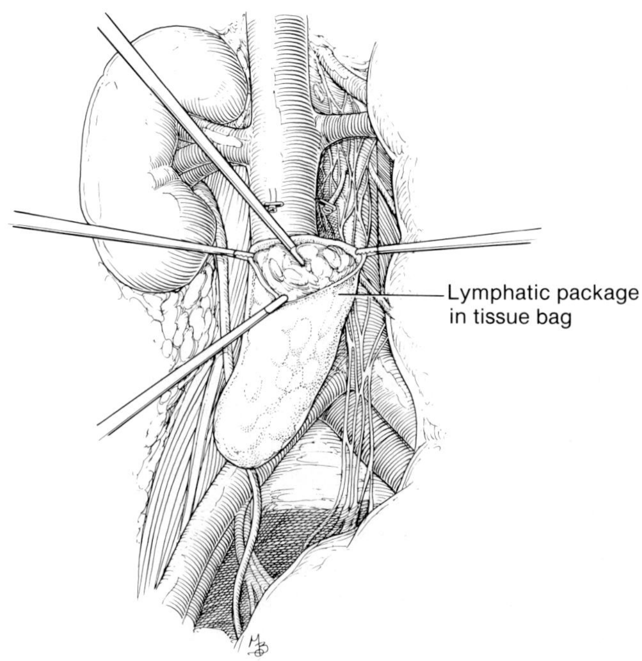

Figure 18–8. Lymph nodal package entrapped in the tissue bag.

REFERENCES

1. Moore, DL: The Developing Human: Clinically Oriented Embryology, 4th ed. Philadelphia, WB Saunders, 1988, pp. 279–281.
2. Crafts, RC: A Textbook of Human Anatomy, 2nd ed. John Wiley & Sons, 1979, pp. 213–345.
3. Lewis, LG: Testis tumor: Report on 250 cases. J Urol 59:763, 1948.
4. Donohue, JP; Maynard, B; Zachary, M: The distribution of nodal metastases in the retroperitoneum from nonseminomatous testis cancer. J Urol 128:315, 1982.
5. Donohue, JP; Foster, RS; Rowland, RG; et al: Nerve-sparing retroperitoneal lymphadenectomy with preservation of ejaculation. J Urol 144:287, 1990.
6. Peckham, MJ: Orchidectomy alone in testicular stage 1 nonseminomatous germ cell tumours. Lancet 2:678, 1982.
7. Donohue, JP: Surveillance or surgery? An update on clinical stage 1 testis cancer. Contrib Urol 3:42, 1991.
8. Rowland, RG; Weisman, D; Williams, S; et al. Accuracy of preoperative staging in stages A and B nonseminomatous germ cell testis tumors. J Urol 127:718, 1982.
9. Fung, CY; Kalish, LA; Brodsky, GL; et al: Stage 1 nonseminomatous germ cell testicular tumor: Prediction of metastatic potential by primary histopathology. J Clin Oncol 6:1467, 1988.
10. Richie, JP; Garnick, MB; Finberg, H: Computerized tomography: How accurate for abdominal staging of testis tumors? J Urol 127:715, 1982.
11. Rukstalis, DB; Chodak, GW: Laparoscopic retroperitoneal lymph node dissection in a patient with stage 1 testicular carcinoma. J Urol 148:1907, 1992.

CHAPTER 19

Laparoscopic Treatment of Lymphoceles

Ermanno Ancona, MD
Paolo Rigotti, MD

Pelvic lymphoceles are collections of lymph fluid in the retroperitoneum. Kidney transplants and pelvic lymph node dissections are the surgical procedures most likely to be complicated by the development of postoperative lymphocele, with an incidence reported to vary from less than 1% to 18% for kidney transplantation[1] and as much as 49% for pelvic lymph node dissection.[2]

A lymphocele is often asymptomatic, but its progressive enlargement can displace or compress adjacent structures. Thus hydronephrosis, deep vein thrombosis, or ipsilateral leg edema can result from compression of the ureter, iliac vein, or lower-extremity lymphatic vessels. Clinical suspicion can be confirmed by ultrasound or computed tomographic (CT) scan, which easily detects the collection of fluid in the extraperitoneal iliac fossa.

Various methods of treatment have been proposed. Simple needle aspiration is considered unreliable because of the high rate of recurrence. Prolonged external catheter drainage[3] carries a serious risk of infection, particularly in immunosuppressed patients. The instillation of sclerosing agents (e.g., tetracycline or povidone-iodine solution) seems to increase the success rate for percutaneous management,[4] but the consequent, marked inflammatory response, resulting in dense scar tissue around the transplanted ureter, can be hazardous in the long-term.

The internal drainage procedure,[5] or marsupialization, is therefore generally considered the most appropriate approach for the treatment of lymphocele, provided there is no evidence of an infected content. The aim of this procedure is to create a free passage for the lymphatic fluid into the peritoneal cavity where it can be reabsorbed. The approach can be through the previous transplant incision or more commonly intraperitoneally through a lower midline laparotomy. A peritoneal fenestration has to be created on the lymphocele cavity and this is accomplished with the excision of an ellipse of peritoneum and lymphocele wall. An adjunctive step is the placement of a portion of omentum in the newly-created peritoneal window. This reduces the risk of closure of the fenestration with consequent recurrence of the lymphocele or of internal bowel loop herniation.

Laparoscopy can be used as an alternative to laparotomy, achieving exactly the same result but with a minimum of trauma for the patient. The various advantages of the laparoscopic technique are particularly significant for the immunosuppressed patient—i.e., wound complications, postoperative ileus, and the need to change the immunosuppressive regimen are all avoided. The patient is immediately mobilized with a theoretically lower risk of thromboembolic complications. The hospital stay is shorter, and there is an early return to activity with associated cost savings.

Finally, the procedure causes less pain and has a better cosmetic result.

TECHNIQUE

The procedure is performed under general anesthesia. Prophylactic antibiotic is administered at the start of the operation. The patient is operated in the standard supine position with the operating table tilted 20° in Trendelenburg position. The surgeon stands on the opposite side from the lymphocele with the assistant facing him or her. A nasogastric tube and a Foley catheter are inserted to decompress the stomach and bladder, respectively. The skin, including that of the abdomen, from the level of the nipple to the symphysis pubis and then to the mid thigh region is prepared with antiseptic solution and the abdomen is draped.

The procedure is the same for lymphoceles secondary to either kidney transplant or pelvic lymphadenectomy, except that in the former condition, more attention should be focused on avoiding injury to the graft and particularly to the ureter.

Laparoscopic Instrumentation

The following instruments are necessary for the procedure:

- Verres needle
- CO_2 automatic electronic insufflator
- Trocars: two 10-mm and one 5-mm
- 10-mm laparoscope with attached video camera
- Retractor rod
- Needle and aspirator
- Cautery hook
- Grasping forceps
- Endoscopic scissors
- Clip applicator
- Needle holder
- Push rod

Creating the Pneumoperitoneum

A small midline supraumbilical stab wound is made, and the Verres needle is inserted. Once the needle is in the peritoneal cavity, CO_2 is insufflated to provide a constant pneumoperitoneum of 15 mm Hg throughout the operation.

The needle is removed, and a 10-mm trocar sheath is inserted through the same site in the peritoneal cavity. This cannula is used to insert the video laparoscope. Additionally, a 10-mm and a 5-mm trocar are inserted in the lower abdominal quadrant on the side opposite the lymphocele. The exact placement of these trocars is selected under direct vision, depending on the location of the lymphocele.

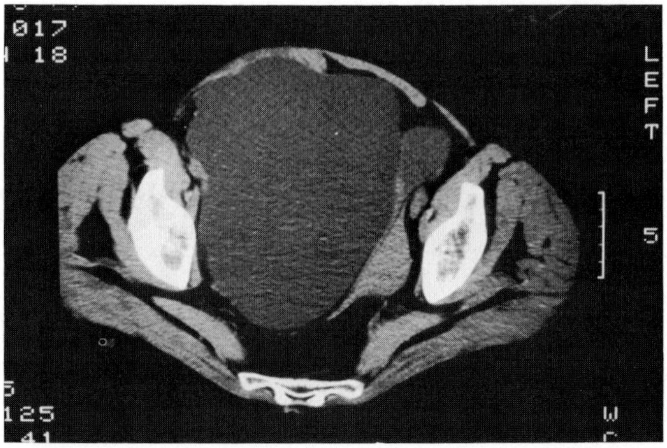

Figure 19–1. Computed tomographic scan demonstrating a large lymphocele in the pelvis.

Locating the Lymphocele

Exact location of the lymphocele is a crucial step in the procedure. The abdominal cavity is carefully inspected, identifying any kidney graft and the collection of lymph in the retroperitoneum.

The lymphocele may be large, bulging into the peritoneal cavity and almost entirely occupying the pelvis (Fig. 19–1), in which case naturally it is easy to locate. But the lymphocele is sometimes small and located posterior to the iliac vessels (Fig. 19–2), so it can be difficult to detect. A soft consistency on probing distinguishes it from the renal transplant. The bladder can be identified by filling it with normal saline through the Foley catheter. Ultrasound or transillumination of the abdominal wall can also help the surgeon to exactly locate the lymphocele.

The final step is to insert a needle through the trocar sheath into the lymphocele cavity and to aspirate the fluid, thus confirming the location of the lym-

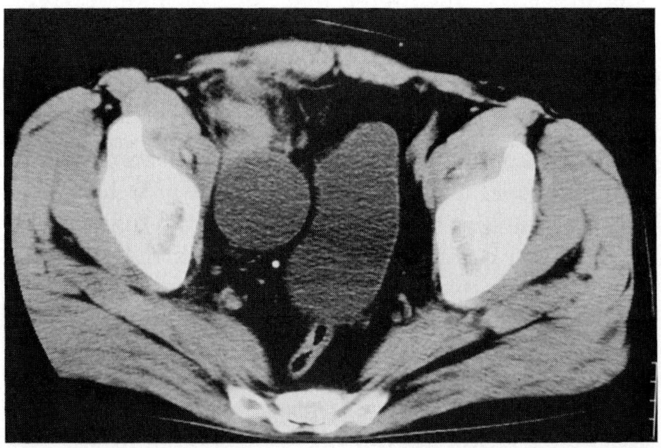

Figure 19–2. Computed tomographic scan demonstrating a small lymphocele located posterior to the iliac vessels.

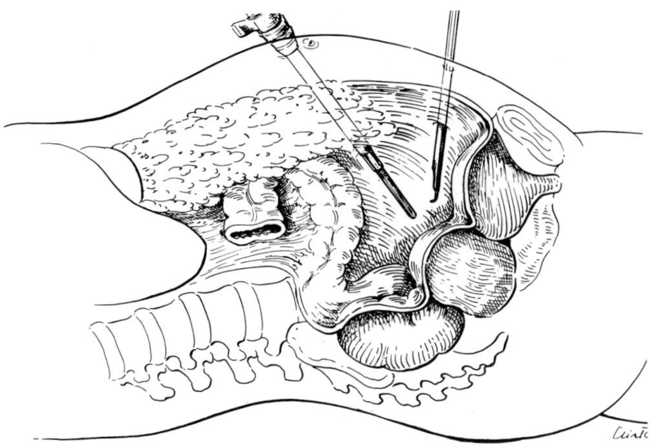

Figure 19–3. Creation of a peritoneal window by incision of the peritoneum over the lymphocele.

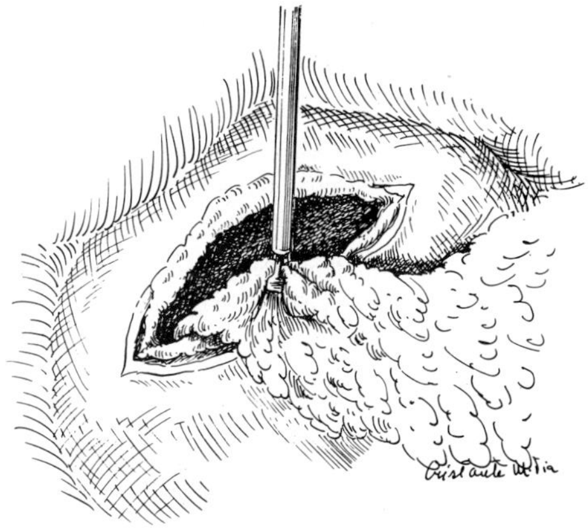

Figure 19–4. Maintaining the patency of the peritoneal window by inserting a flap of omentum in the lymphocele cavity.

phocele. The lymph is analyzed, Gram-stained, and cultured. It is not convenient to completely empty the lymphocele of its fluid contents because this can make the next step more difficult.

Creating the Peritoneal Window

The peritoneum over the lymphocele is incised, using the cautery hook (Fig. 19–3). Two layers are usually visible: the peritoneum and the actual lymphocele wall. After incision of the peritoneum, a 6- to 10-cm incision is progressively performed in the lymphocele wall. If the lymphocele is large, an ellipse can be excised to create a large peritoneal window. Grasping forceps, endoscopic scissors, and the retractor rod can be used at this stage. Particular attention must be given to avoiding injury to a transplanted ureter which may have been displaced by the lymphocele.

The laparoscope is then pushed into the lymphocele cavity. The lymph is completely aspirated, and any internal loculations are lysed bluntly to create a single cavity. If the leaking lymphatic vessel is visible, it can be ligated with clips.

Preventing Recurrence

A flap of omentum can be used to help maintain the patency of the peritoneal window. The inferior free edge of the omentum is drawn into the pelvis with the aid of grasping forceps. Any adhesions are separated with endoscopic scissors to ensure a complete mobilization. The omentum is pushed through the peritoneal window into the lymphocele cavity (Fig. 19–4) and secured in place, fixing it to the edges of the peritoneal window with clips.

When it is not possible to have the omentum drawn into the pelvis, an alternative technique for increasing the patency of the fenestration is to suture the free edges of the peritoneum and lymphocele wall, approximating the two layers together around the peritoneal window. Four or five separate stitches in monofilament suture are applied. The needle is slightly curved to allow entry through the cannula. With the aid of a needle holder, the needle is passed through the peritoneum and the lymphocele wall close to the edge of the window and is regrasped inside the lymphocele cavity (Fig. 19–5). The suture is then withdrawn outside the abdomen and tied with the Roeder slip knot. Using the push rod, the knot is then laid down under direct vision, and the excess suture is cut with the endoscopic scissors. Intracorporeal knotting can be used as an alternative.

After a final inspection to ensure adequate hemostasis, the abdomen is deflated, the sheaths are removed, and the skin incision is closed with sutures.

CONCLUSIONS

To date only 6 cases of lymphocele treated by laparoscopy (3 posttransplant and 3 secondary to pelvic lym-

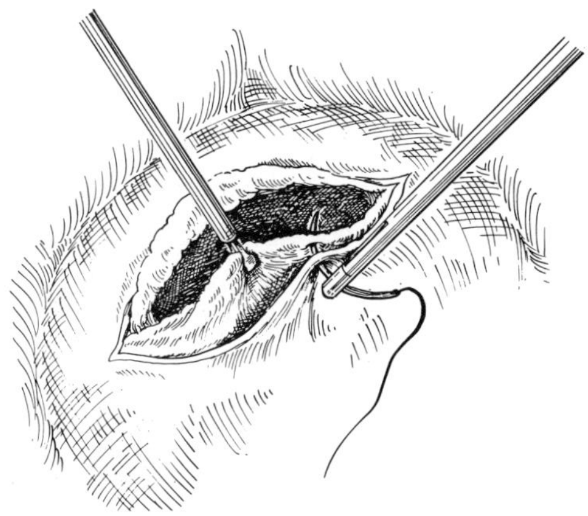

Figure 19–5. Suture of the peritoneum and lymphocele wall around the free edges of the peritoneal window.

phadenectomy) have been reported in the literature, all of which were managed successfully with no complications.[6-10]

The low incidence of lymphoceles makes it difficult to accumulate a large series managed laparoscopically; however, in our opinion, with increasing experience in laparoscopic surgery, laparoscopic internal drainage will soon become the surgical treatment of choice for lymphocele.

REFERENCES

1. Greenberger, BM; Perloff, LJ; Grossman, RA; et al: Treatment of lymphocele in renal allograft recipients. Arch Surg 120:501–504, 1985.
2. Livingston, WD; Confer, DJ; Smith, RB: Large lymphoceles resulting from retroperitoneal lymphadenectomy. J Urol 124:543–546, 1980.
3. White, M; Mueller, PR; Ferrucci, JT; et al: Percutaneous drainage of postoperative abdominal and pelvic lymphoceles. AJR 145:1065–1069, 1985.
4. Teruel, JL; Escobar, EM; Quereda, C; et al: A simple and safe method for management of lymphocele after renal transplantation. J Urol 130:1058–1059, 1983.
5. Schweizer, RT; Bartus, SA; Foster, JH: Treatment of pelvic lymphoceles after renal transplantation by intraperitoneal marsupialization. Am Surg 42:316–318, 1976.
6. Ancona, E; Rigotti, P; Zaninotto, G; et al: Treatment of lymphocele following renal transplantation by laparoscopic surgery. Int Surg 76:261–263, 1991.
7. Bardot, SF; Montie, JE; Jackson, CL; et al: Laparoscopic surgical technique for internal drainage of pelvic lymphocele. J Urol 147:908–909, 1992.
8. Khauli, RB; Mosenthal, AC; Caushaj, PF: Treatment of lymphocele and lymphatic fistula following renal transplantation by laparoscopic peritoneal window. J Urol 147:1353–1355, 1992.
9. McCullough, CS; Soper, NJ; Clayman, RV; et al: Laparoscopic drainage of a posttransplant lymphocele. Transplantation 51:725–741, 1991.
10. Waples, MJ; Wegenke, JD; Vega, RJ: Laparoscopic management of lymphocele after pelvic lymphadenectomy and radical retropubic prostatectomy. Urology 39:82–84, 1992.

CHAPTER 20

Laparoscopic Cystectomy

Raul O. Parra, MD, FACS
Paul G. Hagood, MD

Numerous pathologies of the urinary bladder requiring surgical intervention are amenable to an endocavitary (laparoscopic) approach. Some feasible applications are listed in Table 20–1. Many of these procedures have already been described in case reports and reviews.[1–6] In general, the advances made in laparoscopic surgery in the past 3 years have resulted in notable decreases in patient morbidity and hospital stay.[7–11] Our experience with diverticulectomies[1] and simple cystectomies[2] has demonstrated not only the efficacy but also the comparative advantage of the laparoscopic approach. This chapter examines the indications for and the techniques essential to performing a simple cystectomy. The potential for more complex extirpative bladder surgery is also explored.

SIMPLE CYSTECTOMY

Indications

On occasion supravesical urinary diversion with omission of a cystectomy is performed. Difficult problems such as neurogenic bladder; refractory incontinence; surgically uncorrectable outlet obstruction; and intractable symptoms resulting from tuberculosis, interstitial cystitis, fistula, and radiation have all been treated by diversion without cystectomy.

The defunctionalized bladder deprived of urine can, however, be the source of malignant transformation[12–18] or other significant complications in up to as much as 80% of patients.[19] Eigner and Freiha[19] encountered complications directly related to the bladder in 24 of 30 patients previously diverted without bladder removal. A review of our own experience and a scrutiny of the literature[19–27] provided information on a total of 777 patients with cutaneous urinary diversions done for a variety of conditions. Pyocystitis developed in 164 of the 777 patients (21.1%). Ninety-nine, or 12.7%, required removal of the bladder, despite treatment with assorted medical regimens or more conservative drainage methods. Cystectomy is, however, a major operation associated with significant morbidity and prolonged hospitalization. Decreasing the morbidity is a legitimate concern, especially in this group of patients already familiar with major surgery.

Preoperative Principles

For some laparoscopic techniques such as a varicocelectomy[7] or lymphadenectomy,[10] patients can be admitted the day of surgery. More complex endocavitary procedures must be viewed as major surgery, and proper patient preparation is essential. We prefer a mechanical bowel preparation with 2 to 4 L of GoLYTELY on the day before surgery. If possible, admission the day before surgery will assure compliance with bowel preparation and adequate hydration. A cystogram is useful in detailing the anatomy preoperatively (Fig. 20–1). Possible contraindications to this procedure besides those for general laparoscopy[28] are previous pelvic radiation and the presence of an ongoing bladder or upper tract infection. Sterilization of the bladder and urine is imperative in order to avoid the hazards of spilling infected urine or bladder con-

Table 20–1. LAPAROSCOPIC BLADDER PROCEDURES

Diverticulectomy[1]
Cystectomy (with and without urinary diversion)[2,11]
Partial cystectomy[3]
Colposuspension[4]
Nephroureterectomy with a cuff of bladder[5]
Excision of urachal cyst and fistula[6]
Repair of intraperitoneal rupture
Augmentation cystoplasty

tents intraperitoneally. Furthermore, broad-spectrum prophylactic parenteral antibiotics are routinely administered 2 hours before laparoscopy. In the female, an adequate vaginal preparation is important. This minimizes the risk of infection should the vagina be inadvertently violated while the posterior plane between it and the bladder is dissected.

Finally, a detailed informed consent is obtained. Discussion with the patient should include a review of all alternatives, both surgical and conservative. The patient must be made aware that the procedure is new but is based on sound principles that can be readily applied to his or her own condition. Furthermore, he or she must understand the surgeon's qualifications to perform new or innovative procedures. Also, the complications unique to laparoscopy (including gas emboli, shoulder pain, bowel and vascular injury from trocars, and so forth) should be emphasized. The potential for conversion to an open procedure must be discussed. The best rule of thumb is to first ask "what is in this for the patient," disallowing consideration of surgical satisfaction and economic advantage.[29] Informed consent is less painful for both patient and surgeon if this maxim is followed.

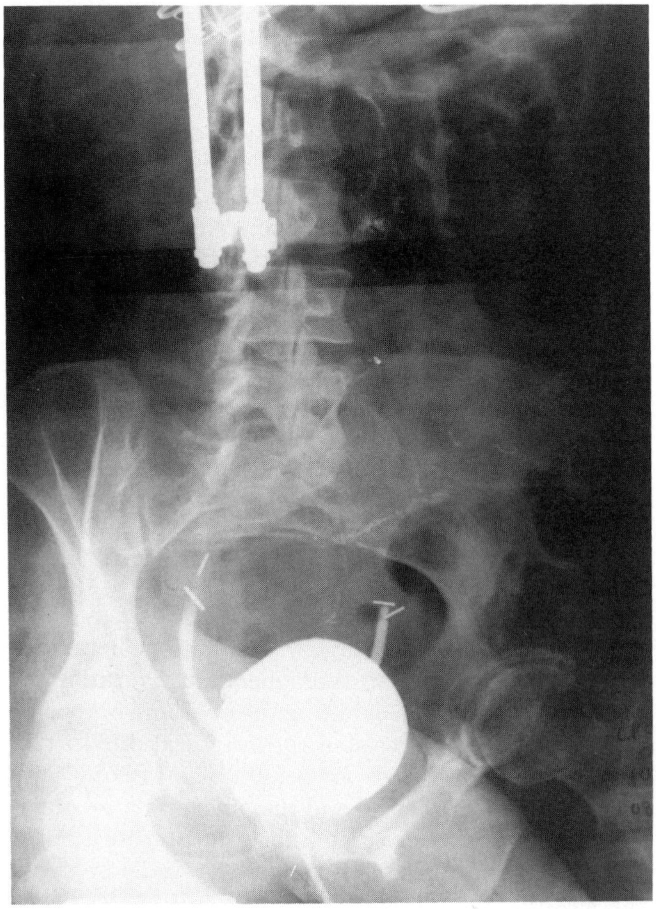

Figure 20–1. Preoperative cystogram.

Patient Positioning

We prefer placing the patient in a modified lithotomy position on Allen stirrups, with the buttocks just at the edge of the operating table. A rolled sheet is placed below the hips to further spread the pelvic girdle. This allows access to the perineum, should cystourethroscopy or elevation of the anterior vaginal wall be necessary. The patient's arms are tucked in at the side to allow free mobility of the operating team.

As effective retraction of intra-abdominal bowel is not yet available for laparoscopy, considerable rotation of the patient occurs during the operation. Extreme lateral and Trendelenburg positions are common, and the patient needs to be secured to the table. Chest straps and shoulder braces should be used. Furthermore, as pressure points will change during the operation, all conceivable points need to be padded. Immediately before induction of pneumoperitoneum, the table is tilted in Trendelenburg position to approximately 20°. This assists in displacing the bowels cephalad. Decompression of the continent pouch or management of an ileal conduit is accomplished by continuous catheter drainage. Gastric decompression is also done by means of a nasogastric tube.

Induction of Pneumoperitoneum

In our experience, establishing a pneumoperitoneum in the virgin abdomen is simple if the Mitchell technique of Verres cannula placement is used.[30] However, the safest and most reliable way is to use a Hasson trocar via a minilaparotomy incision.[31] Once the trocar is in place, it can be secured with sutures and rapid insufflation is accomplished. The laparoscope with the video camera attached can then be passed and additional trocars are placed under direct visual control.

Trocar Placement

The tendency for the neophyte endocavitary surgeon is to think that the more trocars used, the better. The surgeon will, however, find that as experience is gained, a fewer number is superior. An excess of trocars and instruments in the abdomen resembles an overgrown jungle and more often than not impedes rather than augments the procedure. Obviously, fewer trocars also results in less postoperative pain for the patient. We advocate three or four access ports for most pelvic procedures.

Our usual approach is to place a 10.5-mm trocar through which the laparoscope and camera are used at the umbilical area. Two additional 10- to 12-mm ports placed on either side, approximately 2 cm below the navel along the midclavicular line, are all that are customarily needed. In our early experience we tried using smaller ports (5-mm) but invariably needed to upsize them during the operation. As larger and more complex instruments have become available, we have limited our use of 5-mm ports considerably. Disruption of the epigastric vessels can occur with placement of the lateral ports. In addition to being aware of their usual course, the surgeon can often identify them by visualization through the laparoscope or by transillumination.[32] If an additional port is necessary for retraction, this may be a suitable indication for placing a 5- or 10.5-mm trocar in the midline, approximately 2 cm above the pubis.

Postoperative Considerations

Postoperative management begins with the desufflation and closure of the fascia at each trocar location. Some suggest closure of all trocar sites under direct vision from the laparoscope with the pneumoperitoneum intact.[33] Herniation of loops of bowel through trocar sites has been reported, and the surgeon should not be misled by the apparent insignificance of the wounds.[34] We use interrupted figure-of-eight 0 polyglycolic acid (PGA) sutures on the fascia. The skin is closed with subcuticular 4-0 PGA. As the pneumoperitoneum is released, it is helpful to decompress any pneumoscrotum.

Standard surgical practices must be maintained in the care of the patient after laparoscopy. To the surgeon, the practice of instituting full oral intake without assessment of the patient or discharging patients home at a predetermined time are ludicrous notions. In the laparoscopic era, pressure to do just such things is increasing and is to be decried.

As most patients have only minimal pain, severe pain should be considered the result of a surgical complication, until it has been proved otherwise. There are reports to suggest that delayed complications may be more common in laparoscopic procedures than in traditional operations.[35] This may result both from a delayed mechanism of injury (e.g., from thermal injuries to bowel and ischemia from mesenteric vein thrombosis) and from delayed diagnosis. Late thermal bowel injuries usually occur between 4 and 10 days after operation. Puncture wounds to the bowel usually manifest within 48 hours.[36] In particular, unseen needle and trocar injuries are probably much more common than traditionally acknowledged.

Case Studies

The cases described below are those of two patients—a woman and a man. They illustrate the details of the technique and highlight the results.

Case History 20–1
SIMPLE CYSTECTOMY IN A FEMALE

A 27-year-old woman who was paraplegic had an ileocolonic reservoir with a continent stoma. Multiple episodes of pyocystitis ensued, and a cystectomy was recommended. Preoperative preparation was done as outlined previously and included 24 hours of continuous bladder irrigation with neomycin and parental antibiotics.

Results. The total operative time was 130 minutes, and the estimated blood loss calculated from the suction was 115 ml. The patient had an uneventful postoperative course and was discharged on the fifth postoperative day.

Surgical Technique. An 11-mm blunt Hasson trocar was introduced. The forward-viewing 0° laparoscope with an attached video camera was passed through it, and under direct vision, a 12-mm trocar was placed on the right and a 5-mm port on the left. Parietal adhesions were released by sharp and blunt dissection. The urinary reservoir and its conduit were displaced from the operating field by the pneumoperitoneum.

The peritoneal reflection was sharply incised bilaterally, extending from the bifurcation of the common iliac artery to the pubic rami, following the lateral borders of the obliterated umbilical arteries, which were then cauterized and divided. With a combination of sharp and blunt dissection, the space between the lateral wall of the bladder and pelvis was developed as far as the endopelvic fascia. The dissection was continued anteriorly until the prevesical space was entirely opened.

Using grasping forceps and cephalic traction on the bladder permitted the creation of the plane between the posterior vesical wall and the uterus to the level of the cervix. Use of electrocautery, dissecting scissors, or laser is essential here. At this point, further lateral dissection was directed at isolation of the vascular pedicles. The multifire endoscopic GIA 30 stapler* was passed through the right 12-mm trocar. Using this instrument, the vascular pedicles were serially ligated and divided (Fig. 20–2).

The next step consisted of isolation and division of the urethra. Posterior traction on the bladder with forceps facilitated the sharp and blunt dissection of the vesicourethral junction. The endo-GIA stapler was then placed across the urethrovesical angle, and the urethra was divided (Fig. 20–3 *A* and *B*).

*US Surgical, Norwalk, CT.

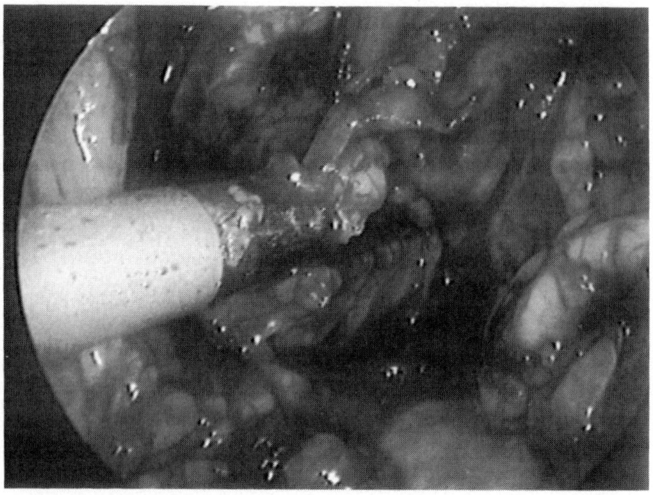

Figure 20–2. GIA endostapler across the vascular pedicle. See also Color Plate 7.

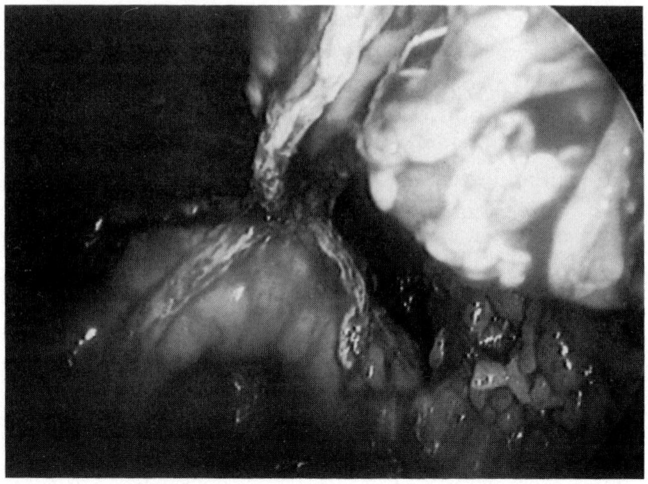

Figure 20–4. Immediately before complete division of vesicovaginal junction. Bladder at top. See also Color Plate 7.

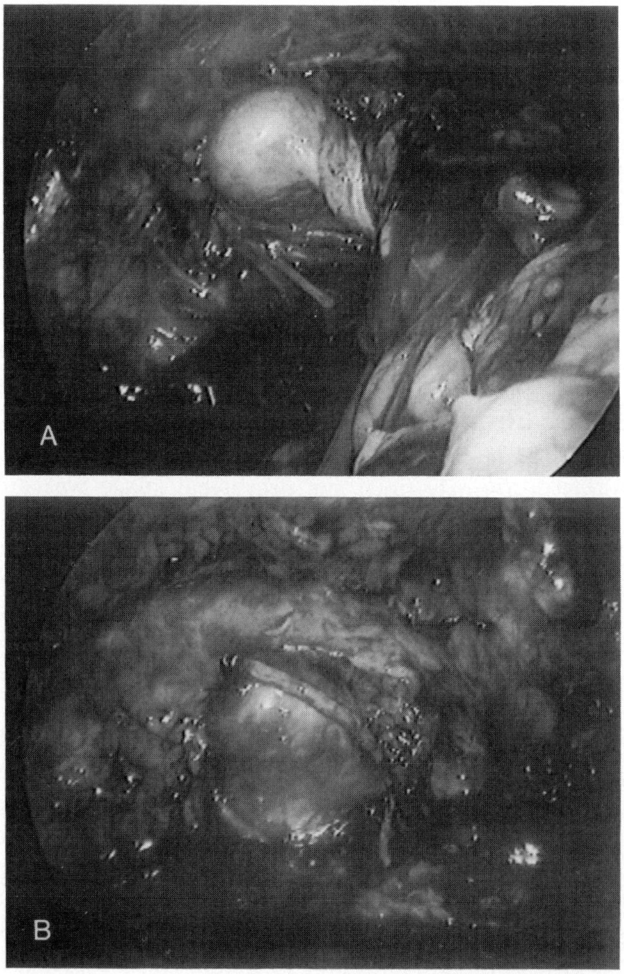

Figure 20–3. *A*, Urethra isolated with transurethral traction. *B*, Stump of urethra after division with endostapler. See also Color Plate 7.

Complete detachment of the bladder from the vagina was performed by three sequential firings of the stapling instrument across the vesicovaginal angle (Fig. 20–4). The specimen was then delivered in toto through the right trocar site. Irrigation and inspection of the pelvis revealed excellent hemostasis, an intact vaginal wall, and no residual bladder tissue. There was no evidence of retained bladder tissue on histopathologic examination.

Case History 20–2
SIMPLE CYSTECTOMY IN A MALE

A 24-year-old paraplegic man had an ileal conduit urinary diversion. Multiple episodes of pyocystitis, frequently complicated by autonomic dysreflexia, became a considerable burden. In the preceding year he had been hospitalized 12 times. The patient had reflex erections and wanted to remain potent; therefore a laparoscopic cystectomy without prostatectomy was performed.

Results. The total operative time was 180 minutes, and the estimated blood loss was 200 ml. The patient had a brief and uneventful postoperative course. The nasogastric tube was removed the next morning (12 hours) and the patient was able to tolerate a regular diet within 24 hours. Postoperative pain was not reported in this paraplegic man. He was discharged home the third postoperative day.

Surgical Technique. An 11-mm Hasson trocar was introduced subumbilically. In total four 10- to 12-mm trocars were placed in a diamond configuration, including a midline suprapubic port used extensively for anterior retraction. Lysis of adhesions was performed, following which excellent visualization of the lower abdominal and pelvic cavity was attained.

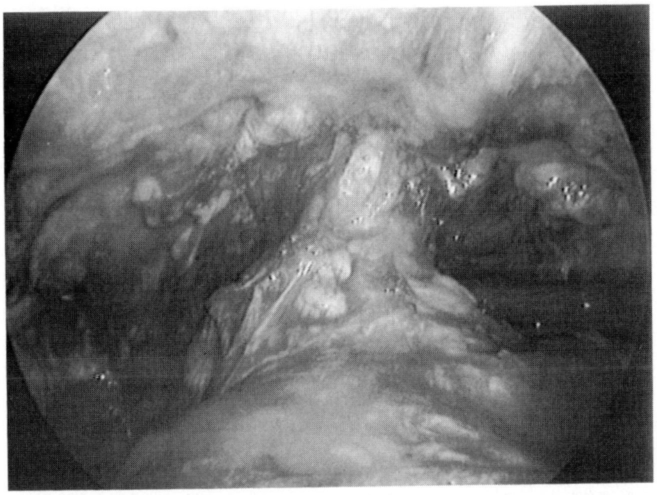

Figure 20–5. Complete anterior dissection in male with endopelvic fascia opened. See also Color Plate 8.

As in the previous case, the conduit was displaced from the operating field by the pneumoperitoneum pressure.

The anterior dissection was similar to the procedure previously described for the woman patient, with the prevesical space developed to the level of the puboprostatic ligaments and endopelvic fascia (Fig. 20–5). Sharp and blunt lateral dissection isolated the vascular pedicles for ligation and division by the endo-GIA stapler. With the aid of grasping forceps, cephalad traction on the bladder was exerted, permitting the creation of a plane between the posterior vesical wall and the rectum to the level of the vesicoprostatic junction. Complete detachment of the bladder from the rectum was performed by sequential staplings along the fascia plane. The next step consisted of isolation and division of the vesicourethral junction. A combination of electrocautery and stapling was used to transect the bladder and to occlude the prostatic urethra. The specimen was then delivered through the right trocar site. On gross inspection, no bladder tissue remained. Irrigation and inspection of the pelvis revealed excellent hemostasis and no evidence of rectal perforation. There was no evidence of retained bladder tissue on pathologic examination.

Comparative Analysis

The medical records of 43 patients who underwent supravesical urinary diversion without cystectomy at our institution over the last ten years were reviewed. The most common indication for diversion was neurogenic bladder disease.[29] A variety of other conditions constituted the indications for the rest: interstitial cystitis (2), radiation cystitis (9), intractable urinary incontinence (2), and vesicovaginal fistula (1).

There were 22 men and 21 women with an age range between 13 and 68 years (mean age, 49 years). Seven of the patients developed vesical empyema (five women and two men), five of whom eventually required cystectomy (three women and two men). One of the men was a T9 paraplegic. Intraoperative blood loss averaged 820 ml (range, 360 ml to 1100 ml). Three of the five patients required blood transfusions, the amount of blood used ranging from 1 to 3 units of packed red blood cells. The mean hospital stay for this group of patients following bladder removal was 20.6 days (range, 13 to 32 days). Three patients developed a wound infection in the postoperative period. The need for pain medication was poorly documented in two of the patients. Accurate records were available for the remaining three patients. Total meperidine hydrochloride use averaged 1330 mg (range, 290 to 2925 mg). The 2925 mg was required by the T9 paraplegic. Acetaminophen with codeine use in these three patients ranged from 2 to 14 tablets. In all instances, the need for pain medication in these individuals was significantly greater than that required by our patients following laparoscopic cystectomy.

CYSTOPROSTATECTOMY AND LAPAROSCOPIC DIVERSION

For pathologies other than a retained bladder, concomitant urinary diversion is necessary. The general indications for cystectomy with diversion are well described for open procedures, and a discussion is not germane to this chapter. We will briefly discuss the specific comparative advantages and disadvantages of laparoscopic cystectomy (simple and radical) with urinary diversion. It should be noted that laparoscopic surgeons are just beginning to attempt such procedures.

A laparoscopic prostatectomy has been performed,[37] and it is conceivable that a radical cystoprostatectomy could be accomplished. Urinary diversion with laparoscopic assistance has been reported by Kozminski and Partamian.[11] The arduous ask of performing the bowel resection and ureteroileal anastomosis was done with the bowel pulled extracorporeally through a trocar site. Many researchers are reporting ureteral surgery (ureterolysis,[38] ureteroureterostomies,[39] and extravesical ureteroneocystostomies,[40]) which suggests the practical application of intracorporeal anastomosis of ureter to ileal conduits. Laparoscopic bowel techniques are also rapidly improving.[41]

Recently, totally intracorporeal bowel resections with ureteral anastomosis have been accomplished.[42] Jordan has performed a laparoscopic Mitrofanoff procedure, with the majority of the bowel work done extracorporeally.[43] Obviously, laparoscopic cystectomy and cystoprostatectomy with ileal conduits may reasonably soon be considered. Despite the reports from Jordan and others, a continent urinary diversion with nonrefluxing ureteral anastomosis through use of the laparoscope still presents considerable problems. An inadequate bowel preparation will compromise a traditional open diversion procedure. In a closed abdomen, gross spillage of bowel contents would probably necessitate conversion to an open procedure.[35] The most pressing technical problem is that of providing adequate exposure for the bowel and ureteral resection and bowel reconstruction.[44] At this point, the surgeons are waiting for the technology.

When considering a new procedure, the pros and cons must be compared on relatively equal ground. First, it is hard to justify a decrease in morbidity when compared with the increased mortality of an unsatisfactory cancer operation. Entrapment systems for tissue removal are in use to limit the intraperitoneal spread of cancer or contagion, but at present their ability to guarantee tissue isolation is not assured. Furthermore, such endobags generally require tissue morcellation, which effectively eliminates the pathologic assessment.[44] Second, for most patients, a standard continent diversion, although presenting more initial morbidity, is more satisfactory in the long run. At this time, the laparoscope has not proved itself equal to standard surgical oncologic techniques, and the minor savings in terms of morbidity should be viewed with circumspection.

CONCLUSIONS

Delayed cystectomy has the disadvantage of being a major operative procedure that can be associated with serious complications and prolonged hospitalization. In the five patients in our series requiring laparotomy for bladder removal, the average hospital stay was 20.6 days, and three developed wound infections.

The usually small volume of a defunctionalized bladder, as well as its disconnection from urinary drainage suggested to us the feasibility of laparoscopic removal. Three obstacles to the procedure included the anticipated presence of adhesions, the risks of bleeding from the vascular pedicle, and the possibility of intraperitoneal spillage of infected material from an open bladder.

The first concern was addressed by use of the Hasson trocar through a minilaparotomy incision. Excision of the bladder from its vascular attachments was made possible by the employment of the multifire endo-GIA 30 stapler. This instrument provided hemostasis and allowed the expedient detachment and removal of the bladder from its urethral, vaginal, and rectal connections or any combination of these in a watertight fashion, thus averting the probability of spilling vesical contents into the peritoneal cavity.

The procedure proved to be quite simple in the female patient. In the male patient, the procedure was only slightly more complex, especially since the patient wanted to maintain potency and a cystoprostatectomy was not done.

We believe there are multiple advantages of laparoscopic cystectomy for a symptomatic bladder. There is no need for a large abdominal incision, making laparoscopy more cosmetically appealing and decreasing the probability of a wound dehiscence and incisional hernia formation.[28] Postoperative pain is reduced, and hospital stay can be markedly shortened, allowing the individual to be discharged more quickly and to return to normal activities sooner. This translates not only into patient benefits but economic advantages as well. One conceivable disadvantage of laparoscopic cystectomy that is inherently common to laparoscopy in general is that significant operator experience is required. However, with appropriate training and guidance, together with the rapid development of improved instruments for urologic laparoscopy, this drawback can be overcome. Our experience suggests that laparoscopic cystectomy be considered in those patients with supravesical urinary diversion and a problematic retained bladder.

Considerable experimental evidence supports the prospect of total laparoscopic management of many bladder pathologies, including those that require radical extirpation and urinary diversion. As technologies are developed for improved retraction of viscera, more complex procedures will be possible. The potential for tumor spillage and specimen procurement needs to be more firmly settled. The surgical efficacy in terms of cancer-free margins and nerve preservation (where indicated) also needs to be critically examined.

REFERENCES

1. Parra, RO; Jones, JP; Andrus, CH; Hagood, PG: Laparoscopic diverticulectomy: Preliminary report of a new approach for the treatment of bladder diverticulum. J Urol 148:869, 1992.
2. Parra, RO; Andrus, CH; Jones, JP; Boullier, JA: Laparoscopic cystectomy: Initial report on a new treatment for the retained bladder. J Urol 148:1140, 1992.
3. Lowe, BA; Novy, MJ; Strang, E: Laparoscopic segmental cystectomy. (Abstract) J Urol 146:408A, 1992.
4. Albala, DM; Schuessler, WW; Vancaille, TG: Laparoscopic bladder neck suspension. J Endourol 6:137, 1992.
5. Chiu, AW; Chen, MT; Huang, WJS; et al: Case report: Laparoscopic nephroureterectomy and endoscopic excision of bladder cuff. Minim Invas Therapy 1:299, 1992.
6. Neufang, T; Ludtke, FE; Lepsien, G: Laparoscopic excision of an urachal fistula—a new therapy for a rare disorder. Minim Invas Therapy 1:245, 1992.
7. Hagood, PG; Mehan, DJ; Worischeck, JH; et al: Laparoscopic varicocelectomy: Preliminary report of a new technque. J Urol 147:73, 1992.

8. Clayman, RV; Kavoussi, LR; Soper, NJ; et al: Laparoscopic nephrectomy: Initial case report. J Urol 146:278, 1991.
9. Parra, RO; Jones, JP; Hagood, PG: Laparoscopic intraperitonal marsupialization: Report on a new technic for lymphoceles. Surg Laparosc Endosc 2:306, 1992.
10. Parra, RO; Andrus, C; Boullier, J: Staging laparoscopic pelvic lymph node dissection: Comparison of results with open pelvic lymphadenectomy. J Urol 147:857, 1992.
11. Kozminski, M; Partamian, KO: Case report of laparoscopic ileal loop conduit. J Endourol 6:147, 1992.
12. Burney, SW; Graves, RC; Friedell, GH: Multiple malignancies in the urinary bladder following a by-pass procedure: Report of a case. Urol Int 26:69, 1970.
13. Silber, SJ: Carcinoma in the bladder left behind. J Urol 110:675, 1973.
14. Rege, PR; Evans, AT: Carcinoma in isolated bladder after ileo-conduit diversion. Urology 5:652, 1975.
15. O'Flynn, JD; Mullaney, J: Vesical leukoplakia progressing to carcinoma. Br J Urol 46:31, 1974.
16. Garvin, DD; Weber, CH, Jr; Polsky, MS: Carcinoma in the defunctionalized bladder: Report of a case and review of the literature. J Urol 117:669, 1977.
17. Melzak, J: The incidence of bladder cancer in paraplegia. Paraplegia 4:85, 1966.
18. Moloney, PJ; Fenster, HN; McLoughlin, MC: Carcinoma in the defunctionalized urinary tract. J Urol 126:260, 1981.
19. Eigner, EB; Freiha, FS: The fate of the remaining bladder following supravesical diversion. J Urol 144:31, 1990.
20. Retik, AB; Perlmutter, AD; Gross, RE: Cutaneous ureteroileostomy in children. N Engl J Med 277:217, 1967.
21. Holland, JM; Schirmer, HKA; King, LR; et al: Pyeloileal urinary conduit: An 8-year experience in 37 patients. J Urol 99:427, 1968.
22. Engel, RN: Complications of bilateral uretero-ileo-cutaneous urinary diversion: A review of 208 cases. J Urol 101:508, 1969.
23. Schmidt, JD; Hawtrey, CE; Flocks, RH; Culp, DA: Complications, results and problems of ileal conduit diversions. J Urol 109:210, 1973.
24. Guerrier, K; Albert, DJ; Persky, L: Experiences with pyocystis. Arch Surg 103:63, 1971.
25. Stewart, WW; Alexander, SC; Ireland, GW: Experience with pyocystis following intestinal conduit urinary diversion. J Urol 109:375, 1973.
26. Richie, JP: Intestinal loop urinary diversion in children. J Urol 111:687, 1974.
27. Stevens, PS; Eckstein, HB: The management of pyocystis following ileal conduit diversion in children. J Urol 47:631, 1975.
28. Borten, M: Laparoscopic Complications. Prevention and Management. Philadelphia, BC Decker, 1986, p. 139.
29. Missen, AJB: New wine—old bottles. Minim Invas Therapy 1:111, 1992.
30. Mitchell, MB; Stiegmann, GV; Mansour, A: Improved technique for establishing pneumoperitoneum for laparoscopy. Surg Laparosc Endosc 1:198, 1992.
31. Hasson, HM: Open laparascopy: A report of 150 cases. J Reprod Med 12:234, 1974.
32. Green, LS; Loughlin, KR; Kavoussi, LR: Management of epigastric vessel injury during laparoscopy. J Endourol 6:99, 1992.
33. Winfield, HN; Donovan, JF: Laparoscopic varicocelectomy. Semin Urol 10:152, 1992.
34. Kavoussi, LR; Sosa, E; Capelouto, CC: Complications of laparoscopic surgery. J Endourol 6:95, 1992.
35. Reich, H; Laparoscopic bowel injury. Surg Laparosc Endosc 2:74, 1992.
36. Penfield, AJ: How to prevent complications of open laparoscopy. J Reprod Med 30:660.
37. Schuessler, WW; Kavoussi, LR; Clayman, RV; Vancaille, TH: Laparoscopic radical prostatectomy: Initial case report. (Abstract) J Urol 147:246A, 1992.
38. Kavoussi, LR; Clayman, RV; Brunt, LM; Soper, NJ: Laparoscopic ureterolysis. J Urol 147:426, 1992.
39. Nezhat, C: Nezhat, F; Green, B; Gonzalez, G: Laparoscopic ureteroureterostomy. J Endourol 6:143, 1992.
40. Urban, DA; Kerb, K; McDougall, EM; et al: Laparoscopic repair of vesicoureteral reflux utilizing the Gregoir-Lich technique in the pig model. (Abstract) Proceedings of 4th International Meeting, Dublin. Minim Invas Therapy 1992, p. 67.
41. Cooperman, AV; Zucker, KA: Laparoscopic guided bowel resection. In: Zucker, KA, ed: Surgical Laparoscopy. St. Louis, Quality Medical Publishing, 1991, p. 344.
42. Kozminski, M: Laparoscopic urinary diversion. In Winfield, HM, ed: Laparoscopy: Surgical Learning Center Syllabus. Dallas, AUA Office of Education, 1992, p. 97.
43. Jordan, G: Laparoscopically assisted Mitrofanoff procedure. Personal communication, 1993.
44. Coptcoat, MJ; Wickham, JEA: Laparoscopy in urology. Minim Invas Therapy 1:337, 1992.

CHAPTER 21

Laparoscopic Reconstructive Surgery of the Urinary Bladder

Inderbir S. Gill, MD, MCh
Sakti Das, MD, FACS
Elspeth M. McDougall, MD, FRCSC

Applications of laparoscopy in urologic surgery are expanding rapidly.[1,2] An everincreasing range of procedures until now requiring open surgery are being approached by this minimally invasive technique. This chapter details the current status of laparoscopy as it pertains to reconstructive procedures on the urinary bladder. Laparoscopic injuries of the urinary bladder are discussed and their management is outlined. Controversy regarding the use of metallic staples in the urinary tract is presented, and relevant literature is reviewed. Finally, speculations on the future prospects of laparoscopy with respect to bladder reconstruction are considered.

BLADDER RECONSTRUCTIVE SURGERY

Bladder Neck Suspension

Female stress urinary incontinence is primarily the result of an abnormal anatomic descent of the proximal urethra and attenuation of the posterior urethrovesical angle.[3,4] Even though the proximal urethral sphincter is inherently intact, its mechanical efficiency is lost because of lack of a firm anchoring to the symphysis pubis.[5] Abnormal descent of the urethra and bladder neck inferiorly and posteriorly prevents transmission of increased intra-abdominal pressure to the proximal urethra; despite the normal urethral sphincter mechanism, the raised intravesical pressure overcomes outlet resistance, resulting in stress urinary incontinence.[6] The aim of stress incontinence surgery is to restore the proximal urethra and the urethrovesical junction to their normal intra-abdominal location, posterior to the symphysis pubis.[7] Laparoscopic bladder neck suspension has recently been offered as a less morbid alternative to the Marshall-Marchetti-Krantz (MMK) procedure.[8] Laparoscopic bladder neck suspension can be performed by either a transperitoneal or a retroperitoneal approach.

Transperitoneal Approach

Technique

The right-handed surgeon performs the procedure standing on the left side of the patient, and vice versa. The patient is positioned either in a frog-leg or a modified lithotomy position with the thighs elevated only minimally from the trunk to allow simultaneous access to the abdominal wall and the perineum. This is necessary for simultaneous transvaginal elevation of the anterior vaginal wall by the surgeon's left hand while laparoscopic sutures are placed between the periurethral fascia and the pubic periosteum with the right hand.[9] Four 11-mm trocars are positioned as follows: one port each at the umbilicus — medial to the left anterior superior iliac spine, medial to the right anterior superior iliac spine, and in the left midclavicular line at the level of the umbilicus.

The procedure is begun by identifying the left medial umbilical ligament. The initial incision is made parallel and immediately medial to the medial umbilical ligament. This incision is extended caudally to the pubic ramus, where it is curved medially for up to 3 to 4 cm beyond the midline. This peritoneal flap is retracted toward the patient's right side, thus exposing the space of Retzius. Meticulous dissection in this area identifies the pubic symphysis, pubic ramii, pubourethral ligaments, bladder neck, proximal urethra, and periurethral fascia that covers the anterior vaginal wall. Manipulation of the Foley catheter will demonstrate the inflated balloon at the bladder neck. With the transvaginally placed, double-gloved left index finger of the surgeon elevating the anterior vaginal wall, the bladder neck is laparoscopically dissected clear of surrounding fatty tissue. A nonabsorbable suture (Dacron 2/0 needle, 36-inch suture) is placed in the endopelvic fascia precisely at the level of the bladder neck on either side and then passed through the highest point on the pubis. A curved needleholder, passed through the left lateral trocar is used to place the suture in the endopelvic fascia; a straight needleholder is used to pass the suture through the pubic periosteum. The suture on the right side is placed first. Transvaginal elevation of the anterior vaginal wall facilitates tying of the knot, which is preferably done by the extracorporeal technique. Only one suture on either side is required to achieve satisfactory elevation of the bladder neck.

The Foley catheter is removed once the patient is fully awake. At this point, ambulation and a clear liquid diet are advised. After the first voiding, residual urine is assessed by straight catheterization. Patients are usually discharged within 24 hours of the procedure. Self-catheterization is continued at home until residues below 100 to 125 ml are noted.

Results

Results in the initial 22 patients reported have been encouraging.[10] Mean operative time was 65 minutes (range, 35 to 175 minutes), and 18 patients were discharged from the hospital within 18 hours of the procedure. Nine patients were catheter-free at the time of discharge, whereas 13 patients wore an indwelling catheter for 3 days. Convalescence was postoperatively complete within 5 days in 19 patients. Stress incontinence was cured in all patients, although follow-up continued for less than 10 months. Three patients required conversion to an open procedure: in one patient, an inadvertent cystotomy that occurred during laparoscopic dissection required open closure. In two patients, the bladder neck suspension sutures could not be placed laparoscopically to the surgeon's satisfaction, and the procedure had to be completed in an open fashion.[10]

Extraperitoneal Approach

Technique

A skin incision is made midway between the umbilicus and the symphysis pubis. The anterior abdominal fascia is identified and is incised sharply. A zero-absorbable suture (e.g., Vicryl) is placed as a tagging suture on either side of the fascia. Blunt finger dissection through this incision allows access into the retropubic space behind the symphysis pubis and placement of the balloon catheter for distention. Following balloon distention, an open cannula port (e.g., Hasson cannula) is inserted in the retropubic space and affixed with the two fascial stay sutures. Laparoscopic examination reveals the bladder neck region and the exposed posterior surface of the symphysis pubis. A minimal amount of additional dissection is required for complete exposure of the endopelvic fascia and the midline cartilaginous notch of the symphysis pubis prior to placement of sutures between the bladder neck and the posterior symphysis (Fig. 21–1). This extraperitoneal technique has been used to perform laparoscopic retropubic bladder neck suspension in 15 patients with stress urinary incontinence (McDougall, EM, personal communication). However, the follow-up to date has been less than 6 months, and therefore clinical results are not yet available to permit comment on the efficacy of this procedure.

The availability of other, less invasive but equally efficacious bladder neck suspension techniques[11,12] makes the current place of laparoscopic bladder neck suspension in the treatment of stress urinary incontinence unclear. The needle suspension techniques mentioned earlier involve either a small incision or none, a postoperative hospital stay of 1 to 3 days, and continence rates approaching 80% to 90%. These compare favorably with long-term success rates following MMK suspension procedure, success rates of which range from 57% to 90% when followed for a period of 5 years.[7]

Advantages of the laparoscopic technique over needle suspension procedures include placement of sutures at the precise area in the endopelvic fascia under vision, suspension from the pubic periosteum as opposed to anterior rectus fascia (as used in needle suspension methods), and elimination of the need for a foreign body such as the pledget or bolster. Further,

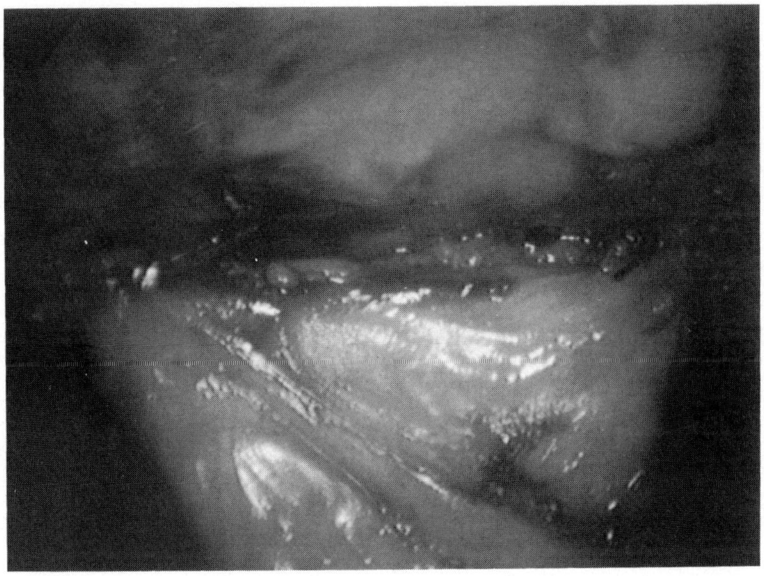

Figure 21–1. Laparoscopic appearance following anterior colposuspension. See also Color Plate 8.

during tightening of the knot, one can actually observe elevation of the bladder neck in relation to the symphysis pubis.[9,10] Recently, laparoscopic colposuspension[13] and laparoscopic placement of a synthetic urethral sling[14] have been reported. Nevertheless, longer follow-up in a larger number of patients is necessary before the efficacy and reliability of laparoscopic bladder neck suspension can be established.

Diverticulectomy

When complicated by stasis, infection, calculi, large size, urinary retention, upper tract obstruction or malignant changes, a bladder diverticulum requires removal.[15–17] The aim of surgical removal is to excise the diverticulum, prevent seeding in cases of malignancy, obtain watertight closure of the bladder, and prevent injury to the ureter and surrounding structures.[17] Until recently, such removal had been effected by open surgical[15–17] or transurethral techniques.[18] Whereas open surgical techniques (extravesical, intravesical, or a combined approach) achieve the preceding aims, dissection is often tedious, and morbidity is not insignificant. Transurethral techniques are limited in scope and are rarely performed. Recently, laparoscopic excision of a bladder diverticulum has successfully been performed.[19,20]

Precise definition of the location and size of the diverticulum and of its relationship to the ureters is obtained preoperatively by an intravenous pyelogram (IVP), a cystogram, and ureteral catheterization if needed.[20] Laparoscopy is performed under general anesthesia, with the patient in the lithotomy position to facilitate simultaneous cystoscopic examination. Ureteral stenting is advisable if the diverticulum is large or is in proximity to the ureter. To facilitate laparoscopic identification of the diverticulum, a cystoscope or a Foley catheter is preoperatively placed in the diverticulum. To place the Foley catheter, its tip is excised, and a cystoscope lens is passed inside the catheter. The sheathed cystoscope is introduced through the urethra into the diverticulum, where the balloon of the Foley catheter is inflated and the lens is removed (Fig. 21–2).[20]

Technique

Following pneumoperitoneum, four ports are positioned, one at each of the following locations: (1) inferior crease of the umbilicus, (2) and (3) 5 to 6 cm inferior to the umbilicus in the midclavicular line bilaterally, and (4) 2 to 3 cm cephalad to the symphysis pubis in the midline. The diverticulum is localized

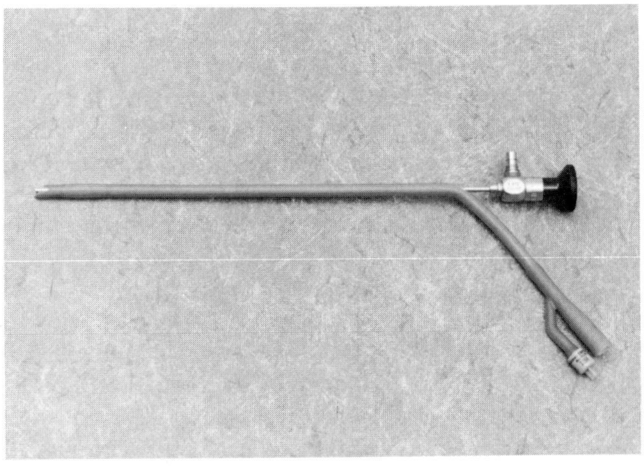

Figure 21–2. A cystoscope lens ensheathed by Foley catheter for placement in the bladder diverticulum.

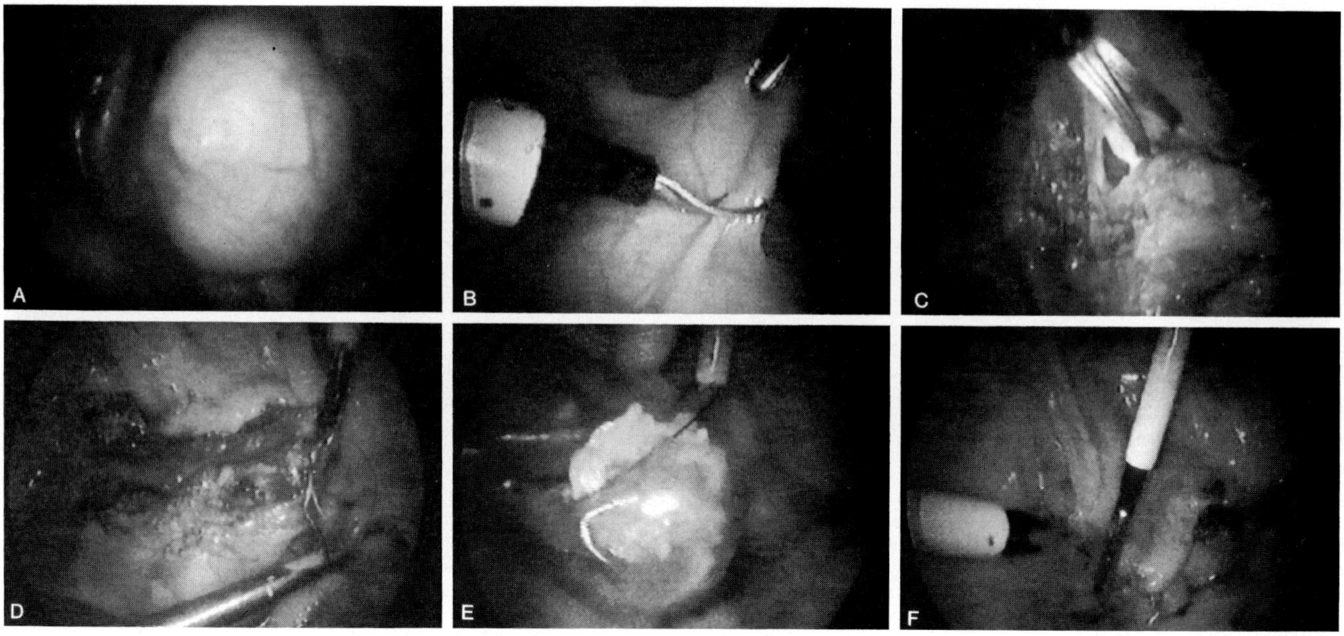

Figure 21–3. *A*, Laparoscopic view of bladder diverticulum with distended Foley balloon. *B*, Dissection of the peritoneum covering the neck of the diverticulum. *C*, Neck of the diverticulum opened anteriorly. *D*, Closure of the bladder opening by intracorporeal suturing. *E*, Excised diverticulum placed in endopouch prior to removal. *F*, Reapproximation of peritoneal edges over the bladder closure. See also Color Plate 8.

laparoscopically by identifying the cystoscope light or the Foley balloon (Fig. 21–3*A*). The overlying peritoneum and perivesical fat are dissected, and the neck and body of the diverticulum are mobilized circumferentially (Fig. 21–3*B*). Care is taken to avoid both ureters. Subsequent operative steps depend on the indication of diverticulectomy. For benign conditions, the neck of the diverticulum is divided with electrosurgical scissors to completely detach it (Fig. 21–3*C*). Bladder closure is obtained by laparoscopic suturing with absorbable sutures. Continuous full-thickness sutures are employed in two layers (Fig. 21–3*D*). If diverticulectomy is being performed for contained malignancy, the diverticular neck is not opened in order to prevent contamination of the operative field by malignant cells. Instead, a laparoscopic stapling device is used simultaneously to close the diverticulum and the bladder and to excise the diverticulum. In order to exclude the staples from contact with urine, horizontal mattress catgut sutures are placed laparoscopically on the bladder aspect of the staple line, under cystoscopic control. The excised diverticulum is removed en bloc through an 11-mm port, or is enclosed in an impermeable sac (Fig. 21–3*E*). Watertightness of the bladder closure is confirmed prior to terminating the procedure. Peritoneal edges are approximated over the bladder closure with sutures or staples (Fig. 21–3*F*). Seven to 10 days later, a cystogram is obtained to ensure healing is occurring, and the Foley catheter is removed. Use of the multifire endostapler (GIA 30) permits speedy bladder closure and hemostasis with simultaneous excision of the diverticulum, thus precluding spillage of diverticular contents.

Excision of Bladder Cuff During Nephroureterectomy

Laparoscopic nephroureterectomy has recently been performed as an extension of the concept of laparoscopic nephrectomy.[21,22] Intact, en bloc removal of the kidney, ureter, and a cuff of the bladder is obtained[21–24] in accordance with oncologic principles for treatment of transitional cell carcinoma of the upper urinary tract.[25]

Technique

At preoperative cystoscopy, a 5-mm ureteral balloon catheter is passed over a 0.035-inch Bentson guide wire and lodged in the intravesical portion of the affected ureter. Using an electrosurgical Orandi knife, the intramural ureter is incised over the inflated balloon. Alternatively, the ureteral tunnel can be circumscribed with the Orandi knife. The balloon catheter is replaced by a 7 Fr, 11.5-mm balloon occlusion catheter which is positioned in the renal pelvis. Laparoscopic ports are positioned, the ipsilateral colon is reflected, and the ureter is identified in the retroperitoneum. The ureter is mobilized caudally up to the ureterovesical junction, where the surrounding perivesical tissue is dissected. The aim is to allow the entire ureterovesical junction to be rolled anteriorly, which facilitates subsequent placement of the GIA endostapler. After the distal ureteral dissection is completed, laparoscopic nephrectomy is carried out.

To obtain the bladder cuff, a (GIA 30) endostapler is inserted through a 12-mm midline suprapubic port. The ureterovesical junction is retracted anteriorly, and the stapler is positioned at the site in order to assess bladder cuff length. The ureteral balloon catheter and the guide wire are removed. A 2-cm bladder cuff is simultaneously stapled and incised with the endostapler. This part of the procedure can be monitored cystoscopically to confirm watertightness of the anastomosis and the patency of the contralateral ureteral orifice. The en bloc specimen, consisting of the kidney, the ureter, and the bladder cuff, is placed in an organ entrapment sac and is removed intact through a suprapubic incision.

An alternative technique for removal of the lower ureter during nephroureterectomy involves transurethral resection of a periureteral mucosal cuff followed by intussusception of the ureter.[26,27] This intussusception ureterectomy combined with transurethral ureteral detachment and pull-through allows for total removal of the intramural ureter and has been employed in both malignant and benign disease.[28] Laparoscopic monitoring of the extravesical aspect of the ureterovesical junction may increase the safety and applicability of this technique.

Results

Analysis of Clayman's first six patients undergoing laparoscopic nephroureterectomy for transitional cell carcinoma of the upper urinary tracts revealed no complications from the transvesical staples (e.g., calculus formation, extravasation, or abscess formation) on radiographic and cystoscopic examination in a follow-up of up to 16 months.[22] An exposed staple was visible in one patient 20 weeks postoperatively, without any evidence of crystal formation. Subsequent follow-up cystoscopy revealed epithelial growth over the staple in this patient.

Partial Cystectomy

Partial cystectomy is indicated for solitary, infiltrating tumors situated on the posterior wall, lateral wall, or dome of the bladder. Partial cystectomy can also be performed for a tumor in a vesical diverticulum, urachal carcinoma, or localized benign lesions that are not amenable to transurethral resection. Additional rare indications of segmental cystectomy include palliation in patients with symptomatic metastases to the bladder or malignant invasion from adjacent organs.

Although it is traditionally accomplished by open surgery, partial cystectomy can be performed by minimally invasive techniques. When operating on malignant lesions, a laparoscopic pelvic lymph node dissection can simultaneously be performed. Preoperative cystoscopic random bladder biopsies to exclude field changes (i.e., carcinoma in situ) are mandatory. Tumor implantation due to spillage of cancer cells during surgery is a serious concern and can be minimized by a short preoperative course of external beam irradiation (2000 roentgens), intravesical photoirradiation by Nd:YAG laser with or without preoperative instillation of intravesical chemotherapeutic agents. Furthermore, especially during laparoscopic excision, the pathology-bearing segment of the bladder must be closed before excision in order to limit tumor spillage.

Recently, a high-grade, invasive transitional cell carcinoma located in the anterior wall of the urinary bladder of a paraplegic patient was treated by laparoscopic segmental cystectomy.[29] Preoperative cystoscopic laser photoirradiation of the tumor was performed. Following placement of laparoscopic ports, a pelvic lymph node dissection was done. Endoscopic GIA staplers and a contact tip laser were used in combination to resect the tumor-bearing segment, which was laparoscopically placed in a plastic bag to further limit its potential for peritoneal contamination. The bladder was closed by laparoscopic suturing techniques, and the plastic bag was retrieved through a minilap incision. The patient was discharged from the hospital on the third postoperative day.

With advances in experience and technology, segmental cystectomy, especially for benign conditions, is a relatively simple procedure that should be routinely amenable to laparoscopic techniques. Further experience to assess the incidence of tumor seeding is necessary before laparoscopic cystectomy for malignant disease can be applied in a more widespread manner.

Urachal Disorders

Surgical excision is the treatment of choice for a variety of urachal abnormalities, including patent urachus, urachal cyst, diverticulum, and fistula. These rare conditions are usually symptomatic from childhood. Preoperative ultrasonography, computed tomography, fistulography, and cystograms may not provide definitive diagnosis. Recently, laparoscopy has been employed for definitive diagnosis and management of a urachal fistula.[30] Care should be taken to vigorously treat any acute infection of the umbilicus with topical and systemic antibiotics before laparoscopic excision; peritonitis[31,32] and even death[33] have been reported from perforation of infected urachal cysts.

Technique

After placing three 5-mm trocars in the hypogastrium, the median umbilical ligament (urachus) was identified. Because the umbilicus is the site of primary pathology, it should not be used either for the Verres needle or for primary trocar placement; instead, a paramedian location is preferred for creating pneumoperitoneum and obtaining laparoscopic access. A boat-tipped probe, passed through the umbilicus into the urachal sinus, was visualized laparoscopically, thus confirming the diagnosis. Dorsal traction on the urachal tract allowed dissection between the anterior abdominal wall and the urachus, thus freeing it ventrally. The urachus was mobilized from its caudal attachment at the bladder and cephalad attachment at the umbilicus. After excision of the urachus, extracorporeally tied catgut endoligatures were placed on either end. The patient was discharged on the third postoperative day, and his presenting complaints of umbilical discharge and periumbilical eczema were completely resolved on follow-up examination.[30]

Laparoscopic Injuries to the Urinary Bladder

The urinary bladder may be inadvertently injured during a laparoscopic procedure. Such injuries can occur as a result of Verres needle puncture, primary trocar insertion, or during dissection and fulguration in the perivesical areas.[34–37] Verres needle injuries of the urinary bladder do not require repair. All trocar injuries require repair by laparoscopic[38] or open techniques. Trocar injuries can usually be recognized intraoperatively, although they occasionally remain undiagnosed until the postoperative period.

Routine preoperative Foley catheterization should decrease the incidence of urinary bladder perforation during laparoscopy. Some gynecologists do not employ routine Foley catheterization but ask the patients to void prior to laparoscopy in order to empty the bladder.[39] Occasionally, however, patients may not be able to void preoperatively because of apprehension about impending surgery and may present with a full bladder, increasing their chances of iatrogenic bladder injury. Furthermore, increasingly complex urologic laparoscopic procedures take at least 2 to 3 hours to complete; absence of a Foley catheter allows bladder distention intraoperatively. The incidence of bacteriuria following transient Foley catheterization is minimal; if the bladder is normal, such bacteriuria is always self-limiting. In our opinion, therefore, a laparoscopic injury caused by a full bladder resulting from absence of a Foley catheter is indefensible.

Evidence of hematuria or pneumaturia[40] through the Foley catheter indicates that the bladder has been violated. To avoid bladder injury, placement of the primary trocar should be directed toward the hollow of the sacrum after obtaining a pneumoperitoneum of 25 to 30 mm Hg; the excess pneumoperitoneum gives an additional safety "air cushion" during insertion of the primary trocar. For the remainder of the procedure, the pneumoperitoneum is decreased to 15 mm Hg. Postoperative inability to void or evidence of an increasing, painless lower abdominal mass (i.e., extraperitoneal extravasation) or generalized abdominal distention (i.e., intraperitoneal rupture) is suggestive of bladder injury and should be investigated with a cystogram.

Peritonitis following laparoscopic injury of an unsuspected vesicourachal diverticulum has been reported.[32] Therefore a preoperative history of umbilical discharge or periumbilical pruritis or eczema should alert one to the possibility of urachal pathology.

Use of Staples in the Urinary Bladder

The primary concern regarding the use of nonabsorbable materials in urinary tract reconstruction centers around their potential to act as a nidus for stone formation.[41] Continued contact of a nonabsorbable suture or staple with urine predisposes to calculus formation. Accordingly, in reconstructive urologic surgery, absorbable suture material is employed. However, because laparoscopic suturing is time-consuming and technically demanding, stapling devices have recently been employed to obtain a secure and rapid closure of the urothelium.

Nonabsorbable staples have been used widely in construction of bowel segments in patients undergoing continent urinary diversion.[41–44] In a review of the use of stainless steel staples in urinary diversion patients, the overall incidence of stone formation was 2.5%, and these calculi occurred 6 to 27 months postoperatively.[45] In continent reservoirs, staple-line calculi occurred in as much as 10% of patients.[44] The efficacy of absorbable and nonabsorbable staples in repairing the urinary bladder in 52 dogs revealed interesting data.[46] At cystoscopy 4 months later, 1 to 2 staples were visible in 8% of nonabsorbable stapled closures and 56% of absorbable stapled closures. However, in both groups, no staple-line calculi were noted, all closures were watertight, and microscopic examination revealed good anastomotic healing.[46]

Of the available nonabsorbable materials, titanium has superior tissue biocompatibility because of its corrosive-resistant properties.[47,48] This has been borne out in clinical studies in patients with titanium endourethral stent placement, in which no calculus formation was noted over a follow-up of 20 months.[49] Laboratory and clinical experience with titanium staples in closing the bladder cuff during laparoscopic nephroureterectomy has not revealed any complications secondary to transvesical staples until now.[45] GIA multifire tissue stapler delivering six 3-cm rows of staples and simultaneously incising between staple rows three and four was used. At 6-month follow-up of cystoscopy in the animal model, no exposed staples were visible, and there was no evidence of bladder stones or extravasation. In the clinical situation, cystoscopy at 10 months did not reveal any visible transvesical staples.[45] Similar staplers have previously been employed during laparoscopic bowel anastomoses.

We continue to believe that, wherever possible, approximation of urothelium should be performed with absorbable sutures. As to laparoscopic procedures on the urinary bladder in benign conditions, laparoscopic suturing with absorbable sutures is preferred. For partial cystectomy or diverticulectomy performed for malignant conditions, both the excised segment of the bladder and the bladder remnant should be closed with multifire endoscopic staplers before division to prevent spillage of malignant cells. The staple line in the urinary bladder remnant should be excluded from urinary contact by horizontal, absorbable mattress sutures, on the bladder side of the staples. Future development of absorbable staples from multifire staplers adapted to laparoscopic use would eliminate the need for laparoscopic suturing in restoring urothelial continuity.

CONCLUSIONS

Commensurate with advances of laparoscopic surgery in other fields, its applications in urology are also expected to increase. Laparoscopic urinary bladder reconstructions of increasing complexity will be attempted. Laparoscopic access to pelvic structures can be obtained either by a transperitoneal or an extraperitoneal approach.[51,52] We believe that the extraperitoneal approach will become the preferred technique of laparoscopic access to the pelvic cavity. Expansion of the extraperitoneal space with a dissecting balloon allows creation of an adequate working space. Advantages of an extraperitoneal laparoscopic approach include the following: It allows immediate direct access to the site of surgical interest, thus decreasing operative time; it prevents transgression of the peritoneal cavity, thus limiting the potential for intraperitoneal bacterial contamination and malignant seeding and minimizing the incidence of abdominal complications such as paralytic ileus, bowel injury, and intraperitoneal adhesions; and the intact peritoneal envelope can be used to retract the loops of bowel, thus enhancing surgical exposure.

Enumerated are our expectations of future advances in this area:

- Reduction cystoplasty
- Augmentation enterocystoplasy
- Autoaugmentation cystoplasty
- Extravesical ureteroneocystostomy
- Repair of traumatic bladder injuries (intra- and extraperitoneal)
- Repair of sliding hernias involving the urinary bladder
- Bladder denervation procedures for neurogenic bladder (cystolysis)
- Sacral rhizotomy
- Intestinal neobladder construction with anastomosis to the urethra
- Combined intra- and extravesical ablation of bladder tumors

The ultimate aim of laparoscopy is to allow optimal surgical management of disease processes while minimizing the extent of and side effects from violation of the physical being. In 1985 DeCherney spoke for both urologists and gynecologists when he wrote, "The obituary of open pelvic reconstructive surgery has been written, it is only its publication that remains."[53]

REFERENCES

1. Gill, IBS; Kerbl, K; Clayman, RV: Laparoscopic surgery: Current applications in urology. AJR, 160:1167, 1993.
2. Das, S: Laparoscopy in pediatric urology. J Endourol 6:151, 1992.
3. Klutke, C; Little, N; Raz, S: The anatomy of stress incontinence. AUA Update Series, 9(39), 1990.
4. Hilton, P; Stanton, SL: Urethral pressure measurement by microtransducer: Results in symptom-free women and in those with genuine stress incontinence. Br J Obstet Gynecol 90:919, 1983.
5. Hodgkinson, CP: Relationship of female urethra and bladder in urinary stress incontinence. Am J Obstet Gynecol 65:560, 1983.
6. McGuire, EJ; Lytton, B; Pepe, V; et al: Stress urinary incontinence. Am J Obstet Gynecol 47:255, 1976.
7. Spencer, JR; O'Connor, VJ; Schaeffer, AJ: A comparison of endoscopic suspension of the vesical neck with suprapubic vesicourethropexy for treatment of stress urinary incontinence. J Urol 137:411, 1987.
8. Parnell, JP; Marshall, VF; Vaughan, ED: Primary management of urinary stress incontinence by the Marshall-Marchetti-Krantz vesicourethropexy. J Urol 127:679, 1982.
9. Vancaillie, TG; Schuessler, WW: Laparoscopic bladder neck suspension. J Laparoendosc Surg, 1:169, 1991.
10. Albala, DM; Schuessler, WW; Vancaillie, TG: Laparoscopic bladder neck suspension. J Endourol 6:137, 1992.
11. Gittes, RF; Loughlin, KR: No-incision pubovaginal suspension for stress incontinence. J Urol 138:568, 1987.
12. Stamey, TA: Endoscopic suspension of the vesical neck for urinary incontinence in female: Report on 203 consecutive patients. Ann Surg 192:465, 1980.
13. Harewood, LM: Laparoscopic colposuspension and stress incontinence. J Endourol 6:5145, 1992.
14. Dickson, C; Boone, T; Preminger, GM: Laparoscopic urethral sling. J Endourol 6:5170, 1992.
15. Fox, M; Power, RF; Bruce, AW: Diverticulum of the bladder-presentation and evaluation of treatament of 115 cases. Br J Urol 34:286, 1962.
16. Gerridzen, JR; Futter, NG: Ten-year review of vesical diverticula. Urology 20:33, 1982.
17. Das, S; Amar, AD: Vesical diverticulum associated with bladder carcinoma: Therapeutic implications. J Urol 136:1013, 1986.
18. Vitale, PJ; Woodside, JR: Management of bladder diverticula by transurethral resection: Re-evaluation of an old technique. J Urol 122:744, 1979.
19. Parra, RO; Jones, JP; Andrus, CH; Hagood, PG: Laparoscopic diverticulectomy: Preliminary report of a new approach for the treatment of bladder diverticulum. J Urol 148:869, 1992.
20. Das, S: Laparoscopic removal of bladder diverticulum. J Urol 148:1837, 1992.
21. Figenshau, RS; Albala, DM; Clayman, RV; et al: Laparoscopic nephroureterectomy: Initial laboratory experience. Minim Invas Therapy 1:93, 1992.
22. Kerbl, K; Clayman, RV; McDougall, EM; et al: Laparoscopic nephroureterectomy: valuation of first clinical series. Eur Urol 23:431, 1993.

23. Rassweiler, JJ; Potempa, DM; Henkel, TO; et al: The technical aspects of transperitoneal laparoscopic nephrectomy (TLN), adrenalectomy (TLA), and nephroureterectomy. J Endourol 6:558, 1992.
24. Chie, AW; Chen, M-T; Huang, WJS; et al: Laparoscopic nephroureterectomy and endoscopic excision of bladder cuff. J Endourol 6:5152, 1992.
25. Cummings, KB: Nephroureterectomy: Rationale in the management of transitional cell carcinoma of the upper urinary tract. Urol Clin North Am 7:569–578, 1980.
26. Ercole, CJJ: Endoscopic removal of lower ureter in nephroureterectomy. Urology 41:49, 1993.
27. Kivist, E: Intussusception ureterectomy. Urol Res 17:389, 1989.
28. Clayman, RV; Garske, GL; Lange, PH: Total nephroureterectomy with ureteral intussusception and transurethral ureteral detachment and pull-through. Urology 21:482, 1983.
29. Lowe, BA; Novy, MJ; Strang, E: Laparoscopic segmental cystectomy. J Urol 147:408A, 1992.
30. Newfang, T; Ludtke, F-E; Lepsien, G: Laparoscopic excision of an urachal fistula—a new therapy for a rare disorder. Minim Invas Therapy 1:245, 1992.
31. Agatstein, EH; Stabile, BE: Peritonitis due to intraperitoneal perforation of infected urachal cysts. Arch Surg 119:1269, 1984.
32. Yong, EL; Prabhakaran, K; Lee, YS; Ratnam, SS: Peritonitis following diagnostic laparoscopy due to injury to a vesicourachal diverticulum. Case report. Br J Obstet Gynecol 96:365, 1989.
33. Akintan, B; Adekunle, A: A fatal case of ruptured infected urachal cyst. Int Urol Nephrol 17:133, 1985.
34. Gregory, FM; Fetterman, HH; Chefetz, MD: Complications of laparoscopy: Two cases of perforated urinary bladder. Am J Obstet Gynecol 120:1121, 1974.
35. Deshmukh, AS: Laparoscopic bladder injury. Urology 19:306, 1982.
36. Homburg, R; Segal, T: Perforation of the urinary bladder by the laparoscope. Am J Obstet Gynecol 13:597, 1978.
37. Sherer, DM: Inadvertent transvaginal cystotomy during laparoscopy. Int J Gynaecol Obstet 32:77, 1990.
38. Reich, H; McGlynn, F: Laparoscopic repair of bladder injury. Obstet Gynecol 76:909, 1990.
39. Akhtar, MS; Beere, DM; Wright, JT; MacRae, KD: Is bladder catheterization really necessary before laparoscopy? Br J Obstet Gynecol 92:1176, 1985.
40. Sia-Kho, E; Kelly, RE: Urinary drainage bag distension: an indication of bladder injury during laparoscopy. J Clin Anesth 4:346, 1992.
41. Brenner, DO; Johnson, DE: Ileal conduit calculi from stapler anastomosis: A long-term complication? Urol 24:537, 1985.
42. Myers, RP; Rife, CC; Barrett, DM: Experience with the bowel stapler for ileal conduit urinary diversion. Br J Urol 54:491, 1982.
43. Karamcheti, A; O'Donnell, WF; Hakala, TR; et al: Autosuture ileal conduit construction: Experience in 110 cases. J Urol 120:545, 1978.
44. Wheeless, CR; Dorsey, JH: Use of the automatic surgical stapler for intestinal anastomosis associated with gynecologic malignancy: Review of 283 procedures. Gynecol Oncol 11:1, 1981.
45. Kerbl, K; Chandhoke, PS; McDougall, EM; et al: Laparoscopic stapled bladder closure: Laboratory and clinical experience. J Urol 149:1437, 1993.
46. Julian, TB; Ravitch, MM: Closure of the urinary bladder with stainless steel and absorbable staples. Ann Surg 204:186, 1986.
47. Williams, DF: Titanium as a metal for implantation. Part 1. Physical properties. J Med Eng Technol 1:195, 1977.
48. Williams, DF: Titanium as a metal for implantation. Part 2. Biological and clinical applications. J Med Eng Technol 1:266, 1977.
49. Parra, RO: Treatment of posterior urethral strictures with a titanium urethral stent. J Urol 146:997, 1991.
50. Parra, RO; Hagood, PG; Boullier, JA: Endocavitary bladder surgery. Urology 41:26, 1993.
51. Ferzli, G; Trapasso, J; Raboy, A; Albert, P: Extraperitoneal endoscopic pelvic lymph node dissection. J Laparoendosc Surg 2:39, 1992.
52. Ferzli, G; Raboy, A; Kleinerman, D; Albert, P: Extraperitoneal endoscopic pelvic lymph dissection vs laparoscopic lymph node dissection in the staging of prostatic and bladder carcinoma. J Laparoendosc Surg (in press).
53. DeCherney, AH: "The leader of the band is tired. . . . " Fertil Steril 44:299, 1985.

CHAPTER 22

Laparoscopic Ureteroileocutaneous Urinary Diversion

Mike Kozminski, MD, FACS

The decade of the 1990s heralds the new era of laparoscopic surgery in the management of urologic maladies. To establish the philosophy of minimally invasive therapy whereby optimal therapeutic results can be achieved with limited surgical injury, urologists are in the process of carrying forward laparoscopic techniques for seemingly its limitless possibilities. Removal or extirpation of each of the intra-abdominal genitourinary organs has been accomplished through the laparoscope at some time. With increasing expertise and technologic innovations, more difficult reconstructive urologic procedures are being perfected at a rapid pace. Similar interest and demand from our general surgical colleagues has led to the development of improved devices and means applicable to laparoscopic intestinal surgeries.

It is inevitable that general understanding and these innovations will be combined in approaching more complex challenges in urology. Laparoscopic construction of ureteroileocutaneous diversion is probably the most formidable of these challenges and can be accomplished in selected cases with proper planning and attention to technical detail. To date, experience is limited, but feasibility has been proved in clinical patients.

INDICATIONS

Despite the recent profusion of continent urinary diversion techniques, ileal loop diversion reported by Bricker[1] in 1950 remains the standard for supravesical urinary diversion. Whether to attempt endoscopically ureteroileal diversion certainly depends on the experience and expertise of the urologist, especially in laparoscopic methods of intestinal anastomosis and advanced suturing techniques. Even in expert hands, the procedure proves extremely time-consuming; therefore it probably is best not to combine it with synchronous removal of the bladder if the latter is necessary.[2] The procedure should not be contemplated if there are specific contraindications to laparoscopy such as coagulopathy, a compromised cardiopulmonary state, multiple prior abdominal surgeries, peritonitis, and so forth. Probably the ideal candidate is the patient with neurogenic bladder requiring only ureteroileocutaneous diversion.

The patient must be counseled extensively about the limited data regarding this new procedure. The early experience of urologists in this novel approach should be discussed candidly. The alternative therapeutic choices should be described, and the significant potential of converting into an open procedure must be explained to obtain detailed consent.

PATIENT PREPARATION

Bowel preparation and antibiotic prophylaxis is necessary in order to lessen potential complications of wound infection and sepsis. Mechanical bowel preparation with propylethylene glycol can be instituted by the patient at home as outpatient or the patient can be admitted the afternoon before surgery. Perioperative broad-spectrum parenteral antibiotics such as ceftriaxone are recommended. The standard perioperative and intraoperative management includes nasogastric tube placement, bladder drainage with urethral Foley catheter, and antiembolic precautions with sequential compression devices placed in both the lower extremities.

It is helpful to have bilateral ureteral catheters placed cystoscopically before surgery as aids in easier identification of the ureters during laparoscopic dissection. The patient should be positioned on a table that has both Trendelenburg and lateral tilting capabilities. To gain exposure to both sides of the retroperitoneum, approximately 10° to 15° of lateral tilting becomes necessary. Before surgery the enterostomal therapist marks the preferred stomal site on the abdomen with indelible ink.

SURGICAL PROCEDURE

The patient is given a general anesthetic with endotracheal intubation. Pneumoperitoneum is created in the standard fashion using the Verres needle through the umbilicus, or, alternatively, open laparoscopy is carried out using the Hasson cannula. The laparoscopic camera with 0° lens is passed through the umbilical port, and additional trocars are placed under camera guidance. It is important to note that endoscopic stapling devices for intracorporeal bowel resection anastomosis require at least a 12-mm trocar. The 12-mm trocar is passed through the future stoma site. Multiple 10-mm trocars allow maximum flexibility for moving the laparoscope camera to various viewing angles and the passage of various instruments such as intestinal clamps and laparoscopic clip applicators. This is essential, since the procedure is conducted on both sides of the retroperitoneum.

The distal ileal segment to be used for construction of the ileal conduit is identified, and the desired segment is marked with long suture tags in its proximal and distal portions. The ends of these differently colored tags are pulled from the trocars on the right side tagged with hemostats.

The cecum and ascending colon on the right side and the descending colon and sigmoid colon on the left side are sequentially dissected and mobilized medially after incision of the peritoneum in the paracolic gutter along the line of Toldt. The ureter is identified by the ureteral stents placed before starting laparoscopy. Manipulating the stiff ureteral guides helps identify the ureter intracorporeally. Following the external iliac vessels proximally to the common iliac bifurcation or looking adjacent to the gonadal vessels are additional ways that can help in identifying the ureter. After the ureter is identified and isolated, a vessel loop or umbilical tape is placed around the ureter and the tape is padded extracorporeally. This tape is used as a handle to lift and pull the ureter for further dissection. The distal ureter is mobilized in the deep pelvis, using both sharp and blunt dissection. Small vessels supplying the ureters are controlled with laparoscopic hemostatic clips. The ureter is then clipped and transected as close to the bladder as possible. By clipping proximal to the transection line, the ureter is occluded, which prevents urine from pooling in the pelvis and allows the ureter to dilate, thereby helping at the time of ureteroileal anastomosis.

After both ureters have been transected and mobilized proximally, the bowel resection is initiated. An adequate length of the bowel should be carefully measured. The pneumoperitoneum often artifically elevates the abdominal wall, giving a false gauge of length needed for the conduit. Holding the proximal and distal ends of the proposed ileal loop up to the abdominal wall and down to the sacral promontory is helpful to determine the appropriate length of ileum needed. One can use an umbilical tape to measure the ileal segment intracorporeally.

While preparing the ileal loop segment during open surgical approach, the mesenteric vascular arrangement is closely examined. This may not be possible during laparoscopic approach, particularly if the patient has extensive fat in the mesentery and if the blood vessels are difficult to visualize. Once the segment of ileum is identified, an endo-GIA 30 or endo-GIA 60 laparoscopic stapling device is placed transversely across the antimesenteric side of the bowel. (see Fig. 22–1) Once the bowel has been stapled and transected, it is important to reassess how much of a mesenteric opening is necessary for reanastomosis of the ileum. Only 1 to 2 cm of mesentery adjacent to the ileum is ligated and divided, using the endo-GIA stapler and thereby minimizing the risk of damaging major vessels in the vascular arcades (Fig. 22–2). A similar procedure is performed on the proximal and distal ends of the ileal loop conduit segment. The conduit is then placed caudally in the pelvis, as it is made certain that the mesentery is not twisted.

The intestinal continuity is re-established by side-to-side anastomosis of the ileal ends (Fig. 22–3). The antimesenteric corner of each staple line is trimmed

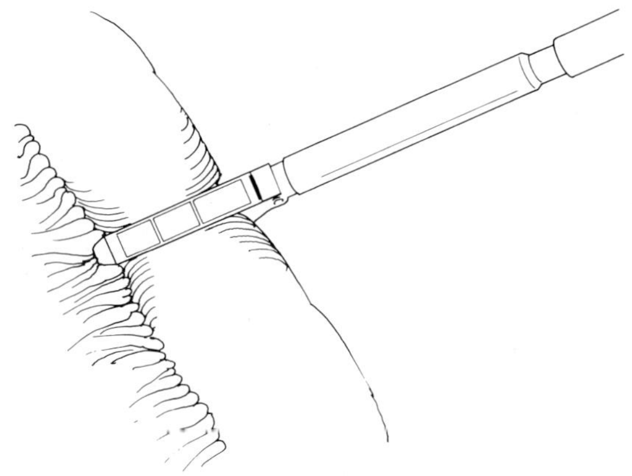

Figure 22-1. Laparoscopic Endo-GIA for stapling and transection of ileal loop.

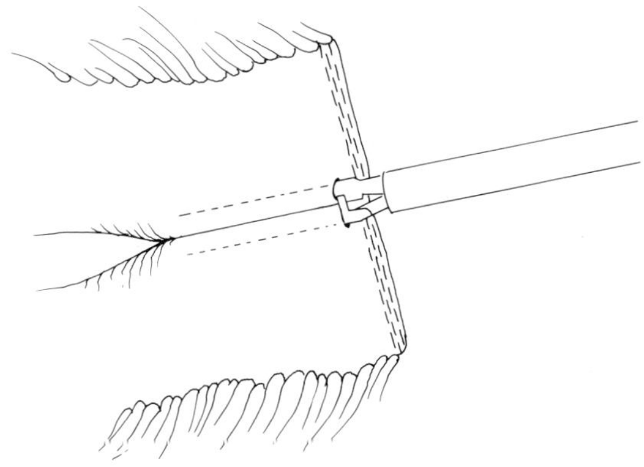

Figure 22-3. Side-to-side anastomosis by stapling the juxtaposed antimesenteric bowel walls.

off with laparoscopic scissors. The ileal ends are stabilized as the jaws of the endo-GIA are passed into the two limbs of bowel. It is critical to check the antimesenteric position of the two limbs of bowel and to verify that nothing is trapped between them before the stapler is fired. Either two endo-GIA 30 loads or one endo-GIA 60 firing is needed to assure sufficient anastomotic lumen. The end of the anastomosis is closed with endo-GIA stapling (Fig. 22-4). The mesenteric window is then reapproximated. However, since such a small mesenteric window was made to create the loop, only a small amount of suture or laparoscopic staples are needed to close the defect.

The left ureter is carefully tunneled with a blunt probe under the sigmoid mesocolon and is carried to the right side of the pelvis. It is necessary to avoid any twisting of the left ureter during this passage. The ureters are then placed next to the site on the ileal conduit to which they will reach without tension. Each ureter can be spatulated with endoscopic scissors. A small enterotomy is made in the ileal segment with laparoscopic scissors at the proposed site of ureteroileal anastomosis. Using intracorporeal suturing techniques, the ureter is anchored to the bowel using an absorbable suture such as 4-0 Vicryl. Two separate strands of sutures are used to run the backside of the anastomosis first. This continuous suture holds the ureter in place until a ureteral stent is passed into the ipsilateral kidney.

The stomal, or distal, end of the loop is brought out through the 12-mm trocar site in the right lower quadrant after the fascial incision is enlarged (Fig. 22-5). A flexible cystoscope is passed through the conduit, and a guidewire followed by diversionary ureteral stent is passed endoscopically through the ileal loop and up the ureter. Once the stent is in a good position, the front side of the ureteroileal anastomosis is completed with the second, running absorbable suture.

In our initial attempt, the ureteroileal anastomosis was performed as an extracorporeal procedure. This was done by pulling the respective ureter and proximal stump of ileal loop out of a trocar site. Using the suprapubic trocar site for the left ureter and the right lower quadrant trocar site for the right ureter, an extracorporeal anastomosis can be performed in a standard fashion. This extracorporeal technique, however, is somewhat cumbersome and time-consuming,

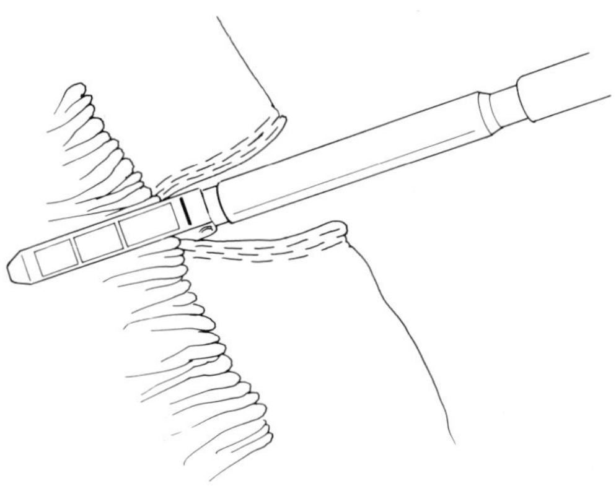

Figure 22-2. Second firing of the GIA stapler to staple and transect 2 cm of mesentery.

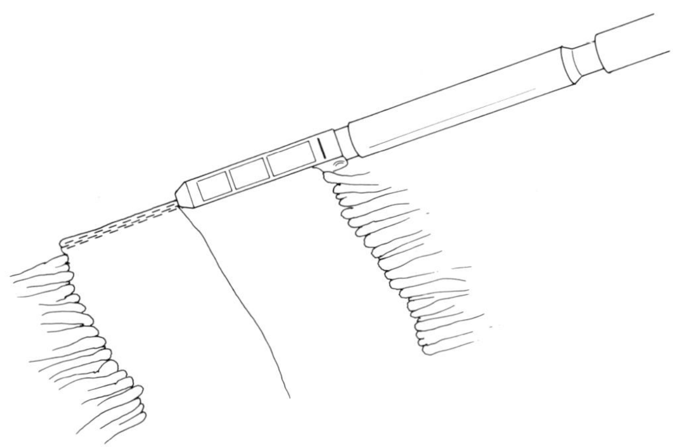

Figure 22-4. Closure of the anastomosis with the stapler.

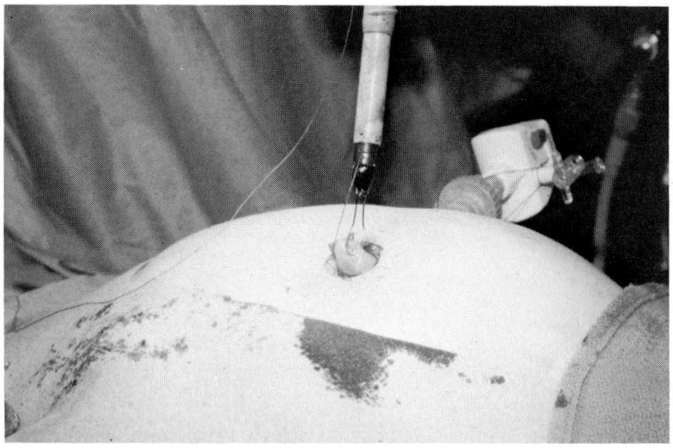

Figure 22–5. Creating the ileal loop stoma at the 12-mm trocar site in the right lower quadrant.

because the pneumoperitoneum has to be deflated and re-created several times. More important, the ureteral anastomosis can be jeopardized by pulling the bowel and ureter in and out of the small trocar openings.

The stoma is secured to the fascia and skin as for standard open ileal conduit diversion. A multi-eyelet red robinson catheter is left in the ileal loop conduit for several days until postoperative ileus is resolved.

Through the lower quadrant trocar sites under direct visual guidance, two closed suction drains are placed in the pelvis adjacent to the ureteroileal anastomosis (Fig. 22–6). The greater omentum is gently repositioned over the bowel in the pelvis. All the trocars are removed under camera guidance, and the small access wounds are closed in the standard manner.

Postoperatively the nasogastric tube suction is removed after resolution of ileus. Pelvic drains can be removed when the drainage is of minimal amount. The ureteral stents are left in place approximately 3 to 4 weeks. Follow-up intravenous pyelogram is done to assess the final result and the condition of the upper tracts several weeks after discharge.

CONCLUSIONS

With the advent of technologic aids and experience in laparoscopy, it is conceivable that virtually all open surgical procedures in the abdomen can be accomplished laparoscopically. Removal of defunctionalized bladder by laparoscopic cystectomy has been reported.[3] Improved containment sacks and tissue removal systems will enable venturing into radial cystectomy for malignant pathologies. In females, such specimens can be conveniently extracted through the vagina. In the near future, it should be feasible to synchronously combine procedures such as cystectomy or anterior exenteration with supravesical urinary division by laparoscopic techniques. Laparoscopic bowel resection procedures are becoming commonplace among general surgeons. Newer devices for vascular control and improved intestinal staplers of various contours and configurations are revolutionizing intestinal surgery through the laparoscope. At the same time, manufacturers are aware of the need for absorbable stapling devices for use on the urothelium. Combination of these intestinal surgical techniques, suitable staplers for urologic purposes, and improved intracorporeal suturing techniques will allow the construction of a continent urinary reservoir entirely through the laparoscope in the not-so-distant future. Research is ongoing to accomplish the full potential of laparoscopic reconstructive surgery in urology. "If it is possible, it has been done; if it is impossible it will be done."

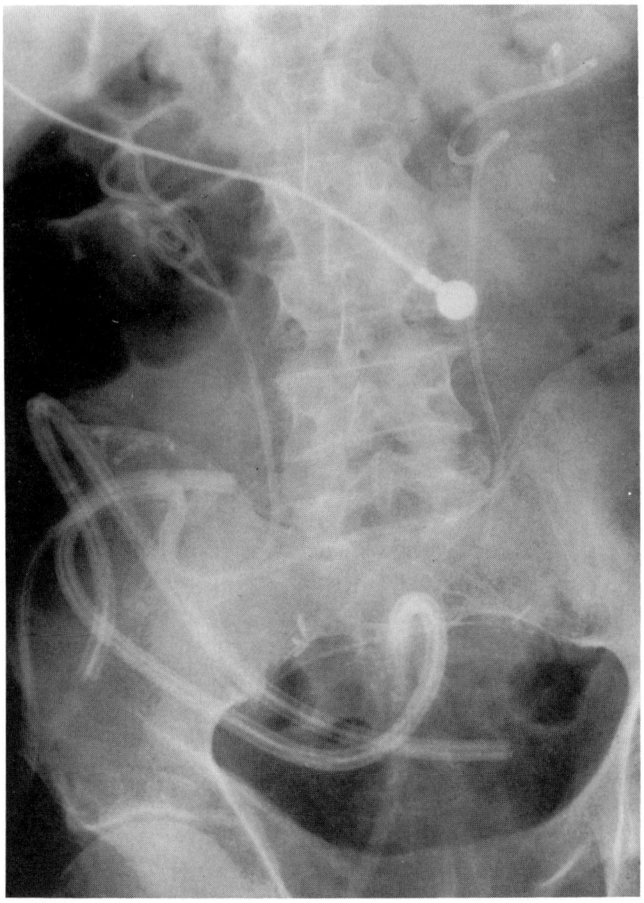

Figure 22–6. An abdominal x-ray, checking the positioning of ureteral stents and suction drains.

REFERENCES

1. Bricker, EM: Bladder substitution after pelvic evisceration. Surg Clin North Am 30:1511, 1950.
2. Kozminski, M; Partamian, KO: Case report of laparoscopic ileal loop conduit. J Endourol 6:147, 1992.
3. Parra, RO; Andrus, CH; Jones, JP; Boullier, JA: Laparoscopic cystectomy: Initial report on a new treatment for the retained bladder. J Urol 148:1140, 1992.

CHAPTER 23

Laparoscopic Surgery for Adrenal Tumors

Kazuo Suzuki, MD
Shinji Kageyama, MD
Daisuke Ueda, MD
Tomomi Ushiyama, MD
Kazuki Kawabe, MD

The surgical approach to the adrenal gland varies widely according to the size and endocrine nature of the tumor to be resected. The anterior, posterior, flank, or thoracoabdominal approaches are preferable in individual cases. The recent progress in medical imaging techniques has made it uncommon to use a bilateral posterior or anterior "chevron" incision for bilateral adrenal exposure. However, the skin incision for adrenalectomy is still large and causes a considerable cosmetic defect. The introduction of high-resolution videoendoscopy systems has permitted surgeons to employ laparoscopic surgery for a variety of procedures. Since laparoscopic cholecystectomy was reported by Mouret in 1987,[1] this technique has rapidly been applied to various diseases requiring cholecystectomy[2,3] and to urologic procedures such as pelvic lymph node dissection,[4,5] varix ligation,[6] nephrectomy,[7-9] ureterolysis,[10] bladder neck suspension,[11] and ileal loop conduit construction.[12] The minimally invasive nature of such surgery is a major advantage. Although adrenal tumors are relatively small and may seem to be suitable for laparoscopic surgery, laparoscopic adrenalectomy has been reported from only a few institutions.[13-16] This may be because adrenal tumors are located in the deep retroperitoneal tissues and are surrounded by abundant perinephric fat. In addition, the adrenal gland is extremely fragile and difficult to grasp at operation. Based on our experience with various newly developed techniques, the latest methods for laparoscopic adrenalectomy are detailed in this chapter, and our clinical experience is presented.

INDICATIONS

Two major points should be considered when determining the indications for laparoscopic adrenalectomy.[13] The first is the size and site of the adrenal tumor, and the second is the type of endocrine dysfunction. Size is an important factor in determining the malignancy of adrenal tumors. The capsule of an adrenal tumor is usually thin and the lesion itself tends to be brittle, so the tumor can easily be ruptured by grasping or pulling during laparoscopic surgery. Accordingly, laparoscopic adrenalectomy for malignant tumors has a potentially high risk of disseminating malignant cells inside the abdominal cavity. Aso and co-workers analyzed 210 patients with incidental adrenal masses and found that all malignant tumors were larger than 6.5 cm in diameter and occurred in patients aged 58 years or younger.[17] Since the tumor should be endoscopically removed en bloc, using an entrapment sac through an 11-mm trocar wound, only lesions to 5 to 6 cm in size are suitable for laparoscopic adrenalectomy. Regarding hormone-producing adrenal tumors, laparoscopic adrenalectomy for pheochromocytoma is controversial. Laparoscopic surgery requires more prolonged tumor manipulation when compared with open adrenalectomy, so the pheochromocytoma patient should be healthy enough to tolerate a prolonged hypertensive period during laparoscopic resection. To prevent intraoperative myocardial dysfunction or cerebral hemorrhage, the patient should have neither previous myocardial injury nor arteriosclerosis. In addition, the blood pressure must be controlled, using alpha-1 and calcium channel blockers before the operation. If the adrenal pheochromocytoma has developed under the liver or inferior vena cava on the right, a laparoscopic procedure should also be avoided. It is necessary to place Cushing's syndrome patients in an appropriate position before operation, because such patients often have systemic osteoporosis, and unexpected pathologic fracture may occur. Additional postoperative care to prevent infection is necessary in such patients. Furthermore, excessive dissection of the perinephric fat must be avoided during laparoscopic adrenalectomy, since unexpected bleeding can occur while separating the tumor from this fatty tissue because Cushing's syndrome patients often have an increased tendency to bleed. Accordingly, careful separation using scissors with clipping or electrocautery is recommended.

EQUIPMENT

Laparoscopic equipment for adrenalectomy consists of special forceps and scissors, a laparoscope incorporating connections to an audiovisual system, surgical ports, and the CO_2 insufflation system.

The surgical forceps and scissors are almost the same as those normally employed for laparoscopic cholecystectomy. Compared with cholecystectomy, however, adrenalectomy is performed at a deeper location, and some special instruments are needed. The authors have devised some new instruments in cooperation with the Olympus Optical Co* to make the procedure more convenient. Since the adrenal gland is relatively fragile, the forceps used should allow meticulous manipulation. In addition to straight forceps, three types of curved forceps were developed, and these have proved useful for freeing the adrenal from the surrounding tissue. An Endo-Babcock† is a useful instrument for grasping the adrenal gland, and an Endoretract† allows easy retraction with virtually no tissue trauma, providing excellent retraction of large structures such as the liver and spleen (Fig. 23–1).

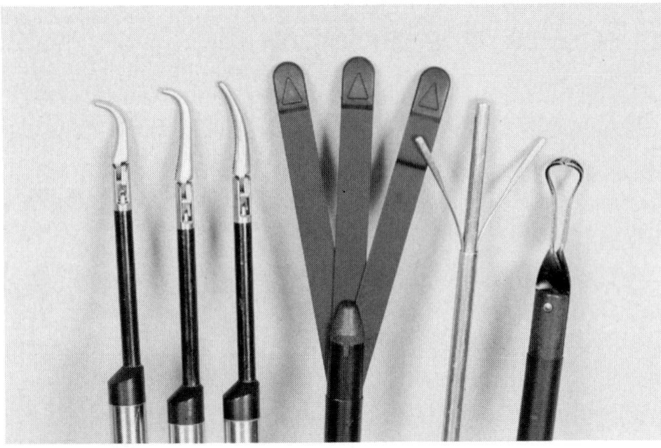

Figure 23–1. Special forceps and retractors used for laparoscopic adrenalectomy.

An ultrasonic endoaspirator* (Fig. 23–2) and an argon-beam coagulator‡ are useful for exposing and dividing the adrenal vessels and surrounding tissues and for controlling hemorrhage from the liver surface. The USU endoaspirator also has many additional functions (irrigation, suction, cauterization, and cutting) combined in one handpiece.

The laparoscope used is 5 mm or 10 mm in diameter, and the 10-mm scope has a 0° or 30° angle. The 30° angle laparoscope is used at deep sites to keep the intestines away from the surgical field. A video guidance system is indispensable for laparoscopic surgery. With a clearer image, surgical manipulation becomes safer, and procedures in a restricted field can be more successfully performed. Accordingly, an elaborate video system is essential for laparoscopic surgery. Three-dimensional imaging systems are currently under development by several companies to replace the charged-coupled device (CCD) camera, and this should enable more rapid progress to be made in laparoscopic surgery in the future.

The working ports are changed according to the patient's position and the tumor location, but three 10-mm trocars and two 5-mm trocars are generally used. Of late, a Hasson-type trocar (a 10-mm blunt-tipped trocar) has been inserted first, without any pneumoperitoneum, through a small incision. In the most recent procedures, a small midline abdominal incision has been made, and two specially designed

†US Surgical Co, Norwalk, CT.
*Olympus Optical Co, Tokyo, Jpn.
‡Bard Co, Covington, GA.

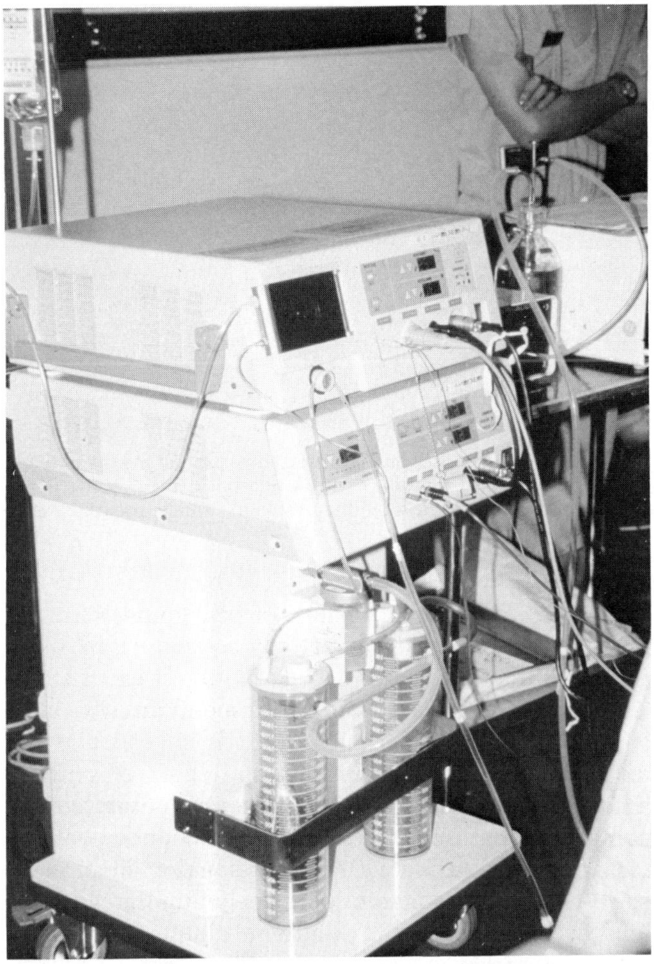

Figure 23–2. Ultrasonic endoaspirator (USU, Olympus Co., Tokyo, Japan).

retractors (Fig. 23–3) have been applied to each side of this incision while another special retractor is inserted in the abdominal cavity. The abdominal wall has then been lifted by raising these retractors, which are hung from a liver retractor.*[18] This allows sufficient working space to be created inside the abdominal cavity without the need for a pneumoperitoneum. This laparoscopy-assisted surgery is a safe method of preventing CO_2 embolism or the other complications of pneumoperitoneum,[19] and it should also be of benefit in patients with poor respiratory function such as those with Cushing's syndrome or elderly individuals.

PROCEDURE

Preoperative Preparation

The preoperative management of hormone-producing adrenal tumors is the same as for open adrenalectomy.

*Heimrich C, Ulrich Co, Ulm-Donay, Germany.

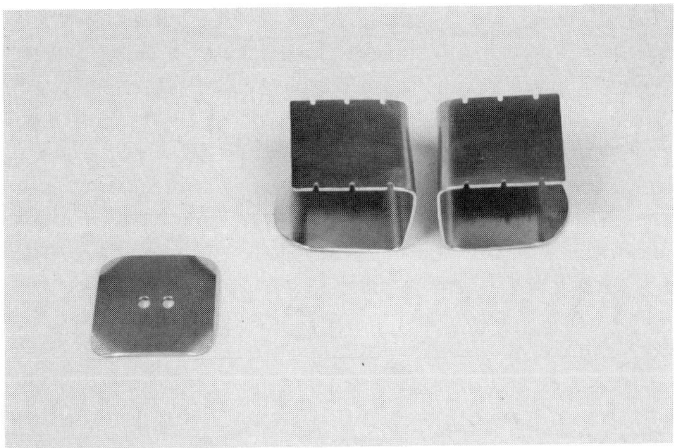

Figure 23–3. Our original abdominal wall retractors used in laparoscopy-assisted surgery. Two 5-cm wide curved retractors are attached to the sides of the small incision and a 5-cm square plane retractor is then inserted into the abdominal cavity.

The most important points regarding laparoscopic adrenalectomy include sufficient bowel preparation to avoid the risk of intestinal damage during laparoscopy and to improve field of view and preoperative respiratory physiotherapy for Cushing's syndrome patients to improve ventilation. Renal and adrenal venography is advisable, because there are many variations in the anatomy of the adrenal vein.

Positioning the Patient and Inserting Trocars

Laparoscopic adrenalectomy is basically performed under general endotracheal anesthesia. Adequate and frequent ventilatory monitoring with arterial blood gas analysis and end-tidal CO_2 determination is required, because some CO_2 retention has to be anticipated owing to exposure of the fatty tissue of the retroperitoneum to the pneumoperitoneum. A nasogastric tube is placed in the stomach, and a Foley catheter is inserted in the urinary bladder. The patient is placed in the semilateral position. In the original procedure, a Verres needle was then inserted at the superior crease of the umbilicus. Recently, we have not blindly inserted a Verres needle and a trocar at the superior margin of the umbilicus for fear of causing intra-abdominal trauma. Instead, a Hasson-type blunt-tipped trocar is inserted into a small skin incision, after which a laparoscope is inserted. A second 5-mm trocar is then placed approximately three fingerbreadths below the xyphoid process. In addition, two 10- to 11-mm trocars are inserted, one in the midclavicular line, 5 cm below the costal margin, and the second in the anterior axillary line, just below the costal margin. After the patient is rotated laterally to displace the small bowel, another 5-mm trocar is inserted in the posterior axillary line just below the costal margin (Fig. 23–4).

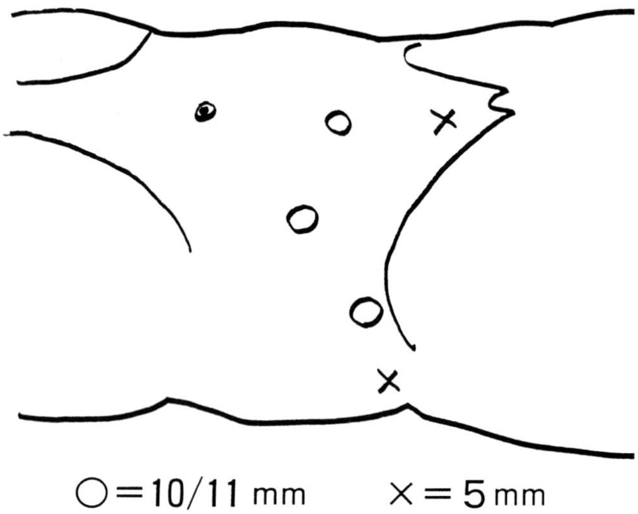

Figure 23–4. Diagram of trocar placement for laparoscopic adrenalectomy.

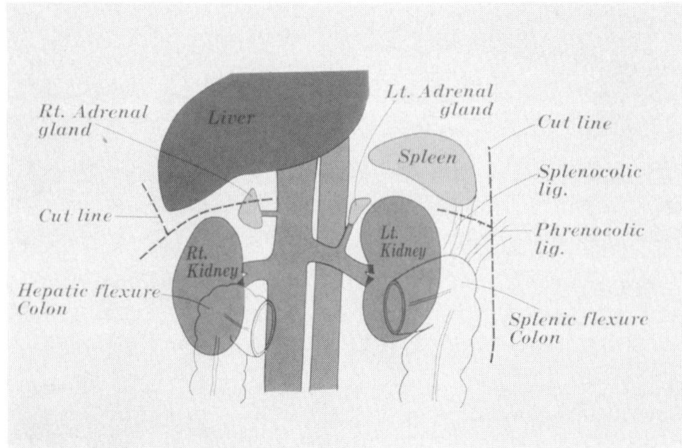

Figure 23–6. Laparoscopic anatomic diagram of the abdominal cavity showing the relation of both adrenal glands to the liver, aorta, inferior vena cava, kidney, spleen, small intestine, and colon.

We have found that elevation of the arterial CO_2 level is inevitable even when the CO_2 insufflation pressure is kept below 8 mmHg. Therefore of late we have tried to perform laparoscopy-assisted surgery without a pneumoperitoneum.[18] Two specially designed retractors are attached to the sides of a small abdominal incision and another special retractor (a 5-cm square metal plane) is inserted in the abdomen (see Fig. 23–3). The abdominal wall is then suspended by raising the retractors, and they are hung from a liver retractor (Fig. 23–5). Sufficient working space inside the abdominal cavity can be created by this technique without the need for a pneumoperitoneum.

Laparoscopic Anatomy

The adrenal gland is located deep in the retroperitoneal tissue and is surrounded by abundant perinephric fat. Laparoscopic adrenalectomy is performed by a transperitoneal approach (Fig. 23–6). With the patient in a semilateral position, the small intestine and colon are reflected medially and inferiorly as a result of the pneumoperitoneum and the effect of gravity, and the peritoneal cavity is observed laterally. By using the laparoscope, we can obtain a closer field of view than is possible with conventional open surgery, so the surgeon needs to be extremely familiar with the laparoscopic anatomy. The adrenal glands do not have similar anatomy on both sides. The right gland lies close to the inferior vena cava and below the liver bed, whereas the left gland nestles close to the tail of the spleen. Each gland is supplied by numerous blood vessels that are independent of the kidney. A detailed knowledge of the anatomy of the adrenal gland is of great benefit during laparoscopic surgery and an understanding of the relevant arteries and veins is most important for achieving hemostasis.

The laparoscopic anatomy of the adrenal and the main variations are described in the following paragraphs.

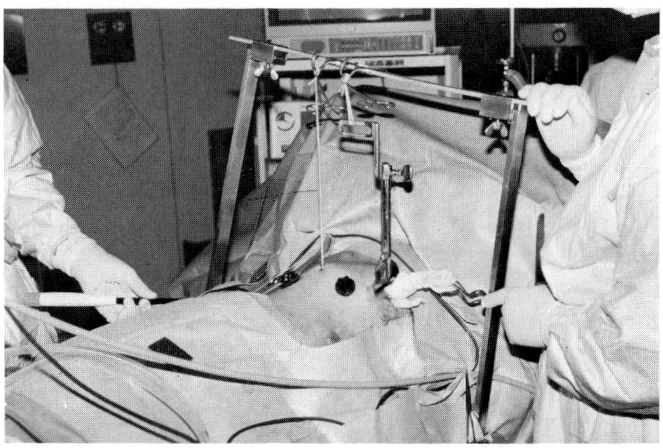

Figure 23–5. The patient is placed in the lateral position, and the abdominal cavity is expanded by lifting the retractors.

Arterial Supply

Hureau and colleagues[20] and Sato[21] demonstrated four sources of blood supply to the adrenal, including branches from the renal artery, the aorta, the inferior phrenic artery, and other arteries (Fig. 23–7). The branch coming from the inferior phrenic artery is commonly named the superior adrenal artery; the branch arising from the aorta is usually named the middle adrenal artery; and the branch from the renal artery is called the inferior adrenal artery. These vessels and the other surrounding arteries are so thin that they are often missed at surgery.

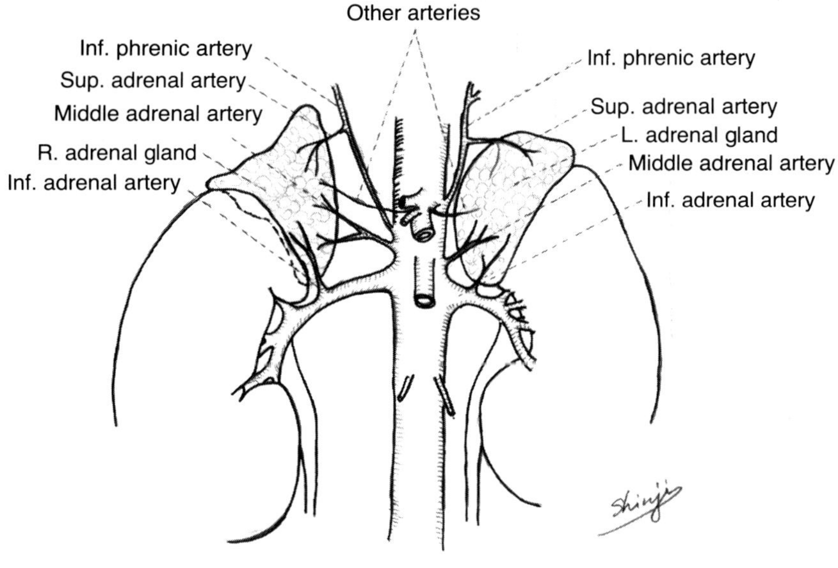

Figure 23–7. Variation of the arterial blood supply to the adrenal gland. Inf., inferior; L, left; R, right; Sup., superior. (Compiled from Hureau, J; Hidden, G; Than, M: The vascularization of the suprarenal glands. Anat Clin 2:127–146, 1980, and Sato, T: Regional anatomy for operative surgery of genitourinary organs: Adrenal gland. Jpn J Clin Urol 45:388–394, 1991.) (In Japanese.)

Venous Supply

Management of the adrenal veins is the most important part of a laparoscopic procedure, because many variations in the venous anatomy may be encountered at surgery. The normal venous drainage is shown in Figure 23–8. The most important variations are the presence of a dilated vein on the right side and variations in the site at which the left adrenal vein enters the renal vein. For that reason, preoperative phlebography is helpful.

On the right side, the adrenal vein drains into the inferior vena cava at a variable level. A dilated vein usually develops at the midportion of the adrenal gland, but it is sometimes encountered near the upper or lower pole. In our experience, the superior adrenal vein drains into the inferior phrenic vein, which sometimes becomes dilated. If the dilated vein is in a high position, the surgical procedure becomes difficult. A vein that is a branch of the renal vein is classically known as the accessory adrenal vein. There are many variations of the numerous small veins in the surrounding tissues.

On the left side, a dilated vein is generally observed at the lower aspect of the adrenal gland and is commonly named the adrenal vein. In some cases, the adrenal vein drains relatively proximally into the renal vein. Since the site of entry is adjacent to the abdominal aorta, surgical procedures must be done extremely carefully. A vein communicating with the inferior phrenic vein may be observed and may be considerably dilated in some cases. A small vein found

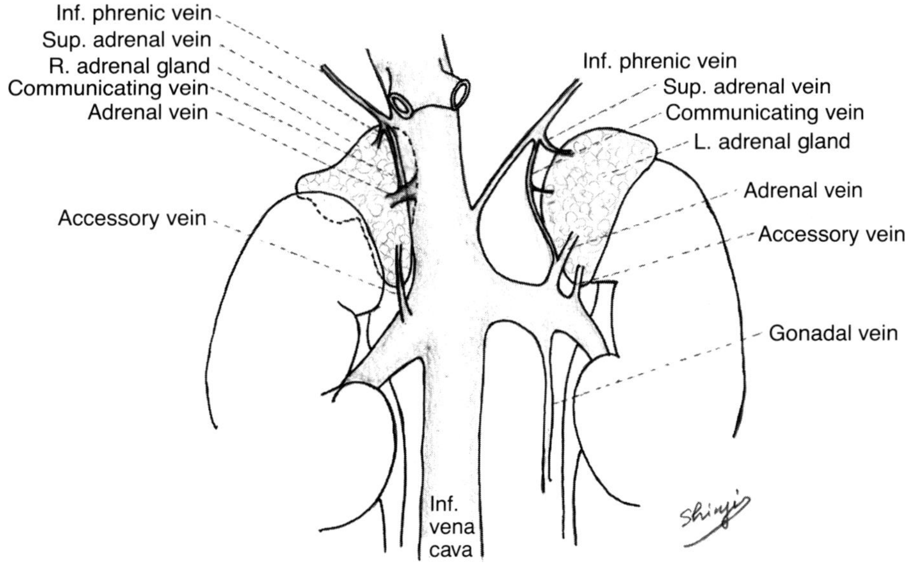

Figure 23–8. Normal venous drainage of the adrenal glands. Inf., inferior; L., left; R., right; Sup., superior. (Compiled from Schwartz, IS: Pituitary and adrenal surgery. In: Principles of Surgery, 4th ed. New York, McGraw-Hill Book Co, 1990, p 1489, and Kumita, T: Über die Lymphgepose der Nieren und Nebennierankapsel. Arch Anat Physiol, Anat Abt Jahrgang, 1909, 49–58, 1939.)

at the lower pole of the adrenal gland usually drains into the renal vein, but it sometimes joins the adrenal vein and is commonly named the adrenal accessory vein.

Surrounding Organs

In the case of right adrenalectomy, the upper pole of the adrenal is sometimes strongly adherent to the inferior surface of the liver. In addition, the adrenal gland is positioned so deeply that special forceps are needed to lift the lobe of the liver during surgery. In the case of left adrenalectomy, great care must be taken to avoid injury to the spleen and pancreas.

Technique

The adrenal gland exhibits a different anatomic structure on each side. The blood supply and its relationship with the surrounding organs are quite different on the right and left sides. Therefore different surgical techniques are required for each side. The view of the abdominal cavity obtained at laparoscopic surgery is somewhat different from that at open surgery. Open adrenalectomy through the transperitoneal approach is usually performed in the supine or semilateral position as opposed to the lateral position for laparoscopic adrenalectomy. The small intestine and colon are already reflected medially, and the kidney can be detected behind the retroperitoneum at the start of laparoscopic surgery.

Right Adrenalectomy

The line of the peritoneal incision is shown in Figure 23–9. The area for making this incision is clearly found by raising the liver (Fig. 23–10). However, sharp dissection of the large omentum and the peritoneum from the liver is often necessary because of adhesions. Incision of the posterior peritoneum is made from the hepatic flexure of the colon to near the duodenum and is extended along the lateral margin of the liver. The vena cava and the perinephric fat are disclosed by incision of Gerota's fascia. Dissection of the anterior surface of the adrenal gland should be commenced just below the diaphragm, because separating the diaphragm from the adrenal gland, which is covered with perinephric fat, is important for determining the correct plane of dissection. Next, the vena cava and the right renal vein are exposed. Recently, we have used an ultrasonic endoaspirator and an argon beam coagulator for exposing the adrenal vessels and stopping bleeding from the liver surface. In a case with pheochromocytoma, the adrenal vein should be separated and clipped before tumor manipulation. Although this procedure is extremely difficult on the right side, the introduction of an ultrasonic endoaspirator makes it easy to prepare the adrenal vein. The accessory adrenal vein draining into the right renal

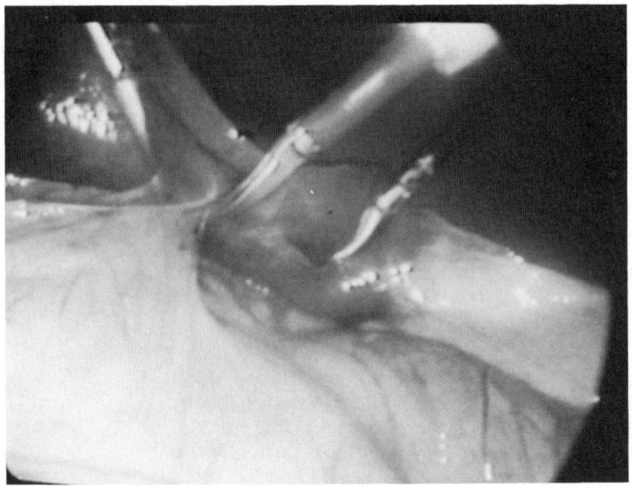

A

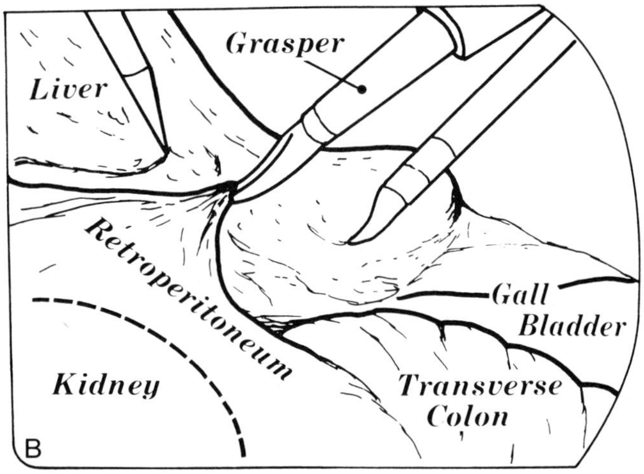

B

Figure 23–10. *A* and *B*, By raising the liver and the gallbladder, the site for making the incision is exposed.

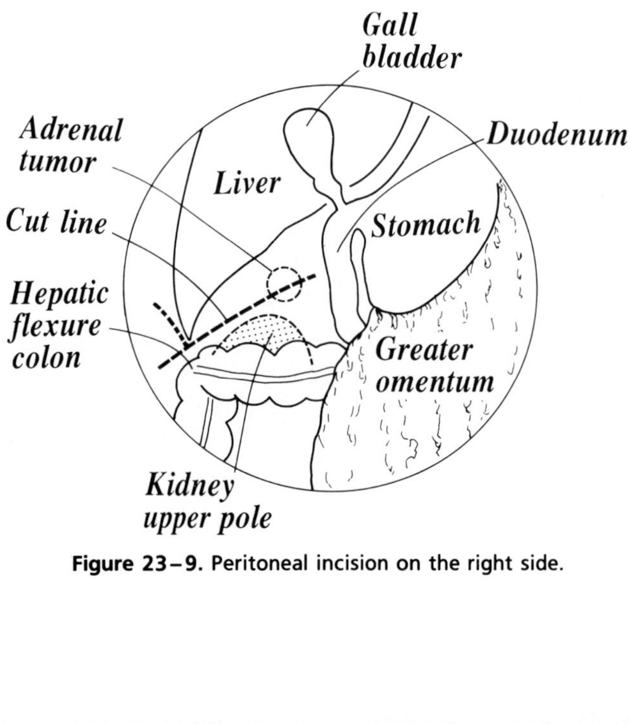

Figure 23–9. Peritoneal incision on the right side.

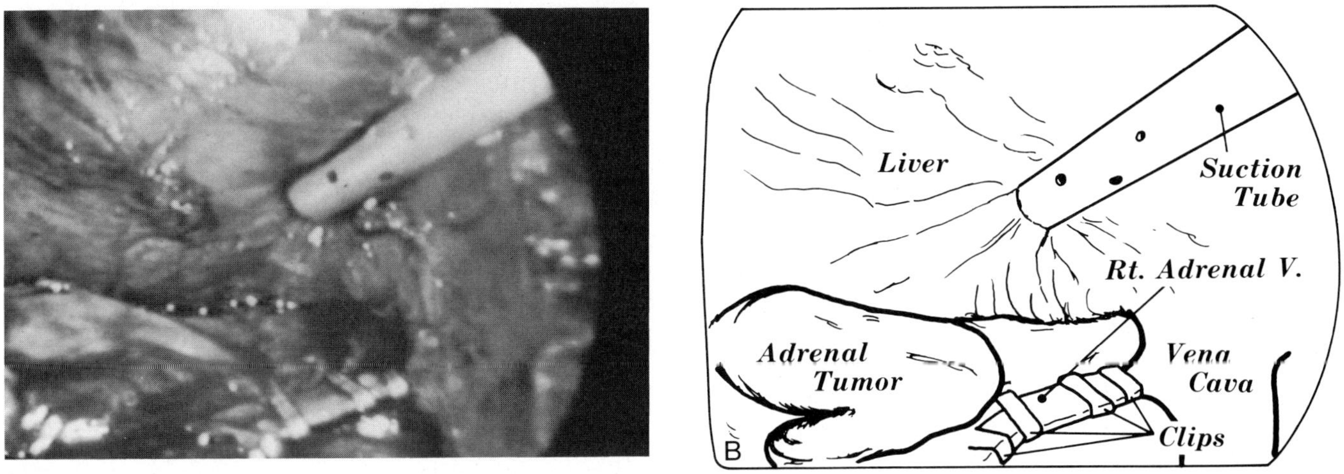

A

Figure 23–11. *A* and *B*, The right adrenal vein is exposed after careful dissection of the inferior vena cava and the psoas muscle. Rt., right; V, vein.

vein and the inferior adrenal artery are exposed, clipped, and cut. Then the lateral side of the vena cava is dissected with the ultrasonic endoaspirator, and the surface of the psoas muscle is exposed. After upward dissection along the psoas muscle, the adrenal vein is identified (Fig. 23–11). In early procedures, we pulled the adrenal tumor laterally to expose the adrenal vessels (Fig. 23–12). However, tugging on the adrenal vein is dangerous, because it is short and fragile. Accordingly, preparation should be careful, using an ultrasonic endoaspirator. After complete exposure, the adrenal vein is transected. A multiple-load clip applier is used to place two clips on the proximal end and one or two clips on the distal end of the adrenal vein. After preparation of the adrenal vein, the lower pole of the gland is lifted, and the several small arteries and veins in this region are dissected with the ultrasonic endoaspirator, electrocautry, and clipping. Next, the lateral side of the adrenal gland is separated from the perinephric fat, which is followed by separation of the upper pole from the diaphragm in the same way. Finally, the upper medial part of the adrenal gland is separated from the vena cava and liver. The superior adrenal vein, which drains into the inferior phrenic vein, is sometimes dilated in patients with a right adrenal tumor. Dissection of this vein can also be dangerous but is extremely important. In about one third of the patients with a right adrenal tumor, the upper pole of the adrenal gland is embedded in the liver, and dissection is difficult. Although we had to leave a small portion of normal adrenal tissue in early cases, following the introduction of an argon beam

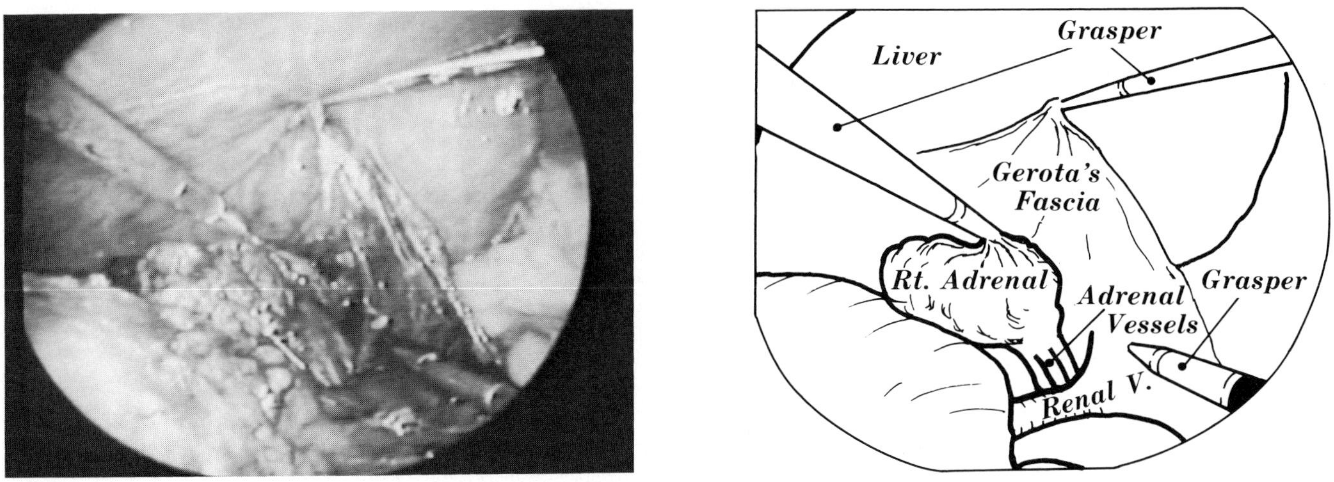

A B

Figure 23–12. *A* and *B*, By pulling the adrenal tumor laterally, the right adrenal vessels come into view. Rt., right; V, vein.

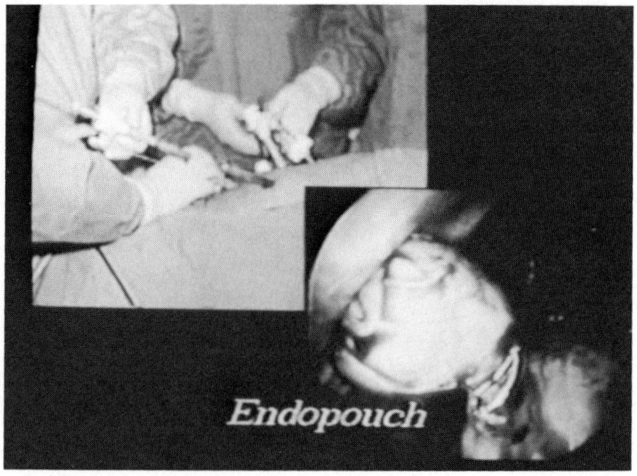

Figure 23–13. The adrenal tumor is enclosed with an Endopouch and removed through the trocar wound.

coagulator, we can now completely remove the gland along with a margin of the adjacent liver tissue.

When the adrenal tumor is completely freed, it is enclosed in an Endopouch* and removed through the 11-mm trocar wound (Fig. 23–13). In our early cases, an approximately 2-cm long wound extension was needed for en bloc removal. After we began to perform open laparoscopy to avoid the complications of blind trocar puncture, almost all the adrenal tumors could be extracted en bloc through the laparoscopy incision. More recently, we have performed laparoscopy-assisted adrenalectomy for patients with ventilatory complications, pheochromocytoma, or both as mentioned previously. This method also allows the adrenal tumor to be removed en bloc through the abdominal incision. After adrenalectomy, the trocars are safely removed under laparoscopic observation. A Penrose drain is not usually inserted. However, when there is minor bleeding from the liver surface, slight oozing, or both, a Penrose drain should be left in overnight. The retroperitoneal space is covered by the colon without suturing the peritoneum. The nasogastric tube is removed after wound closure.

Postoperatively, all patients are allowed to begin oral intake on the night of surgery and are walking by the next morning. Postoperative management of hormone-producing adrenal tumors (i.e., steroid replacement for Cushing's syndrome and the like) is the same as with conventional open adrenalectomy.

Left Adrenalectomy

A laparoscopic view of the left upper abdominal cavity in the lateral position is demonstrated in Figure 23–14. If the patient is not obese and has no omental or bowel adhesions, the phrenocolic ligament and the splenocolic ligament are clearly observed at laparoscopy.

The incision in the retroperitoneum is made from the phrenocolic ligament and extended in two directions, transversely beside the transverse colon and vertically along the spleen and the descending colon (Fig. 23–15). The descending colon and the transverse colon are then separated from Gerota's fascia. Next, Gerota's fascia is incised and spread out medially and superiorly together with the retroperitoneum. For the same reason as for the right side, the anterior surface of the adrenal gland should initially be dissected just below the diaphragm. The left renal vein is then dissected carefully, and the small arteries and veins crossing the renal vein are electrocauterized. The adrenal vein is identified where it joins the proximal part of the left renal vein (Fig. 23–16). This point differs

*Ethicon Co, New Brunswick, NJ.

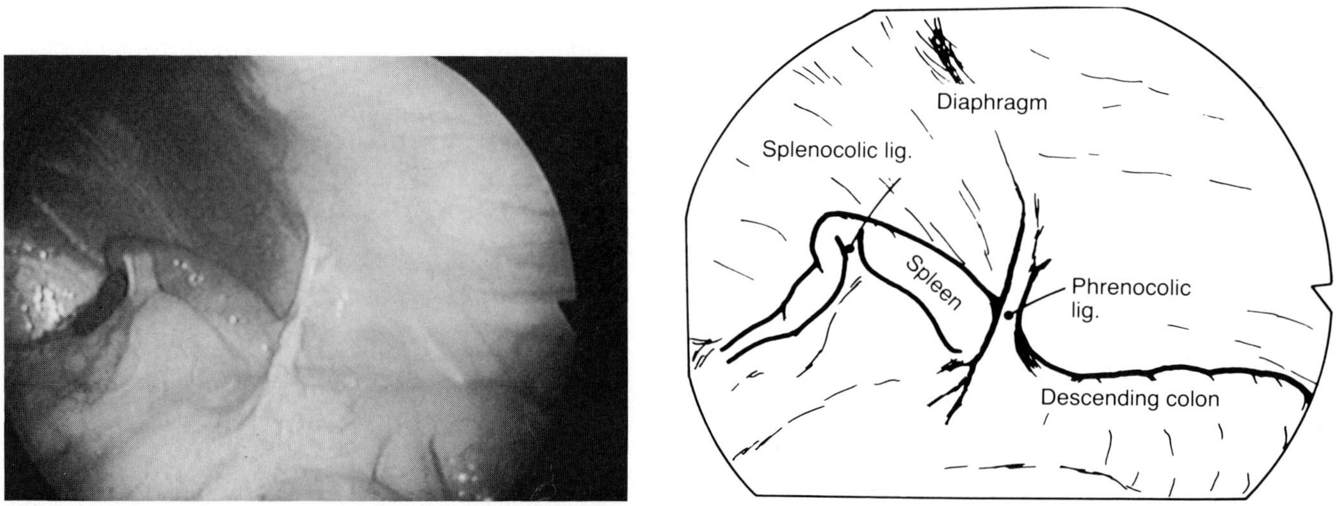

A B

Figure 23–14. *A* and *B*, If the patient is not obese, the phrenocolic and splenocolic ligaments are clearly observed. Lig., ligament.

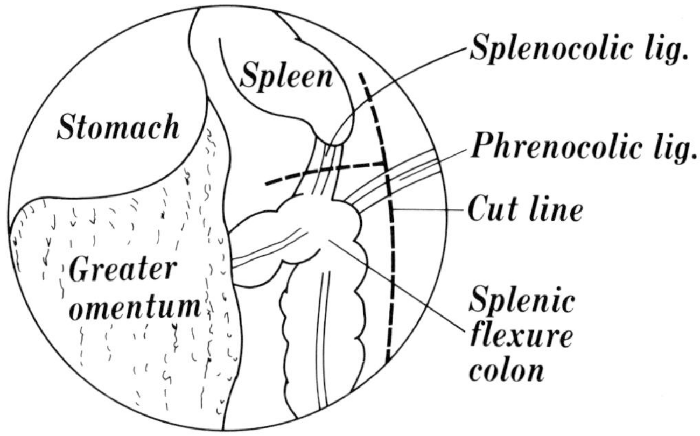

Figure 23–15. Peritoneal incision on the left side. Lig., ligament.

slightly among individuals, and various anomalies of the left renal, gonadal, or adrenal veins can be observed in a few cases (Fig. 23–17). Therefore, to confirm the locations of these veins, preoperative adrenal venography is most important. A small adrenal acces-

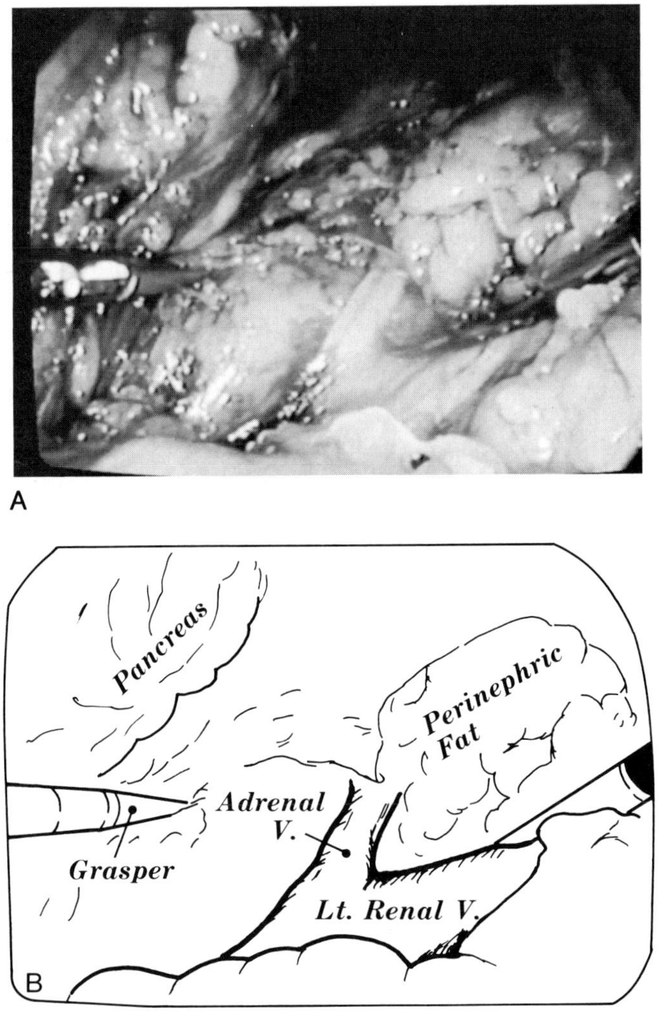

Figure 23–16. *A* and *B*, The left renal and adrenal veins are clearly observed. Lt., left, V, vein.

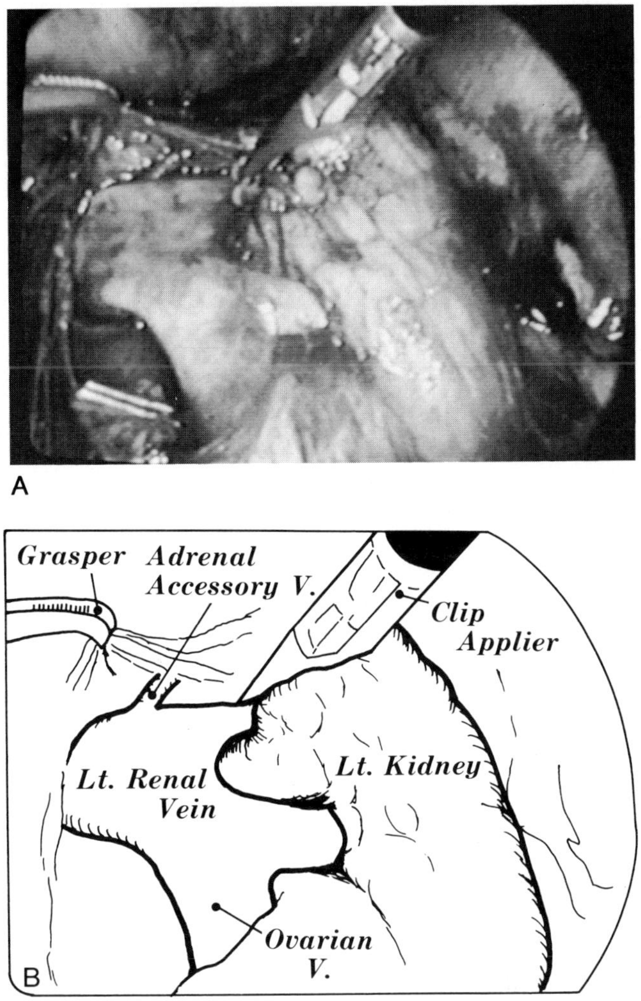

Figure 23–17. *A* and *B*, Anomaly of the left renal vein. The left adrenal vein enters the renal vein more proximally and is not yet exposed in this figure. Lt., left; V., vein.

sory vein that runs to the left renal vein is usually located distal to the adrenal vein. After dissection of this accessory vein, the adrenal vein is clipped and cut in the usual fashion. The subsequent procedures for left adrenalectomy are performed in the same manner as on the right side. The superior adrenal vein that drains into the inferior phrenic vein should be handled carefully. Separation of the upper pole of the left adrenal gland is relatively easy compared with a similar separation on the right side. If the retroperitoneum is widely incised, two or three metal clips should be placed in it adjacent to the splenic flexure of the colon.

RESULTS AND COMPLICATIONS

Since February 14, 1992, we have performed laparoscopic adrenalectomy in 19 patients (11 males and eight females, ages 26 to 64 years) with various endocrine disorders. The clinical diagnosis was primary aldosteronism in eight patients, pheochromocytoma in

Table 23–1. RESULTS AND COMPLICATIONS OF LAPAROSCOPIC ADRENALECTOMY IN 19 PATIENTS

Result	Average	Range
Operating time	253 minutes	182–470
Estimated blood loss	295 ml	60–2100
Weight of specimen	12.9 g	6.2–34.8
Complication	**No. of Patients**	
Hemorrhage (>500 ml)	4	
Blood transfusion	3	
Wound infection	1	
Paralytic ileus	1	
High fever (>38°C)	5	
Shoulder pain	1	

three, Cushing's syndrome due to a solitary adrenal adenoma in three, pre-Cushing's syndrome in one, and nonfunctioning adrenal adenoma in four. Seven tumors were located on the right side and 12 on the left. There were no malignancies among these tumors. The patients with pheochromocytoma had neither myocardial impairment nor arteriosclerosis, and their blood pressure was controlled by alpha-1 and calcium channel blockers before the operation. All operations were performed with the informed consent of the patient.

The mean operating time (from Verres needle puncture to wound closure) was 253 minutes (182 to 470 minutes), and the mean blood loss was estimated to be 295 ml. Massive intraoperative bleeding occurred in four patients, of whom three required blood transfusion. The cause of hemorrhage was injury to a capsular artery of the left kidney in one patient with Cushing's syndrome, bleeding from small left adrenal vessels in one patient with pheochromocytoma, bleeding from the right upper adrenal vein in another, and bleeding from the left adrenal accessory vein following detachment of a clip in the last patient. The blood pressure of the pheochromocytoma patients was controlled with nitroglycerin, phentolamine, and adenosinetriphosphate during the operation.

Although several minor complications (wound infection, mild paralytic ileus, and so forth) were observed, there were no significant operative or postoperative complications apart from massive bleeding (Table 23–1). The incidence of intraoperative hemorrhage should be reduced as the surgical technique is improved and new laparoscopic instruments are introduced.

Table 23–2 shows a comparison of our 19 laparoscopic patients and our last 11 patients who underwent open adrenalectomy. Compared with open adrenalectomy, a longer operating time was needed for laparoscopic surgery. However, the postoperative recovery period (first oral intake, ambulation, and time for convalescence) was significantly shorter after the laparoscopic procedure. Thus laparoscopic adrenalectomy shortens the convalescence period and avoids large skin and muscle incisions and the need for rib resection. With further experience, both the complication rate and operating time should decrease.

CONCLUSIONS

Laparoscopic adrenalectomy is a new surgical procedure for the treatment of adrenal tumors. Although adrenal tumors are relatively small and may seem suitable for laparoscopic surgery, this procedure is actually extremely difficult because of the anatomic location. In our series, laparoscopic adrenalectomy was generally successful, although massive bleeding occurred in about 20% of the patients. This problem should be overcome as the technique is improved and new laparoscopic instruments are introduced. In addition, the indications for this procedure in patients with pheochromocytoma and relatively large tumors needs to be established in the future.

Table 23–2. COMPARISON BETWEEN LAPAROSCOPIC AND OPEN ADRENALECTOMIES

	Laparoscopic (N = 19)	Open (N = 11)	
Operation time (minutes)	253.3 ± 69.8	157.7 ± 60.9	P <0.01
Estimated blood loss (ml)	295.2 ± 547.5	297.4 ± 157.8	NS
Weight of specimen (g)	12.9 ± 7.1	18.7 ± 25.6	NS
First oral intake (days)	1.5 ± 0.84	2.6 ± 0.66	P <0.01
Ambulation (days)	1.4 ± 0.87	3.4 ± 2.1	P <0.05
Return to preoperative activity (days)	10.1 ± 3.9	23.1 ± 5.8	P <0.01

N, number; NS, not significant; P, probability.

REFERENCES

1. Mouret, P: From the first laparoscopic cholecystectomy to the frontiers of laparoscopic surgery: The future prospectives. Dig Surg 8:124–126, 1991.
2. Reddick, EJ; Hertzmann, P: A briefer history of laparoscopic general surgery. Course notes in laparoscopic general surgery. Reddick EJ, Nashville, EJR Enterprise and Laparoscope, 1990.
3. Stoker, ME; Vose, J; O'Mara, P; Maini, BS: Laparoscopic cholecystectomy—a clinical and financial analysis of 280 operations. Arch Surg 127:589–595, 1992.
4. Schuessler, WW; Vancaillie, TG; Reich, H; Griffith, DP: Transperitoneal endosurgical lymphadenectomy in patients with localized prostatic cancer. J Urol 145:988–991, 1991.
5. Winfield, HN; Donovan, JF; See, WA; et al: Laparoscopic pelvic lymph node dissection for genitourinary malignancies: Indications, techniques, and results. J Endourol 6:103–111, 1992.
6. Donovan, JF; Winfield, HN: Laparoscopic varix ligation. J Urol 147:77–86, 1992.
7. Clayman, RV; Kavoussi, LR; Soper, NJ; et al: Laparoscopic nephrectomy: Review of the initial 10 cases. J Endourol 6:127–132, 1992.
8. Suzuki, K; Ihara, H; Kurita, Y; et al: Laparoscopic nephrectomy for atrophic kidney associated with ectopic ureter in a child. Eur Urol 23:463–465, 1992.
9. Ono, Y; Sahashi, M; Yamada, S; Ohshima, S: Laparoscopic nephrectomy without morcellation for renal cell carcinoma: Report of initial two cases. J Urol 150:1222–1224, 1993.
10. Kavoussi, LR; Clayman, RV; Brunt, LM; et al: Laparoscopic ureterolysis. J Urol 147:426–429, 1992.
11. Albala, DM; Schuessler, WW; Vancaillie, TG: Laparoscopic bladder neck suspension. J Endourol 6:137–141, 1992.
12. Kozminski, M; Partamian, KO: Case report of laparoscopic ileal loop conduit. J Endourol 6:147–150, 1992.
13. Suzuki, K; Kageyama, S; Ueda, D; et al: Laparoscopic adrenalectomy: Clinical experience with 12 cases. J Urol 150:1099–1102, 1993.
14. Sardi, A; McKinnon, W: Laparoscopic adrenalectomy for primary aldosteronism. JAMA 269:989–990, 1993.
15. Gagner, M; Lacroix, A; Bolte, E: Laparoscopic adrenalectomy in Cushing's syndrome and pheochromocytoma. N Engl J Med 327:1033, 1992.
16. Higashihara, E; Tanaka, Y; Hiroe, S; et al: Laparoscopic adrenalectomy: The initial 3 cases. J Urol 149:973–976, 1993.
17. Aso, Y; Homma, Y: A survey on incidental adrenal tumors in Japan. J Urol 147:1478–1481, 1992.
18. Suzuki, K; Ihara, H; Kurita, Y; et al: Laparoscopy-assisted radical nephrectomy without pneumoperitoneum. Eur Urol (in press).
19. Wittgen, CM; Andrus, CH; Fitzgerald, SD; et al: Analysis of the hemodynamics and ventilatory effects of laparoscopic cholecystectomy. Arch Surg 126:997–1001, 1991.
20. Hureau, J; Hidden, G; Thanh, M: The vascularization of the suprarenal glands. Anat Clin 2:127–146, 1980.
21. Sato, T: Regional anatomy for operative surgery of genitourinary organs: Adrenal gland. (in Japanese). Jpn J Clin Urol 45:388–394, 1991.
22. Schwartz, IS: Pituitary and adrenal surgery. In Principles of Surgery, 4th ed. New York, McGraw-Hill Book Co., 1990, p. 489.
23. Kumita T: Uber die Lymphgefasse der Nieren und Nebennierenkapsel. Arch Anat Physiol, Anat Abt Jahrgang., Berlin, 49–58, 1939.

SECTION V

SUTURING, STAPLING, AND CLIPPING

CHAPTER 24

Laparoscopic Suturing: Principles and Techniques

Zoltan Szabo, PhD, FICS
David W. Bowyer, MD

Manual suturing and knot tying in the laparoscopic surgical field are fundamental and necessary skills for most advanced endourologic reconstructive procedures. If more and more open procedures are to be brought under the laparoscope this can only be accomplished with deft suturing skill, not only for reconstruction but also for repairing iatrogenic injuries and improving the psychologic comfort level of surgeons.

A plethora of devices have surfaced over the initial phase of laparoscopic surgery to avoid the difficulty of suturing by hand and to find easier alternatives, such as stapling, absorbable clip applications, silver beads,[1] pretied loops, prelooped sutures, lasso loops, extracorporeal knots, knot pushers, tissue welding (or gluing) techniques, all of which may have a place in tissue approximation. However, the simple, time-honored technique of manual suturing is still the standard. Without intracorporeal suturing and knotting skills the endourologic surgeon is limited in range of procedures, and when sophisticated suturing is required, he or she must convert to laparotomy, thereby eliminating the much desired patient benefit of the laparoscopic approach. Having instruments that allow good maneuverability and suture materials that are easily visualized and handled would aid in reducing suturing difficulty; however, technical skill and motivation are by far the most critical factors.

LAPAROSCOPIC CHALLENGES

Since most surgical procedures need some form of tissue reconstruction, laparoscopic suturing is important. Critical factors in its performance include (1) formal training (and supervised practice), (2) the appropriate mental approach, (3) proper strategy, (4) meticulous technique, and (5) suitable instrumentation and suture materials.

Laparoscopic hand suturing, intracorporeal knot tying, and anastomosis are considered to be among the most challenging techniques any surgeon encounters. Manual and mental dexterity (tenacity, patience, and motivation) are prime qualities. For those who are naturally so inclined, the skill acquisition path is relatively straightforward; for others, more effort is required.

Laparoscopic suturing involves precision surgical technique and is based on a two-handed application of microsurgical principles, strategies, and techniques.[2,3] Of the two techniques, laparoscopic suturing is the more difficult because of the following factors:

- Limited access
- Remote manipulation of tissues with long, rigid instruments
- Significantly reduced tactile feedback from use of long instruments

- Indirect visualization provided by a laparoscope coupled to a closed circuit television system, resulting in
  - reduced resolution (involving clarity, illumination, and distortion)
  - monocular view (two-dimensional image) and lack of depth perception
- Magnification of 2 to 15 times
- Altered eye-hand coordination
- Lack of experience resulting from the early evolutionary phase of this modality

TRAINING

The technical microsurgical skills necessary to perform advanced laparoscopic surgery must be developed in the laboratory with steplike progression to video-laparoscopic technique.

Intracorporeal suturing, being severalfold more difficult than microsurgical suturing (Fig. 24–1), requires approximately 40 to 80 hours of formal hands-on training to develop competence. This training includes work at different training stations that gradually lead to increasing complex techniques. Established standards of skill are used objectively to assess the rate of progress. Each station is designed to provide insight and skill as foundation for the next station's training exercises. Training stations include microsurgical, video-microsurgical, and video-laparoscopic. The goals include (1) magnified eye-hand coordination in the limited access surgical field, (2) the special choreography involved with needle passage and intracorporeal knot-tying techniques, and (3) learning to interpret a two-dimensional image as a virtual three-dimensional image. Exercises use various models from the inanimate to live small animals to fresh large-animal tissue, and finally live large animals. This initial training builds up visual memory and experience and increases a surgeon's confidence.

This series of exercises provides (1) a systematic progression of training steps enabling the surgeon to develop confidence and meaningful skills and (2) resource containment. Although the novice might prefer to use the large animal model early in training, it is a costly way to practice simple basics. Cost-effectiveness mandates that the surgeon first develop fundamental skills and meet minimum skill level criteria before progressing to the large animal model and then the clinical arena.

PRINCIPLES

Visual Perception

To work successfully in the magnified surgical field, it is important to understand the underlying principles of visual perception and eye-hand coordination as they relate to laparoscopic suturing skills. In the magnified surgical field, speed of movement increases in proportion to magnification. Although motion is defined as the rate of change of distance with respect to time, this does not clearly define how motion is perceived.[4] As movements become rapid, the brain becomes overwhelmed and sluggish in processing and interpreting the volume of retinal stimuli generated by the video image. The perception of motion (particularly skilled, precisely controlled motion) and the exertion of exact force, using two hands becomes too complex to be rapidly guided solely by retinal stimuli. Since the normal human brain is compelled to construct and interpret an image as quickly as possible, it will do so with the least amount of visual information available. This presents a problem for beginners, who

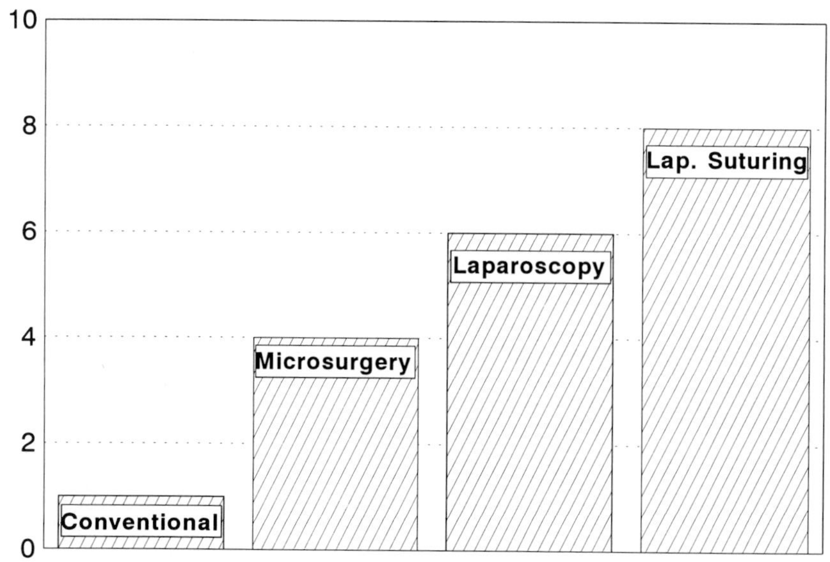

Figure 24–1. Surgical skill, relative levels of difficulty (10 is represented by suturing with closed eyes).

do not have experience to rely on or to augment this sketchy information.

The surgeon must concentrate on somatosensory inputs, using all the available clues to control movement and make correct decisions. The initial learning phase is the most demanding[5] and is often overwhelming. The immediate solution is to slow down one's movements to enrich the visual stimuli. Also, reasoning and the use of visual memory are required to augment the available visual clues and create a more informed visual perception. Microsurgical training provides the key by "training the eye." As good habits and repetitious patterns develop, the pressure gradually diminishes; however, maintaining concentration is always necessary.

A properly trained surgeon's effort during laparoscopic suturing is estimated to be expended as follows: 50%, video-visual perception; 40%, thought processing; and only 10% on actual instrument movement (Fig. 24–2). (For others, i.e., the less trained and experienced surgeons, the latter two percentages are often reversed.) Each movement made laparoscopically costs the surgeon a great deal of energy, of which a limited amount is available in a given time period. It is therefore recommended that the surgeon be in top physical and mental condition comparable to that required for competitive athletes. Alcohol and caffeine should be avoided 24 hours before surgery, because they will have a detrimental effect on performance.

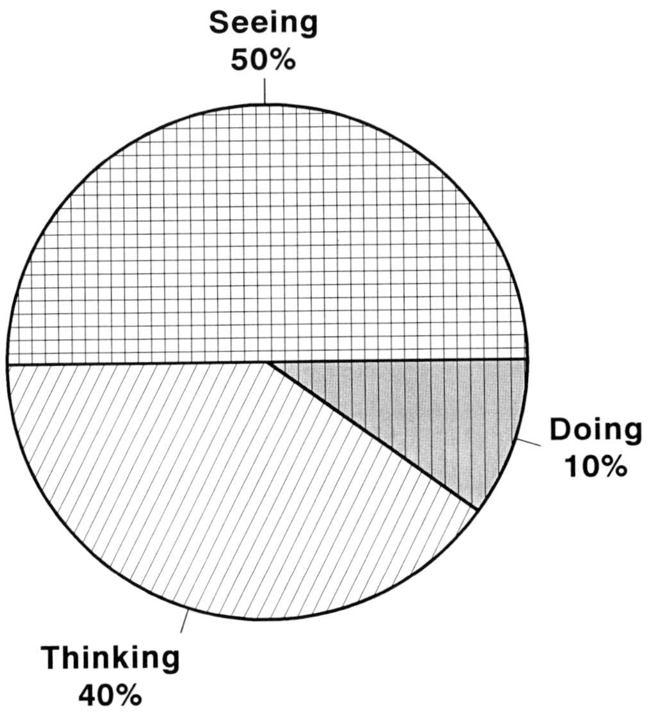

Figure 24–2. The proper proportion of surgical effort required in laparoscopic suturing and intracorporeal knot tying.

Macular Vision

Macular vision is perceived in the central portion of the retina and enables one to see a sharp image, rich in details, with good color discrimination. However, it can only be focused on a small region (comparable to the size of a full moon in the night sky). It is macular vision that is relied on to judge the critical aspects, such as the position of the needle tip or the identification of various tissue layers.

Such benefits come at a cost, because an eye-hand coordination imbalance occurs here. The harder a surgeon concentrates, the more the macular vision and the less the peripheral vision is used. As the area of acute vision narrows, the surgeon can track the activity of only one instrument tip at a time. Therefore while the assisting grasper holding adjacent tissues goes untracked, it can move in an erratic fashion, potentially causing "unattended" trauma. The normal tendency is to "lean," or push down, as can frequently be observed in novices. Calm suggestions or warnings must be issued by the assisting surgeon or camera operator to prevent disaster. Training and practice are necessary to develop two-handed coordination in which the untracked assisting grasper either releases the tissue and pulls it out of harm's way or stays steadily in position.

One's vision should be frequently checked and corrected accurately to 20/20. Corrective eyewear must be worn during laparoscopic surgery. In the unaided operative field $\pm$ 0.5 to 1 diopter, distortion may go unnoticed; however, in the videoscopic setting, the video image already has borderline resolution, so that further deterioration[6] can make suturing impossible. The eyes should be well rested preceding a case since the uncommon stress placed on vision during videoscopic surgery can rapidly exhaust the limited metabolic reserves. Development of visual memory during training helps tremendously to augment the retinal stimuli and to reduce stress on the visual system.

Reasoning and mentally rehearsing the steps of a procedure are also important in aiding visual perception. For example, when looking for "lost" instrument tips, one should look directly at the instrument ports, and from the angle of the instrument, one can estimate and calculate the direction and extent of movement needed to bring the tips back into view.

Using contrasting colors (e.g., for backgrounds and stents) helps to reduce visual clutter, provides a reference point for vision, and focuses attention on the pertinent anatomy. In the future, high-definition and three-dimensional video might benefit the laparoscopic surgeon, making manual suturing easier.

Optimizing the image quality by frequently adjusting and fine-tuning the monitor controls (aperture, contrast, and brightness), sharp-focusing the camera (as well as cleaning it and the laparoscope lenses) are *small details that make a big difference.* Creating comfortable ambient lighting in the operating room minimizes eye fatigue, as does eliminating glare from the video screen. These controls should be ideally handled by a qualified biomedical technician.

Balance in Eye-Hand Coordination

In open surgery, a well-developed balance in eye-hand coordination exists. Skilled movements are employed as the eye guides and checks hand movement. When an error is detected or when it may be imminent, movement can be stopped in time and corrected. In magnified surgery, eye-hand coordination must be relearned because normal hand movements will appear to be much faster, on a larger scale, and rather difficult to control. The simplest and most effective technique is to slow one's movements down, proportional to the degree of magnification. The more critical the movement is, the more it needs to be slowed to (1) calculate movement trajectory and (2) allow error detection and prevention. Such movement calculations require time, and with skilled movements, reducing the speed of movement allows the correct decision making. Beginners in particular should slow down, but even experienced surgeons should start slowly and seek the optimum pace.

During the various steps of suturing it is often desirable to have the magnification changed. This can be accomplished by moving the laparoscope closer to the tissue or further away (zooming in and out). Changes in the magnification should be accompanied by a comparable change in the speed of movement; that is, as magnification is increased, movements should be significantly slowed. This enables the surgeon to (1) collect his or her thoughts, (2) examine and recognize new or altered visual clues, (3) gradually regain his or her eye-hand coordination, and (4) make good decisions along the way.

Economy of Motion and a Flawless Technique. The economy of motion principle refers to using only necessary movements to consistently accomplish a procedure or technique successfully. As with this principle, a flawless technique also requires avoiding movements that do not contribute to the progress of a procedure. Further, it requires the avoidance of short cuts that violate surgical principles. *A flawless, fluent performance minimizes the expenditure of energy, stress, and operating time.*

Among the many benefits of slowed movements is the reduced amount of waste involved with making errors; that is, saving the time and effort spent to (1) first make the error, (2) then realize and undo it, and (3) correct it.

More subtle, although equally important in a cumulative sense, is the savings of time, effort, and frustration when the surgeon works efficiently, that is, making only accurate, fruitful movements. The most common "small errors" are often not even regarded as mistakes; however, they are wasted motions. Examples include failing to grasp the target structure on the first attempt, whether this is the needle, suture, or tissue. When working slowly, the surgeon is able to detect whether his or her efforts will succeed, and if it is doubtful, can alter the course before it is too late. Moving rapidly may be equivalent to moving thoughtlessly. Mistakes and frustration are waiting to happen.

Other small errors include losing hold of targeted tissues — for example, the tissue falls off the needle after making the entrance bite or one simply lets go of tissue being held by the assisting grasper. These errors are the result of loss of concentration, poor coordination, or lack of anticipation.

In short, this concept involves precision performed at a pace that is conducive to error-free, efficient performance.

Reducing Operating Time. Laparoscopic suturing, with its inherent limitations, requires more time. To counteract the lengthening of operating time resulting from slowed movements, a tight choreography of movements improves productivity. The surgeon, working slowly but accurately, can complete the procedure more rapidly by avoiding mistakes and making calculated movements, thereby reducing the overall operating time.

Choreography. Certain components of laparoscopic suturing involve repetitious steps. It would therefore be logical that such steps be organized into an efficient series or pattern, ideally with one movement flowing naturally into the next. Such is the concept of choreography for suturing and knot tying. Similar choreography can be extended to other processes as well.

Quality of Repair. Despite the difficulty of laparoscopic suturing, the quality of repair cannot be less than that obtainable with open surgery; in fact, it is possible to obtain a superior repair, since the magnified image facilitates greater precision. Certain procedures can be done better laparoscopically than in open surgery, particularly when access and visualization is normally difficult. An example is the laparoscopic vesicourethral anastomosis following laparoscopic radical prostatectomy.[7]

With all the preceding factors in place and with sufficient experience, it is even possible to acquire a degree of skill in which laparoscopic suturing feels almost "natural" and easy. After a long absence, one may get a bit "rusty," but this skill returns quickly after placing the first few stitches. Failing to prepare a good setup causes the most disruption in the performance of laparoscopic suturing.

SETUP

Setup is everything, and the main issue is no longer whether suturing is possible but how it can be made easier. Suturing and camera port locations are determined by the position and axis of the proposed suture line. Although an optimal setup cannot always be fully accomplished, the goal should be to approximate it as closely as possible. Furthermore, even if ports cannot be placed perfectly, the assistant can move tissues into a more favorable position to favor the suturing surgeon's ideal instrument stroke.

The optimal suturing direction is from approximately 1 o'clock to 7 o'clock for the right-handed surgeon. For the left-handed surgeon, it is 11 o'clock to 5 o'clock (Fig. 24–3). Since tissues cannot always be positioned exactly for the surgeon's dominant hand, the solution is to employ an ambidextrous suturing technique.

For example, when the setup up calls for a left-handed stitch, the accomplished right-handed but ambidextrous surgeon can deftly place the appropriate stitch.

For port setups, the natural position of the eyes and hands are the best starting points; that is, vision or camera port is in the center, dominant and assisting hands are on either side in their respective places (Fig. 24–4). Placing the viewing port elsewhere—to either side of the suturing instruments—would make this process awkward and more difficult by disturbing the natural eye-hand coordination. Sometimes this is unavoidable; care should therefore be taken not to place the laparoscope and suturing instruments too close to each other in the same plane. Placing the camera directly opposite the suturing instruments causes further deterioration of eye-hand coordination, and instrument control becomes erratic. Working upside down is still possible; however, the mirror image reversal creates an impossible obstacle. The use of 0° or angled laparoscopes is a factor in determining the proper setup.

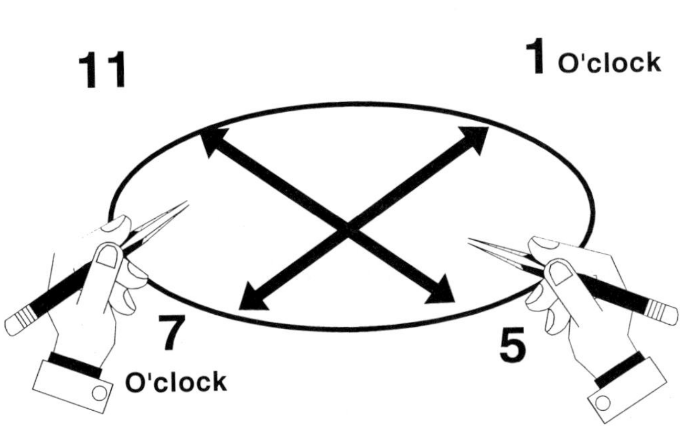

Figure 24–3. Optimal laparoscopic hand-suturing directions: for the right-handed, 1 to 7 o'clock; for the left-handed, 11 to 5 o'clock; for the ambidextrous surgeon: both directions.

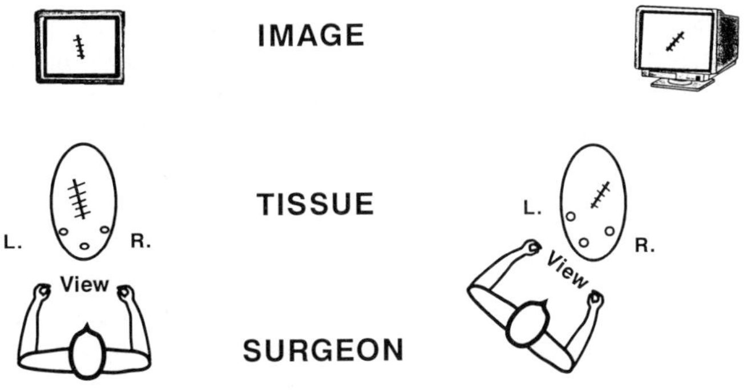

Figure 24–4. Operating room setup: coaxial alignment. The surgeon, tissue, and video screen are all in a straight line.

Scope Holders

Frequently, the camera operator's position interferes with that of the suturing surgeon with the result that either the procedure cannot be tracked properly or the operator must maintain an awkward position for a long period of time without fatiguing.

Erratic camera operation greatly increases the difficulty and stress of laparoscopic suturing. Mechanical,* pneumatic,† or robotic‡ camera holders are useful in remedying this problem. Once setup and exposure, which requires a great deal of camera and laparoscope movement, has been accomplished, suturing follows in a relatively stable field. The extent of the camera positioning is usually limited to zooming in or out to better see the needle-driving or knot-tying activity. A mechanical attachment that will accomplish this useful function, with a mechanical pedal hard-wired to the scope holder has been developed.†

Teamwork

Laparoscopic suturing succeeds best with a well-rehearsed, harmonious team.[8,9] It is not surprising that the best performance is obtained when three skilled surgeons work together in this manner. This allows rotation of the various roles between the primary surgeon, assisting surgeon, and camera operator, minimizing the fatigue and error rate that is inherent when one surgeon works in the same position for too long. Also, this rotation allows a different perspective and greater insight into the reconstructive procedure underway. Despite the benefits of this approach, it may not be economically feasible. The next best team

*OmniTract Surgical, St. Paul, MN.
†Leonard First Assistant, Huntingdon Valley, PA.
‡AESOP, Computer Motion, Goleta, CA

would be a well-rehearsed two-surgeon and camera person (nurse or operating room technician) team.

The primary surgeon sets the pace of surgery and concentrates on the immediately pertinent details of suturing to the exclusion of the rest of the procedure, and other important details need to be tracked by the assistant surgeon. Visual concentration on small areas can cause one to lose sight of adjacent structures or to lose focus on the instrument tip (especially the assisting instrument), leading to "unattended trauma" of tissues.

The assistant surgeon's primary task is to provide immediate support to the primary surgeon and to position the tissue being sutured into the optimal position for needle passage and also to keep the overall procedure in sight and to comment calmly on the work in progress. (This support includes keeping track of the suture tail and preventing the occurrence of unattended trauma.)

The camera operator needs to have intimate knowledge of the procedures to provide optimal image and magnification. Also he or she must comprehend the primary surgeon's needs and create a smooth visual path by anticipating the primary surgeon's imminent moves. This is a difficult job, and "drifting arm fatigue" often results in serious impairment of the speed, efficiency, and fluency of the procedure. The use of laparoscope holders with simple-to-use adjustments can be of great help, especially when a steady, magnified image is critical.

NEEDLE DRIVING

Instrumentation

Suturing instruments are the direct link between the surgeon's hands and the tissues. Two interfaces are involved: (1) the hand-to-instrument interface (handle) and (2) the instrument-to-tissue interface (tip).

Most laparoscopic suturing instruments currently on the market are minor modifications of conventional dissectors or graspers. Some instruments feature new tip designs with conventional laparoscopic handles or new handle designs with traditional instrument tips, but both result in restricted maneuvering, limiting the overall performance and comfort level. Whether they have a ring handle, U-shaped pistol grip, knob grip, or pruning shears grip, all are somewhat cumbersome to use for complex suturing and reconstruction.

The ideal laparoscopic suturing instruments should easily accommodate a fluently choreographed two-handed series of movements. These instruments require a careful design of the handle, stem, and tips (Fig. 24–5). The recently developed Szabo-Berci instrument pair* is a matching set specifically designed to meet these requirements.

Coaxial Handles. The traditional, angled, pistol grip limits the instruments' rotatability. Further, ring handles can cause compression nerve damage (the numb thumb syndrome). Ideally, the handle should be fitted to one of a surgeon's natural hand grips; for delicate, precision surgery this is the pencil grip.[10] A coaxial stem-to-handle relationship allows for the greater maneuverability and rotation necessary for laparoscopic suturing. Maintaining a straight-line relationship all the way reduces the complexity of movement coordination. Modification of the handle into a cylindrical shape allows for smooth and repeated 360° rotation and maximum dexterity.

*Karl Storz Endoscopy America, Culver City, CA.

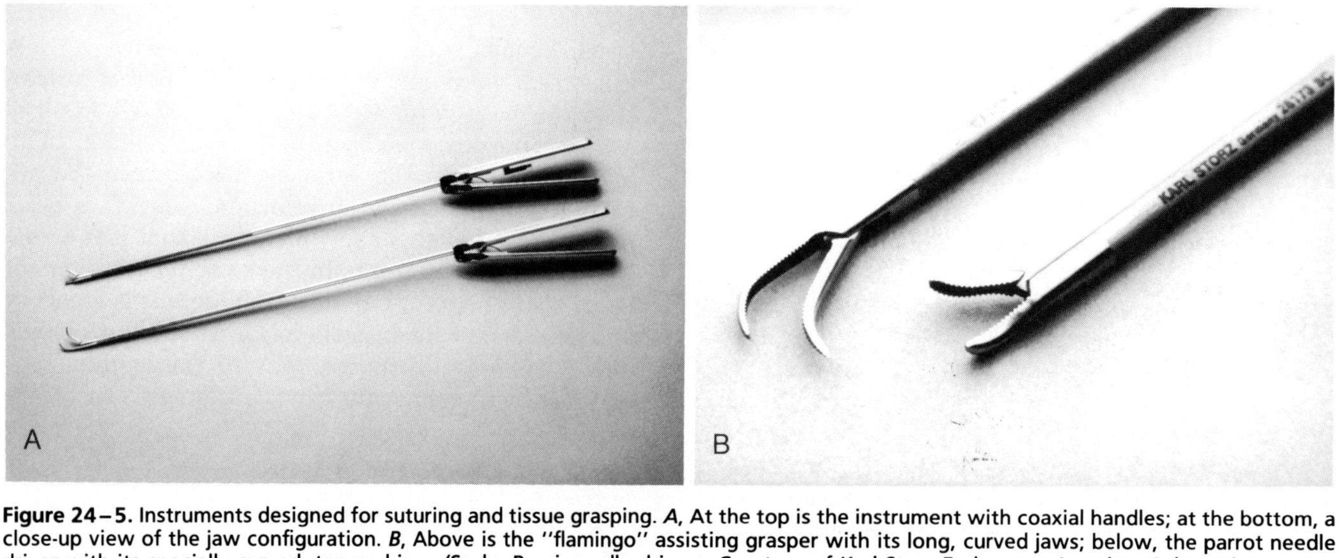

Figure 24–5. Instruments designed for suturing and tissue grasping. *A*, At the top is the instrument with coaxial handles; at the bottom, a close-up view of the jaw configuration. *B*, Above is the "flamingo" assisting grasper with its long, curved jaws; below, the parrot needle driver with its specially curved, tapered jaw. (Szabo-Berci needle drivers, Courtesy of Karl Storz Endoscopy America, Culver City, CA.)

Grips. Since the skin surface of the fingers are rich in nerve endings, the instrument handle should be grasped, or rather delicately held, in the "precision end grip." This is somewhere between a pencil grip and a watchmaker's screwdriving grasp. (It is also similar to fine-tuning a radio.) This grip allows delicate, minute movements to be transmitted using a combination of finger, wrist, and forearm to guide the instruments. This is the preferred grip for laparoscopic suturing, because it enhances the sensory input over an otherwise limited tactile feedback. These features, as well as the grip's unlimited rotatability, allow the precision control necessary for sophisticated maneuvers and complex suturing.

Stems. An instrument stem 5 mm in diameter provides adequate rigidity for suturing and dissection, but it must be at least 33 cm in length to reach the lower urinary tract. For laparoscopic microsurgery, the stem portion near the jaws should be reduced to 3 mm.

Tips. The limited access inherent in laparoscopic suturing essentially requires that both the needle driver and assisting instrument have multipurpose tip designs. A dedicated needle driver or assisting grasper design limits the application to a single function, which can result in increased instrument exchange activity, thus reducing operating efficiency and fluency and diluting concentration. Tips of both instruments need to be designed not only for their primary function but also for their secondary multifunction role, taking into account the delicate tissue handling and precision suturing that are required.

Multipurpose Use. There should be enough multipurpose function in the design to allow sufficient interchangeability to facilitate ambidextrous use. The needle driver must have the ability to (1) handle tissue, (2) firmly grasp and drive the needle (in a reversible locking grip), and (3) handle the thread.

Needle Driver. The needle driver, operated by the dominant hand, holds the needle with its sturdy curved and pointed tip. It fits through a 5-mm port, and its curvature allows multidirectional positioning and easy looping of the thread, while its pointed tip can easily retrieve the suture from wet tissue surfaces. A simple, smoothly functioning lock mechanism allows the needle to be secured in position while suturing, lessening the concentration needed to keep the jaws closed.

Assisting Grasper. The assisting grasper, held by the nondominant hand, is designed to complement the needle-driving instrument. Its jaws are long and curved, like the beak of a flamingo, and it requires a 10-mm port with a 5-mm reducer. These long jaws, when opened wide, can easily scoop up the suture, thus requiring a less precise three-dimension estimation of spatial relationships between the instrument jaw and the thread. The sharp angle of its fine tips provides the surgeon with the necessary agility (1) to position tissue for entrance and exit bites, (2) to pick up the suture from wet tissue surfaces, and (3) to pick up tissues by their serosal and adventitial layers and minimize trauma. This assisting grasper also allows the surgeon to easily grasp the exiting needle as it is placed through the tissue by the needle driver. Although its design is not intended as a needle driver, it could in fact function as one, thereby allowing the ambidextrous approach. This instrument's handles are "free-action"; i.e., it has no locks.

For both instruments, the required closing pressure of the handles (stiffness) is set at a relatively firm tension to approximate the target tissue's resisting force. This is also intended to match the force required to drive a needle through various types of tissues in the laparoscopic field and to prevent the instrument from inadvertently slipping out of the surgeon's hand. The two-handed approach, possible with these suturing instruments, allows the surgeon to place a stitch in any position in the body cavity with confidence.

Suture Materials

Selecting the ideal suture material for laparoscopic suturing can mean the difference between struggling, then failing, or simply succeeding. The main concerns are (1) the match of proper suture selection to the target anatomy and (2) the suture's visibility and handling characteristics. The latter issue is important, because currently the suture industry uses color to identify various suture materials. The color black, which is easiest to see, is used for identifying permanent silk sutures and monofilament nylon only. Gore-tex* suture, which is fluorescent white in color, has high visibility in the laparoscopic field. If one must use an absorbable material, he or she is left to struggle with light violet-colored Vicryl† and Polysorb‡ or dark purple monofilament PDS (polydiaxinone)† that is difficult to distinguish in the busy, often bloody, surgical field. Also of concern are (1) tissue trauma caused by various needle tip designs and (2) tissue response to various threads (absorbable vs permanent sutures).

To confirm whether suture visibility significantly influences the surgeon's stress level, a simple experiment was conducted in which "day-glow" dye was used to color suture thread in an animal experiment. The results indicated that this fluorescent dye dramatically increased visibility, and when multiple sutures were used, they were easy to distinguish from each other, leading to increased surgical efficiency.[11]

*W.L. Gore, Inc., Flagstaff, AZ.
†Ethicon, Inc., Somerville, NJ.
‡US Surgical Corporation, Norwalk, CT.

Needles

Needle shape and size need to be carefully selected for each procedure, with consideration given to anatomy and physiology of the tissue. Most popular laparoscopic needles are the ski-shaped needles, composed of a straight shaft and curved tip; however, one can also use straight or various curved needles. One needle shape that seems particularly useful is a needle combining two different curvatures. Double-armed sutures are sometimes handy, offering the easier exit bite on both proximal and distal lumen of a small conduit during anastomosis. One interesting configuration is a needle with both ends sharpened and the suture swaged in the middle. A fish hook–type of needle with compound curves eases the performance of a retroperitoneal anastomosis in a confined, funnel-like space, such as that in the vesicourethral anastomosis.

The needle tip can be tapered (atraumatic, round), cutting, or a combination of the two. The latter is preferred because it has a round body armed with a small cutting tip. The cutting tip is the reverse cutting form, lessening the chance for cutting through the tissue edge meant to be included in the bite. The actual body of the needle should be carefully contoured to provide a sure grip for the needle driver, with either a triangular or flattened round body and longitudinal ribbing.

The color of needles is also a consideration; primarily a needle should be easily distinguishable from the thread.

Loading and Driving

Straightforward techniques can be used to efficiently introduce the suture into the laparoscopic field and load the needle into the needle driver. As with suturing, the economy of motion principle and movement choreography come into play to facilitate this procedure. The assisting grasper is threaded through a 5-mm reducer with the thread grasped about 1 inch behind the needle. Working with short suture will result in the most direct progression. If a longer suture is used, it needs to be folded into halves or fourths, grasped in the middle, and introduced through the port.

To load the needle efficiently into the needle driver, the thread is grasped about 1 inch away from the needle end, lifted up and dangled so that the needle tip touches the tissue surface (Fig. 24–6*A*). Then it can be swiveled or "pirouetted" into a position that would be ideal for the needle driver to begin suturing. (For the right-handed surgeon, the needle should be angled in a 1 o'clock to 7 o'clock position, with the needle pointing at 7 o'clock). Then the driver grasps the needle in this position with the needle driver approaching the shaft of the needle in a perpendicular fashion (Fig. 24–6*B*,*C*). Minor adjustments of the needle can be made before locking it into position.

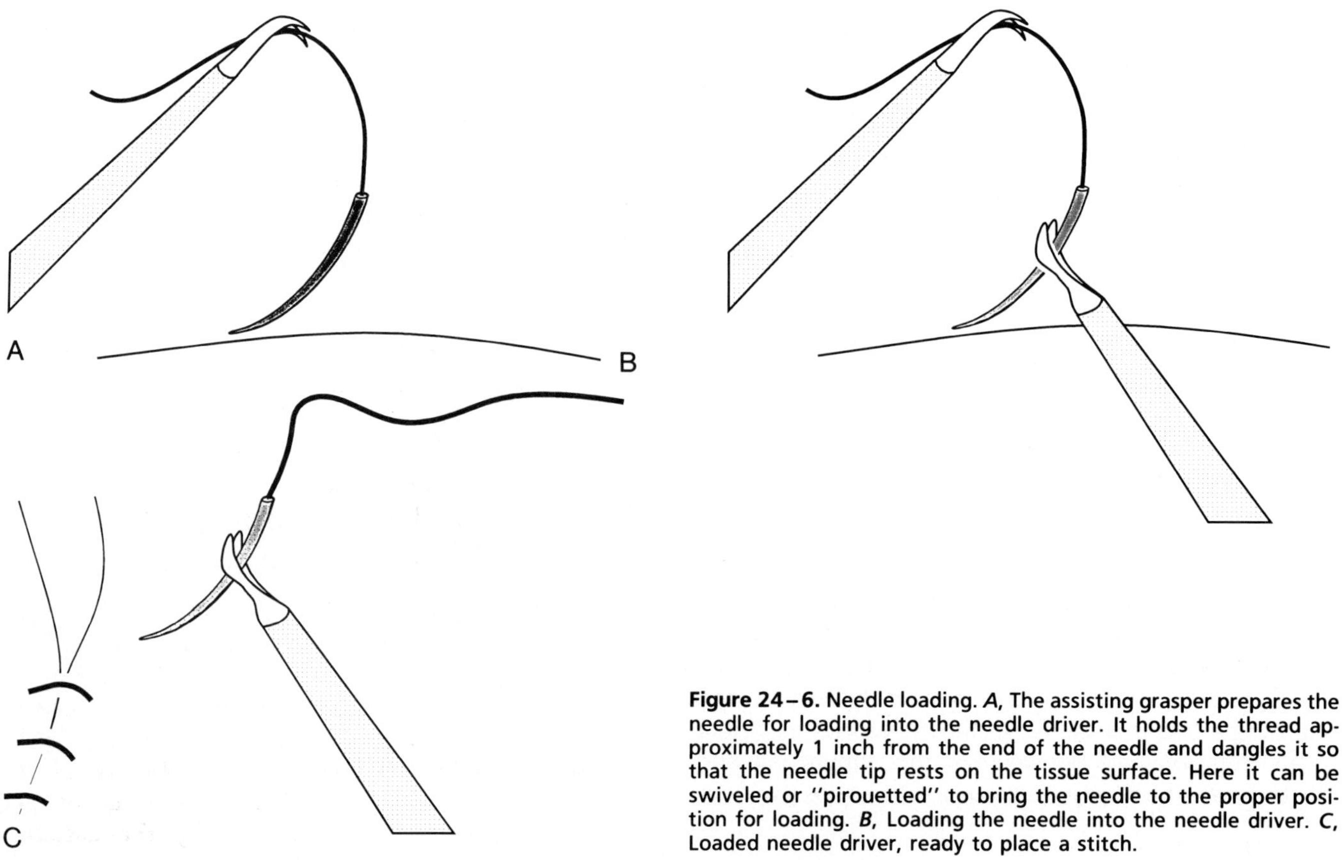

Figure 24–6. Needle loading. *A*, The assisting grasper prepares the needle for loading into the needle driver. It holds the thread approximately 1 inch from the end of the needle and dangles it so that the needle tip rests on the tissue surface. Here it can be swiveled or "pirouetted" to bring the needle to the proper position for loading. *B*, Loading the needle into the needle driver. *C*, Loaded needle driver, ready to place a stitch.

Deflection. Needle deflection is the most annoying and frustrating problem when one attempts to pass the needle through tissue. Not understanding the principles of proper needle grasping, driving, and overall control leads to deeper problems. The natural response is to seek a strong grasping driver, which is potentially dangerous, because the needle can act like a scalpel if inadvertent movements are made with it. Single-purpose needle drivers are more likely to be involved with such iatrogenic injuries, since they have no inherent fail-safe capability.

Needle passage is controlled by a combination of forces acting in accordance to the laws of vector physics (i.e., tissue resistance versus driving force). The concept of atraumatic needle passage requires that the force pushing the needle must be precisely aligned on the same axis as the needle driver (i.e., the point of grasp [fulcrum]), and the needle driving direction must be in direct opposition (head-on) to tissue resistance (Fig. 24–7). The path of least resistance (and the shortest path) for needle passage is perpendicular to the tissue surface. When diverting from this path, the surgeon will discover how tough even delicate tissue can be. It is a matter of technique.

Needle deflection simply results from the needle not being pushed (or driven) head-on (perpendicular) against tissue resistance. Proportional to the diverting angle, the driving force will be used to push the needle further sideways, deflecting it in the needle driver from the correct jaw grip (Fig. 24–8). When held in the jaws of a strongly grasping needle holder, especially if locked in, the needle will be forced sideways, resulting in a traumatic needle passage. The needle would naturally follow the direction of its point, but if the driving force pushes it another direction, it can and will follow (or rather, create) a broader, more traumatic path by lacerating the entrance or exit points.

Tissue Handling

It is vital that tissues be handled in an institution with laparoscopic instruments with great care and gentleness. Tissue bruising can easily occur when excessive force is applied by the surgeon, resulting in crushing trauma; and retraction by less experienced surgeons can easily lead to battered tissues. Collateral trauma, adhesion formation, and scarring lead to poorer postoperative results.

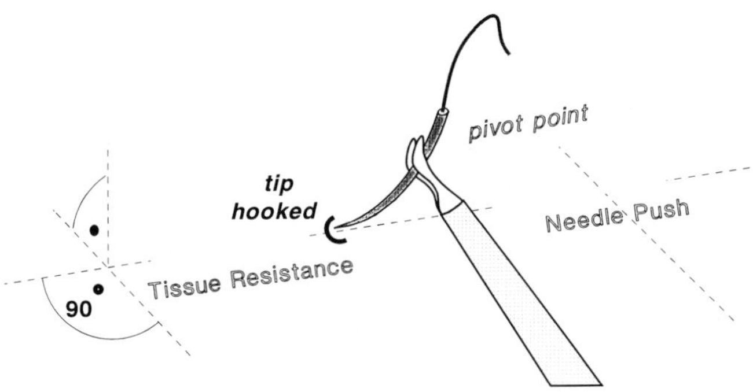

Figure 24–7. Vector physics involved with needle driving and tissue resistance. The needle must be driven head-on against (perpendicular to) tissue resistance.

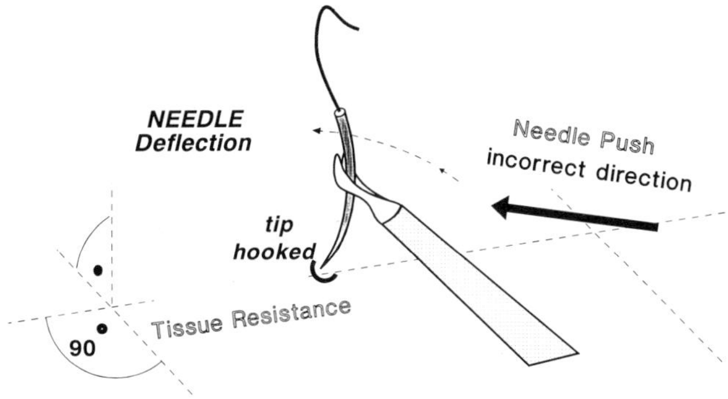

Figure 24–8. Incorrect direction of needle driving, resulting in needle deflection.

During needle passage delicate tissue handling is absolutely essential. Counterpressure from the assisting grasper should routinely be provided immediately adjacent to the entrance and exit points of the needle.

Entrance and Exit

Amount of Bite. The amount of bite refers to the distance from the point of needle penetration to the tissue edge and also the amount of tissue that is included in the suture loop. Bites that are too small do not provide adequate seal or strength and require the placement of more stitches to compensate. This results in wasting time and inflicting additional trauma. On the other hand, bites that are too large gather excessive tissue, resulting in a bulky suture line and the potential for stenosis or suture necrosis. The amount of bite must be accurately calculated for each structure, bearing in mind its function and the reconstructive goal.

Selection of Entrance Points. Selection of the first entrance point sets the stage for the remaining stitches and should be carefully studied and calculated to create the ideal suture line. Considerations depend on function and potential complications (e.g., whether a watertight suture line or inverted edges are needed). Errors often involve the inappropriately sized bites, too small, too large, or both, resulting in a tortuous suture line.

Exit Bite. Generally, the exit bite should be the same size as the entrance bite when coapting tissues of the same caliber; they may be smaller if stenosis is a concern. To make the exit, the needle tip is rotated upward to tent up the tissue. Adjustments can be made if this point appears to result in a bite that is too large or small. When the desired point is located, counterpressure must be applied by the assisting

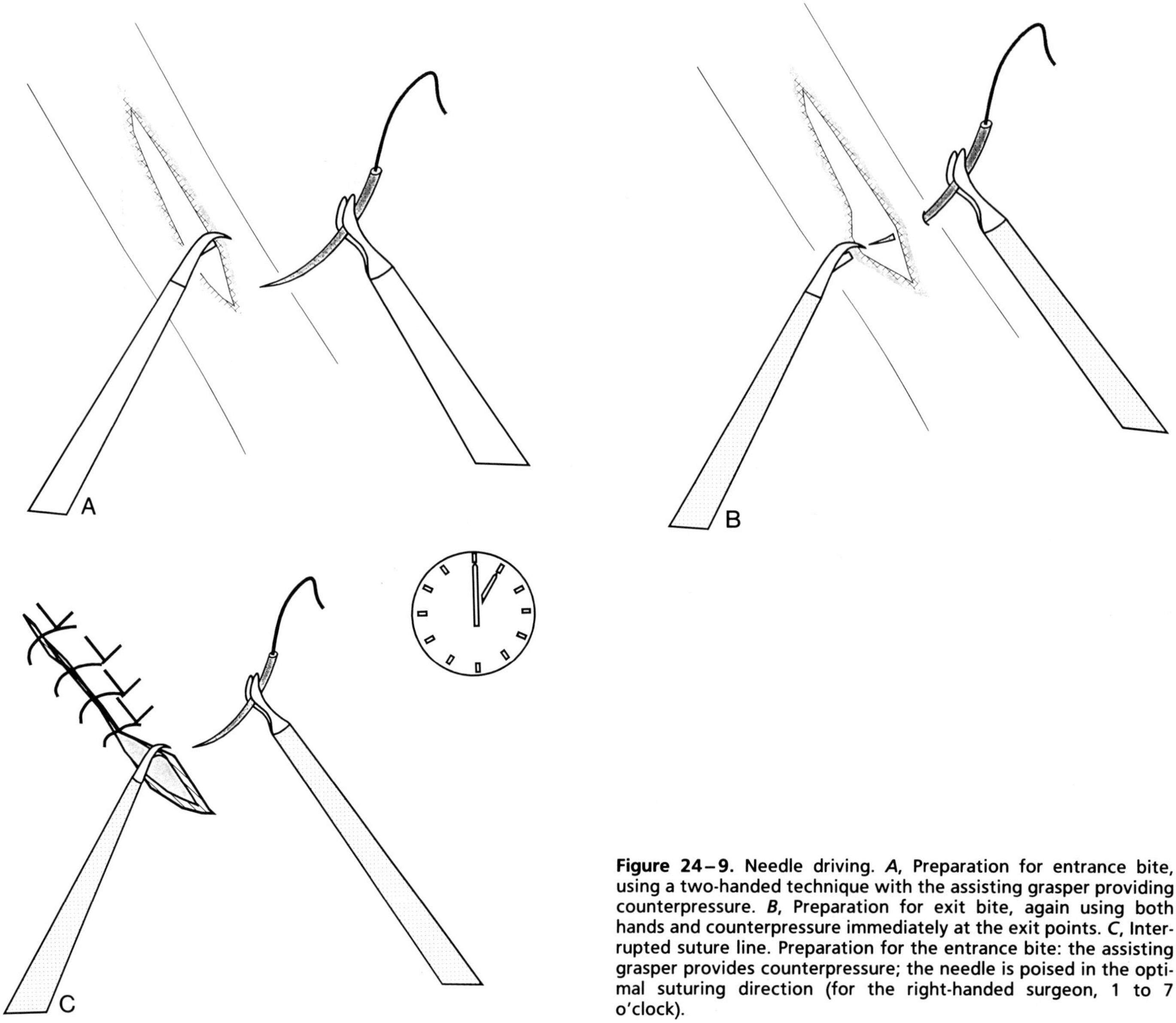

Figure 24–9. Needle driving. *A*, Preparation for entrance bite, using a two-handed technique with the assisting grasper providing counterpressure. *B*, Preparation for exit bite, again using both hands and counterpressure immediately at the exit points. *C*, Interrupted suture line. Preparation for the entrance bite: the assisting grasper provides counterpressure; the needle is poised in the optimal suturing direction (for the right-handed surgeon, 1 to 7 o'clock).

grasper right at the exit point to maintain atraumatic technique; this, of course, is also required of entrance bites (Fig. 24–9*A*–*C*). The needle should carefully be extracted by the needle driver or assisting grasper to avoid undue trauma. Ideally, the needle should be pulled out following its curvature.

Since the exit bite is easier to perform than the entrance bite, double-armed sutures (i.e., a thead with a needle on each end) would be useful, especially for difficult anastomoses. This technique avoids the potential of snagging the posterior wall of the anastomosed duct (most frequently occurring during or immediately following the entrance bite). This technique is therefore considered safer, although it is less economical.

KNOT TYING

Shortcuts

Often shortcuts offer a simple solution to otherwise tedious procedures, but there are simply no shortcuts or substitutes for skill. Shortcuts can be a time and effort saver for the experienced surgeon; however, novices or those with limited experience rarely benefit from their use and contrary to the intended goal, shortcuts can easily result in complications.

The difficulty of intracorporeal knot tying was found to be even greater than suturing, so many innovations have been tried. For example, a silver bead much larger than the needle diameter crimped to the end of the suture, was devised to anchor the suture in the tissue. In some cases, absorbable clips can be used in place of the silver bead. This anchoring technique is often used in transanal endoscopic microsurgery,[1] which falls into the intraluminal laparoscopic approach, with a narrow working channel no more than 5 cm in width. Although intracorporeal knotting is possible, it is somewhat tedious, requiring the use of special instrumentation specifically designed for transanal microsurgery. There the silver bead technique is acceptable in this circumstance, although it is less than satisfactory in most other procedures.

Clipping Two Ends. After placing entrance and exit bites the short and long tails can be held together with a hemoclip or similar device by clamping both ends of the clip. In effect this provides a mechanical loop. The apparent advantage is time savings; however, it has limitations, requires considerable skill, and gives a sloppily secured first stitch. Nonetheless, there are situations, such as in temporary stay sutures, in which it is a satisfactory method.

Lasso Loop. A loop is tied on the end of this suture extracorporeally by the surgeon, forming a lasso loop. After the entrance and exit bites are made, the needle is threaded back through this loop. When pulled taut, the lasso will bring the tissue edges together. The drawback is the loose approximation, and as tension is released, the edges can easily slip apart.

Jamming Anchor Knot (Fig. 24–10). The problem with the lasso loop can be addressed with the jamming anchor knot. In a similar manner, a loop must be tied externally with a slip knot and then introduced through a port. The bites are made; the needle is threaded through this loop and tightened. The short and long tails are then pulled in opposite directions, further tightening and securing the knot. This knot can slip again if left on its own, and requires tying at a minimum a square knot on top, which will secure the loop, preventing it from slipping back when tension is released. This is acceptable for starting a continuous suture line but cumbersome for use with interrupted stitches, unless considerable tension of tissues is encountered.

Pretied Loop. The pretied loop is a practical method for ligation purposes. A loop is formed and secured by a pretied Roeder knot. The loop, contained within an applicator tube, is introduced, the open loop encircles the target tissue, and the knot is cinched down by pushing with a hollow applicator stick (knot pusher) (Endoloop* or Surgiwhip†).

Prelooped Suture. A needle and prelooped suture is loosely secured at the end of an applicator (Suture Applier‡). It is introduced into the operative area, and the needle is then grasped, the driver pulling enough thread to place the entrance and exit bites. The needle is then threaded through the double loops and pulled taut; the applicator plunger is pushed down, pulling

*Ethicon Endo-Surgery, Cincinnati, OH.
†US Surgical Corporation, Norwalk, CT.
‡Laparomed, Irvine, CA.

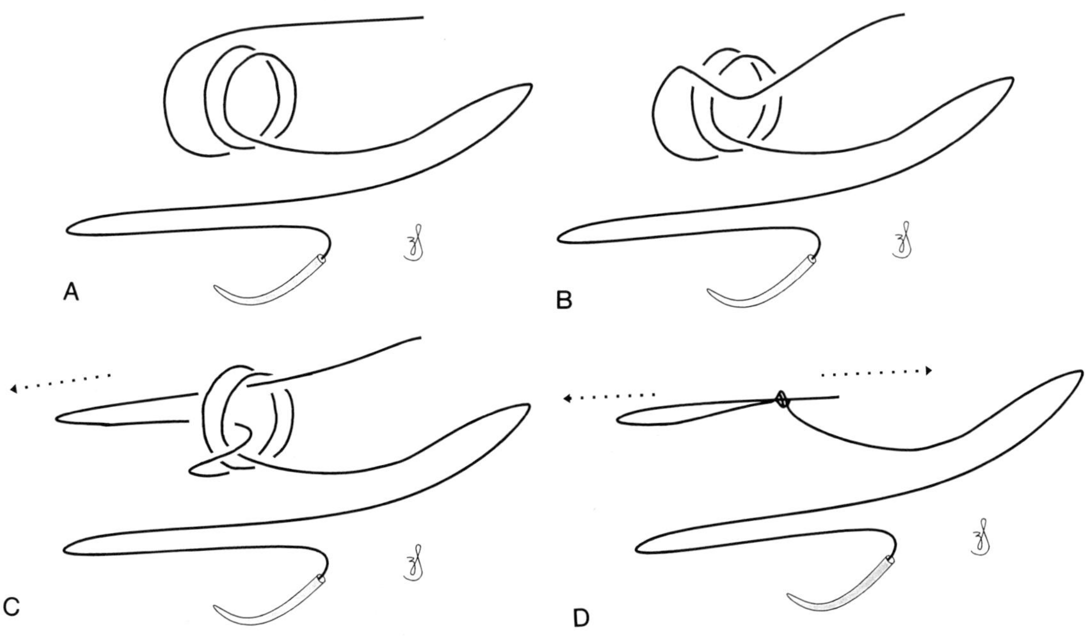

Figure 24–10. Jamming anchor knot, a semiextracorporeal knot used for continuous suturing. *A*, Extracorporeally, a two and one-half revolution coil is prepared and positioned so that the end of the thread is on the top position and the needle end rests on the surface. *B*, The thread end is the active member and is brought in front of the coil; a loop is formed and . . . *C*, is backed into the coil. *D*, The coil is then cinched down onto the loop.

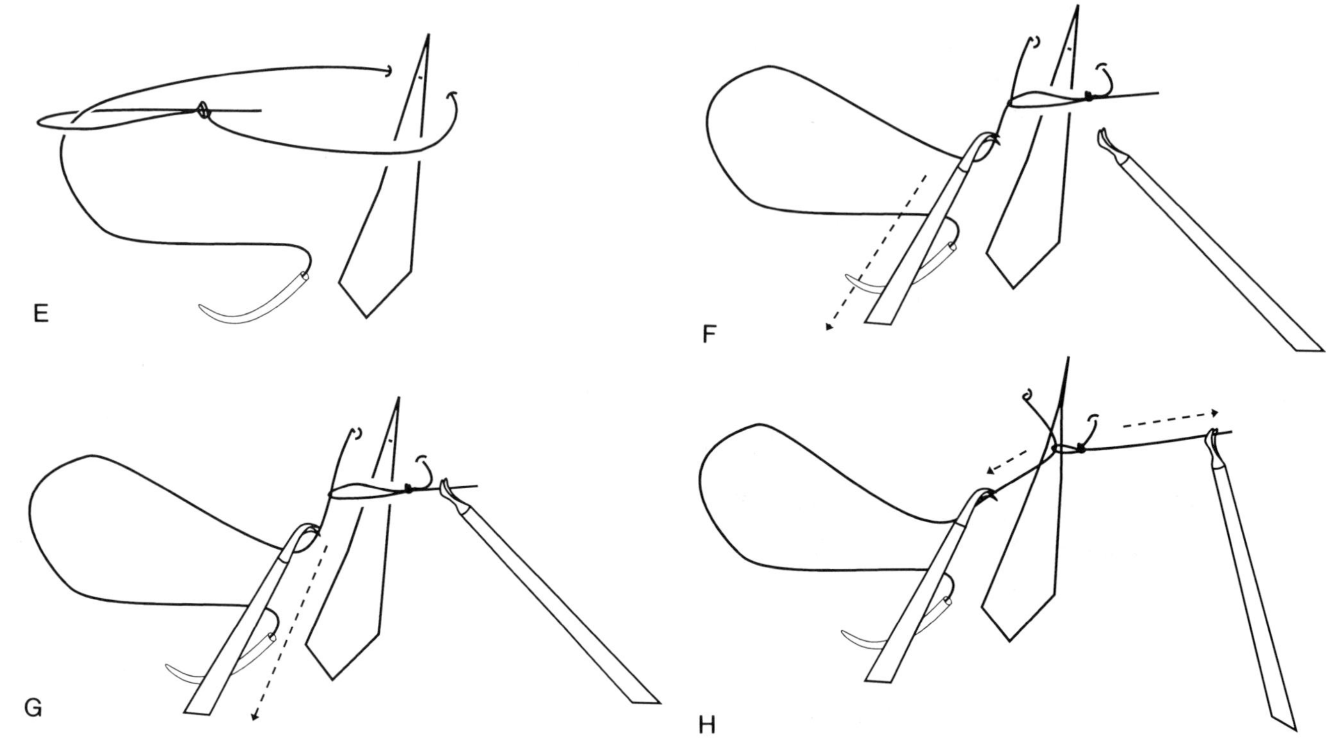

Figure 24–10 *Continued. E,* The suture with loop is then introduced through the trocar, entrance and exit bites are made, and the needle is passed through the loop. *F,* The assisting grasper pulls on the thread with the needle; *G,* the needle driver grasps the thread tail with the loop. *H,* The two instruments pull horizontally in opposite directions to cinch down the stitch and approximate the tissue edges. The assisting grasper releases its hold, and the needle driver grasps the needle in preparing to proceed with the continuous suture line.

the prelooped thread and tightening the knot. The knot is a form of slip knot. While reasonably simple, it involves a disposable single use device and therefore has cost disadvantages.

Laser Welding. [12] In microsurgery the laser welding technique was advocated for microvascular, vas deferens, and fallopian tube repair anastomosis, but it never has become a mainstream technique. In certain situations, it can probably be a solution, but it is likely to complement rather than replace suturing.

Tissue Gluing. [10] Again, fibrin and other glues have often been tried but have been slow to gain popularity. Gluing may be used in combination with other tissue approximation techniques as an augmenting technique, perhaps providing hemostatic or hydrostatic seal.

Undoubtedly other ingenious methods will emerge as the boundaries of laparoscopic surgery expand; however, the traditional, "low-tech" concept of hand suturing and square or surgeon's knot method of securing two suture ends will remain the most popular and enduring for reasons that have kept it as a standard for centuries.

Extracorporeal Knotting

Extracorporeal knots are not appropriate for delicate tissues because the tension on the tissues is quite strong and will cause tissue trauma. However, extracorporeal knotting can be used (1) in sturdy tissue, e.g., muscular or fibrous tissues, (2) when the intracorporeal space is too tight for the instrument tips to maneuver, (3) in procedures in which only a few knots are needed, or (4) if the surgeon lacks the skill to perform intracorporeal knotting.

The process of extracorporeal knotting is considerably slower than the choreographed intracorporeal technique because it requires exiting the operative site (and body cavity), tying the knot, and reintroducing it to the operative site. It is like climbing out of a swimming pool to adjust one's bathing suit, and then climbing back in. Increased operating time results.

These knots work best with slippery monofilament suture materials. Braided suture has a tendency to lock up too soon; that is, the knot locks before it is in the proper place, and the tissues are left without adequate approximation.

Roeder Knot (Fig. 24–11). A long suture is introduced through a port, leaving the end outside the port. The needle is then driven through the entrance and exit points and brought outside through the same port. The two suture ends are held together, following which (1) an overhand flat knot is tied, (2) one end is wrapped around the main leads several times, and (3) the end is pulled back through the last loop and tightened. A knot pusher holds the lead thread, and the

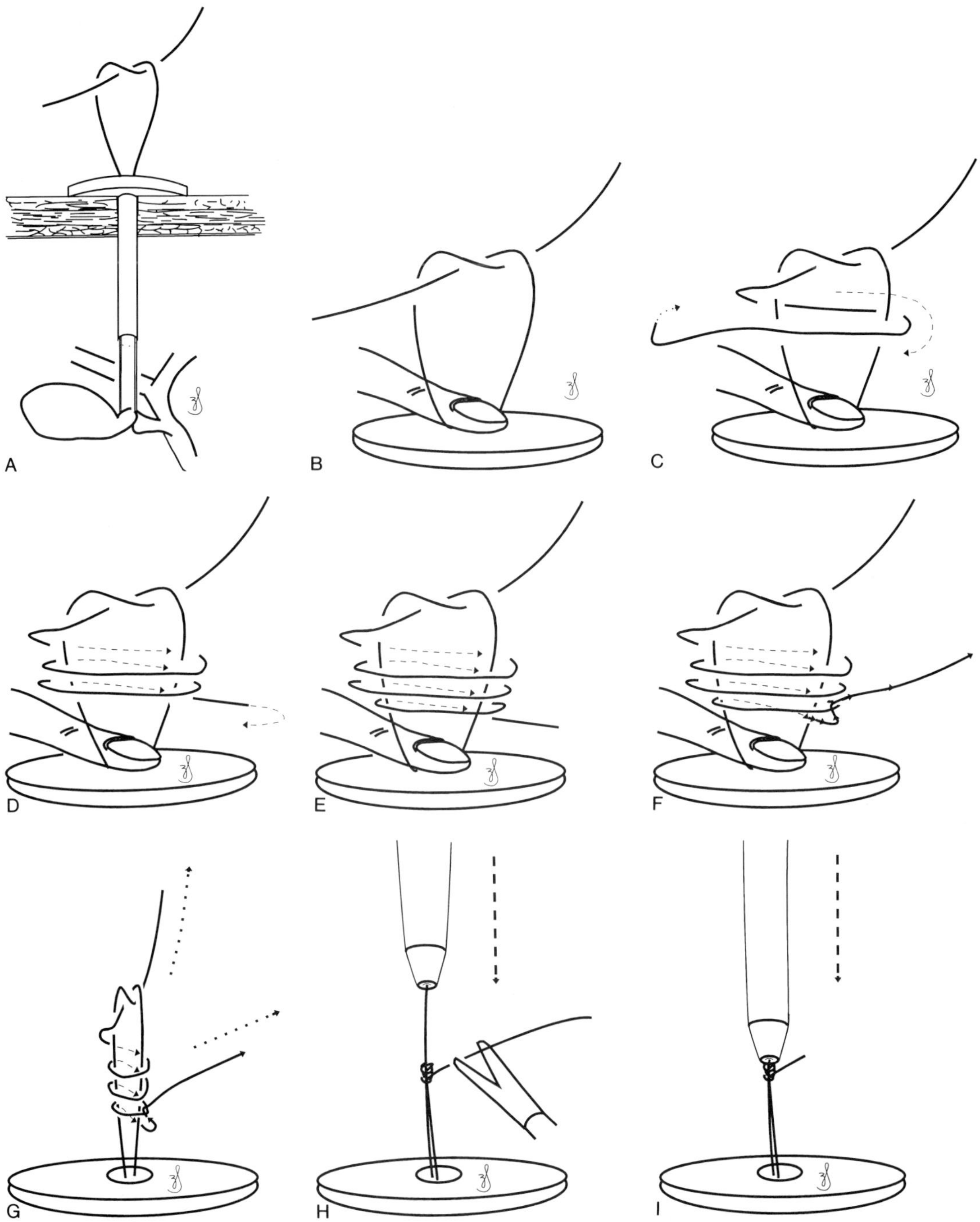

Figure 24–11. Roeder knot. As with all types of extracorporeal knots, the needle is threaded through the trocar, leaving the thread ends outside the trocar. The needle is passed through the tissue and is then brought outside again through the trocar. *A,* A flat knot is loosely made extracorporeally; *B,* then a finger is placed on top of the trocar between the two threads. *C–E,* The thread with or without the needle is coiled around the flat knot loop three and one-half times in a downward spiral (toward the trocar). The active tail is now on the same side of the knot (i.e., both tails are on the right side). *F,* After this has been completed, the same tail is threaded back through the last (bottom) coil. . . *G,* and is pulled taut; simultaneously the other thread (top) is also pulled taut, forming the knot.

H, The top thread is threaded through a knot pusher (a hollow tube with a tapered end facing the knot). The lower thread is cut short.

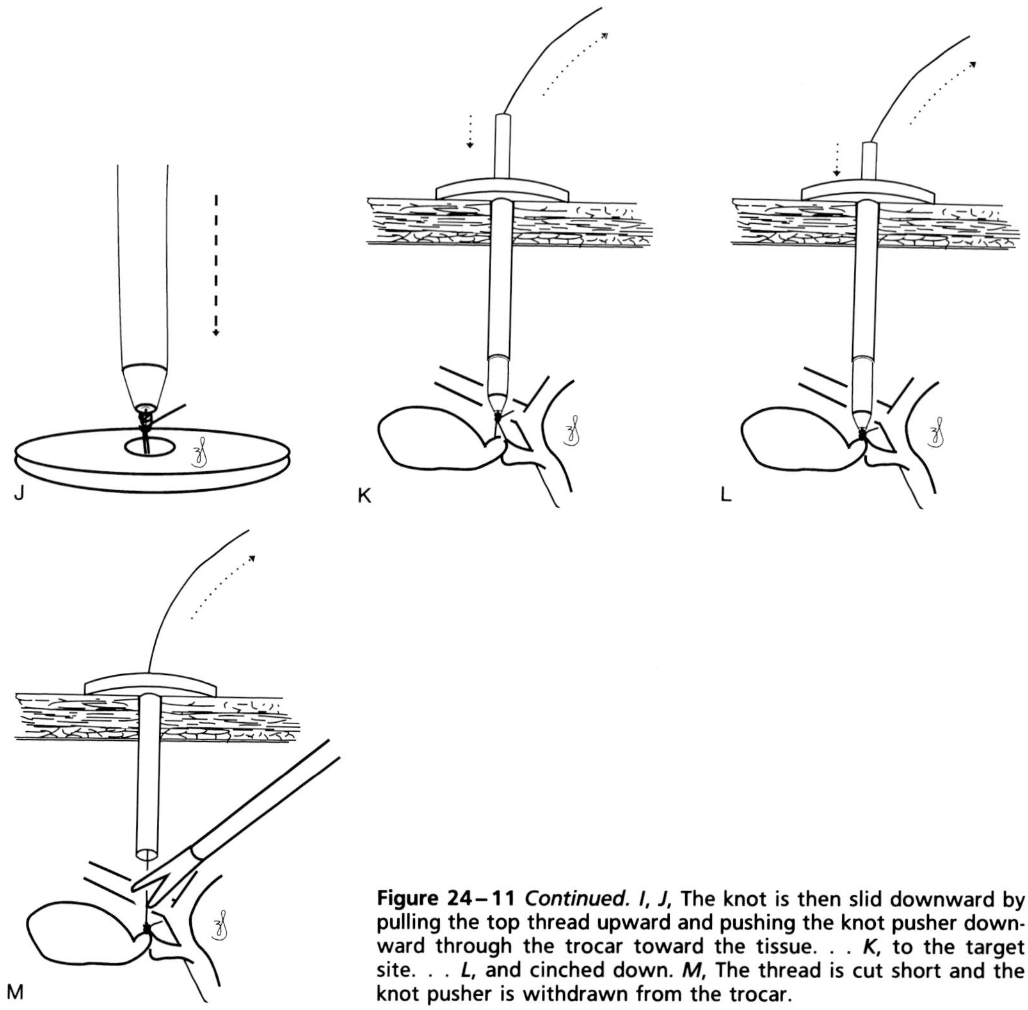

Figure 24–11 *Continued. I, J,* The knot is then slid downward by pulling the top thread upward and pushing the knot pusher downward through the trocar toward the tissue. . . *K,* to the target site. . . *L,* and cinched down. *M,* The thread is cut short and the knot pusher is withdrawn from the trocar.

knot is pushed down to its correct position. This is a cumbersome and complicated process not suitable for delicate tissues. However, this was the most widely used knot until recently, when intracorporeal knot-tying techniques were demonstrated to be feasible in laparoscopic surgery.[13]

Sliding Knot. For the sliding knot, the suture is placed in the previously described manner, a half-hitch is tied and with a special knot pusher is pushed down through the port into the intracorporeal position. The second, third, and fourth knots are tied and pushed down, one on top of the other. The knot is relatively simple; however, it is cumbersome and minimizes the surgeon's control.

Intracorporeal Knotting

An intracorporeal square or surgeon's knot is the purest way of maintaining the tried and true simplicity of open knot-tying technique. It is also an important step in learning sophisticated suturing skills for reconstructive procedures. The precise choreography of square-knot tying serves as a focus for learning laparoscopic suturing and an easy-to-follow pattern for novice and expert alike. Not only does this technique provide a small triumph when successfully accomplished, it also teaches good habits and increases dexterity. As one's skills improve one seeks shortcuts surpassing the initial accomplishment. However, if things go wrong or a difficult situation arises, the exact technique described below is the best system to fall back on.

Square-Slip Knot (Fig. 24–12). Although initially difficult to learn and requiring considerable practice to master, this technique is the most flexible, practical, and economical way to secure two suture ends and approximate tissue edges. The knot is the traditional, instrument-tied *square knot,* which can be converted to a *slip knot,* adjusted for ideal position and tension, then reconverted to the locking square configuration. If stiff monofilament suture is used, a third or fourth throw may be placed for additional security. If the proper choreography is followed, it is an elegant technique.

Because of this knot's convertibility between a

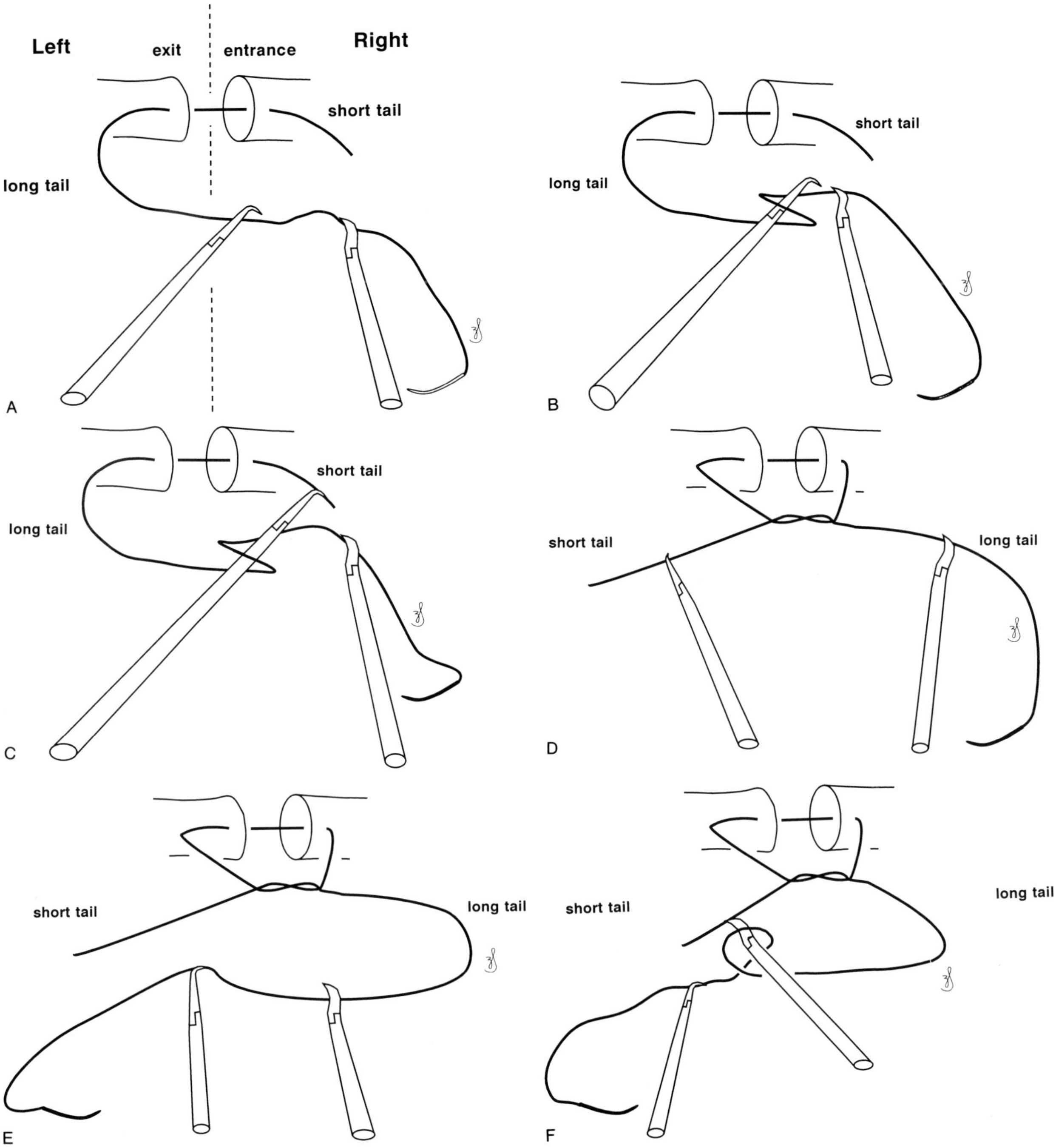

Figure 24–12. Square or slip knot, an intracorporeal convertible locking/slip knot for interrupted and continuous suturing. This knot can be tied tight (beginning with the first flat knot) or left loose in the case of the suspension slip-knot technique. For continuous suturing, the last loop is pulled up and is treated like the short tail in the procedure described as follows: *A–D*, First flat knot; *E–H*, second, opposing, flat knot; *I–L*, converting the locked square knot into its sliding configuration and reconverting it back to its original locking configuration.

A, After the needle has passed through the tissue, the needle driver crosses over to the opposite side of the field and grasps the long tail (with the needle), and positions it below the short tail in a C configuration. (If using monofilament suture, it is imperative that the needle driver be rotated counterclockwise until the C-loop is laid in a horizontal plane). *B*, The assisting grasper is placed over the C-loop, and the needle driver wraps once over and under the assisting grasper. *C*, The assisting grasper grasps the short tail of the thread. (This process is facilitated by bringing *both instruments* toward the short tail.) *D*, The instruments pull in opposite directions to cinch down the first flat knot. The assisting grasper releases its hold, and the needle driver, while still holding the thread, crosses over and hands its thread to the assisting grasper.

E, A reversed C-loop has now been created. (If using monofilament suture, the assisting grasper should rotate the thread clockwise until a horizontal plane for the reversed C-loop is created.) The needle driver is placed over this loop; *F*, the long tail is wrapped around it once, over then under the needle driver, and reaches to grasp the short tail.

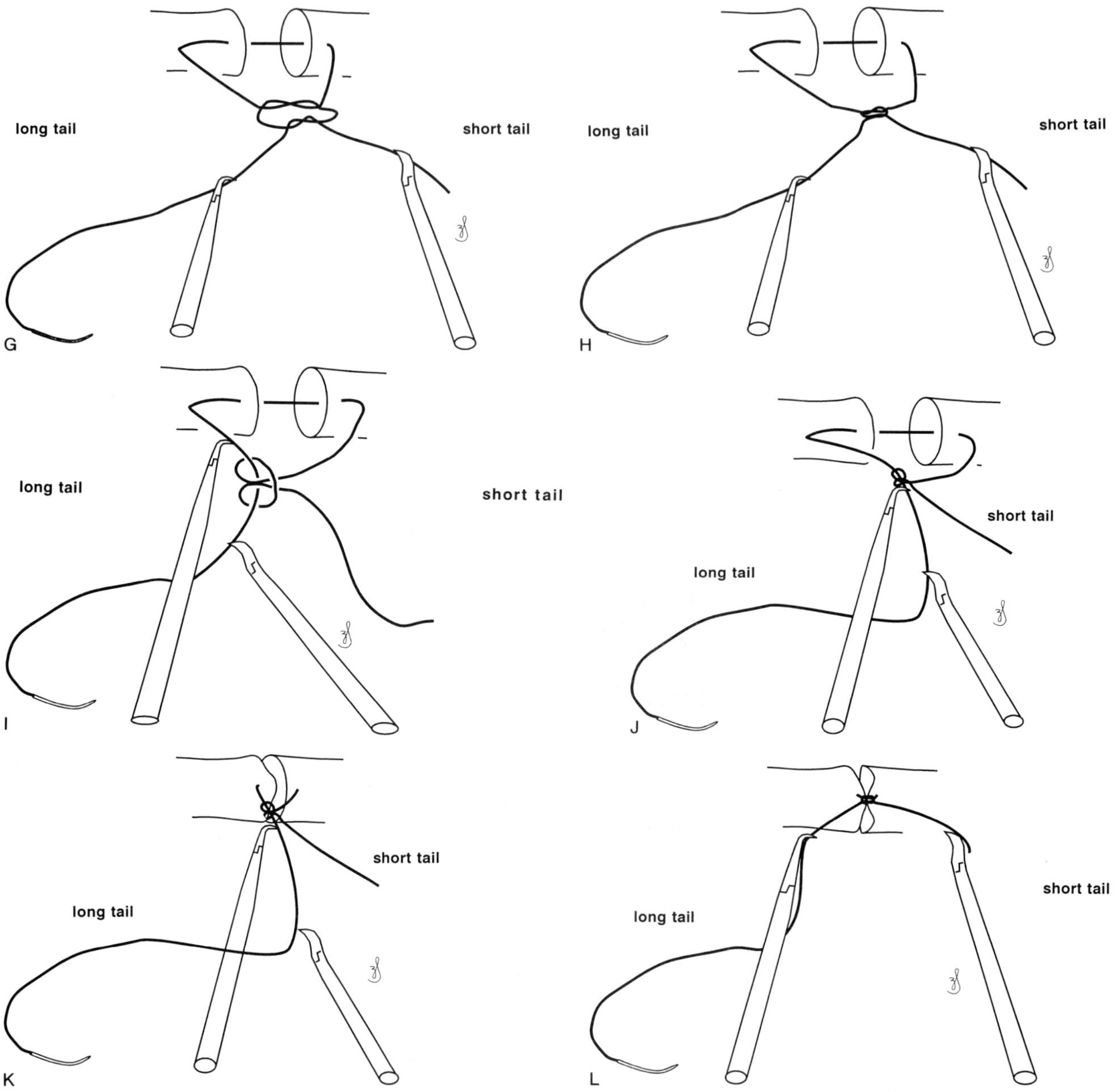

Figure 24–12 *Continued. G,* The instruments pull the tails in opposite directions. . . *H,* and cinch the knot downward into a locking configuration.

I, To convert the (locking) square knot to its sliding configuration, the knot should first be divided mentally into left and right sides. Using the left side, the assisting grasper grasps the loose suture loop above the knot (between the knot and the tissue), and also on the left side, the needle driver grasps the long tail (with the needle) below the knot. The two instruments pull the thread vertically in opposite directions and do not release the thread. *J,K,* The needle driver maintains its hold, and the assisting grasper repositions below the knot with a gentle grasp, pushes the knot toward the tissue, and cinches the knot downward to the desired position and tension. Again, the instruments should maintain their hold on the threads. The knot can be shifted so that it stays centered rather than locking against the exit (or entrance) point. *L,* To reconvert the slip knot to the locking square knot, the assisting grasper grasps the thread near the needle driver and the needle driver is repositioned on the short tail (on the right side). The two instruments pull horizontally in opposite directions. The locking square knot has been recreated. A third, opposing, flat knot can be added if desired but is optional. (This is accomplished in the same manner as the first flat knot.)

locking and sliding configuration, it can be used for the "suspension slip knot technique."[3,9] This is desirable for use in difficult anastomoses when the tissue edges and lumen need to be visualized for the critical first few stitches so that technical errors can be avoided. In this technique, the locking square knot is tied as described but in a loose loop with the tissue edges loosely approximated, so that identification of the lumen and tissue layers is possible for the subsequent stitches. After the critical stitches have been placed, the square knot that was previously tied is converted to a sliding configuration, and the knot can be pushed down, approximating the tissue to its final position. The knot is then reconverted to its original locking configuration and is secure. An additional flat knot can be added if desired.

Surgeon's Knot. If moderate tension exists at the tissue edges to be approximated, the first single throw easily reopens, and so a double throw is recommended for a better hold. The knot is secured with an opposite single throw. The advantage is obvious, but the disadvantage is that this becomes a permanent knot that cannot be reopened. If adjustment is necessary, the knot has to be cut out and replaced. Considering the difficulty of this process, the square-slip knot is clearly the best choice whenever possible. Furthermore, if significant tension exists, increased tissue trauma could result at the first few knots.

Granny Knot. The granny knot is composed of two half-hitches placed one on the other in the same direction. This is an unpredictable knot—sometimes it slips and other times it jams. This knot usually is the result of a randomly, or incorrectly tied square knot and is an indication of novice level knot-tying ability.

Twist Knot. The twist knot was promoted because it avoids the complex choreography required by the square knot. The long tail is grasped by the needle driver instrument and rotated 3 or more times around its axis, then the short tail is pulled through the created loops, pulled tight, creating a knot. Although it seems simple, it takes considerable skill to accomplish the tying correctly. It may seem that an extra pair of hands is needed, so that the traditional square or surgeon's knot may as well be used. Without the technique of the choreographed square knot, this method is a feasible means of intracorporeal knot tying.

Aberdeen Knot (Fig. 24–13)**.** Securing a continuous suture line can be accomplished in two ways. In one method, the last loop is loosened, and the ends are tied in a traditional square or surgeon's knot. Another method uses the needle driver; reaching through the loosened loop, the long tail is grasped 5 to 10 mm from its exit from the tissue and is pulled through, creating a new loop. This loop is shortened, the needle driver tip, passed through it again, grasps the long tail, which is pulled through, creating another loop. After repeating this two or three times, the full thread with the needle is pulled through the loop, completing a secure knot. This is also known as the crochet, or French, knot. Although this knotting technique requires minimal rotation of the instruments it still needs considerable skill.

SUTURE LINE

Interrupted Suturing Technique

Whether approximation consists of interrupted, continuous, or a combination of both types of sutures, tissues should be prepared and positioned so that minimal tension exists.

Considerations in constructing a linear suture line include length of the defect, type of tissues to be approximated, and the function of those tissues. Besides choosing the appropriate suture material and needle, the thread must be trimmed to the shortest possible length for the repair in order to avoid tangling in the field. The instrument port locations should be positioned so that the needle driver port is parallel with the suture line and it and the assisting grasper port are 45° to 90° and at least 6 inches apart. The needle should be positioned perpendicular to the suture line. The surgeon's position should be such that the entrance and exit scooping motions follow a 1 o'clock to 7 o'clock direction relative to the surgeon's frontal plane (Fig. 24–14). Intracorporeal knot-tying technique must be second nature to the surgeon.

Interrupted sutures can be used in this suspension slip knot technique[3] if the tissues are under considerable tension or if the tissues' edges need to be visualized for the critical first few stitches. This technique involves a loose suture loop tied with a square knot, which is later converted to its sliding configuration and cinched down, then is reconverted to a locking square knot. Stitches must be placed to approximate the tissues without excessive tension or misalignment of the layers.

Continuous Suturing Technique

Continuous suturing is a more rapid technique than interrupted suturing, but it is also more difficult to accomplish well. Continuous suturing begins and ends with an anchoring knot; the latter can be tied with the loop of the last stitch. It is necessary to identify the tissue edges, carefully adjusting the tension on the suture loops as the approximation progresses.

Suture consideration is important since monofilament and braided thread behave differently. The

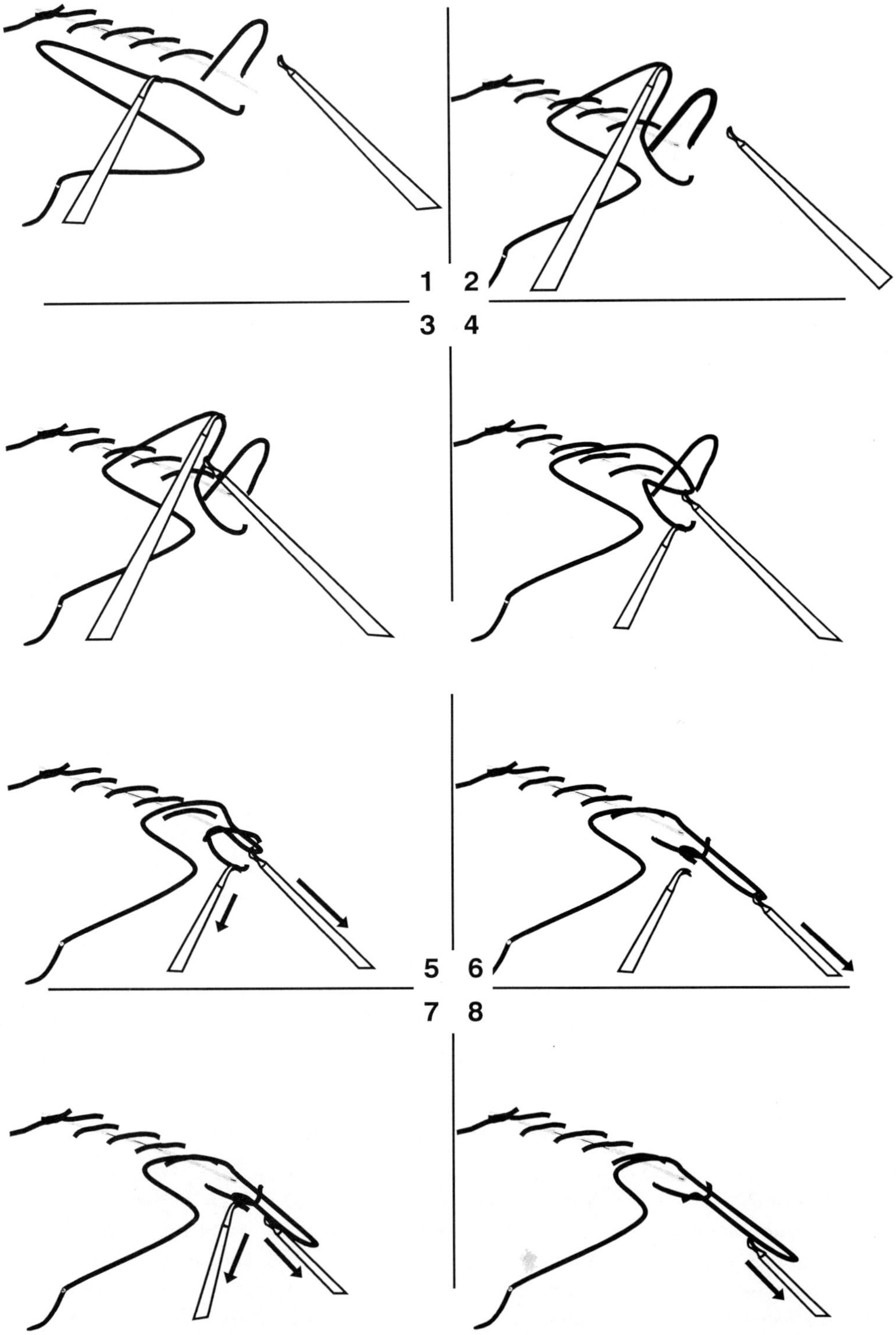

Figure 24–13. Aberdeen knot, an intracorporeal knot for continuous suturing. This is a type of crocheting knot popularized by Cuschieri. *1,* The last stitch is pulled up to form a loop. The assisting grasper grasps the long tail. . . *2,* and lifts it up, positioning it on the left side (or "behind" the loop). *3,* From the right side, the needle driver enters the loop and grasps the thread held by the assisting grasper. *4,* It then pulls it through partially downward (and toward the right); *5,* meanwhile, the assisting grasper pulls downward (and towards the left). *6,* The result: the original loop is cinched down, and a new loop is formed. *7,8,* The assisting grasper helps cinch down the original loop by advancing the thread through the tissue.

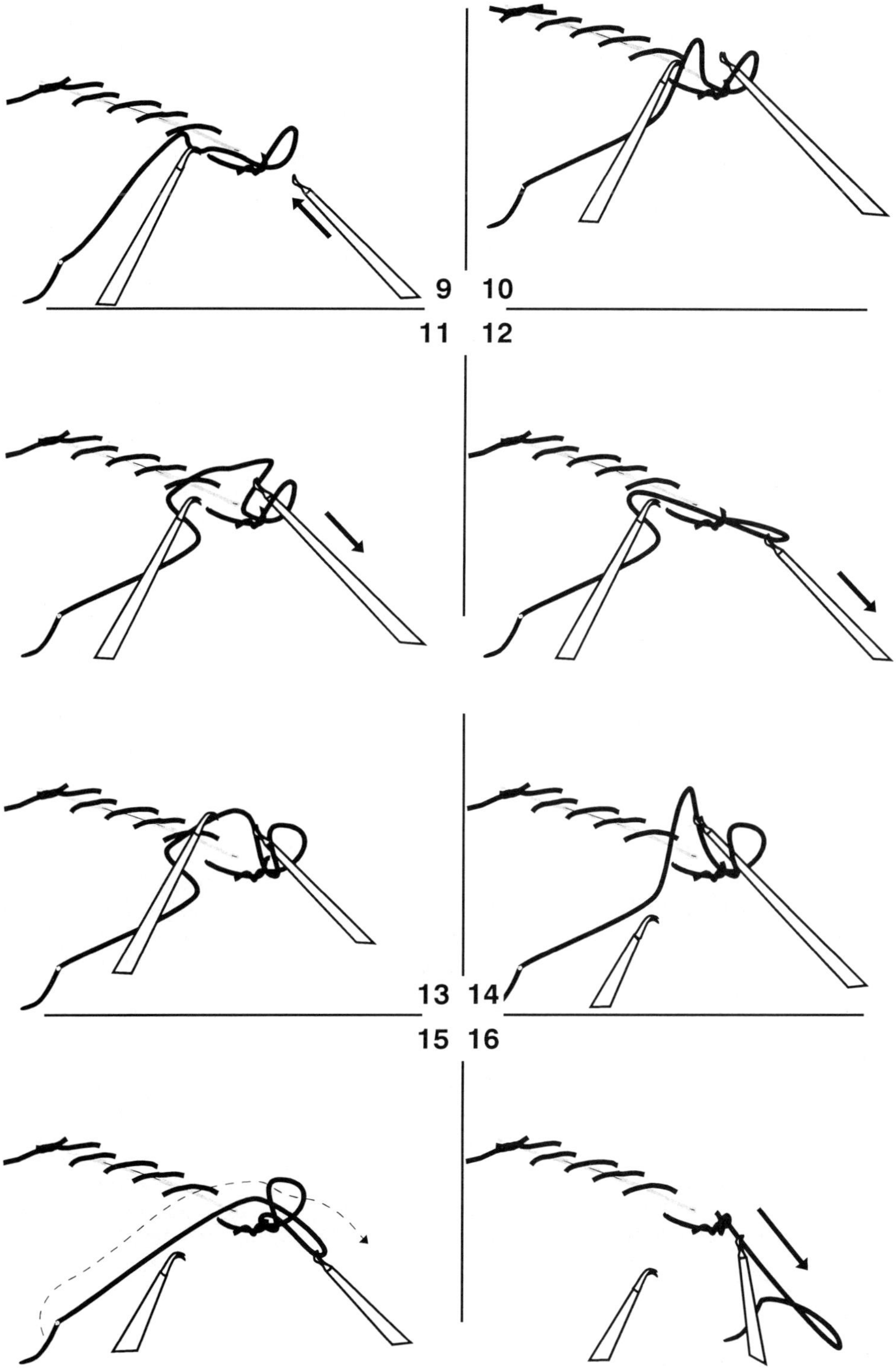

Figure 24–13 *Continued. 9*, The new (2nd) loop is lifted up, and *10–12*, the same procedure is repeated. *13–16*, The same procedure is repeated a third time with one exception: instead of creating another loop, the entire thread, needle and all, is pulled through and cinched tight.

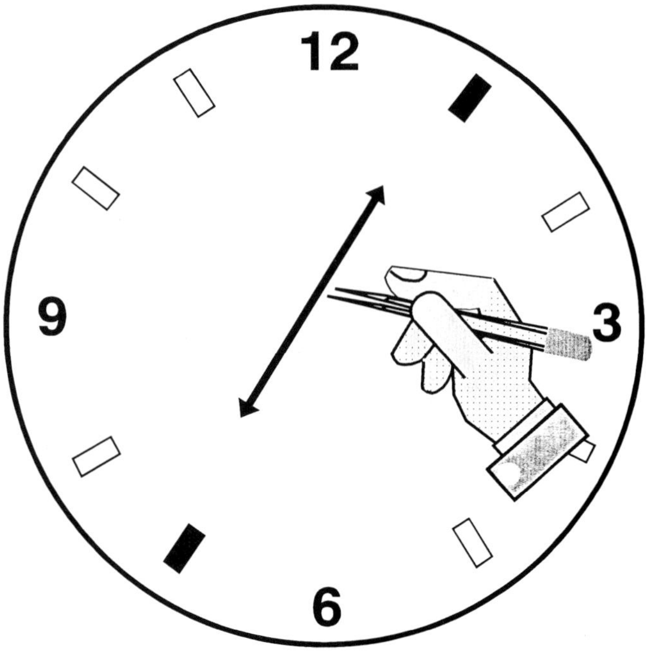

Figure 24–14. The optimal suturing position for the right-handed surgeon: from one o'clock to seven o'clock.

former is stiff and springy and can be run rapidly in a noninterlocking manner, but this is often results in an uneven suture line. Woven thread sutures have a tendency to drag, lock the suture line, and are more cumbersome to handle, since each stitch has to be placed with the tension it is intended to be left with.

ANASTOMOSIS

Ductal Anastomosis. Currently anastomosis of ducts can be accomplished laparoscopically using methods based on the demanding techniques of microvascular anastomoses. It can be accomplished with end-to-end, end-to-side, or side-to-side anastomoses. A laparoscopically hand-sutured vesicourethral anastomosis technique (an end-to-end anastomosis) following laparoscopic radical prostatectomy has already been proved feasible and successful in an experimental canine model in which a watertight seal and proper mucosal approximation were necessary. To maximize efficiency, a redesign of the anastomosis technique would be necessary, considering the difficulty of approach.

End-to-End Anastomosis. This is the method of choice for approximating ducts of equal caliber and wall thickness. The number of stitches, their configuration, and the size of the bites depend on the function of the structure. Either interrupted or continuous sutures can be used. The former provides better precision and control; the latter is more rapid but less forgiving.

End-to-Side Anastomosis. Conduits with disparate lumens and wall thicknesses can be joined with the end-to-side technique which is easier to achieve than end-to-end anastomosis. Further, it is less invasive since only part of the recipient's circumference is involved in the procedure.

Side-to-Side Anastomosis. This technique is a practical method of approximating conduits that normally lie side by side and is similar in technique to the end-to-side anastomosis.

REFERENCES

1. Bueβ, G; Kipfmüller, K; Hack, D; et al: Technique of Transanal Endoscopic Microsurgery, Surg Endosc, 1988.
2. Buncke, HJ; Chater, NL; Szabo, Z: Manual of Microvascular Surgery. Danbury, CT, Davis & Geck, 1975.
3. Szabo, Z; Stellini, L; Rose, EH; et al: Slip-knot suspension technique: A fail-safe microanastomosis technique for small-caliber vessels. Microsurg 13:100–102, 1992.
4. Caelli, T: The perception of motion, in visual perception theory and practice. Oxford, Pergamon Press, 1981, pp. 147–169.
5. Seitz, RJ; Roland, PE; Bohm, C; et al: Motor learning in man: A positron emission tomographic study. NeuroReport 1:17–20, 1990.
6. Marr, D: From images to surfaces, in vision: A computational investigation into the human representation and processing of visual information. San Francisco, WH Freeman, 1982, pp. 99–253.
7. Bowyer, DW; Moran, ME; Szabo, Z: Laparoscopic suturing in urology: A model for vesicourethral anastomosis following radical prostatectomy. Min Invas Ther 4(2):165–170, 1993.
8. Airan, MT; Ko, ST: Personal communication, November 1991.
9. Sandridge, DA: Personal communication, June 1992.
10. Casanova, R; Herrera, GA; Engels, BV; et al: Microarterial sutureless anastomosis using polymeric adhesive: An experimental study. J Reconstr Microsurg 3:201–207, 1987.
11. Bowyer, DW; Moran, ME; Szabo, Z: Laparoscopic suture materials. Presented at the Western Section of the American Urological Association, Kauai, HI, October 1992.
12. Treat, MR; Bessler, M: Personal communication, August 1992.
13. Advanced Laparoscopic Skills Course, Laser Institute, University of Utah Department of Surgery, Salt Lake City, July 1991.

CHAPTER 25

Laparoscopic Intracorporeal and Extracorporeal Suturing

Leslie A. Sharpe, MD, FACOG

Suturing and knot tying remain the traditional standard of care at laparotomy, augmented in some areas by cautery, clips, staples, or elastic bands. Laparoscopic suturing and knot tying are no less valuable, although until recently they have been rather neglected because of technical difficulty. Recent enhancement of instrumentation and technique has made suturing practical for the fully trained laparoscopic surgeon. Advances in knot-tying technique allow rapid placement of standard surgical knots equivalent to those made at laparotomy. More extensive procedures may be converted to laparoscopy when the suture method is applied.

CLINICAL APPLICATION

The suture method allows ligation of arteries and control of bulky tissue bundles not readily managed by other methods of hemostatis. It allows accurate repair of tissues in a wide variety of applications with precise control of forces applied during tissue approximation. It extends laparoscopy beyond tissue extirpation into the broad range of reparative procedures. The suture method also offers greater flexibility in the planning of surgical treatment for a variety of conditions. A surgeon proficient in the suture method can adapt to laparoscopy many of the skills acquired in the practice of traditional surgery and can therefore more rapidly convert a significant proportion of procedures to the laparoscopic approach. The well-trained surgeon knows how to perform organ repair by suturing. The challenge is to accomplish such suturing laparoscopically. Careful planning, adequate instrumentation, and an organized approach favor success. Table 25-1 lists some procedures amenable to laparoscopic surgery by the suture method.

INSTRUMENTATION

Instrumentation for laparoscopic suturing was initially propagated by Semm, who used 3-mm and 5-mm needle holders in conjunction with 1-inch straight needles swaged with catgut suture through 5-mm access ports. He used Roeder knots to secure the ligatures. The straight needles were relatively difficult to maneuver through solid tissues, and the weak grasp of the needle holders made needle slippage commonplace. Curved needles twisted too easily to be of any practical use (Fig. 25-1). The more recently developed ski needle has a curved tip and a flattened body section to resist some of the tendency to twist (Fig. 25-2).

The Reddick-Saye needle holder offers enhanced grasping power, a secure locking mechanism, slender

Table 25–1. PROCEDURES AMENABLE TO LAPAROSCOPIC SUTURING

Urology	General Surgery	Gynecology
Renal cyst marsupialization	Cholecystectomy	Hysterectomy
Nephrectomy	Bile duct repair	Metroplasty
Nephropexy	Nissen fundoplication	Myomectomy
Pyeloplasty	Enterotomy repair	Ovarian cystectomy
Ureteroureterostomy	Bowel resection	Salpingoplasty
Ureteral anastomosis	Bowel anastomosis	Salpingo-oophorectomy
Ureteral implantation	Omentectomy	Enterocele repair
Urinary diversion	Appendectomy	Uterine suspension
Cystotomy repair	Herniorrhaphy	Vaginal suspension
Diverticulectomy		
Cystectomy		
Retropubic urethropexy		

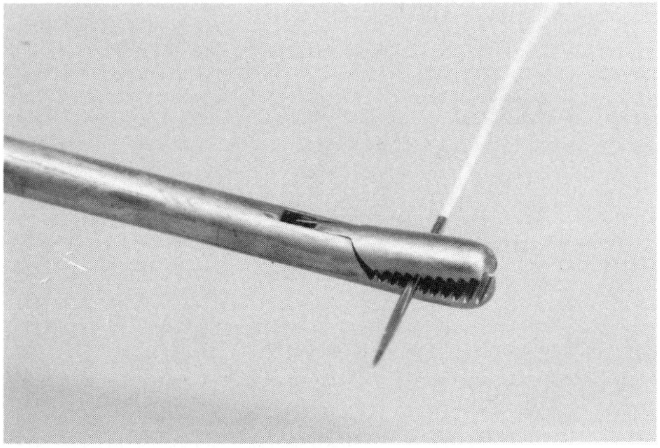

Figure 25–1. A Semm 5-mm needle holder grasping a 1-inch straight needle swaged to catgut suture.

jaws for delicate work, and a diamond-patterned jaw surface for grasp of straight or curved needles.

The Cook needle holder* works well with straight or curved needles and is designed to turn a curved needle into perpendicular orientation automatically. It grasps strongly and resists twisting of the needle. Its unique mechanism requires protrusion of the instrument tip beyond the needle to an extent that it may at times interfere with needle placement in tissues (Fig. 25–3). The mechanism may cut or damage sutures, therefore it cannot be used to grasp a suture for instrumental knot tying or needle passage through an access port. A separate introducer 10 mm in diameter is necessary to load suture and needle for insertion through the access port.

The Sharpe needle holder† has vertically oriented viselike jaws with diamond-patterned teeth to provide secure grasp of needles or suture. There is no tip protrusion to interfere with use, and a curved needle can be held either upright or inverted for flexible application. When used with curved needles having square or flat-sided profiles, it preferentially orients them to perpendicular and then strongly resists their twisting. The 7-mm tip size allows application of greater grasping force, for maximum needle stability when suturing bulky tissues or using large needles. The 10-mm shaft diameter eliminates need for adapters. Its firm needle grasp aids intracorporeal knot tying, and its ability to grasp a suture speeds needle introduction and withdrawal when used with the 10- to 11-mm access ports most suitable for use with large curved needles. When used in conjunction with the Sharpe hemostat, it also speeds needle orientation and manipulation internally (Fig. 25–4).

Laparoscopic suturing is enhanced when the needles and suture products in use have been conceived for a particular use or to match a specific needle holder. The Ethicon Endonaht‡ suture system works well with Semm style needle holders. The ski needle

*Cook OB/GYN, Spencer, IN.
†Sharpe Endosurgical Corp, Minneapolis, MN.

‡Ethicon, Inc, Somerville, NJ.

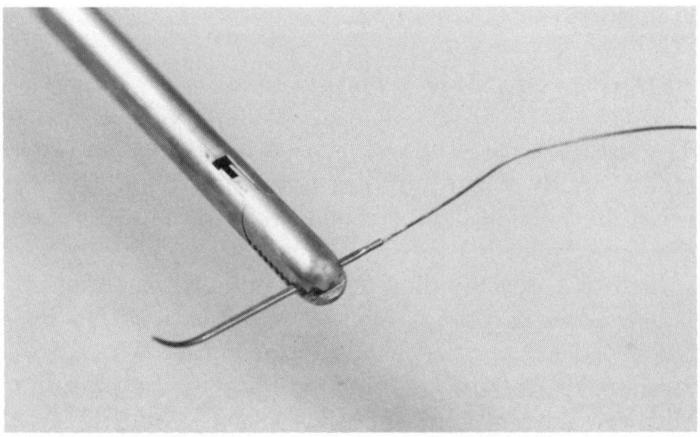

Figure 25–2. A Semm 5-mm needle holder grasping a ski needle swaged to 3-0 Vicryl suture.

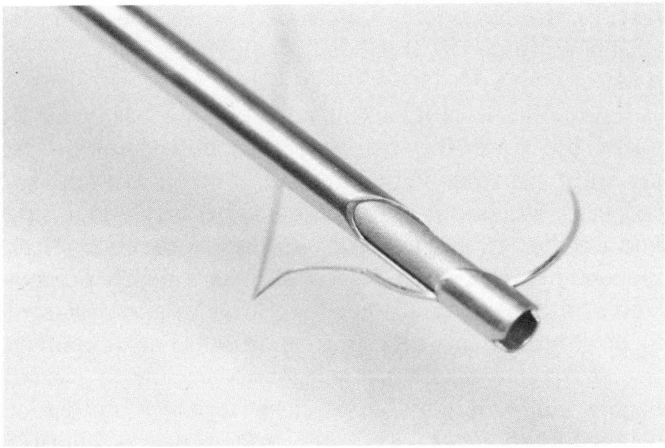

Figure 25–3. A Cook 5-mm needle holder grasping a G.I. needle swaged to 3-0 Vicryl suture.

design tracks through solid tissue more easily, and works well with Semm or Reddick-Saye type needle holders. Stronger, longer curved needles with square or flat-sided profile (Ethicon EN-2) are optimal for use with the Sharpe needle holder.

A high-resolution video system is required for clear view of suture and needles. To compensate for unavoidable gas losses while handling suture through access ports, an automatic CO_2 insufflator with 9 to 15 l/minute flow capacity is advisable. Access ports with ball valve or trumpet style gas seals tend to snag or cut sutures and should not be used. Access ports having trap door or rubber flap style gas seals are compatible with manipulation of sutures. Size 10- to 11-mm ports allow passage of larger curved needles that are useful in most applications. Greatest flexibility and speed in suturing are achieved when the needle will fit through any port in use. Large ports also allow movement of the laparoscope as needed for a better view.

ORIENTATION TO VIDEO-MONITORED SURGERY

The challenges of accurate suture placement and smooth needle retrieval are compounded when they are performed with two-dimensional video monitoring. With practice the surgeon learns to use parallax effects as a partial corrective for the lack of true depth perception. Any subtle movement of the laparoscope produces greater apparent movement of objects nearer the lens. Any given amount of instrument movement appears less in those farther away from the lens; advancement of the scope produces more rapid increase in size of the images of nearer objects. Moving the scope in close compresses the depth of field and enhances apparent depth perception.

Rotation of the video camera from the horizontal plane produces disorienting rotated images on the video monitor and confusing movements in the up-down and left-right directions. The surgeon is best oriented when standing behind a horizontal video camera that faces its video monitor (Fig. 25–5).

The assistant, who usually faces the video camera at a 90° angle, manipulates instruments entering from one side of the camera's field of view and faces a video monitor with confusing images. Up and down motions remain as expected, but left-right and in-out become confused (Fig. 25–6).

Whenever confusion occurs, camera rotation should first be eliminated; then the video image is interpreted from the video camera's frame of reference. Proper direction of hand motion can be reasoned out, initiated slowly, and then can more easily be completed by fine adjustment of hand motion while underway. Since laparoscopic suturing involves delicate hand motions and multiple grasping operations, careful attention to orientation is essential to avoid frus-

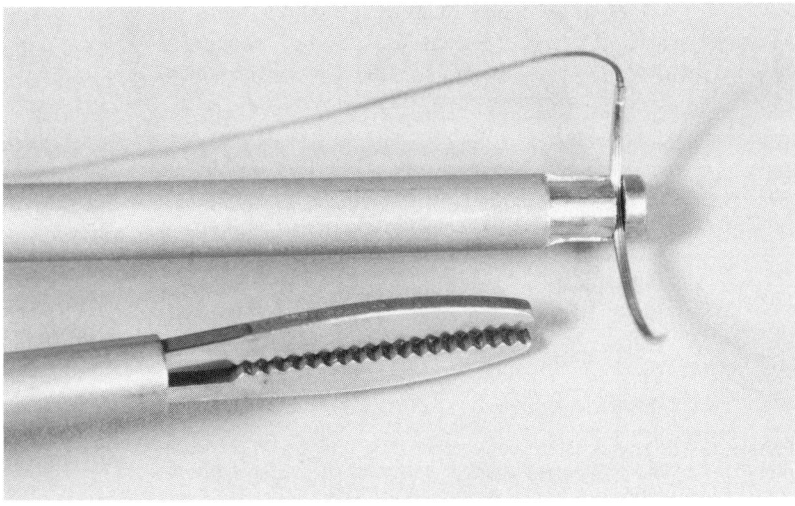

Figure 25–4. A Sharpe needle holder grasping an Ethicon EN-2 needle swaged to 0 Vicryl suture. A Sharpe hemostat aids needle manipulation.

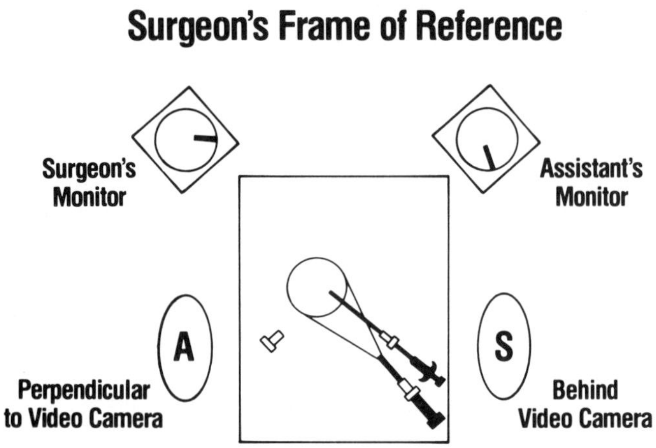

Movements

Instrument Handle	Image of Tip
Inward	Smaller
Outward	Larger
Right	Left
Left	Right
Up	Down
Down	Up

Figure 25–5. The surgeon behind the video camera views well-oriented images on the video monitor.

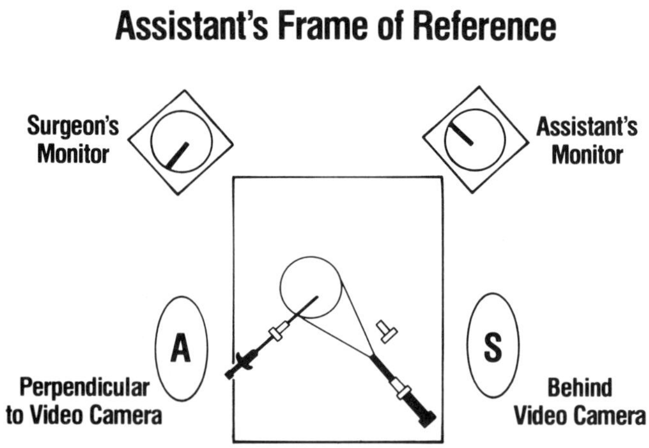

Movements

Instrument Handle	Image of Tip
Inward	Right
Outward	Left
Right	Smaller
Left	Larger
Up	Down
Down	Up

Figure 25–6. The assistant views confusing images on the video monitor and must interpret them in terms of the video camera's frame of reference.

tration, needless delay, or tissue trauma due to application of force on the needle contrary to its proper path.

The delicate motions of suturing are best coordinated by a surgeon working with both hands. The assistant provides exposure and controls the laparoscope. A wide-angle view is best for stitch planning and needle orientation; a close view is best for stitch placement and needle retrieval, where depth perception and fine grasp are needed. Surgeon and assistant must communicate clearly to coordinate movement of the laparoscope with the surgeon's actions. A loaded needle holder is capable of catastrophic puncture or laceration of vital structures and must be handled with great care. Insertion, manipulation, and retrieval of needles must be done at all times *in full view.*

PROCEDURE PLANNING

The surgeon should mentally visualize the operative anatomy, then plan the size and number of access ports in order to assure adequate visualization, exposure, and access for suturing. Suturing is most easily done when the shaft of the needle holder lies parallel to the tissue planes being approximated, so that the needle is perpendicular to the suture line. Careful port placement therefore contributes to success. Port placement should also allow assisting instruments to function without colliding or crossing (Fig. 25–7). In general, access is optimal when two working ports can be brought to bear on all sides of the target organ.

SUTURING TECHNIQUE

A stout, curved needle may be inserted into the abdomen by grasping the suture 1 cm away from it with the needle holder, which then carries it heel first through a 10- to 11-mm access port. Once inside, the needle is first stabilized by grasping its tip end in a hemostat; it is then turned to the desired orientation by pulling on the suture with the needle holder (Fig. 25–8). The well-oriented needle is easily loaded into the needle holder.

Depth perception challenges and restricted range of needle holder movement force the surgeon to use extra care in stitch placement. The needle is kept in view for safety. It is helpful to touch the needle tip lightly to the intended point of tissue entry, then carefully adjust needle angle until it can be driven through the tissues as desired. The assisting hemostat can exert counterpressure to clear the needle tip and then grasp the needle to stabilize it before release from the needle holder (Fig. 25–9). The unsecured needle too readily turns out of view, forcing a time-consuming repeat of the entire process. The secured needle is usually

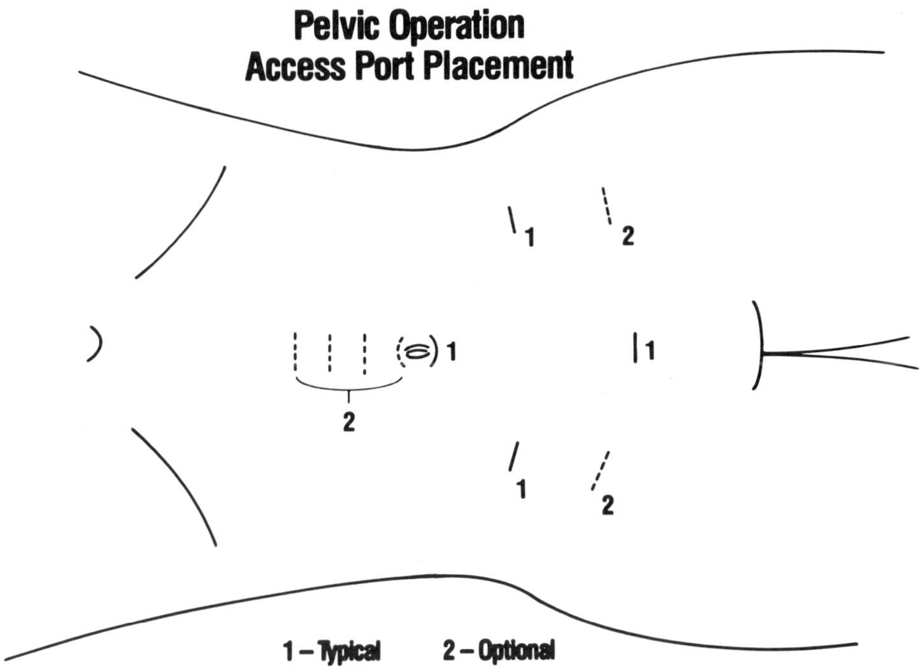

Figure 25–7. Port locations to provide optimal angles of access for pelvic suturing procedures.

pulled through without difficulty to complete the stitch. The needle holder then grasps the suture near the needle in order to retrieve it (Fig. 25–10). The needle is pulled heel first through the access port while the gas seal is held open to prevent snagging. A typical stitch can be completed in less than 60 seconds.

Continuous suturing proceeds as above, but the needle is left on as the anchoring knot is tied. The surgeon places each succeeding stitch as previously described, using care to avoid entanglement in slack suture. Slack suture is most readily managed by the assistant outside the access port and is pulled through by the surgeon after completion of each stitch. Knot tying is simplified if a second suture is placed at the end point to tie onto or if two continuous sutures meet and are tied together. Three-stranded knots are difficult to tie laparoscopically and should be avoided.

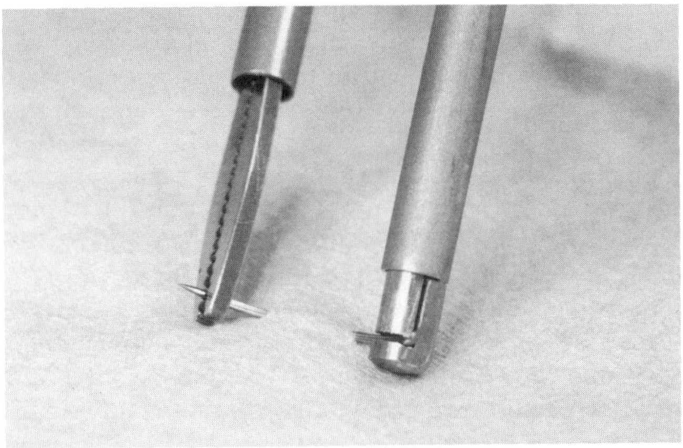

Figure 25–9. The stitch is placed as desired, and the needle is stabilized by grasping its tip with a hemostat before its release from the needle holder.

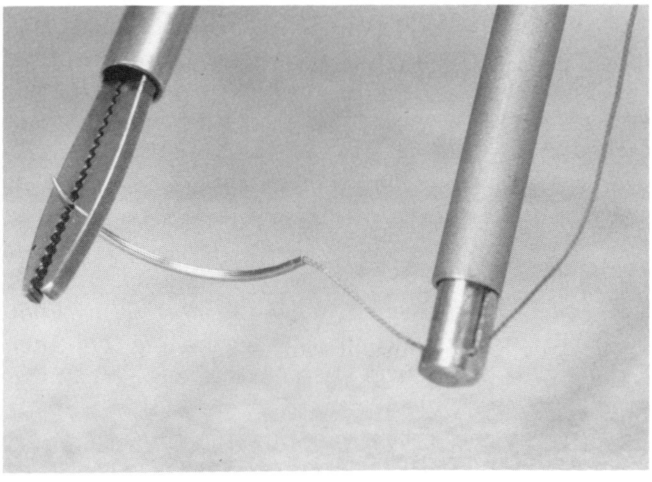

Figure 25–8. The hemostat stabilizes the tip of the needle; then traction on the suture turns it to the desired orientation to load in the needle holder.

INTRACORPOREAL KNOT TYING

Instrument tying involves the wrapping of one or two loops of one end of a suture strand around a clamp, which then pulls the other suture end through the loops to form a knot. Using one laparoscopic instrument to wrap such loops around another is difficult, since the loops are often lost when the nearly parallel

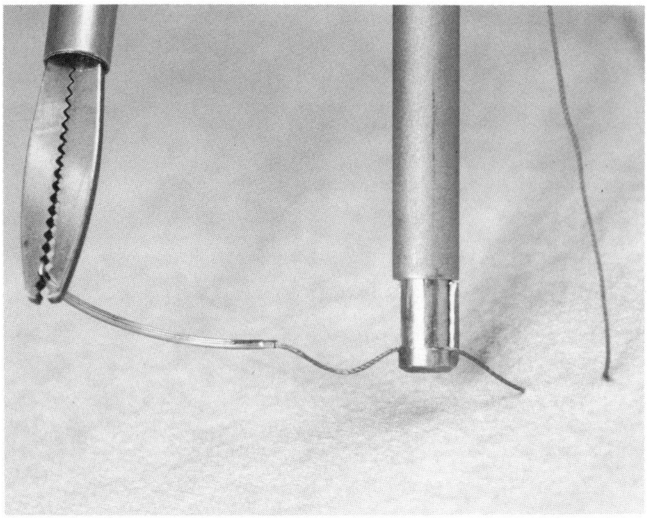

Figure 25–10. A hemostat pulls the needle through, and the needle holder grasps the suture to retrieve the needle through the access port.

tips pass each other. The traditional method of instrument tying can be adapted to laparoscopy, however, if a powerful needle holder is available. The needle is held by its tip end in the needle holder and is used to help form the knots. The heel end of the needle wraps loops of suture around the assisting clamp well above its tip, where they are easily retained as the clamp grasps the other end of the suture to pull through and form the knot (Fig. 25–11). Knots are tied most rapidly when the assistant holds the free suture end and hands it to the surgeon's hemostat after loops have been wrapped around it. This method is simple and rapid and can be used to form surgeon's or square knots as desired. Knot tension is limited by the strength of swaged suture attachment to the needle and grasping power of the assisting clamp.

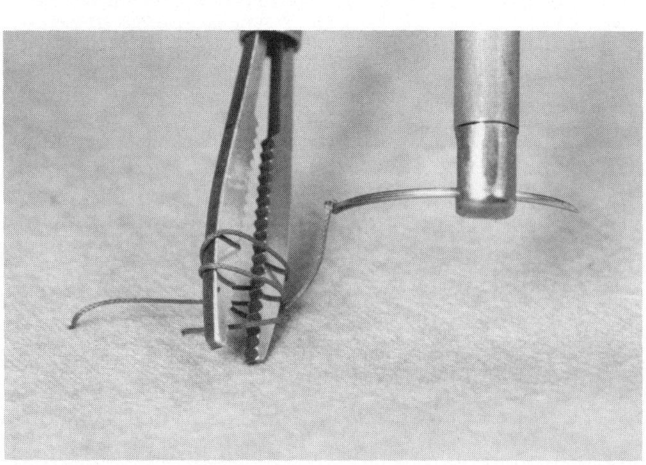

Figure 25–11. The needle wraps two loops above the tip of the hemostat, which then pulls the suture end through to form a knot. (From Sharpe, LA: Laparoscopic suturing techniques. In: Gomella, LG; Kozminski, M; Winfield, HN; eds.: Laparoscopic Urologic Surgery. New York, Raven Press, 1994, p. 102.)

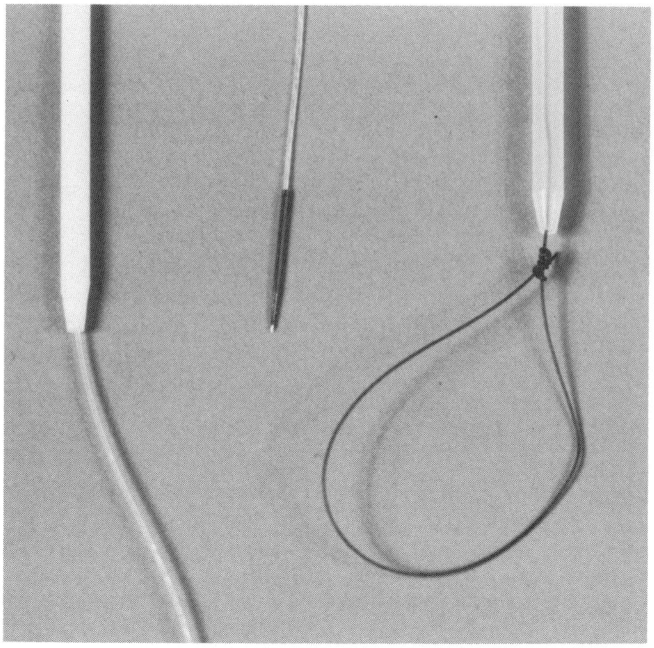

Figure 25–12. The knot-pusher sleeve and the straight needle of endosuture are shown on the left; on the right is an endoloop with a pretied Roeder knot.

EXTRACORPOREAL KNOTTING

The Roeder knot or variations of it can be used to form a snare loop that closes when the knot is pushed along the suture by an elongated hollow push rod. As the loop is drawn tight upon tissue, the knot jams and then resists loosening. All jam knots are more complex than traditional surgical knots, must be tied correctly to assure proper function, and do not work equally well with all suture types. They require redundant ligations for vascular pedicle security, and they cannot be used to terminate a continuous suture line. Pretied Endoloops* and also Endosuture with a 1-inch straight needle swaged onto catgut suture and a preattached knot pusher sleeve are available (Fig. 25–12). The surgeon should know how to tie a jam knot in order to use the Endosuture system (Fig. 25–13, *A* to *D*).

The figure-of-eight loop is a true slip knot, which is easily and rapidly formed, and is the most secure knot available to initiate a continuous suture line. The knot forms a collapsible loop at the suture end. When the needle and suture are passed through this loop, it closes and anchors the suture line (Fig. 25–14 *A* to *F*).

*Ethicon, Inc, Somerville, NJ.

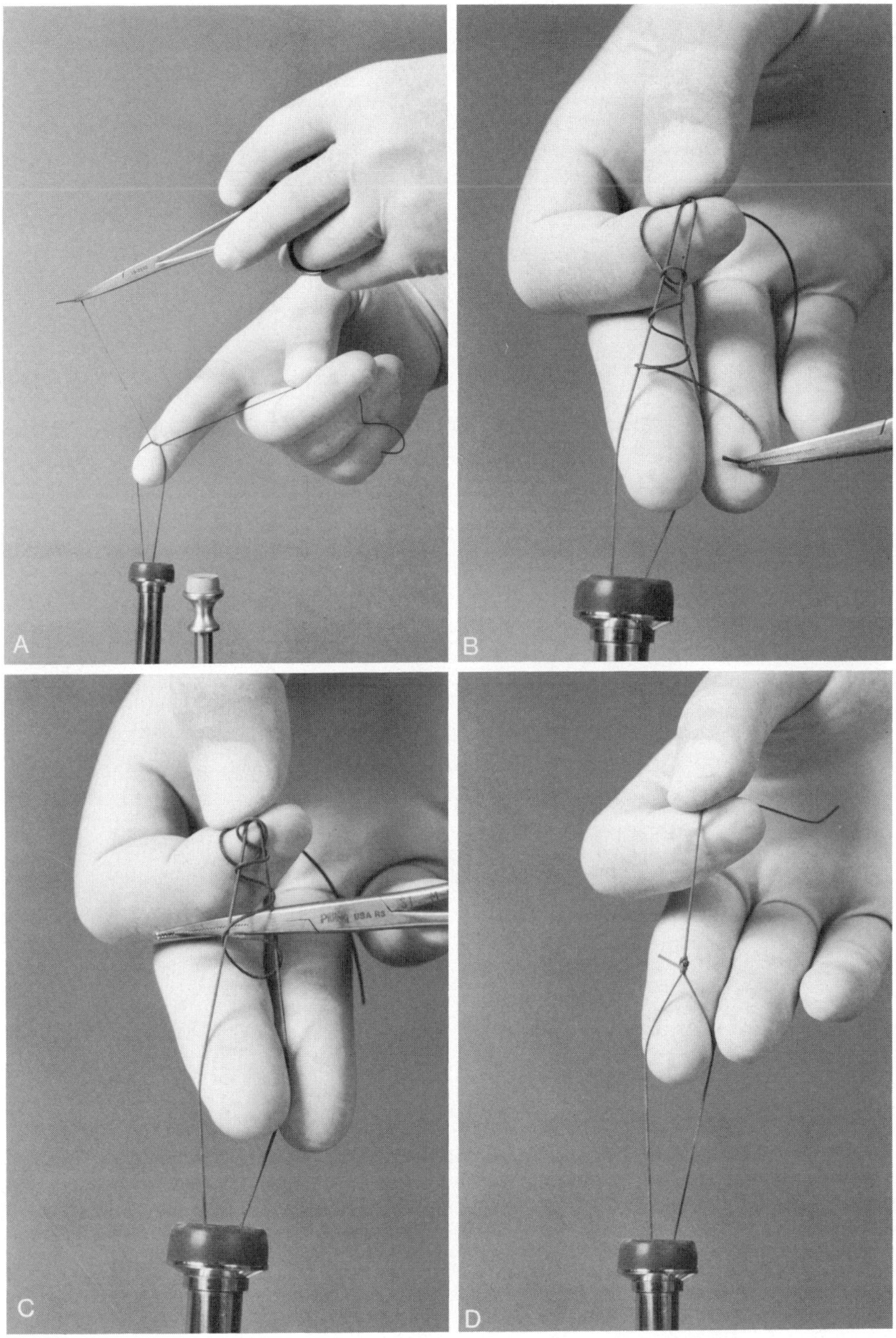

Figure 25–13. *A*, Roeder knot begins with a single hitch, using a clamp to control the free end of suture. *B*, The first hitch is held between thumb and finger, as a clamp passes the free end three times around both strands. *C*, The clamp passes the free end between strands above the last turn, far enough so that it remains there when released. *D*, The knot is drawn tight, and the free end is cut short. The knot-pusher sleeve may push it into place (not shown). (From Sharpe, LA: Laparoscopic suturing techniques. In: Gomella, LG; Kozminski, M; Winfield, HN; eds.: Laparoscopic Urologic Surgery. New York, Raven Press, 1994, p. 103.)

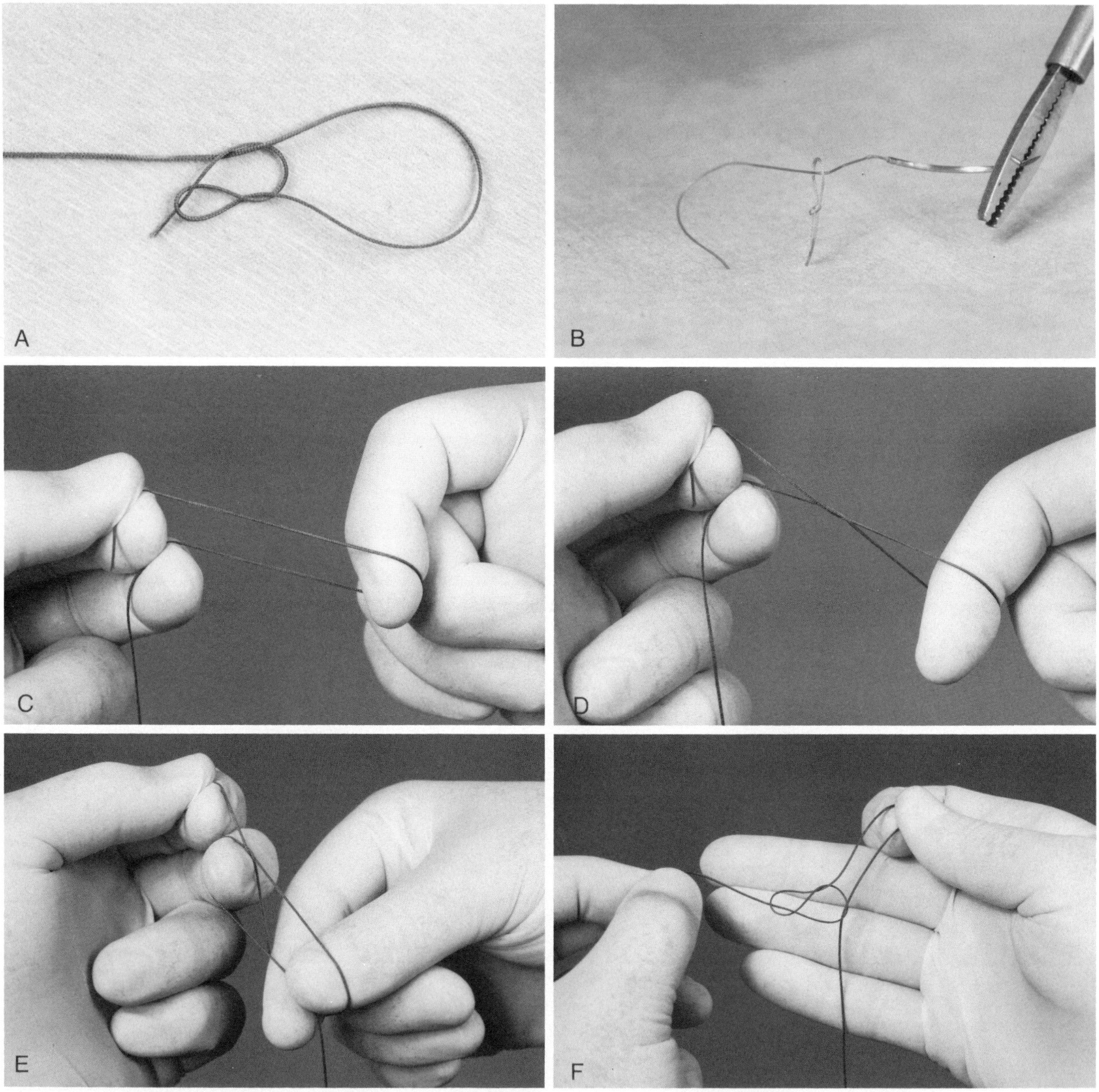

Figure 25–14. *A*, Figure-of-eight loop. A loop of suture is pulled through the stable figure-of-eight knot. *B*, Needle and suture pass through the figure-of-eight loop, which closes and anchors the suture as it is pulled tight. *C*, A figure-of-eight loop is begun by looping the suture around a finger as shown. *D*, The finger turns the loop counterclockwise one full turn. *E*, Thumb and finger reach through the loop and grasp the long strand. *F*, The long strand is pulled through to form the figure-of-eight knot and sliding loop.

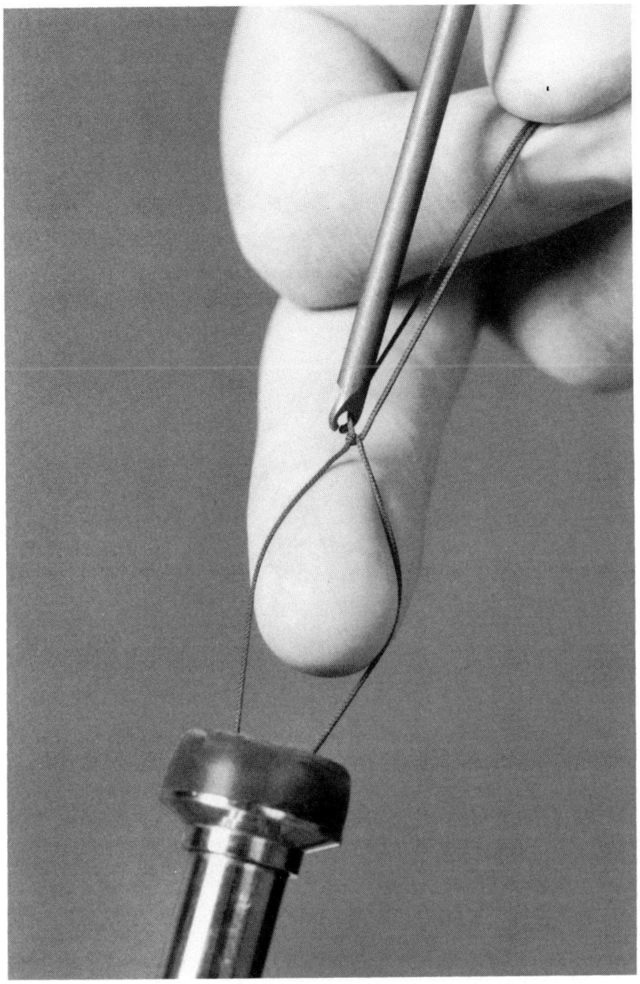

Figure 25–15. A Clarke knot pusher engages one strand above the knot, then pushes it in place as both strands are held taut.

The Clarke knot pusher is used to place internally standard surgical square knots that have been formed externally. After each square hitch is formed, the surgeon holds both strands taut, engages one strand with the knot pusher and then slides the knot into place internally. If it is held too tautly, the knot tends to jam and may fray or break the suture. If it is too slack, the suture may disengage from the knot pusher. Internal knot friction makes a double-throw surgeon's knot difficult to use. Twisting of the strands around each other may be difficult to detect and if present will impair knot quality. When used carefully with proper attention to detail, the Clarke knot pusher is a significant addition to laparoscopic surgical technique (Fig. 25–15).

The Sharpe knot pusher,* lately added to the laparoscopic armamentarium, has significant advantages. It is held in one hand throughout the ligation, increasing speed and efficiency, and minimizing risk of suture twisting. Its closed tip continuously engages one suture strand, which is made captive by a clamp and can be controlled by the knot pusher. One-handed square knots can be rapidly formed, then carried internally, and tied securely (Fig. 25–16 *A* to *C*). The closed tip allows each hitch to be carried loosely into place, minimizing risk of fraying or unwarranted breakage, even when using a fine suture. It easily places a double-throw surgeon's knot with proper tension, maximizing integrity of the first knot. Twisting of the loose suture strands is easily detected, readily corrected, and does not recur unless the surgeon loses control of a suture strand. The knot pusher exerts linear forces across the knot and accurately transmits knot tension to the surgeon's hand, so that any size or type of suture can be tied with confidence (Fig. 25–16 *D* to *E*). A surgeon's knot and four square knots can be formed in less than 60 seconds.

CONCLUSIONS

With the development of more powerful needle holders and clamps, improved suture products, and more effective knot-tying techniques, the suture method has become a practical skill for any well-trained laparoscopic surgeon. With experience the surgeon learns to plan ahead in each situation the optimal direction of needle rotation through the tissues, which port will allow proper orientation of the needle holder to achieve such needle rotation, and through which port to insert the assisting instrument so that the stitch can be placed and the needle can be retrieved without crossing instruments or losing control of the needle. Facility with suturing and knot tying allows the surgeon to adapt many more traditional techniques to laparoscopy and further to extend its application in a variety of reparative procedures. The patience, perserverance, and careful planning necessary for success are amply rewarded by enhanced patient outcomes and satisfaction with care.

*Sharpe Endosurgical Corp, Minneapolis, MN.

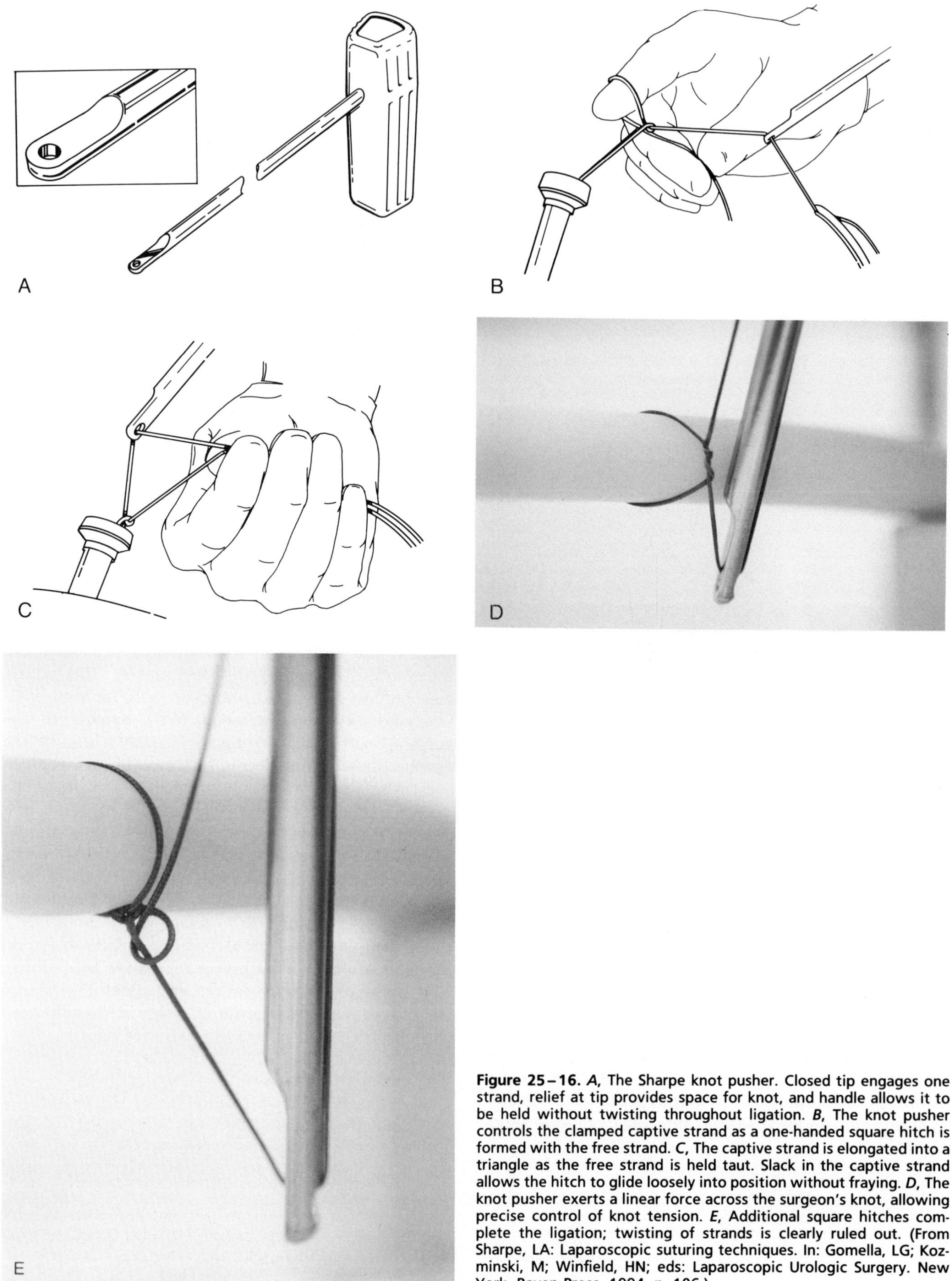

Figure 25–16. *A,* The Sharpe knot pusher. Closed tip engages one strand, relief at tip provides space for knot, and handle allows it to be held without twisting throughout ligation. *B,* The knot pusher controls the clamped captive strand as a one-handed square hitch is formed with the free strand. *C,* The captive strand is elongated into a triangle as the free strand is held taut. Slack in the captive strand allows the hitch to glide loosely into position without fraying. *D,* The knot pusher exerts a linear force across the surgeon's knot, allowing precise control of knot tension. *E,* Additional square hitches complete the ligation; twisting of strands is clearly ruled out. (From Sharpe, LA: Laparoscopic suturing techniques. In: Gomella, LG; Kozminski, M; Winfield, HN; eds: Laparoscopic Urologic Surgery. New York, Raven Press, 1994, p. 106.)

CHAPTER 26

Laparoscopic Clipping and Stapling Techniques

Michael E. Moran, MD
Roger K. Low, MD

Clipping and stapling devices are currently routinely used during laparoscopic surgery. Numerous devices are making their way into the market and it behooves the urologic laparoscopist to understand the implications of these increasingly sophisticated instruments, including their application and limitations. In this section we briefly review the historical foundations of clipping and stapling in surgery, discuss the theory for their utilization in laparoscopy, and detail the current clinical applications of these devices.

Surgical stapling has its foundations in the large, cumbersome prototypes investigated and utilized in the Soviet Union during the 1950s.[1] In the United States, these instruments were investigated and rapidly achieved widespread surgical utilization in the 1970s.[2] A large number of metallic stapling devices have since been developed and incorporated into the newer laparoscopic techniques. Limitations imposed by a closed laparoscopic environment favor a quick mechanical system to achieve hemostasis or reconstruct an organ. A linear stapler was initially utilized in laparoscopic surgery for intracorporeal bowel resections and reconstruction with a functional end-to-end technique.[3,4] Urologic adaptation for controlled hemostatic renal pedicle division during nephrectomy and for the distal portion of a nephroureterectomy has been reported.[5,6] The device has also been used to aid in the formation of laparoscopic ileal conduits.[7,8] The exact ramifications of these instruments and their potential for the future remains uncertain. Metallic staples within the urinary tract provide a foreign body nidus with well-recognized risks of encrustation and stone formation.[9] To overcome this problem, absorbable staples have been developed for investigational purposes.[10–12] Biofragmentable rings have been developed for sutureless intestinal anastomoses.[13,14]

An intriguing stapling device has been developed by Avant and Starr[15] that consists of a four-component end-to-end stapling system structurally applied over a balloon anvil. The staple fasteners are subsequently removed after the anastomosis becomes watertight. Inherent advantages include a removable metallic stapling fastener so there is no foreign body, potential quick reconstruction of a difficult sutured anastomosis, and a reliable method of laparoscopic reconstruction. Avant and Starr mention that the balloon anvil system inflates and stretches the apical urethra, dilating it for maximal incorporation of length into the urethrovesical anastomosis, perhaps diminishing the risk of incontinence.[15]

THEORY OF LAPAROSCOPIC HEMOSTASIS

Hemostasis in the closed environment imposed by minimal access surgery is one obstacle blocking progression to more complex intracorporeal techniques.

Table 26–1. METHODS OF LAPAROSCOPIC HEMOSTASIS EXCLUDING AUGMENTING PERIPHERAL CLOTTING PARAMETERS

Mechanical
Pressure
Clamping
Thermal
Radiofrequency electrocautery
monopolar
bipolar
Endothermal
Argon beam coagulator
Lasers
Cryoprobe
Radiofrequency energy
Microwave energy
Chemical
Fibrin glue
Calcium-impregnated swabs
Endo-Avitene
Suture or ligation
Stapling or clipping

The ability to maintain a clear surgical field allows complex tasks such as suturing to be performed.[16,17] Some of the instruments discussed in this chapter are essential components to the surgeon's hemostatic equipment. There are five basic modalities at the surgeon's disposal for the augmentation of local hemostasis (Table 26–1). Those particularly germane to this discussion are stapling and clip application.

Vascular pedicles have been safely ligated and divided by autostaplers for two decades.[18] The concern for arteriovenous fistula development is certainly worth consideration, especially if both structures are taken en bloc.[19] Vascular autostapling devices are theoretically designed to separate the artery and the vein before fixing the staple delivery mode. The laparoscopic autostaplers have few clinical data to support their widespread applicability as yet. Laboratory studies indicate that it is crucial to anticipate the trajectory necessary for delivering the 12-mm device to the targeted pedicle vasculature. The wrong approach results in untoward tension on the vessels during the engagement process. During transperitoneal laparoscopic nephrectomies, anterior axillary line portals both cranial and caudad to the laparoscope portal were effective in autostapling the renal artery and vein.[20] The amount of blood lost during a laparoscopic nephrectomy was also minimized during autostapled pedicle ligation compared with that lost during individual clip applications. Studies concerning the amount of load these vascular staples can withstand also indicate that they maintain hemostasis at superphysiologic pressures (1137 to 1551 mm Hg).[19] During the same study, 20% of the animals developed an arteriovenous fistula during long-term follow-up.

Clip application during pedicle dissection has been addressed in the general surgical literature.[21,22] There are proponents for loop ligation and for titanium clipping. Urologically, the laparoscopic nephrectomy animal model indicated that clips were associated with more blood loss than autostapling techniques.[20] One investigation of the two major manufacturers of laparoscopic clip appliers studied the pressures necessary to dislodge each type of clip in vitro and in vivo.[23] Both types had an unusually high rate of distraction during the in vivo studies.[23] The surgeon should be aware that these clips can become dislodged during the course of subsequent dissecting if either radial or horizontal traction is applied near or at the clip.

THEORY OF LAPAROSCOPIC TISSUE REAPPROXIMATION AND HEALING

The ability of the laparoscopic surgeon to reconstruct the genitourinary tract is fundamentally the same in the closed compared with the open abdomen. The five techniques available for tissue reapproximation are listed in Table 26–2. As previously mentioned, Avant's ingenious device combines both crimping and splinting in an end-to-end anastomotic device.[15] The surgical literature is replete with arguments for and against suturing compared with stapling for gastrointestinal reconstruction.[25–27] Much research in the mechanisms of tissue healing following various reconstruction techniques has been fostered.[25] However, the integrity of the intrinsic blood supply is paramount to the ability of mucosa-to-mucosa sealing.[25]

Anastomosis and complex enteric-uroepithelial composite appositions are the rule for urologic reconstruction. A number of synthetic, autograft, and xenograft materials have been sought to further diminish the trauma of urologic reconstruction.[28] Methods of laparoscopically reapproximating these and native bowel segments to the bladder are being investigated. Stapled and sutured bladder resections and closures have been described.[5,29–31] Bladder diverticula have been removed, and partial cystectomies with and without nephroureterectomy have been described.[3,10,32] Both clinical study and animal work on the use of metallic autostapling instruments suggest that this

Table 26–2. THE FIVE METHODS OF TISSUE REAPPROXIMATION*

Suturing
Stapling
Crimping
Thermal welding (laser)
Gluing

*Each can be applied alone or in combination with the others.

technique is successful.[33] Delayed complications, specifically encrustation on the nidus of the foreign body have not been observed to date. This probably reflects the investigator's method of careful apposition, trying to keep the staple line from direct contact with the urine. Upper tract reconstructions have also been reported. Dismembered pyeloplasties,[34] anterior pyelocaliceal diverticulectomy with omental patch,[35] and partial nephrectomies[36,37] all have been performed. The reconstructions to date have been hampered by constraints of limited instrument technology; lack of stereoscopic imaging; and closed, fixed, operative access to the urologic areas of interest.

LAPAROSCOPIC EXTRACORPOREAL STAPLING

The first use of surgical stapling technology in laparoscopic surgery was for the resection of bowel. The development of large abdominal trocars allowed the surgeon to deliver the isolated bowel segment extracorporeally for stapled resection after classic "open" techniques. These trocars were specially designed in sizes approaching 30 and 40 mm (Fig. 26–1). In experimental models, the bowel could be easily mobilized on its vascular mesentery, opening intracorporeally a window for the resected segment. The segment could then be grasped with endoscopic Babcock-type clamps and delivered through the large working trocar. Standard functional end-to-end anastomoses with the use of linear cutting staplers and TA staplers have been performed (Fig. 26–2). Urologically, this technique was first used by Kozminski and Partamian to perform an ileal conduit urinary diversion.[7] Once the resected bowel segment was mobilized and mesentery was closed intracorporeally with biting clips, then the ureteral anastomoses were accomplished extracorporeally after mobilizing the ureters, by suturing techniques. Securing the conduit to the retroperitoneum was again accomplished by biting clips applied intracorporeally.

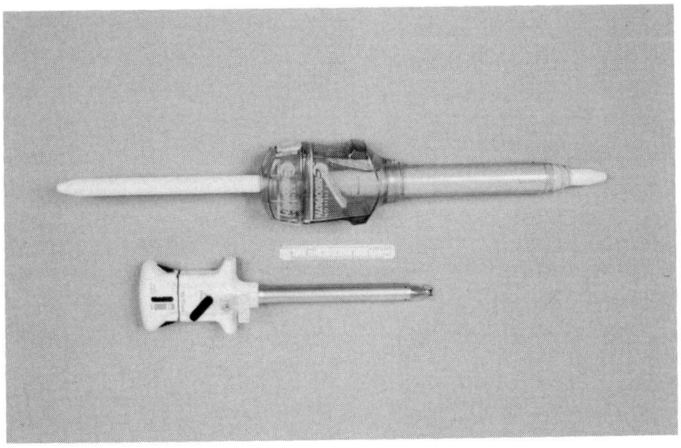

Figure 26–1. Large laparoscopic portals allow the colon to be delivered to the anterior abdominal wall. Extracorporeal stapling can then be performed.

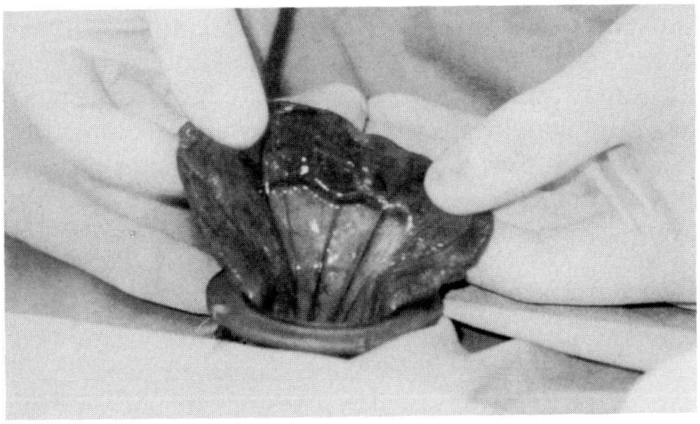

Figure 26–2. Small bowel delivered for extracorporeal stapling techniques.

End-to-end anastomoses have been accomplished with a variety of techniques using extracorporeally assisted (EEA) circular staplers. The esophagus and colon have been the prime organs resected in this fashion. Following colon resection, a purse-string suture is placed to secure both luminal ends, one to secure the open stapler and one to fix the anvil. An alternative to EEA staplers is the biodegradable anastomotic ring (BAR) device. This instrument has been utilized for laparoscopic-assisted colon anastomoses through small celiotomies. Purse-string sutures are again necessary before applying the anastomotic ring; however, special purse-string applicators are being devised.[38] These instruments have compared favorably with standard stapler reconstruction in comparative clinical trials.[13] This may have significance, especially with increasing concerns regarding the devascularizing effects of triple-stapled, functional side-to-side anastomoses that result in long-term luminal narrowing.[25]

LAPAROSCOPIC INTRACORPOREAL STAPLING AND CLIPPING

The primary applications of intracorporeal stapling and clipping have been discussed along with the theory of laparoscopic hemostasis and tissue reapproximation. Now attention is focused on the use of intracorporeal staples and clips. As with almost every laparoscopic instrument there are the considerations of reusable versus disposable devices. Clip appliers come in both forms, but as of this writing, the automatic staplers are single-patient use items. One primary problem with these devices is the lack of research data regarding their reliability, problems commonly encountered during utilization, tissue reactivity, and ease of use. Because of the extensive use of their open counterparts, staples and clips have become instantly popular amongst laparoscopic surgeons. Because of the many barriers to intracorporeal suturing, clip appliers and automatic staplers have become routine instruments on many operating room tables.

Clip Appliers

Clip appliers have several crucial features warranting careful scrutiny by the surgical consumer (Fig. 26–3; Table 26–3). The size, shape, and security of the applied metallic clips must initially be discussed. Titanium clip sizes range from 6.0 to 11.0 mm. Each company's laparoscopic clip has a characteristic "footprint" (Fig. 26–4). Investigations imply that all laparoscopic clips are capable of being distracted.[23] Dislodgement should be a feature recognized by all laparoscopists. Once applied, further dissection around the clips is capable of transversely dislodging them. Nondisposable clip appliers require multiple passages through the entrance trocar for multifiring. The only cost is the initial purchase price of the instrument and the reloadable cartridges, whereas each disposable clip applier must be purchased. However, the disposable clip appliers have additional features not currently available on the reusable instruments (Fig. 26–5). Disposable devices are capable of multifire (20 clips) and have rotatable shafts. The pistol grip can comfortably rest in the surgeon's palm as the angle of application can be adjusted 360°. At present, all clip appliers are designed for placement through 10-mm portals. When a clip is deployed, the vessels should be carefully positioned by assisting graspers for alignment perpendicular to the jaws. Using multifire, disposable clip appliers, the clip should be loaded intracorporeally to avoid inadvertent dislodgement during passage through the flapper valves of the trocar. By gently squeezing the trigger, the clip applier more firmly grasps the clip so that the exact deployment site can be selected. The trigger is then firmly squeezed. If too much force is used, or too much tissue is taken, the delicate autoloading mechanisms can malfunction, precluding its further use.

Table 26–3. ENDOSCOPIC CLIP APPLIERS

	Disposable Types	
	Endoclip	***Endopath***
Manufacturer	US Surgical	Ethicon
No. of clips	20	20
Port size	10 mm	10 or 11 mm
Clip size	Medium, 6.0 mm Medium large, 8.9 mm Large, 11.0 mm	Medium large, 8.8 mm
Shaft	360°	360°

Research has also studied the tissue reactivity of various types of clips.[10] All clips can potentially cause adhesion formation.[39] In studies comparing metallic and absorbable types of clips, no significant difference could be found between types. Other studies have been concerned about the reliability of these clips for maintaining hemostasis.[19] We have already discussed loss by distraction of these laparoscopic clips.[23]

The technique of vascular pedicle application deserves further discussion. Most investigators mention that more than one clip is necessary on major vascular structures. In addition, the clips are probably most secure if placed so that the open jaws face opposite directions. Electrocautery should not be used when dividing clipped vessels, because conductance to these metallic structures can occur. Necrosis can result in sloughing of the vessels within the occluding clips. Finally, studies have been performed on the ability to perform computed tomography and magnetic resonance imaging following titanium clip application. Although they produce more artifacts than absorbable ones, they do so less than other steel clips.

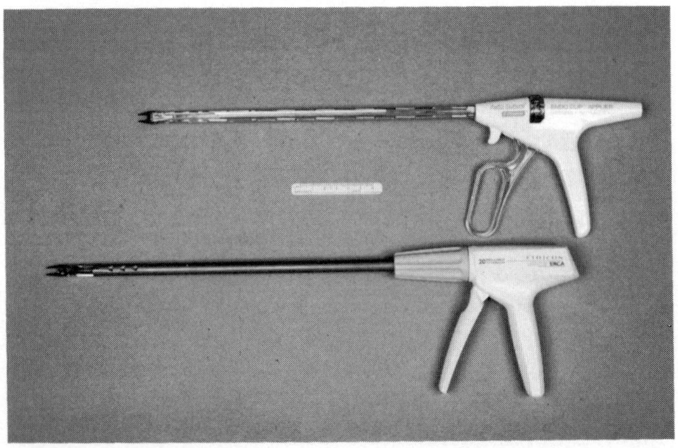

Figure 26–3. Two manufacturers' disposable clip appliers: U.S. Surgical, above; Ethicon, below.

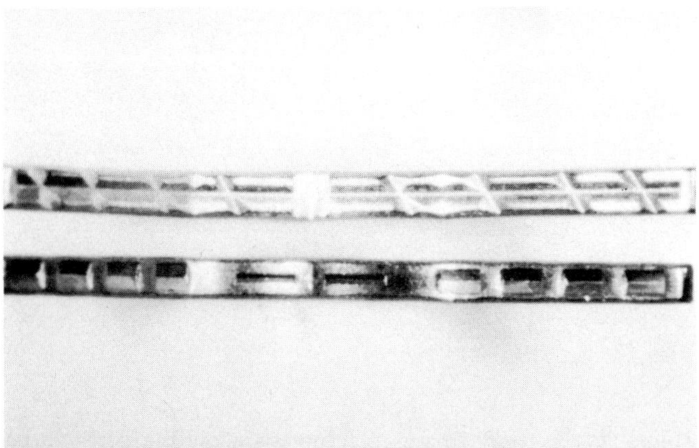

Figure 26–4. "Footprints" of laparoscopic clips. Ethicon above; U.S. Surgical below.

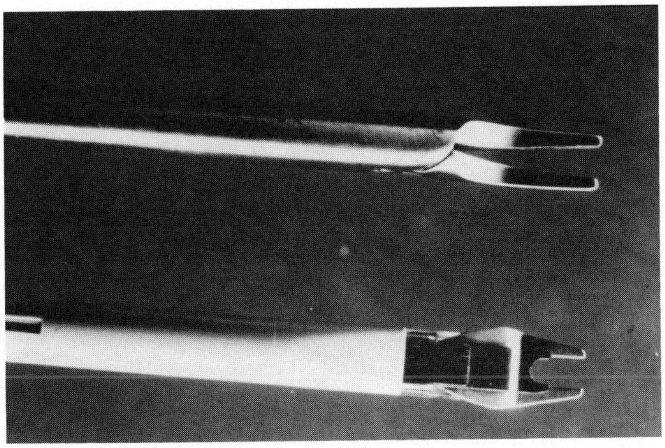

Figure 26–5. Comparison of disposable (above) and reusable (below) laparoscopic clip appliers. (Courtesy of Ethicon Endosurgery, Cincinnati, OH.)

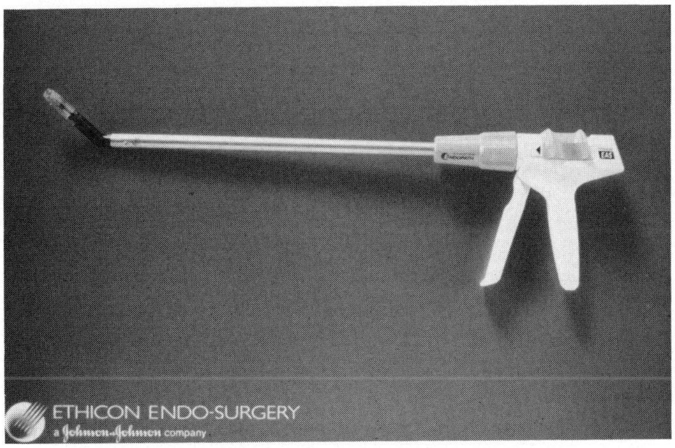

Figure 26–6. Biting, reticulated clip applier.

Biting Clips Appliers

Clip appliers were specifically designed to occlude and control vascular structures. The need to reapproximate and hold tissues together in fixed positions prompted the development of biting clip appliers. The surgeon's interest in laparoscopic herniorrhaphy was the primary driving force for the availability of both reusable and disposable instruments.[40] These must be applied carefully to take full advantage of the biting ends (Table 26–4). Initially, the surgeon should approximate the two opposing tissue edges with graspers. Next, the clip applier's trigger is pulled so as just to expose the biting ends. Each tip is carefully positioned to centrally locate the clip across the tissue edges. Finally, further tension on the trigger produces the "B" configuration in an ideal location of the tissues to be approximated. These devices have been used in reperitonealization following transabdominal bilateral pelvic lymphadenectomy, fixation of mesh for hernia repairs,[40] retraction of viscera from the pelvis with mesh for high-dose radiation therapy,[41] fixation of vesicourethral slings,[42,43] and closure of mesenteric defects after bowel resection.[44] Another refinement of the biting clip applicator is the addition of a distal articulating segment. This additional degree of motion allows angulation upward to 40° (Fig. 26–6). The surgeon can thus fixate materials such as mesh to the anterior abdominal wall or deep pelvic recess (i.e., Cooper's ligament) from a fixed access trocar.

The disposable multifire biting clip appliers come with either 10 or 20 clips per instrument with a 360° rotatable shaft and a distal articulating feature. One investigation compares sutures to these clips for security following placement. Prolene sutures resulted in higher burst pressures than the clips.[45]

Table 26–4. TYPES OF BITING CLIP APPLIERS

	Endo Hernia	Endopath EMS
Manufacturer	US Surgical	Ethicon
Port size	12 mm	10 or 11 mm
No. of clips	10	20
Reloadable	yes (×4)	no
Shaft	360°	360°
Depth of bite	3.0 mm	2.59 mm
Special features	Reticulation (0° to 40°)	(nondisposable) Reticulation

Automatic Staplers

Automated stapling devices allow the rapid deployment of multiple metallic staples to facilitate division and reapproximation of visceral structures (Fig. 26–7). These devices are available for laparoscopic, intracorporeal use and have a variety of features. Linear cutting, manual; linear cutting, powered; linear noncutting, manual; and linear noncutting, powered multifire disposable staplers are currently marked (Table 26–5). Each stapler has a specific size trocar limitation. The endo-GIA 30* is the original mechanical linear cutting device. It requires a 12-mm laparoscopic portal for placement. The endo-GIA 60 requires a 15-mm trocar. The Endopath 30† and Endopath 60† require a 12-mm and an 18-mm trocar, respectively. All automatic staplers have a 360° rotatable shaft. There is no articulated autostapler at present, although prototypes are being investigated.

The laparoscopic staplers deploy two triple rows of staples from the 30-mm blades. The staples are available in reloadable, color-coded cartridges: white, 2.5 mm; blue, 3.8 mm; and green, 4.8 mm. Staple size depends on the thickness of tissues being reapproxi-

*US Surgical Co, Norwalk, CT.
†Ethicon, Cincinnati, OH.

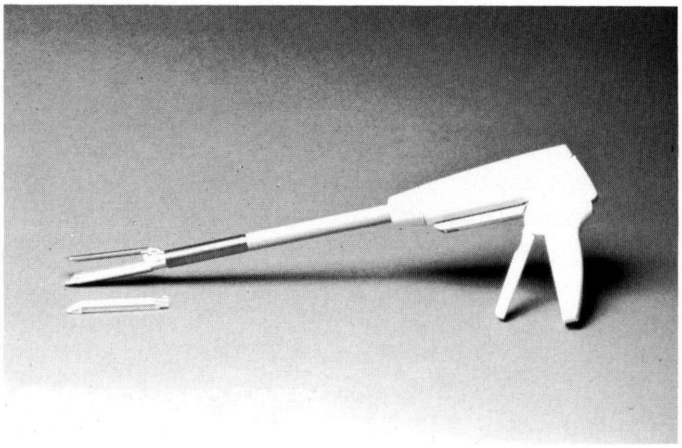

Figure 26–7. Intracorporeal automatic stapler. (Courtesy of Ethicon Endosurgery, Cincinnati, OH.)

mated or divided. The white 2.5-mm staples are usually used on vascular structures because of their compressibility. The larger blue 3.8-mm and green 4.8-mm staples are ideal for thicker visceral structures such as thickened ureter, small bowel, large bowel, or the bladder. An endoscopic sizer is available for tissue compression that will indicate which size staples will produce the best anastomosis or occlusion.

Linear cutting staplers usually deploy 3 rows of staples on either side of the cutting blade. An important consideration in using automated staplers is that the knife cuts short of the end of the staple line. Also, the staples are not loaded to the ends of the cartridges, making deployment length shorter than the 30 or 60 mm of the instrument. For this reason, when applying a linear cutting stapler, the ends should be seen protruding beyond the distal side of tissue before engaging the firing mechanism. The actual placement and firing of an endoscopic stapler is similar to that for the open surgery stapler. Once placed in an intracorporeal cavity, the release mechanism allows the jaws to be opened. Graspers guide the targeted visceral structure into the opened jaws. The graspers then align the tissues so that they provide a straight, smooth staple line without tissue bunching. The safety is disengaged, and the trigger is pulled, firing the staples and moving the knife that separates the tissues. The manufacturers have provided a safety lockout mechanism to prevent the knife from cutting tissue if the staple cartridge is empty or if a misfire should occur. In addition, these disposable staplers can multifire reloaded cartridges up to three additional firings (a total of four).

Linear noncutting staplers are available in both 30- and 60-mm lengths, deploying three or four rows of staples. Theoretically, these staplers reapproximate tissues with less incorporation of tissue mass. The staples on all of the noncutting instruments are identical to their cutting relatives.

Linear cutting staplers have had a wide variety of general surgical, thoracic, gynecologic, and urologic applications. As previously mentioned, the 30-mm long, 2.5-mm stapler has been used to divide vascular pedicles. The larger linear cutting staplers can be used for intracorporeal gastrointestinal resections and reconstructions. Small-bowel resections, partial colectomies, laparoscopic-assisted low anterior resections, gastric resections, gastrojejunostomies, esophageal resections, pulmonary wedge resections, lobectomies, and pneumonectomies have been facilitated with linear cutting staplers. Solid viscera, including the spleen, kidney, and uterus, have also been removed with the aid of these devices. Urologic reconstructions, including ileal conduit formation and distal and partial cystectomy, have been accomplished intracorporeally with the aid of these staplers. The noncutting staplers were originally developed for thoracoscopic purposes but are useful for closing enterotomies.

The major drawback of using these automated staplers other than the nonabsorbable foreign bodies (staples) within the urinary tract is cost. Estimates for linear cutting staplers are from $250 to $350 per instrument. Reloadable cartridges can currently be placed for no more than four applications. Each car-

Table 26–5. ENDOSCOPIC LINEAR CUTTING STAPLES

	Endo-GIA 30	Endo-GIA 60	Endopath 30	Endopath 60
Manufacturer	US Surgical	US Surgical	Ethicon	Ethicon
Port size	12 mm	15 mm	12 mm	12 mm
Length of staple line	30 mm	60 mm	30 mm	60 mm
Staple pattern	2 triple rows	2 triple rows	2 triple rows	2 double rows
Staple size (cartridge color)	2.5-mm (white) 3.8-mm (blue) 4.8-mm (green)		3.85-mm (blue) 4.85-mm (green)	
Reloads per instrument	3	3	3	3
Shaft	360°	360°	360°	360°
Special features	None	Pneumatic	Without cutting knife (4 rows)	Without cutting knife (4 rows)

tridge costs from $100 to $130. To date there are no circumferential end-to-end anastomotic, intracorporeal staplers. Currently, no absorbable staples for automated, intracorporeal staplers are available. Despite these drawbacks, the ability to rapidly, hemostatically, and reliably separate viscera and reapproximate them intracorporeally is a major advance for laparoscopic urologic reconstruction.

UROLOGIC LAPAROSCOPIC APPLICATIONS

Clinical applications of metal clips and automated staplers in laparoscopic urologic surgery focus on methods of securing hemostasis of vascular pedicles, resection or reconstruction of the bladder, and bowel segment exclusion for urinary diversion. Although metal clips and automated staplers facilitate the ability to perform laparoscopically many urological procedures, their long-term safety and efficacy has yet to be determined.

Securing the renal pedicle with metallic clips and automated staplers during laparoscopic nephrectomy and nephroureterectomy has been described.[6] When these two modalities were compared with open suture ligation of the renal pedicle in a porcine animal model, all three methods were found to be equally efficacious at preventing arterial leakage at physiologic pressures. At superphysiologic pressures (average, 1364 mm Hg), five or six pigs had leakage from renal arteries secured with staples.[19] The multifire vascular stapler cuts between two triple-staggered rows of 2.5-mm staples. Application of three 9-mm titanium clips and suture ligation with a 2-0 silk stick and 0 silk free tie both prevented leakage even at renal artery burst pressures (average, 1821 mm Hg). Moran similarly found renal artery branch vessel ligation with three clips transversely placed in opposing directions and linear stapling equally efficacious in a porcine animal model.[20] En masse occlusion of the renal pedicle without separation of the artery and vein, using a 12-mm vascular stapler, has also been examined in animals. One of three animals followed for 6 months demonstrated an arteriovenous fistula on aortography.[19] The true risk of arteriovenous fistula formation from en masse renal pedicle ligation may be even higher, given previous studies documenting their formation 5 months to 40 years after surgery.[46–48] Currently, recommendations are to use 9-mm titanium clips to secure renal vessels. A total of five clips, three placed proximally and two on the specimen side, placed transversely in opposing directions before vessel division is recommended.

Automated staplers have a wide application for laparoscopic procedures involving the bladder. The multifire linear cutting stapler has been used to divide the vascular pedicles and urethra during a laparoscopic cystectomy in 27-year-old woman with recurrent pyocystis and previous urinary diversion.[31] The endostapler has also been used to close bladder defects following diverticulectomy and distal ureterectomy for upper tract transitional cell carcinomas.[5,6] Parra and co-workers reported the first laparoscopic bladder diverticulectomy in an 87-year-old man with a superiorly positioned, narrow-necked diverticulum and chronic urinary tract infections. Adequate healing without urinary extravasation was documented by cystography 8 days after surgery.[32] In addition to expediting surgery, automated staplers may have an added benefit during excision of bladder diverticula containing urothelial malignancies by preventing potential spillage of tumor cells into the peritoneum. Neoplastic changes in the lining of diverticula occur in approximately 0% to 13.5% of cases.[49–52]

Laparoscopic division of a bladder cuff during nephroureterectomy and ureterectomy in porcine experiments and humans has been described by Kerbl and associates. After cystoscopically incising the ureteral orifice and submucosal tunnel, a 2-cm juxtaureteral bladder cuff is dissected laparoscopically. A linear cutting, multifire stapler is then used to close and excise the cuff of bladder.[33]

Segmental bowel excision and reconstruction using automated staplers has been practiced during open surgery for many years. Bohm and colleagues described the technique of laparoscopic intestinal resection and intraperitoneal reanastomosis.[53] After mobilization of the selected intestinal segment and isolation of the vascular pedicle, the linear cutting stapler is inserted into enterotomies on the antimesenteric border of afferent and efferent limbs of the future anastomosis. Two consecutive firings of the 3- or 6-cm stapler creates a 5- to 11-cm anastomosis. A cotton umbilical tape encircling the bowel close to the anastomosis provides countertraction and prevents spillage of intestinal contents into the peritoneum. Firing the linear stapler across both loops of bowel near the corner of the anastomosis transects the specimen and completes the anastomosis. Kozminski and Partamian reported the first urologic application of automated stapling for laparoscopic bowel resection and intracorporeal ileal conduit formation.[7] Their initial clinical case involved performing a palliative supravesical diversion in an 83-year-old man for unresectable fibrosarcoma of the prostate. Intracorporeal ureteral and bowel mobilization was accomplished through six 10- to 12-mm trocars. Bowel resection and reanastomosis were performed extracorporeally with linear stapling devices after evacuating the pneumoperitoneum and pulling the bowel through the 12-mm port site. Two subsequent patients have had ileal loop diversion with entirely intracorporeal bowel resections and reanastomosis using these staplers.[7] In all three patients, the ureteroileal anastomoses were sutured extracorporeally. This same technique has been repeated by others.[8] Other applications for these techniques may be urologic reconstructions with other gastrointestinal segments. Augmentation cystoplasty can be performed with harvested gastric, small-bowel, or large-bowel segments. Ureteral interposition or replacement can theoretically be performed. Finally, supravesical diversions with ileal conduits represent only one of many methods of noncontinent and continent heterotopic or orthotopic bladder replacement techniques. Automatic, linear cutting staplers have the potential to make such urologic reconstructions possible.

The lithogenic properties of metallic staples used for urinary tract reconstruction are well known. Stone formation attributed to exposed steel staples occurs in 3.2% to 4.2% of patients with ileal conduits and 4.9% to 10% of patients with Kock pouches.[54–57] The lithogenic potential of titanium staples exposed to human urine is not known. Kerbl and associates have used a linear titanium stapling device to excise a bladder cuff during nephroureterectomy in six adult humans.[33] Three patients have been followed more than a year without complication and endoscopic evidence of staple exposure. Endoscopic verification of lack of exposed staples and oversewing the staple line are recommended by some authors. Prototypic automated staplers using dissolvable staples are currently under study. Julian and Ravitch compared stone formation on exposed stainless steel and absorbable staples used to close the bladder in dogs. Although staple exposure was much higher in bladders closed with absorbable staples (56% compared with 2%), crystal formation more commonly occurred on exposed stainless steel staples (25% compared with 7%).[58]

Finally, the correction of vesicoureteral reflux using laparoscopic biting clips to reapproximate the muscularis over the distal ureter and to create a nonrefluxing tunnel has been described for the porcine model.[29,59]

CONCLUSIONS

Clipping and stapling intracorporeally have predominant utility for hemostasis and reconstruction. There are other purposes for these techniques and instruments, including marking the margins of a resection. Metallic sphere clips are available to affix sutures intracorporeally.[60] Laparoscopic absorbable locking clips are also available for the same purpose. Absorbable stenting materials may allow other techniques to replace suturing and stapling for tissue reconstruction. By precisely aligning tissue margins, laser welding systems may be capable of rapidly accomplishing intracorporeal end-to-end anastomoses. Superphysiologic burst pressures have been reported for ureteral laser welds.[61] This technique will probably remain a research technology for some time, although manufacturing firms are investigating devices that could rapidly facilitate widespread application.[62] A simpler solution would be a chemical or biologic substance that would reliably "glue" tissues together.[25,63] Entire symposia for investigating such materials have occurred, yet there are no available substances that produce the necessary adherence safely. It is thought that microrobotics will allow simple insect-like behavior to accomplish these tasks from remote control.[37] Despite the realistic probability that technology will develop solutions to complex problems encountered in the closed environment of the laparoscopic surgeon, intracorporeal suturing, clipping, and stapling techniques currently remain essential skills.

REFERENCES

1. Petrovsky, B; Perelman, M; Kuznichev, A: Resection and plastic surgery of bronchi (Transl from Russian). Mir Publishing, 1968, pp 202–221.
2. Steichen, FM; Ravitch, MM: Contemporary stapling instruments and basic mechanical suturing techniques. Surg Clin North Am 64:425–440, 1984.
3. Fowler, DL; White, RA: Laparoscopic-assisted sigmoid resection, Surg Laparosc Endosc 1:183, 1991.
4. Meljer, D-W; Bannenberg, JG; Klopper, P-J: The laparoscopic construction of an intestinal anastomosis. Surg Endosc 2:244A, 1993.
5. Chiu, AW; Chen, MT; Huang, WJS; et al: Case report: Laparoscopic nephroureterectomy and endoscopic excision of bladder cuff. Min Invas Therap 1:299, 1992.
6. Clayman, RV; Kavoussi, LR; Figenshau, RS; et al: Laparoscopic nephroureterectomy: Initial case report. J Laparosc Surg 1:343, 1991.
7. Kozminski, M; Partamian, KO: Case report of laparoscopic ileal loop conduit. J Endourol, 6:145, 1992.
8. Thorbeck, CV; Sanchez de Badajoz, S; Toscano, R: Laparoscopic ileal conduit. Surg Endosc 2:257A, 1993.
9. Bisson, J; Vinson, RK; Leadbetter, GW: Urolithiasis from stapler anastomosis. Am J Surg 137:280, 1989.
10. Grainger, DA; Meyer, WR; DeCherney, AH; Diamond, MP: Laparoscopic clips: Evaluation of absorbable and titanium with regard to hemostasis and tissue reactivity. J Reprod Med 36:493, 1991.
11. Klein, RD; Jessup, G; Ahart, F; et al: Comparison of laparoscopic titanium and absorbable polymeric ligating clips. Surg Endosc 7:124A, 1993.
12. Ravo, B; Rosales, C; Serino, F; Castagneto, M: The use of absorbable staples for construction of a bladder tube. Surgery 173:29, 1991.
13. Corman, ML; Prager, ED; Hardy, TG; Bubrick, MP; and the Valtrac Study Groups: Comparison of the Valtrac biofragmentable anastomosis ring with conventional suture and stapled anastomosis in colon surgery. Results of a prospective, randomized clinical trial. Dis Colon Rectum 32:183, 1989.
14. Smith, AD; Bubrick, MP; Mestitz, ST; et al: Evaluation of the biofragmentable anastomotic ring following preoperative irradiation to the rectosigmoid in dogs. Dis Colon Rectum 31:5, 1988.
15. Avant, LO; Starr, GA: Vesicourethral reanastomosis by mechanical stapling and transurethral deep dorsal venous ligation: A new technique for radical retropubic prostatectomy. Personal communication, May, 1991.
16. Kirker-Head, CA; Steckel, RR; Schwartz, A; Williams, R: Eval-

uation of surgical staples for ligation of the renal pedicle during nephrectomy. Urol Res 16:63, 1988.

17. Low, RK; Moran, ME: Argon beam coagulation and laparoscopic reconstruction. Min Invas Therapy 2:75, 1993.
18. Sugarbaker, DJ; Mentzer, SJ: Improved technique for hilar vascular stapling. Ann Thorac Surg 53:165, 1992.
19. Kerbl, K; Chandhoke, PS; McDougall, E; et al: Laparoscopic clips and staples: Vascular application. J Endourol 6:S142, 1992.
20. Moran, ME: Theory of vascular pedicle hemostasis during laparoscopic nephrectomy. Min Invas Therap 1:A69, 1991.
21. Nathanson, LK; Easter, DW; Cuschieri, A: Ligation of the structures of the cystic pedicle during laparoscopic cholecystectomy. Am J Surg 161:350, 1991.
22. Nathanson, LK; Nathanson, PDK; Cuschieri, A: Safety of vessel ligation in laparoscopic surgery. Endoscopy 23:206, 1991.
23. Nelson, MT; Nakashima, M; Mulvihill, SJ: How safe are laparoscopically placed clips? An in vitro and in vivo study. Arch Surg 127:718, 1992.
24. Dziki, AJ; Duncan, MD; Harmon, JW; et al: Advantages of handsewn over stapled bowel anastomosis. Dis Colon Rectum 34:442, 1991.
25. Jansson, OK; Zilling, TL; Walther, BS: Healing of colonic anastomoses: Comparative experimental study of glued, manually sutured, and stapled anastomoses. Dis Colon Rectum 34:557, 1991.
26. Moritz, E; Achleitner, D; Holbling, N; et al: Single vs. double stapling technique in colorectal surgery. A prospective randomized trial. Dis Colon Rectum 34:495, 1991.
27. West of Scotland and Highland Anastomosis Study Group: Suturing or stapling in gastrointestinal surgery: A prospective randomized study. Br J Surg 78:337, 1991.
28. Griffith, DP; Gleeson, MJ: The prosthetic bladder—perhaps the technology has arrived. Scan J Urol Nephrol 142:109, 1992.
29. Clayman, RC; McDougall, E; Chandhoke, PS; et al: Laparoscopic ureteral reimplantation: Laboratory studies. J Endourol 6:S144, 1992.
30. Das, S: Laparoscopic removal of bladder diverticulum. J Urol 148:1837, 1992.
31. Parra, RO; Andrus, CH; Jones, JP; Boullier, JA: Laparoscopic cystectomy: Initial case report on a new treatment for the retained bladder. J Urol 148:1140, 1992.
32. Parra, RO; Jones, JP; Andrus, CH; Hagood, PG: Laparoscopic diverticulectomy: Preliminary report of a new approach for the treatment of bladder diverticulum. J Urol 148:869, 1992.
33. Kerbl, K; Chandhoke, PS; McDougall, E; et al: Laparoscopic stapled bladder closure: Laboratory and clinical experience. J Urol 149:1437, 1993.
34. Schuessler, WW; Vancaillie, TG; Preminger, GM: Laparoscopic dismembered pyeloplasty. Min Invas Therapy 1:A68, 1992.
35. Stoller, ML; Irby, PB; Carroll, P; Osman, M: Laparoscopic renal cyst resection. J Endourol 6:S56, 1992.
36. Baniel, J; Schein, M: Partial nephrectomy using a linear stapling device. Br J Urol 698:218, 1992.
37. Winfield, HN; Donovan, JF; Godet, AS; Clayman, RV: Human laparoscopic partial nephrectomy. J Endourol 6:S59, 1992.
38. Hill, ADK; Chambler, AFW; Querechi, A; et al: Laparoscopic hemicolectomy using the biodegradable anastomotic ring. Surg Endosc 6:232A, 1993.
39. Ling, FW; Stovall, TG; Meyer, NL; et al: Adhesion formation associated with the use of absorbable staples in comparison to other types of peritoneal injury. Int J Gynecol Obstet 30:361, 1989.
40. Ger, R; Monroe, K; Duvivier, R; Mishrick, A: Management of indirect inguinal hernias by laparoscopic closure of the neck of the sac. Am J Surg 159:370, 1990.
41. Azziz, R; Murphy, AA; Rosenberg, SM; Patton, GW: Use of an oxidized, regenerated cellulose, absorbable adhesion barrier at laparoscopy. J Reprod Med 36:479, 1991.
42. Dickson, C; Boone, T; Preminger, GM: Laparoscopic urethral sling. Min Invas Therapy 1:A105, 1992.
43. Moran, ME; Radomski, SB; Stone, AR: Laparoscopic pubo-bladder neck sling: An animal model. Min Invas Therapy 1:A46, 1991.
44. Jacobs, M; Verdeja, JC; Goldstein, HS: Minimally invasive colon resection (laparoscopic colectomy). Surg Laparosc Endosc 1:144, 1991.
45. Dion, YM; Gharara, J; Guidoin, R: Bursting strength evaluation of an experimental hernia repair using prolene mesh attached to tissue with EMS stapler or with US Surgical Endopath. Surg Endosc 7:124A, 1993.
46. Feldman, SL; Presman, D; Kandel, GL: Renal arteriovenous fistula following nephrectomy. Br J Urol 57:592, 1985.
47. Goldstein, AG; Delaurentis, DA; Schwarz, AJ: Postnephrectomy arteriovenous fistula. Br J Urol 98:44, 1967.
48. Lacombe, M: Renal arteriovenous fistula following nephrectomy. Urology 25:13, 1985.
49. Geridzen, GR; Futter, NG: Ten-year review of vesicle diverticula. Urology 20:33, 1982.
50. Kelalis, PP; McLean, P: The treatment of diverticulum of the bladder. J Urol 98:349, 1967.
51. Kutzmann, AA: Diverticulum of the urinary bladder: An analysis of 100 cases. Surg Gynecol Obstet 56:898, 1933.
52. Peterson, LJ; Paulson, DF; Glenn, JF: The histopathology of vesical diverticula. J Urol 110:62, 1973.
53. Bohm, B; Milsom, JW; Stolfi, VM; Kitigo, K: Laparoscopic intraperitoneal anastomosis. Surg Endosc 7:194, 1993.
54. Brenner, M; Johnson, DE: Ileal conduit calculi from stapler anastomosis: A long-term complication? Urology, 26:537, 1985.
55. Ginsberg, D; Huffman, JL; Lieskowsky, G; et al: Urinary tract stones: A complication of the Kock pouch continent urinary diversion. J Urol 145:956, 1991.
56. Lieskovsky, G; Boyd, SD; Skinner, DG: Cutaneous Kock-pouch urinary diversion. Probl Urol 5:268, 1991.
57. Myers, RP; Rife, CC; Barrett, DM: Experience with the bowel stapler for ileal conduit urinary diversion. Br J Urol 54:491, 1982.
58. Julian, TB; Ravitch, MM: Closure of the urinary bladder with stainless steel and absorbable staples. Ann Surg 204:186, 1986.
59. Atala, A; Goldstein, DS; Kavoussi, LR; et al: Laparoscopic correction of vesicoureteral reflux. J Urol 149:453A, 1993.
60. Andrews, A; Lewis, JL: Minimal access suturing: An assessment of knot substitutes. Min Invas Therap 1:309, 1992.
61. Schlossberg, SM; Poppas, DP: Tissue welding with lasers. Semin Urol 9:206, 1991.
62. Sauer, JS; Hinshaw, JR: A fiber optic exoscope for laser tissue welding. Lasers Surg Med 6:219, 1986.
63. Levinson, AK; Greskovich, FJ; Swanson, DA; et al: Fibrin glue for partial nephrectomy. Urology 38:314, 1991.
64. Flynn, AM: GNAT robots. Am Surg 57:192A, 1991.

SECTION VI

COMPLICATIONS

CHAPTER 27

Laparoscopic Complications and Management

Diane M. Hartman, MD
Paramjit S. Chandhoke, MD, PhD

For laparoscopic urology to become widely accepted and practiced, it is essential that complications of the procedure be minimized. Laparoscopic surgery has a steep learning curve. Unlike other endourological procedures, such as transurethral resection of the prostate, percutaneous nephrolithotomy, and ureteroscopy, in which much of the procedure is done by a single surgeon, laparoscopy necessitates a team approach. Often, two or three urologists work in concert during laparoscopic urologic procedures. Therefore not only do all the team members need to be trained in laparoscopic surgery but they all have to learn to work together. Until the team gains adequate experience with a particular laparoscopic procedure, the complications rate may be painfully high.

In a recent multiinstitutional survey, the overall complications of laparoscopic pelvic lymph node dissection were noted to be as high as 15% in the first 372 patients undergoing this procedure at eight medical centers.[1] Similarly, nine complications occurred in the first ten patients undergoing laparoscopic nephrectomy.[2] To minimize complications early in their experience, it is prudent that urologists attempt simple laparoscopic procedures before undertaking the more extensive surgeries, such as laparoscopic nephrectomy.

The first step in planning a laparoscopic procedure is proper patient selection and informed consent. It is necessary to disclose to the patient the surgeon's experience with laparoscopy and the potential complications. Alternatives to laparoscopy should be discussed. Furthermore, the necessity to convert the laparoscopic procedure to an open conventional one should the need arise must be made clear. It is important to have a patient's family member present during the informed consent. Should a complication arise, the family member may be the first person consulted and the one with whom patient management decisions can be made in the postoperative period. Examples of informed consent for specific urologic procedures have been published elsewhere.[3]

PREVENTION OF COMPLICATIONS

Patient Selection

Early in the laparoscopic experience, it is wise to select patients who need simple procedures and in whom prior abdominal surgery has not been performed. As a surgeon gains experience, more extensive procedures in more complicated patients can be undertaken.

Absolute contraindications to laparoscopic surgery are

- Active peritonitis or bowel perforation
- Marked bowel distention or bowel obstruction
- History of extensive bowel adhesions
- Coagulopathy that is not corrected
- Hypovolemic shock
- Sepsis
- Abdominal wall infection

Relative contraindications to laparoscopic surgery are

- Obesity
- Abdominal aortic aneurysm
- Severe pulmonary or cardiovascular disease
- Large intra-abdominal masses
- Ascites
- Umbilical hernia

It is recommended that patients receive general intubated anesthesia for laparoscopic urologic surgery. Patients who are not candidates for general anesthesia, such as those with significant pulmonary or cardiovascular disease, are considered unsuitable for laparoscopic surgery. Preoperative bowel preparation is essential for most of the laparoscopic urologic procedures. If this has not been achieved satisfactorily preoperatively, it is not unreasonable to reschedule the surgery.

The risks of infection and bleeding are present with laparoscopy just as for any other surgical procedure. Both of these factors need to be treated or controlled prior to surgery. Any acute bowel pathology is a contraindication to laparoscopy. Bowel distention and adhesions increase the risk for bowel injury during trocar placement and interfere with adequate visualization of the surgical field. With obesity, the weight of the abdominal wall limits the intraperitoneal working space that can be generated at a pneumoperitoneum of 15 mm Hg. The presence of an abdominal aortic aneurysm increases the risk of vascular injury at the time of primary trocar placement. Although laparoscopy may be adequate to sample tissue from large abdominal masses for diagnosis, this technique may not be able to safely remove such masses from the abdomen. There may be an increased risk of developing peritonitis postoperatively in an ascitic abdomen. The presence of an umbilical hernia precludes placement of the primary trocar at the umbilicus. Also, there may be associated bowel adhesions that increase the risk of bowel injury during trocar placement.

Proper Instrumentation

The current success of laparoscopic urologic surgery is in part due to the development of new instrumentation. For the surgeon, this translates to keeping abreast with new technology and being aware of its potential complications. The nursing staff should also be familiar with the instrumentation and should be able to trouble-shoot problems as they arise.[4] The instrumentation used for laparoscopic surgery can be divided into three parts: video equipment, insufflation apparatus, and surgical instruments.

As for all endoscopic procedures, adequate visualization of the surgical field is paramount. The camera should be focused and white-balanced before inserting it into the abdomen. The laparoscope should be kept warm, and the lens should be kept clear with defogging solution as necessary. The assistant working the camera must anticipate what the surgeon wants to see during the procedure: to pull the camera back when instruments are moving in and out of the ports and to bring the camera in close to a particular area to facilitate dissection. The surgeons should be aware of the position of all instruments within the abdomen at all times, even those not in direct view of the laparoscope.

It is the responsibility of the surgeon not only to secure proper pneumoperitoneum but to maintain it safely throughout the procedure. For this the surgeon should periodically monitor the intraperitoneal pressure and keep it below 15 mm Hg. Preferably, the insufflator gas flow and pressure gauges should be kept in direct view of the surgeon during the procedure. How does the surgeon know that the insufflator monitor is registering the intraperitoneal pressure accurately? In most cases, it is not possible to calibrate the pressure readings before the procedure. However, once the insufflator is connected to the Verres needle prior to its insertion into the abdomen, it is helpful to ensure that (1) the pressure reading is not higher than 2 to 3 mm Hg and (2) the pressure on the monitor rises above 30 mm Hg if the tubing is occluded. This test reassures the surgeon that the pressure monitor is working adequately. The CO_2 tank should have sufficient gas to last the length of the surgery. Losing the pneumoperitoneum at a critical part of the procedure can lead to significant complications.

All surgical instruments should be inserted in the abdomen under direct vision and should be aimed upward (toward the ceiling) to minimize inadvertent bowel injury. All insulated instruments should be carefully checked for cracks before inserting them in the abdomen. The entire noninsulated portion of the instruments should always be kept in view when activating the electrocautery to avoid inadvertent burn injury to the bowel or other organs. The surgeon should be familiar with new clipping and stapling devices before inserting them in the abdomen. Once the tissue is engaged with these devices, misuse of the instrument can lead to significant complications.

INTRAOPERATIVE COMPLICATIONS

Intraoperative complications of laparoscopy encompass a wide variety of injuries, from insignificant to potentially lethal problems. These include complications during insufflating needle and trocar placement and injuries to vascular, gastrointestinal, and genitourinary systems. Complications resulting from electric injuries are discussed later in this section. Anesthetic complications have been considered in Chapter 4. Ultimately, timely diagnosis of all intraoperative complications allows the laparoscopic surgeon the best possible outcomes.

Complications of Needle and Trocar Placement

An adequate pneumoperitoneum is necessary for all laparoscopic procedures. This pneumoperitoneum is obtained either by blind placement of a spring-loaded Verres needle or by placement of a Hasson trocar through a minilaparotomy. The proper technique for access to the peritoneum is reviewed in Chapter 7. Placement of the insufflating needle in the improper space can cause technical difficulties or even the necessity to abort the procedure.[5] A favorable sign indicating correct position of the Verres needle during insufflation is dullness over the liver.

The Verres needle must traverse two tissue planes in the midline before entering the peritoneal cavity. These are the anterior rectus fascia and the peritoneum. If during needle placement the needle does not penetrate the rectus fascia, subcutaneous emphysema will result on insufflation (Fig. 27–1). This can be recognized by high insufflation pressures and subcutaneous crepitus over the abdomen and thorax. As much of the insufflated CO_2 as possible should be evacuated, and needle placement should resume.

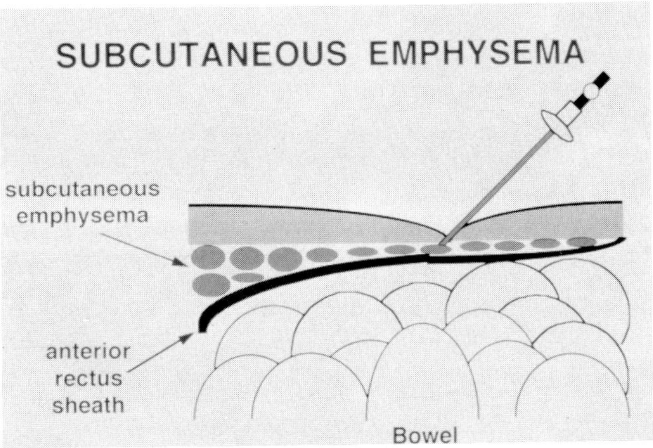

Figure 27–1. Subcutaneous emphysema. The tip of the Verres needle has not traversed the rectus muscle. The insufflating gas tracks within the subcutaneous space, which may result in crepitus over the abdomen and thorax.

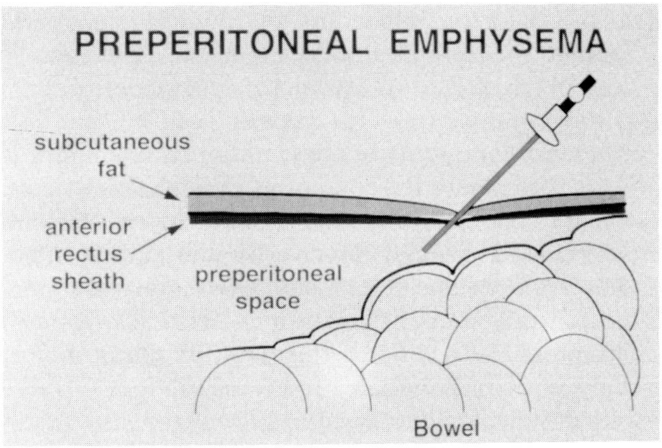

Figure 27–2. Preperitoneal emphysema. The Verres needle has traversed the anterior rectus sheath but not the peritoneum, resulting in accumulation of the insufflating gas within the preperitoneal space.

A more difficult problem is misplacement of the Verres needle in the preperitoneal space, which creates preperitoneal emphysema (Fig. 27–2). This is more difficult to diagnose, since insufflation pressures may remain relatively low and abdominal wall tympany can occur; creation of a pneumoscrotum or pneumopenis should alert the surgeon of preperitoneal insufflation.[6] Pneumopreperitoneum may make it impossible to continue with the procedure for two main reasons. First, the distention of the preperitoneum causes the peritoneum itself to be deflected toward the intraperitoneal contents. Therefore the effective space between intra-abdominal organs and the peritoneum is markedly decreased. This is why puncturing through the peritoneum from the preperitoneal space should be avoided. The second reason a pneumopreperitoneum may make the laparoscopic procedure unwise is that it distorts the peritoneum, making it difficult to identify normal landmarks.[5] If a large amount of CO_2 has been insufflated into the preperitoneal space, as much as possible should be allowed to escape. A minilaparotomy and Hasson cannula placement are the best way to create a pneumoperitoneum at this point.

Insufflation of the omentum can also occur with the Verres needle. If the omentum is so distended that it obscures view of the intra-abdominal contents, the procedure should be aborted.

Complications of Pneumoperitoneum

Once the Verres needle or Hasson cannula is correctly placed, a pneumoperitoneum is created by insufflation of CO_2 gas. It is important to monitor the intra-abdominal pressure at all times to ensure that it stays below 15 mm Hg. A tension pneumoperitoneum (intra-abdominal pressures greater than 30 mm Hg) occurs most commonly in obese patients in whom it is difficult to evaluate the abdominal distention. A tense, distended abdomen, difficulty ventilating the patient, and decreased vascular return with subsequent hypotension are the signs of a tension pneumoperitoneum.[7] A tension pneumoperitoneum may occur if intraperitoneal pressures are not being carefully monitored or if there is a malfunction of the insufflator. Adverse respiratory or circulatory effects are rare if the intraperitoneal pressure is kept below 20 mm Hg.[8,9] New insufflation devices now often have pressure-regulated gas flow that prevents this complication.

Pneumothorax, pneumomediastinum, and pneumopericardium have all been described as complications of laparoscopic surgery.[10,11] The insufflating gas may have access to the thorax through defects or weak points in the diaphragm.[11] A pneumothorax can also occur if a lateral port is placed through the pleura above the twelfth rib. Once the gas is in the thorax, it can dissect along tissue planes and can result in pneumomediastinum or pneumopericardium. If unrecognized, tension pneumothorax or tension pneumopericardium will cause cardiovascular collapse. If a pneumothorax or pneumopericardium is identified, the procedure should be aborted. Keeping the insufflation pressure low and promptly investigating acute changes in ventilatory pressures or hypotension will help prevent this complication.

Gas embolus is a well-documented, rare, and life-threatening complication of laparoscopy.[12–14] The most common cause of this is direct insufflation into a vessel; however, some hypothesize that gas under pressure may embolize through small vessels traumatized during dissection. The gas embolus causes a right ventricular outflow obstruction as the bubble produces an air lock in the pulmonary outflow tract. Pulmonary perfusion and subsequent left ventricular filling are markedly decreased, leading to cardiovascular collapse. The amount of gas necessary to produce this scenario depends on the solubility of the gas. Since CO_2 is soluble in blood, a larger volume can be tolerated, whereas a small volume (as little as 20 ml) of room air can create these symptoms.[15] The classic precordial "mill wheel" murmur, severe hypotension, hypoxia, and a precipitous drop in the end-tidal CO_2 are the signs of gas embolus. Early diagnosis and aggressive treatment are mandatory to prevent a lethal event. Immediate cessation of the procedure, desufflation, and placing the patient in a head-down, right-side-up position will help minimize the right ventricular outflow obstruction.[16] A central venous catheter can be passed to the right atrium to evacuate the gas. The incidence of gas embolus during laparoscopic procedures is estimated at 1 in 65,000 cases.[17]

Vascular Injuries

Vascular injuries are among the most common complications sustained in laparoscopic procedures.[1] The injuries range from insignificant small vessel hemorrhage to lethal lacerations of the major retroperitoneal vessels.[18] In one large study, the incidence of injury to the major vessels during laparoscopy was 3 in 10,000 procedures.[9] These injuries can occur from needle or trocar placement or during dissection. Vessels of the abdominal wall are common sites of lacerations. Superficial subcutaneous vessels, especially the superior epigastric artery, may be traumatized with needle or trocar placement. This may result in significant postoperative ecchymosis (Fig. 27–3) or a subcutaneous hematoma (Fig. 27–4). If direct pressure does not stop the bleeding, a small cut down to the proximal and distal vessels, with subsequent ligation, may be necessary. Beneath the fascia, the inferior epigastric vessels are also subject to injury. This can often be diagnosed from a continuous drip from a trocar site during laparoscopy; the resulting rectus hematoma can conceal a significant volume of blood. Electrocauterization at the trocar site can be attempted to stop the hemorrhage. An abdominal wall suture on a Keith needle can also be used to control the bleeding.[1] Direct visualization of trocar placement and use of the laparoscope light to delineate the subcutaneous and subfascial vessels helps to avoid trauma to the abdominal wall vasculature.

Except for anesthetic complications, injury to the major retroperitoneal vessels is the most common cause of death during laparoscopic procedures.[20] Although it is a rare occurrence, the dire consequences of this complication make it mandatory for all laparoscopic surgeons to fully understand the prevention,

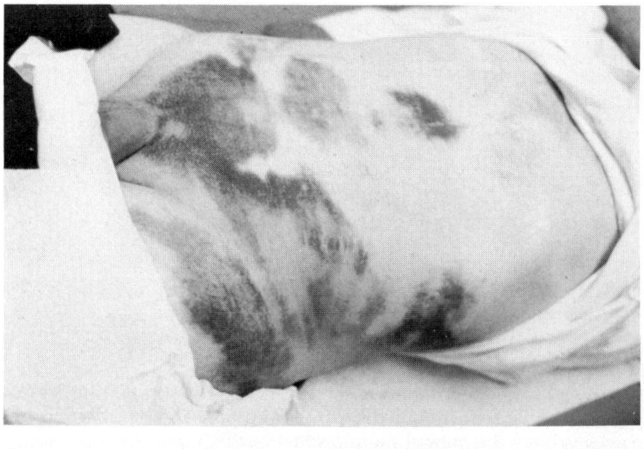

Figure 27–3. Postoperative ecchymosis in a patient following laparoscopic pelvic lymph node dissection.

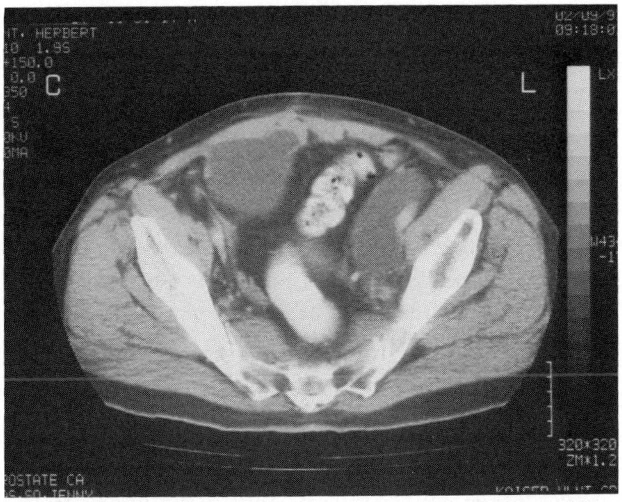

Figure 27–4. Postoperative abdominal computed tomographic scan of a patient following laparoscopy. Note the right anterior abdominal wall hematoma caused by vessel injury as well as left pelvic lymphocele.

diagnosis, and expedient treatment of this complication. If the Verres needle is initially placed in a vascular structure and blood is withdrawn, it should be left in place for tamponade, and a laparotomy should be performed. Large-vessel injuries from a trocar or laparoscope with a large amount of hemorrhage in a short period of time are typically much more significant. If possible, the trocar or laparoscope should be left in place, and an emergent laparotomy should be performed. Maintaining the pneumoperitoneum facilitates access into the abdominal cavity. The immediate necessity for laparotomy is why all operative suites performing laparoscopy must have a laparotomy set in the room during the procedure. Direct compression of the aorta gives immediate vascular control while resuscitation takes place. As long as the hemorrhage is controlled, definitive treatment of the injury should only proceed, with the aid of a vascular surgeon, after the patient is stabilized.

Minor intra-abdominal vessels can also be injured during the course of laparoscopy. Although laparoscopic control by hemoclips, coagulation, or ligation is usually sufficient, in some cases laparotomy is required to control hemorrhage.[1] A significant vascular injury to the mesentery may also occur with needle or trocar placement.[21] At the end of each laparoscopic procedure, the patient should be placed supine and the intraperitoneal pressure should be lowered to 5 mm Hg. A full examination of the abdomen and of each trocar site should then be performed.

Gastrointestinal Complications

Injuries to the gastrointestinal tract are a significant complication of laparoscopy. The true incidence of bowel injuries is unknown, because many small punctures are self-limited and therefore are not recognized. Recognition of all bowel injuries at the time of laparoscopy is the single most important factor in minimizing the morbidity and mortality from gastrointestinal injuries.[22]

The small bowel is the gastrointestinal structure that is most commonly traumatized during laparoscopy.[1] The integrity of the small bowel can be violated with Verres needle or trocar placement, dissection, or electrical injuries.

Intra-abdominal adhesions, previous laparotomy, distended bowel, disseminated cancer, or peritonitis increase the risk of direct injury to the bowel by a trocar or needle.[23] Minor needle punctures of the small intestines will likely heal with little consequence and require no treatment. Larger injuries (from a trocar or laparoscope) do require repair. With the advancement of laparoscopic techniques for bowel surgery, a skilled laparoscopic surgeon may be able to repair reasonable injuries through the laparoscope. If this is not possible, a laparotomy is required. In most cases a primary repair is possible; however, if there is any question of the vascular supply to the injured bowel segment, resection and primary anastomosis is recommended.

Electrical burns of the small bowel during laparoscopy are a more troublesome problem. These injuries may be a result of operator inexperience; however, the burns can also occur out of the vision of the laparoscope. Because of this, many of the electrical injuries manifest themselves 2 to 5 days later with fever, abdominal pain, an ileus, and peritoneal signs. If an electrical injury is recognized at the time of surgery, an attempt should be made to evaluate the extent of the injury. The full extent of the injury may be much greater than what can be seen superficially. Electrical current is propagated along the subserosal blood vessels, and a large injury can be produced with little serosal change. It is for this reason that bowel sustaining an electrical burn needs repair, either through the laparoscope or by an open laparotomy.

Gastric perforation is a rare, and often preventable, complication of needle or trocar placement. Placement of a nasogastric tube and decompression of the stomach before access to the peritoneum will prevent most injuries. A common cause of this distention is through forced masked ventilation by the anesthesiologist.[24] As long as there is no significant bleeding, small gastric injuries will heal themselves; larger lacerations or hemorrhage necessitate laparotomy for formal repair.[25]

Large-bowel injuries are far more uncommon than small-bowel injuries during laparoscopy. Because of the high bacterial count in the large bowel, any injury with peritoneal contamination requires laparotomy and repair. Primary repair or segmental resection with primary anastomosis provides adequate treatment for most injuries. Only extremely extensive injuries should require a diverting colostomy.

Injuries to solid organs in the abdomen such as liver and spleen can occur with needle or trocar placement or dissection. If adequate hemostasis can be achieved through the laparoscope, no laparotomy is necessary.

Genitourinary Injuries

Trauma to the urinary bladder occurs with trocar placement and to a lesser extent with Verres needle placement. Bladder injuries are usually seen with the failure to place a urinary catheter to decompress the bladder before abdominal access or in patients with congenital abnormalities or previous pelvic surgery, which alters the anatomy.[26] A urachal diverticulum or urachal cyst can easily be lacerated because of its midline intraumbilical position. Injuries to any urachal structure should be treated by excising the abnormality in an open procedure.[27] Most minor bladder injuries can be treated with catheter drainage. A cystogram should be performed to assure that the cystostomy has closed, because intraperitoneal bladder disruptions may not spontaneously heal with drainage alone.[1] Closure of a cystostomy using laparoscopic clips can also be performed.[1]

The ureters are also at risk of injury during laparoscopy. These injuries usually occur from dissection, transection, or electrocautery. Any intraoperative indication of minor ureteral injury should be managed with transurethral stenting of the ureter.[28] If this is not possible, open repair is necessary. Many ureteral injuries are not noted at time of laparoscopy, and they can manifest themselves with unilateral flank pain, fever, or urinary ascites. All of these injuries require open repair. There have been case reports of electrical burns of the ureters caused by electrical sparking, even when the cautery itself is not in proximity to the ureter.[29,30] A good working knowledge of the course and anatomic relationships of the ureters is the key to avoiding ureteral injuries.

Electrical Injuries

The use of electrical current for coagulation is not unique to laparoscopic procedures; however, the limited field of vision and ability of the trocars and laparoscopes to store electrical energy make electrosurgical injury a significant complication of laparoscopy. Burns of the skin commonly occur at the site of the dispersion electrode, such as "bovie pads." If the plate does not have good contact with the patient's skin, the small contact points can build up heat and cause a burn. The electroradiographic pads can conduct electricity and act as dispersion pads if they are proximal to the dispersion pad.[31]

Electrical injury to the intra-abdominal structures is a serious complication of laparoscopy. Many of these injuries are not diagnosed at time of laparoscopy. They may occur as a result of direct contact or an intraperitoneal arc of sparks from the structure being cauterized to another structure. Direct contact with intra-abdominal structures that are not intended to be cauterized must be avoided. Care must be taken in activating the electrocautery if the instrument is out of the field of vision. Arcing of sparks occurs as the electrical current seeks the dispersion pad. As tissue is being cauterized, its resistance increases. As the resistance increases, the electrical current has more difficulty reaching the dispersion pad, and sparks can occur.[32] Cases of ureteral and bowel injury have been described when electrocautery was used for tubal ligation.[29,33] A nonconducting tube that contains an active electrode can store energy and can become an active electrode itself. This is a worrisome problem, since the laparoscope may not be recognized as an electrode, and it can inadvertently touch many structures in the abdomen, causing electrical burns. Conductive trocars can disperse the energy along their entire sheath and can therefore reduce the chance of inadvertent bowel injury.[32]

When burn injury of bowel or ureter is suspected, a careful examination should follow to assess the full extent of the injury. The electrical current travels along vasculature, and the injuries may be much more extensive than the serosal burn would indicate. These injuries should be treated as previously described. The use of bipolar electrocautery (in which the electrical current is dispersed only between the two forceps) or an ultrasonic "harmonic scalpel" can prevent many of these electrosurgical injuries.

With the use of electric current in a closed space containing a combustible gas mixture, there is some small chance for an explosion. Because of this hazard, CO_2 is ideal for laparoscopy, because it does not support combustion (unlike oxygen or nitrous oxide, which do support combustion). The intraluminal bowel gases of methane and hydrogen are volatile, especially if mixed with oxygen. If a bowel injury allows sufficient bowel gas to escape intraperitoneally, there is a chance of explosion with the use of electrocautery. This is probably of little concern when the pneumoperitoneum is created with CO_2; however, the mixture of nitrous oxide, methane, and hydrogen is an extremely combustible mixture.[34] This is one reason nitrous oxide is not used to create a pneumoperitoneum.

POSTOPERATIVE COMPLICATIONS

Some of the complications that manifest in the postoperative period are preventable if recognized during the intraoperative period. Injury to vascular, gastrointestinal, and genitourinary systems, discussed in the previous section, may be noted only in the postoperative period. One important step in preventing these complications is to make a systematic and orderly exit from the abdomen at the end of the procedure. The steps for exiting the abdomen have been discussed in Chapter 7.

Delayed Hemorrhage

Significant bleeding is usually noted intraoperatively if it occurs within the surgical field. However, there are three situations in which significant bleeding may be missed intraoperatively. The first is a major vessel injury (e.g., external iliac arterial injury during pelvic lymph node dissection) that bleeds into the retroperitoneal space. The expanding retroperitoneal hematoma may be discovered only with imaging studies in the postoperative period. The second situation is that of solid organ injury (e.g., laceration of liver, kidney, spleen) that is obscured by overlying bowel during surgery. The Trendelenburg position allows the accumulated blood to pool underneath the liver intraoperatively. It is important that while going through the steps of exiting the abdomen, the patient be placed supine so that this complication can be discovered. The third situation is bleeding of an abdominal vessel from a trocar site. If proper steps are followed at time of exiting the abdomen, this injury is discovered when the trocar is removed and can be repaired appropriately (Chap. 7). If significant delayed hemorrhage from the abdominal wall is noted in the postoperative period, open surgical repair is recommended.

In most instances of significant delayed hemorrhage within the abdomen, embolization of the bleeding vessel is initially recommended. If the vascular injury is severe enough that the patient is hemodynamically unstable or the embolization is clinically hazardous, open surgical repair is recommended.

Hollow Organ Injury

Either bladder or bowel injury may be noted only in the postoperative period. Usually these are injuries related to trocars or electrical burns. Verres needle injuries to a hollow organ are usually clinically insignificant. Trocar injuries leave tissue edges that usually heal well if the edges are closely approximated. Electrical burns on hollow organs are more devastating, since the burn results in tissue necrosis with a poor healing potential. Such injuries may be missed intraoperatively, because all that may be noted then is a discoloration of the serosa and the depth of injury is underestimated. These burn injuries usually occur with the noninsulated portion of an instrument that lies outside the visual field. Another complication that may occur is the incorporation of bowel within the fascial closure of 10-mm or larger trocar sites. With direct laparoscopic monitoring of the fascial closures through another port, this complication can be avoided.

With bowel injuries, the patient may present with nausea, vomiting, abdominal pain, and signs of an intra-abdominal abscess. Such a presentation can occur as early as the day after surgery or as late as several weeks after the laparoscopic procedure. In most cases, laparotomy is necessary to repair the bowel injury. With bladder injury, hematuria or pneumaturia may be noted in the immediate postoperative period, or the patient may present with signs of a pelvic abscess. Because the bladder perforation may be intraperitoneal, the patient may also present with vague abdominal pain, nausea, and vomiting. Small bladder injuries may heal spontaneously with prolonged bladder catheter drainage. Larger injuries need open surgical repair.

Ureteral Injury

Inadvertent injury to the ureter may be recognized only in the postoperative period. The ureter may have been transected, clipped, or fulgurated during the procedure. The patient may present with ureteral obstruction or urinary extravasation at the site of the injury. Once the injury has been confirmed by an imaging study, ureteral continuity may be established with endourologic techniques. If the endourologic approach fails, the ureter should be repaired using open surgery.

Incisional Hernia

There is a possibility of an incisional hernia occurring at 10-mm or larger trocar sites if the fascia is not closed separately from the skin. Incisional hernia at the 5-mm trocar sites, where the fascia is usually not closed, is rare. The patient may present postoperatively with localized abdominal pain, a bulge over the incisional site, or both (Figs. 27–5 and 27–6). Open surgical repair of the hernia is recommended.

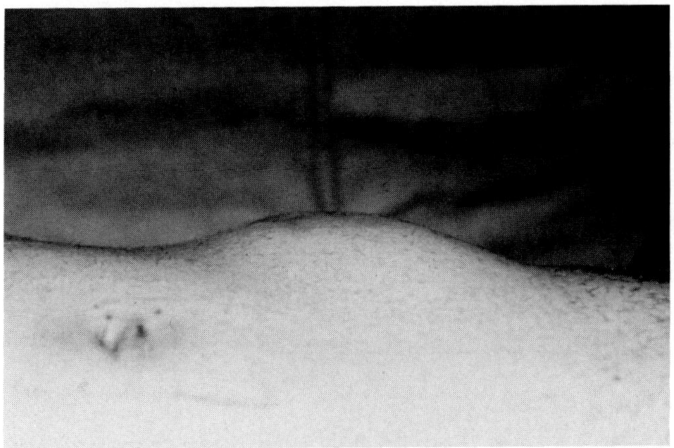

Figure 27–5. Incisional hernia. Photograph of a patient's abdomen with a bulge noted over the area of the 10-mm trocar site following laparoscopic pelvic lymph node dissection.

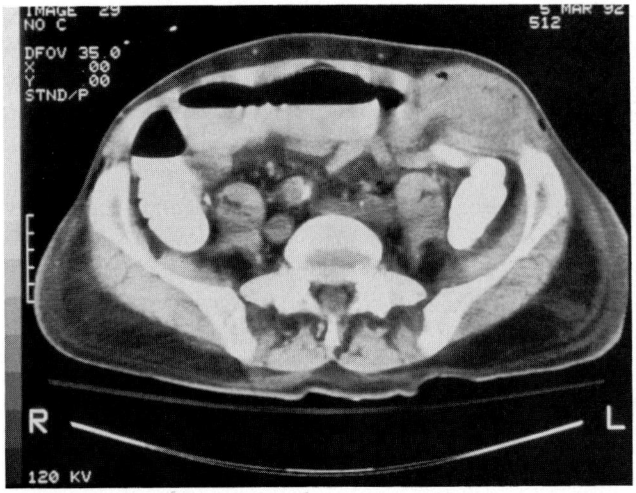

Figure 27–6. Incisional hernia. Abdominal computed tomographic scan of the patient represented in Figure 22–5 showing herniation of the bowel through the fascial defect.

Peripheral Nerve Damage

Special consideration must always be given to patient positioning at the beginning of the procedure and at any time the patient or operating table is moved during the procedure. This complication may be prevented by proper patient positioning and padding of bony prominences.[35] Peripheral nerve damage occurs because of abnormal stretching or compression of a nerve with a neurologic deficit noted in the immediate postoperative period. The brachial plexus is the most common nerve involved in positioning injuries. Little can be done when the nerve palsy is noted in the postoperative period. It is important to document the deficit by formal nerve conduction studies. Minor nerve injuries may resolve within 4 to 6 weeks, whereas the severe injuries may result in a permanent deficit.

Deep Venous Thrombosis

The risk of a deep venous thrombosis from laparoscopic urologic surgery is thought to be greater than from open surgery, although adequate data are as yet unavailable. Two factors that may increase this risk are prolonged pelvic venous stasis (from the pneumoperitoneum) and an increased length of the procedure (e.g., with more extensive urologic surgery such as nephrectomy). This complication can be minimized by the use of intermittent pneumatic compression of the lower extremities or the perioperative use of low-dose coumadin.[36] The treatment of deep venous thrombosis is prolonged anticoagulation therapy.

Lymphoceles

It was initially thought that with the intraperitoneal approach, any lymphatic leak following a pelvic lymph node dissection will drain into the peritoneal cavity, preventing lymphocele formation. However, this is not true; lymphoceles do occur with the intraperitoneal approach.[1] The lymphocele can cause debilitating lower extremity edema and mechanical venous obstruction. Diagnosis is usually made in the postoperative period by ultrasound imaging or computed tomography (see Fig. 27–4). The preferred treatment of a pelvic lymphocele is intraperitoneal marsupialization using a laparoscopic approach (Chap. 20).

CONCLUSIONS

Although laparoscopic urologic surgery is new, most of the complications that occur with this procedure have been known for quite some time from the gynecologic experience.[13] Laparoscopic surgery has a steep learning curve with an increased rate of complications in the first few cases. With careful preoperative planning, intraoperative adherence to laparoscopic principles, and vigilance, these complications can be minimized.

REFERENCES

1. Kavoussi, LR; Sosa, E; Chandhoke, PS; et al: Complications of laparoscopic lymph node dissection. J Urol 149:322–325, 1993.
2. Clayman, RV; Kavoussi, LR; Soper, NJ; et al: Laparoscopic nephrectomy: Review of initial ten cases. J Endourol 6:127–132, 1992.
3. Chandhoke, PS; Clayman, RV: Informed consent documents. In: Clayman, RV; McDougall, eds: Laparoscopic Urology. St. Louis, Quality Medical Publishing, 1993, pp. 426–435.
4. Kavoussi, LR; Sosa, E; Capelouto, C: Complications of laparoscopic surgery. J Endourol 6:95–98, 1992.
5. Winfield, HN; Donovan, JF; See, WA; et al: Urologic laparoscopic surgery. J Urol 146:941–948, 1991.
6. Ahn, HW; Leach, JA: A comparison of subcutaneous and preperitoneal emphysema arising from gynecologic laparoscopic procedures. J Reprod Med 17:335–337, 1976.
7. Kashton, J; Green, JF; Parson, EQ; Holcroft, JW: Hemodynamic effects of increased abdominal pressure. J Surg Res 30:249–255, 1981.
8. Kelman, GR; Swapp, GH; Smith, I; et al: Cardiac output and arterial blood-gas tension during laparoscopy. Br J Anaesth 44:1155–1161, 1972.
9. Motew, M; Ivankovich, AD; Bieniarz, J; et al: Cardiovascular effects and acid-base and blood gas changes during laparoscopy. Am J Obstet Gynecol 115:1002–1011, 1973.
10. Kalhan, SB; Reaney, JA; Collins, RL: Pneumomediastinum and subcutaneous emphysema during laparoscopy. Clev Clin J Med, 47:639–642, 1990.
11. Pascval, JB; Baranda, MM; Tamero, MT; et al: Subcutaneous emphysema, pneumomediastinum, bilateral pneumothorax, and pneumopericardium after laparoscopy. Endoscopy 22:59, 1990.
12. Yacoub, OF; Cardona, I; Coveler, LA; Dodson, MG: Carbon dioxide embolism during laparoscopy. Anesthesiology 57:533–535, 1982.
13. Bradfield, ST: Gas emboli during laparoscopy. Anaesth Intensive Care 19:474, 1991.
14. DePlater, RMH; Jones, ISC: Non-fatal carbon dioxide embolism during laparoscopy. Anaesth Intensive Care 17:359–361, 1989.
15. Graff, TD; Arbegast, NR; Phillips, OC; et al: Gas embolism: A comparative study of air and carbon dioxide as embolic agents

in the systemic venous system. Am J Obstet Gynecol 78:259–265, 1959.

16. See, WA; Monk, TG; Weldon, BG: Complications of laparoscopy. In: Clayman, RV; McDougall, E; eds: Laparoscopic Urology. St. Louis, Quality Medical Publishing, 1992, pp. 183–206.
17. Borten, M: Complications of pneumoperitoneum. In: Borten, M, ed: Laparoscopic Complications, Prevention and Management: Philadelphia, BC Decker, 1986, pp. 265–284.
18. Peterson, HB; Greenspan, JR; Org, HW: Death following puncture of the aorta during laparoscopic clip sterilization. Br J Obstet Gynecol 90:480–482, 1983.
19. Mintz, M: Risks and prophylaxis in laparoscopy: A surgery of 100,000 cases. J Reprod Med 18:269–272, 1977.
20. Borten, M, ed: Vascular Injuries in Laparoscopic Complications: Prevention and Management. Philadelphia, BC Decker, 1986, pp. 298–326.
21. Karam, KS; Hajj, SJ: Mesenteric hematoma: Meckel's diverticulum: A rare laparoscopic complication. Fertil Steril 28:1003–1005, 1977.
22. Peterson, HB; DeStefano, F; Rubin, GL; et al: Deaths attributable to tubal sterilization in the United States. Am J Obstet Gynecol 146:131–136, 1981.
23. Borten, M: Gastrointestinal injuries. In: Borten, M, ed: Laparoscopic Complications: Prevention and Management, Philadelphia, BC Decker, 1986, pp. 317–329.
24. Reynolds, RC; Pauca, AL: Gastric perforation , an anesthesia-induced hazard in laparoscopy. Anesthesiology 38:84–85, 1973.
25. Endler, GC; Moghissi, KS: Gastric perforation during pelvic laparoscopy. Obstet Gynecol 47(s): 40–42, 1976.
26. Deshmukh, AS: Laparoscopic bladder injury. Urology 19:306–307, 1982.
27. Yong, EL; Prabhakaran, K; Lee, YS; Ratnem, SS: Peritonitis following diagnostic laparoscopy due to injury to a vesicourachal diverticulum. Br J Obstet Gynaecol 96:365, 1989.
28. Grainer, DA; Soderstrom, RM; Schiff, SF; et al: Ureteral injuries at laparoscopy: Insights into diagnosis, management and prevention. Obstet Gynecol 75:839–941, 1990.
29. Irvin, TT; Goligher, JC; Scott, JS: Injury to the ureter during laparoscopic tubal sterilization. Arch Surg 110:1501–1503, 1975.
30. Cheng, YS: Ureteral injury resulting from laparoscopic fulguration of endometrial implant. Am J Obstet Gynecol 126:1045–1046, 1976.
31. Becker, CM; Malhotra, IV; Hedley-White, J: The distribution of radiofrequency current and burns. Anesthesiology 38:106–122, 1973.
32. Borten, J: Electrical complications. In: Borten, M, ed: Laparoscopic Complications: Prevention and Management. Philadelphia, BC Decker, 1986, pp. 317–329.
33. Freilich, TH: Possibility of burns during laparoscopic tubal sterilization. Am J Obstet Gynecol 129:708–709, 1977.
34. Drummond, GB; Scott, DB: Laparoscopic explosion hazards with nitrous oxide. Br J Med 1:586, 1976.
35. Britt, BA; Joy, N; Makay, MB: Positioning trauma. In: Orkin, FK; Cooperman, LK; eds: Complications in Anesthesiology. Philadelphia, JB Lippincott, 1983, pp. 646–670.
36. Chandhoke, PS; Gooding, GAW; Narayan, P: Prospective randomized trial of coumadin vs. sequential compression stockings as prophylaxis for postoperative deep venous thrombosis in major urologic surgery. J Urol 147:1056–1059, 1992.

SECTION VII

FUTURE PERSPECTIVES

CHAPTER 28

Future Perspectives in Laparoscopy

Michael E. Moran, MD

Technology and microelectronics are revolutionizing every aspect of our society. Polymer science, microcomputerization, optical engineering, bioengineering, and many other technologic innovations are being focused on advanced health care delivery. Surgery has not been immune to such technologic advancement. The precise extent and overall impact of new, minimal access urologic surgeries has doubled in the past 12 months and it is anticipated to double again within 6 months. This logarithmic growth in laparoscopic urologic surgery is being driven by patient demand. With the rapid dissemination of knowledge by mass media, an increasingly informed society is seeking alternative therapy for the heretofore conventional open operations.[1] *Minimal access surgery* is a redefinition of the term for technologically advanced surgery originally coined by Wickham in 1987, as the "new surgery, or minimally invasive surgery."[2] These terms merely quantify the degree of surgical trauma. Laparoscopic surgery has been correctly pointed out by Cuschieri to produce minimal access trauma but still imparts surgical trauma.[3] Minimal invasive surgery is the next echelon vis-à-vis further reduction of risk and trauma for patients. True minimally invasive surgery may ultimately minimize trauma by eliminating direct organ dissection and removal by the "classic" methods. Thermal ablation and chemoprecipitant infarction represent such futuristic modalities that are already in clinical trials.[4,5,6]

The aim of this "new age" surgery is to minimize the trauma that the patient experiences. Average patients are unwilling to submit to the classic treatments if less invasive, even though often more speculative, alternatives exist. Laparoscopic urologic surgery represents that alternative to many patients. The procedures must still be viewed as experimental, yet the patients are willing to sign up for the protocols with little thought of the consequences. As investigators and clinicians, we must weigh the technical limitations of training and skill versus the classic traumas of standard therapy.[1]

MINIMAL ACCESS SURGERY

Surgical progress has been a series of quantum leaps based on technological advances.[7] Wickham identifies five sequential eras of surgery: the preanesthetic era, the postanesthetic era, the era of supportive medicine, the era of conservative surgery, and the era of minimally invasive surgery. Each era is characteristically diminishing in the timed constraints for progression to successive levels. It is ironic that the laparoscopic techniques devised today will probably be replaced by technologic wonders of tomorrow within our lifetimes. Despite this prediction, minimal access surgery has just begun to affect surgical practice. Laparoscopic urologic surgery is not merely a new fad for the urologists. It is a serious method of systematically eliminating "classic" methods of open urogenital surgeries.

No area of urologic surgery is immune to the invasion of this endoscopic surgery. Methods of surgical extirpations for oncologic processes and inflammatory diseases of the urinary tract are being increasingly reported. Recent attention has been focused on laparoscopic urinary reconstruction. The development of equipment and technology are lagging behind the skill and prowess of pioneers in this burgeoning field. There is no question that many of the classic urologic operations can be performed with laparoscopic techniques; the doubt remains — are the operations producing equivalent or better results? The electronic imaging systems available allow the surgeon an unprecedented anatomic view of the urinary tract. The magnification inherent in the imaging system is both an advantage and a disadvantage. The brightly illuminated fields produce a two-dimensional effect that makes the neophyte laparoscopist appear clumsy and uncoordinated. Movements tend to be sporadic and jerky. Finesse comes with patience and practice. By slowing movements to the point of control, economy of motion and fluid movements result. This operating environment is similar to that of microsurgery. Ultimately, the precision of microsurgical dissection and reconstruction is a potential advantage of this type of surgery.

TRAUMA OF SURGERY

Most of us have lived through two revolutionary eras of urologic practice: the endoscopic treatment of prostatic disease and the abdication of open stone surgery. Wickham has chosen the latter to represent the traumas inflicted upon our patients and the result of technology on reducing them.[2] Progressing from open stone surgery through percutaneous nephrostolithotripsy, and first- and second-generation shock-wave lithotripsy therapy, patients are subjected to less and less interventional trauma. The results are dramatically reduced hospital stays and faster return to normal activities. In one decade, urologists have progressed in the treatment of stone disease further than any other surgical specialty. However, general surgeons are rapidly reclaiming superiority in the realm of advanced laparoscopic procedures. It has been estimated that three fifths of all cholecystectomies performed in the United States this year will be done laparoscopically (more than 300,000 cases).

Accomplishing the functional equivalence of previously open procedures is the goal of pioneering laparoscopic surgeons. Avoidance of the trauma of the abdominal incision is just one of the advantages of this type of surgery. Psychologically, the patient feels less violated by several small stab wounds than by an incision. Anesthesia requirements are reduced as our technical capacity becomes more refined. The therapeutic procedure becomes less traumatic because of the inherent precision derived from the magnified field of dissection allowed by the electronic imaging systems.

FUTURE OF MINIMAL ACCESS SURGERY

What the ramifications of this type of surgery will eventually have on urologic practice is speculative. Wickham has, perhaps, the most radical view: that technology will pervasively alter the face of medical practice in the future. Hospitals will need to be redesigned as therapeutic centers. Medical care will be allocated and integrated to include an endoscopic surgical specialist. Note that this is not a urologist or a general surgeon, but one specially trained to perform high-technology, minimal access surgery. Wickham still designates the need for an open surgeon in his future medical practice. The decision who is to operate and when is no longer in the treatment paradigm of the urologist.[8]

One thing is certain — amid this change patients will benefit. Currently, an increasing number of urologic operations are being attempted laparoscopically.[9,10] Any tabulated list is bound to be obsolete by the time of publication. The spectacular accomplishments of pioneering surgeons in this field reflect substantial technologic support. It can be expected that as the prudence of laparoscopic urologic procedures becomes established, clinical acceptance of these techniques will follow. The advancements in the various facets of laparoscopic technology are outlined in the following sections.

OPTICS AND IMAGING SYSTEMS

Lens systems are being modified by optics engineers to produce visualization of unparalleled detail. One such system is the Olympus compensating telescope, which gives a clear, wide-angled field of view with inherent advantages for the laparoscopist. Light transmission systems are becoming more advanced, delivering up to 20% more light than previous noncoherent bundle systems. Liquid light cables have been available for years, and the new laparoscopic systems are now capable of taking full advantage of their superior light delivery. High-intensity light sources utilizing the halide elements produce less color distortion and brighter illumination. Charged electronic coupling device (CCD) miniature television cameras have become the standard modality for monitoring the laparoscopic procedure. Integrated systems can also produce hard-copy documentation for patients' records, provide in-line simultaneous radiographic images, plus incorporate super VHS recording.[11] The number and size of the CCD chips affect the color and resolution of the video image. At the high end of the market,

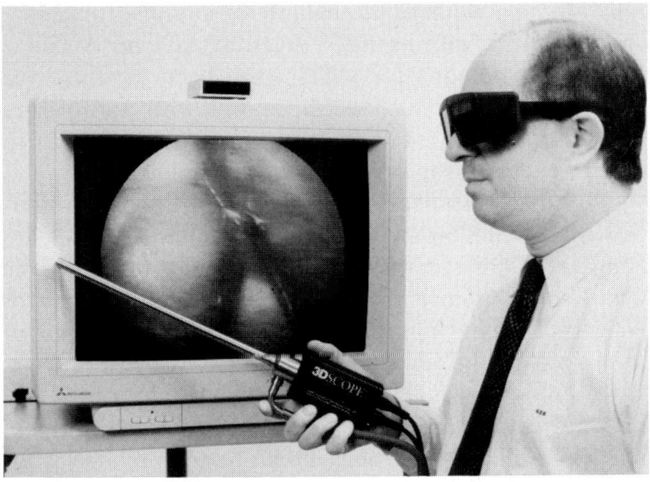

Figure 28–1. One of several prototypic laparoscopic 3-dimensional imaging systems, 3-D Scope. An infrared sensor provides the feedback necessary to integrate the angled input from the CCD chips. (Courtesy of American Surgical Technologies Corp., Chelmsford, MA.)

three CCD chip cameras provide optimal imaging in the red-spectrum range, crucial for advanced laparoscopic surgery. The newest optical system actually obviates the lens system by providing the video camera at the working end of the laparoscope. There is less distortion of the imaging and less inherent light loss, resulting in improved resolution (over 900 lines). Micro-CCD chips are being developed that will provide two proximally angled arrays that can be integrated with specially coated glasses to provide depth-of-field imaging (Fig. 28–1). Flexible videolaparoscopes are also being devised to allow more adaptability within the closed intraperitoneal environment (Fig. 28–2). These types of endoscopes will allow an increased ability for stereotactic maneuverability within the confines of the closed laparoscopic environment.

Integrated computerized imaging systems that visualize wavelengths outside of the human visible spectra were utilized in the recent Gulf War with devastating accuracy. Such systems are now finding applications with medical imaging systems. Laparoscopic lymph node dissections might easily become crude procedures compared with image-directed lymphatic sampling. These are already described for breast, lung, and prostatic carcinomas. Electronic integration is already possible with current electronic chains commonly used in the operating room. With the addition of a video mixer, control of image placement and image-on-image viewing are possible. Split-screen imaging can allow simultaneous visualization of several input systems (three-dimensional ultrasound images, infrared, ultraviolet, etc.). Systems that have dual image capability will allow the surgeon an unprecedented degree of visual control. For complex urologic reconstructive efforts, the ability to see with a flexible endoscope through a visceral structure can be performed synchronously with laparoscopic intraperitoneal maneuvers and endoluminal-assisted surgery.

The future belongs to systems designed to overcome the major drawback of current monocular imaging systems. There are two developments indicating that depth perception is soon to be a reality for imaging systems. The first is light amplification by stimulated emission of radiation (laser) holography. Computerized interpretation of laser holographic images is already a reality.[12] The expense and amount of equipment necessary for clinical application relegate its use to the future. The second development is already financially and practically available. Newer lens systems have been modified by advanced computer design to provide binocular depth perception. These will be modified for electronic imaging systems and represent the precursor to holographic imaging systems.

Laparoscopic Doppler and two-dimensional ultrasound systems are already in use (Fig. 28–3). Applications are currently limited, yet the number and complexity of these devices are increasing rapidly.[13] Doppler devices can identify vascular structures during laparoscopic dissection. Direct, intracorporeal ultrasonography may be useful for many purposes such as measurement of tumor extent, mapping at-risk regions for synchronous tumors, identification of calcar-

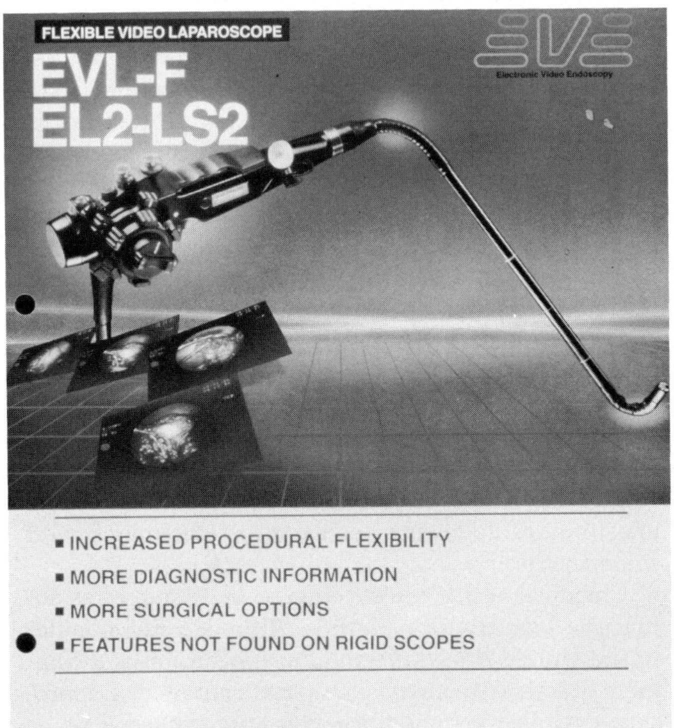

Figure 28–2. Flexible video laparoscope. CCD chip is positioned on the distal tip of this flexible laparoscope.

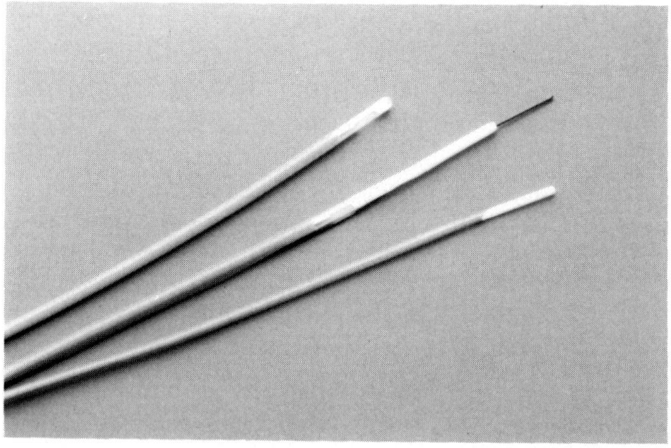

Figure 28–3. Small endoluminal ultrasound probes. Sizes vary from 1 to 5 mm and can provide tissue penetration from 2 to 4 cm. (Courtesy of Boston Scientific, Watertown, MA.)

eous deposits (stones, plaques, etc.), and monitoring directed sampling procedures.

LAPAROSCOPIC HEMOSTASIS SYSTEMS

In order to ascend the evolutionary ladder of complex endoscopic abdominal surgery, the capacity to achieve hemostasis rapidly and safely is a prerequisite. To this end, older devices are being redesigned for laparoscopic purposes.[14] Hemostatic devices may utilize mechanical (e.g., staples, sutures, clamps), chemical (e.g., collagen, thrombin), or thermal (e.g., microwave, cautery, argon-beam coagulator, laser) properties to attain the desired effect.

Automated suturing devices are already in use intra-abdominally in Europe. Modifications and newer designs promise to obviate the frustration of current hand-suturing techniques. Simple exercises and modeling of complex endoscopic-suturing situations are critical to the mastery of intracorporeal suturing techniques.[15] Stapling devices are being modified to such an extent that suturing may be entirely obviated. Laparoscopic autostapling devices are already available. Bowel, stomach, esophagus, lung, kidney, and bladder have already been the subjects of endoscopic stapling without difficulty. Urologic reconstruction, especially involving ureteral or urethral anastomoses, requires noncalculogenic or absorbable staples. Such a device has been used for urethrovesical anastomoses following radical prostatectomies with some success.[16]

Chemical agents are also increasingly sought as adjunctive hemostatic materials. Although not popular in the United States, fibrin glue application is a common practice in many European centers.[17] Laparoscopic applicators and fibrin glue spray guns are being marketed throughout much of Europe. Beyond the applicability as a hemostatic agent, such material can also act as a watertight sealant for complex uroanastomoses and lymphatics.[18] Agents such as Avitene, known to surgeons for years, have been modified for laparoscopic utility. Special clamps and applicators are now capable of delivering such biomaterials to operative areas for endoscopic hemostasis.

Thermal hemostatic mechanisms offer the potential for future laparoscopic utility. The argon-beam coagulator has recently been adapted for laparoscopic use. It offers many advantages over standard electrocautery for the laparoscopic surgeon, since it effectively clears the field, simultaneously providing thermal hemostasis.[19] The superficial penetration of the thermal cauterization produces little tissue charring, and the ability to identify tissue planes makes it an ideal method of hemostasis during laparoscopic reconstruction.[20]

Laser technology may find its long-awaited promise in complex laparoscopic procedures. Pinpoint energy application with "new age" lasers such as a circumferentially arrayed Eximer laser and the energy characteristics of the midinfrared lasers may make them the instruments of choice for combined hemostasis and tissue ablation. Thulium-holmium-chromium:YAG lasers have a 2-μm wavelength, providing a large absorption peak in water and making application for endoscopic tissue ablation possible. The erbium:YAG represents yet another doped YAG system with potential for cutting and tissue ablation.[21] There exists a growing need for transportable, less expensive, more compact, and more reliable laser systems. Solid-state microprocessor electronics may solve this problem by the availability of diode lasers.[22] Most available systems currently lack the power of the Nd:YAG or KTP lasers, but a growing number of manufacturers are actively seeking to solve these drawbacks.

Probes for laparoscopic laser use have been one major drawback for their clinical utility. The need to provide some method to control the heating process at the tips of these instruments has been a concern. Untoward sequelae have aroused the suspicion that gas emboli may occur from direct-contact laparoscopic laser dissection.[23] Newer synthetics have allowed laser application with a variety of instrument configurations that no longer require flowing gas or iced saline application (Fig. 28–4). There are indications that laser energy can also be applied from bipolar devices, producing even greater control of this thermal energy. Another device, recently approved by the Food and Drug Administration, is the laser-assisted scalpel (Fig. 28–5).[24] It can be predicted that the number of laser applications will grow steadily as our knowledge of laser-tissue interactions increases. Devices that allow rapid cutting and maintenance of hemostasis are likely to result in streamlining surgical laparoscopic procedures. The number and wavelengths of surgical

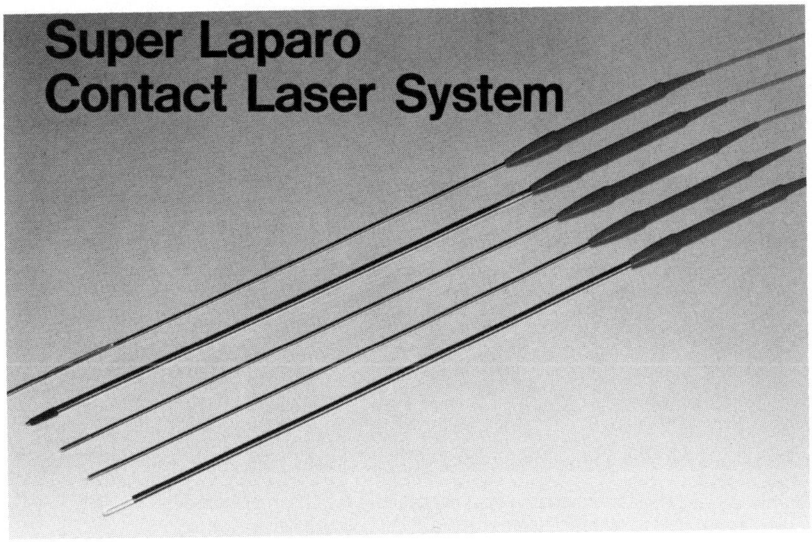

Figure 28–4. Laparoscopic contact laser probes. (Courtesy of SLT Japan, Tokyo, Japan.)

lasers are increasing rapidly. The exact role of the lasers in controlled hemostatic dissection remains an exciting unknown.

Laser sealing and approximation combined with absorbable tissue stents may represent the anastomosis of the future. Tissue welding has been used in open procedures for such diffuse connections as vascular, urethral, ureteral, and bowel anastomoses. Recently, laparoscopic laser welding has been accomplished with a special laser laparoscope and computerized feedback from infrared thermal sensors.[25] Lower power settings are possible with the use of tissue solders.[26] Solders vary according to the wavelength of light utilized for laser welding, producing anastomoses with superphysiologic burst pressures (above 200 mm Hg).[27] Performing these advanced laser anastomoses may seem inordinately complex and the equipment may seem costly, but the alternatives for laparoscopic reconstruction are not much better. A system for accomplishing a laser-welded anastomosis has been prototyped. Consisting of an absorbable stent used to lock the tissues into predetermined configurations, the ExoScope performs an automated anastomosis using circumferentially arrayed laser fibers to weld tissues in an end-to-end fashion.[28]

Microwave scalpels represent yet another modality of achieving hemostasis.[29] These devices have predominantly been employed for open hepatobiliary surgery, and little is yet known about their utility in laparoscopic surgery. The exact role and capacity of microwave dissectors for laparoscopic purposes are not known; however, the characteristic deep thermal effects may make difficult intraparenchymal surgery possible. Scalpels are also being marketed for cutting hemostatically by ultrasonic oscillation, such as the Harmonic Scalpel (Fig. 28–6). The risk of conductance problems associated with electrosurgery would be eliminated. Claims by the manufacturer that no tissue charring occurs are encouraging, but the ability to control hemorrhage from larger vessels is uncertain.

LAPAROSCOPIC INSTRUMENTS

Access and the safe introduction of the laparoscope are continuing problems the urologist must overcome. The Verres needle has become the standard instrument for insufflation; however, it should also be kept in mind that increasing numbers of surgeons are moving to open Hasson cannula placement in order to avoid any risk of blind access. This, plus expanding the realm of laparoscopy to include patients who have had previous open explorations, produces a need for

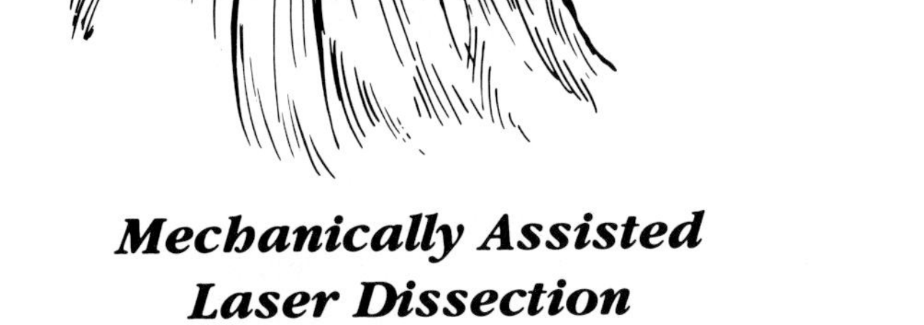

Figure 28–5. Blunt dissecting probe with a dual feature of laser-assisted lysis. (Courtesy of MicroSurge Inc., Brookline, MA.)

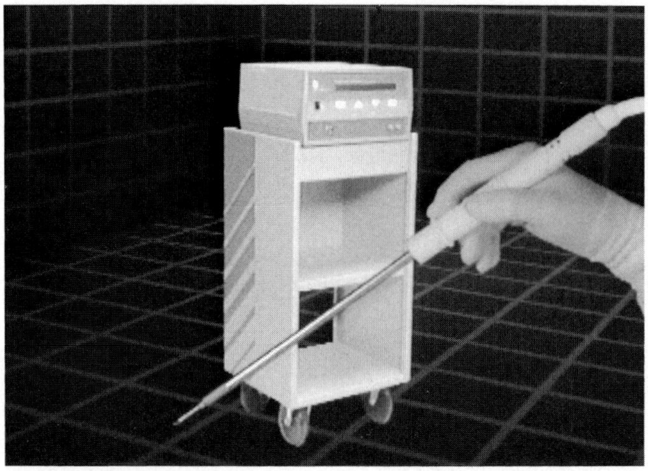

Figure 28–6. Ultrasonic energy can be utilized for thermal hemostasis as in the Harmonic Scalpel. (Courtesy of Ultracision, Inc., Smithfield, RI.)

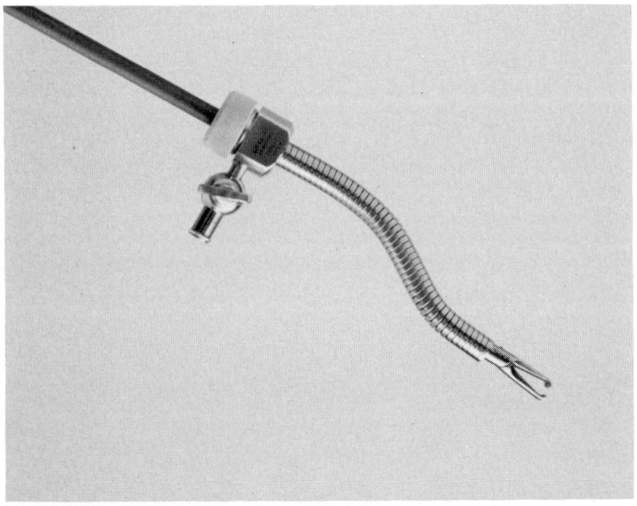

Figure 28–8. Flexible access portals allow the passage of variously configured instruments. (Courtesy of Karl Storz, Culver City, CA.)

improved access mechanisms. A growing literature expounds the ability of ultrasound to successfully identify and map abdominal adhesions before laparoscopic access.[30] Others have developed fine-needle access techniques.[31] The ultimate method of safe access would be visualized avoidance of vessels and viscera prior to the insufflation of the peritoneum. This requires a needle scope for success. All the advantages of the open Hasson technique plus the speed of closed Verres techniques would result.[32] Several manufacturers are attempting to fill the need for such a device; however, currently there exists no specifically built laparoscopic visual access system (Fig. 28–7).

The exact method of approaching the genitourinary organs of interest is not standard. One institution's method of accomplishing a given operation varies significantly from another's, unless the training programs have fostered similarity. The portals for access are round and rigid. There are no particular reasons for these manufacturing parameters except that they have always been designed in this way. Investigators have begun to question this dogmatic approach. In response, there are now malleable access portals available (Fig. 28–8). The flexibility of the shaft allows placement of instruments that are not straight. The advantage of curved instruments resides in their greater flexibility to work around various fixed structures that impede access to an area targeted for surgery.[33] Curved instruments also allow better visualization of the area where the instrument is placed, because it can be angled away from the line of sight. Finally, curved instruments change the fulcrum point of a rigid instrument from the trocar site on the anterior abdominal wall to the area of curvature. By making smaller moves, more work can be accomplished with a given device (Fig. 28–9).

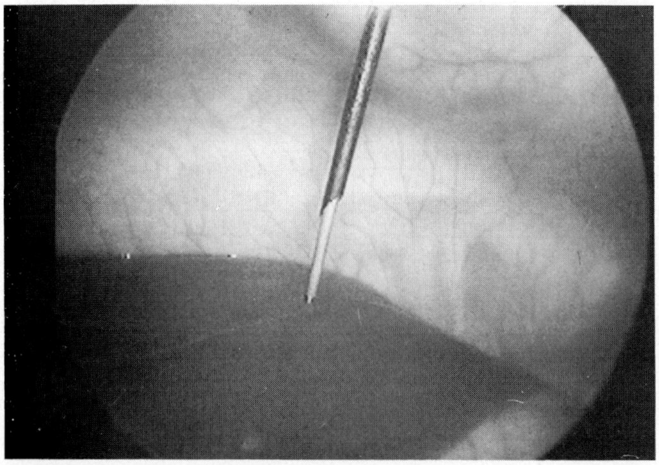

Figure 28–7. Visualized needle access utilizing microendoscopes. (Courtesy of Boston Scientific, Watertown, MA.)

LAPAROSCOPIC RETRACTION DEVICES

Retraction devices represent the next major technologic revolution that must occur before complex laparoscopic procedures can evolve. Many simple mechanical devices are already available, but they provide a minimal amount of retraction. By any open-procedure standard for providing the required assistance of controlled visualization, these are crude.

An entirely new concept of retraction is needed in order to proceed with complex retroperitoneal surgery. Employing a crude intra-abdominal balloon retractor, we have been able to safely and expeditiously perform retroperitoneal lymph node dissections in the porcine model with little trauma to the adjacent viscera.[34] Inflatable balloons that perform as multitask workstations are currently being designed. Pseudoelastic

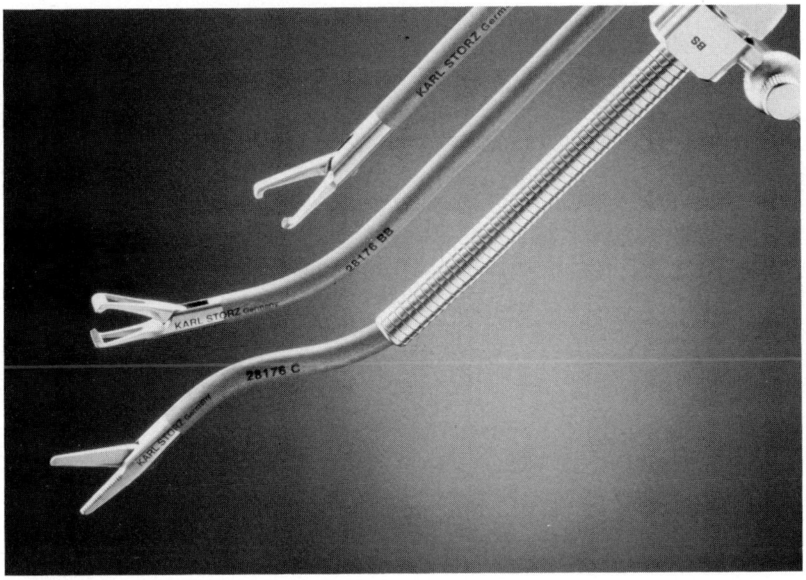

Figure 28–9. Curved grasping instruments. (Courtesy of Karl Storz, Culver City, CA.)

nickel-titanium alloy (Tinel) has been prototypically developed for shape-memory laparoscopic instruments.[35] It is conceivable that every area within the abdominal cavity will be accessible for safe surgical intervention.

One method of avoiding retraction of intraperitoneal viscera is to approach the urinary tract in its retroperitoneal space. Initial attempts at this approach were difficult.[36] Others have developed techniques to place open laparoscopic trocars in these potential spaces and begin the dissection either manually or with the aid of a balloon device before insufflation. It has been speculated that insufflation of these preperitoneal or retroperitoneal spaces is associated with the development of hypercapnia.[37] In actual clinical performance of a wide variety of urologic laparoscopic cases this has not been supported.[38–42] The ability to access these potential spaces should allow for the dissection of the urinary organ of choice and prevent the need to retract visceral structures. Reconstructive urologic procedures that use bowel segments will still require transperitoneal access and the attendant need for retraction.

ENVIRONMENTAL CONTAINMENT AND TISSUE REMOVAL SYSTEMS

Advanced laparoscopic urologic procedures cannot realistically be minimally invasive if the abdomen must be opened at the conclusion of the procedure in order to remove a diseased organ. Tissue morcellation has been a reality for years, primarily spurred by the efforts of neurosurgeons and orthopedists interested in rapidly removing bone and cartilage. Coptcoat and associates recently devised a method of liquefaction employing a modified morcellator device that they termed ELSA (endoscopic liquidization and surgical aspiration).[43] Their primary interest was removing prostatic tissue transurethrally by a robotic process. It took no leap of the imagination to find alternative methods of using the device that subsequently was used to perform percutaneous lithotripsy. Clayman has taken the concept a step beyond with a newer design. By placing the motor-driven morcellation elements within a housing outside the body, he can safely remove the entire kidney from the laparoscopic access portal.[44] The major drawback of this device is that the specimen appears to have been "food-processed," making certain pathologic interpretations difficult. It is probable that tumor volume, margins, the presence of synchronous lesions and the identification of capsular penetration would be impossible to determine. These are significant problems for the management of malignant diseases. Newer designs for the safe and rapid removal of solid masses are the next hurdle for the progress of complex laparoscopic surgery.

ROBOTICS

Automation represents the most advanced capacity for minimal access intra-abdominal surgery. Pneumatic robotic-arms are already available for holding the laparoscope better than can the trusted medical student (Fig. 28–10).[45] Precision, computerized response devices that interact with the human hand-eye coordination capacity are employed by the military for weaponry. Children's games are already using this same technology for amazing games of video skill.[46] It is foreseeable that this same capacity will evolve into microrobotic intra-abdominal devices that will work

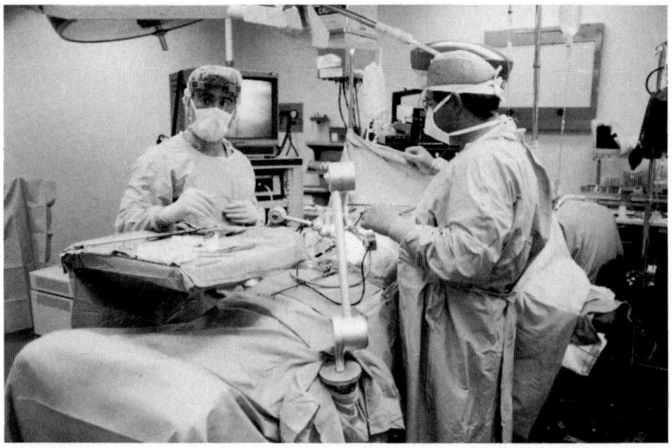

Figure 28–10. Pneumatically controlled laparoscopic robotic assistants. (Courtesy of Leonard Medical, Huntingdon Valley, PA.)

on remote radio-signal commands. Such systems for surgical intervention are already being developed.[47] Complete, remote surgical interaction with the endoscopic camera and robotic instruments coupled with computer-mediated feedback (auditory, visual, and tactile) provides a near-virtual reality for the surgeon (Fig. 28–11). Technology is being rapidly brought to surgical application. Robodoc is one such computer-controlled, robotic, interactive orthopedic device (Fig. 28–12). It can rapidly and reproducibly make total joint replacement a precision-tooled, automated procedure. But this represents just the initial surgical application of a whole panoply of robotic technology. The Massachusetts Institute of Technology is proposing new computerized intelligence chips that allow small, mobile robotic devices to learn and interact.[48] Such GNAT robots combine distributed real-time control with sensor-triggered behavior. Currently, insectlike mobile robots have been constructed but are limited in their capacity to perform dexterous surgical maneuvers by inadequacies of the microengines. The University of California, Berkeley and AT&T Bell Laboratories are independently investigating microengines that could power small robotic devices. Nippondenso, one of the world's largest auto manufacturers, has devised an electromagnetic wave engine, using microwave energy "beamed" into it from a distance. Where this technology will lead, no one can quite predict. These microrobotic, computer-controlled, intra-abdominal surgical devices are sure to become more advanced. Utilization of this technology to help conventional surgical procedures seems inevitable. The cost must be weighed against the potential benefits to the patients. Perhaps Wickham is correct; since this type of surgery is sure to involve mechanical engineers, artificial intelligence laboratories, optical engineers, microrobotics, and communications experts, the surgery of tomorrow may become limited to an endoscopic surgical specialist working for a corporate sponsor.

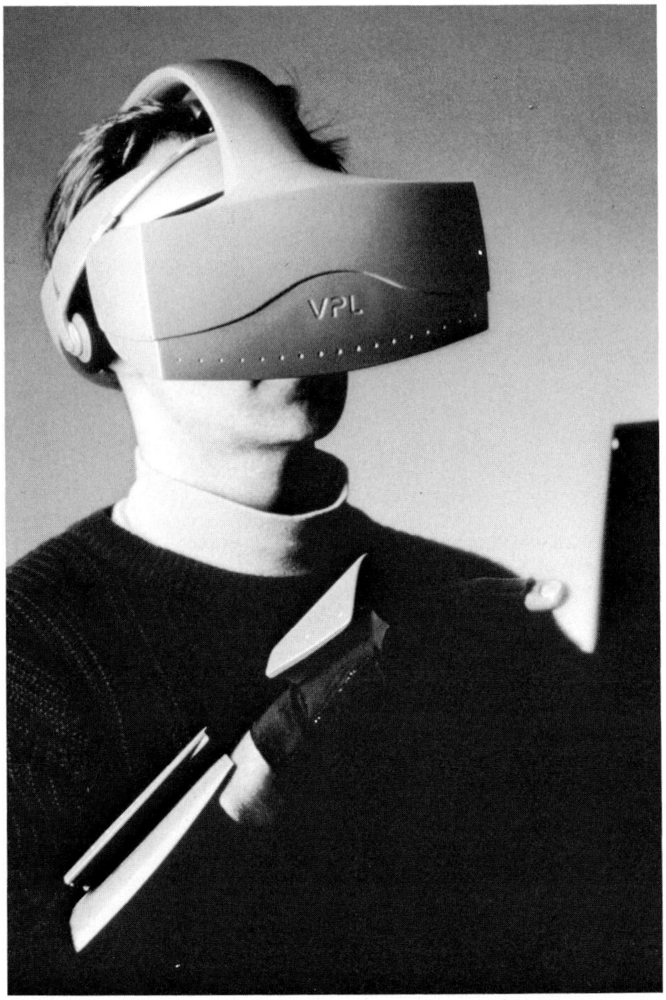

Figure 28–11. Virtual reality system. (Courtesy of Dr. Satava, Monterey, CA.)

CONCLUSIONS

I have managed to go far into the realm of futuristic urologic surgery. That is one of the innate features of a realm with no significant past—a tabula rasa on which technology has but to write the coming chapters. It is a future that none can truly anticipate. It requires fertile minds with pioneers' capacity to proceed. Patients are demanding to be minimally invaded. The close cooperation of manufacturers with clinical urologists is a *must* to rapidly move forward. Physicians who wish to learn techniques must seek courses where advanced technology is available. One says to oneself, "I will not practice long enough to see this technology affect the way I perform surgery!" Yet it has already changed the practice of surgery. It is no longer a question of what will be performed but a question of when it will be performed.

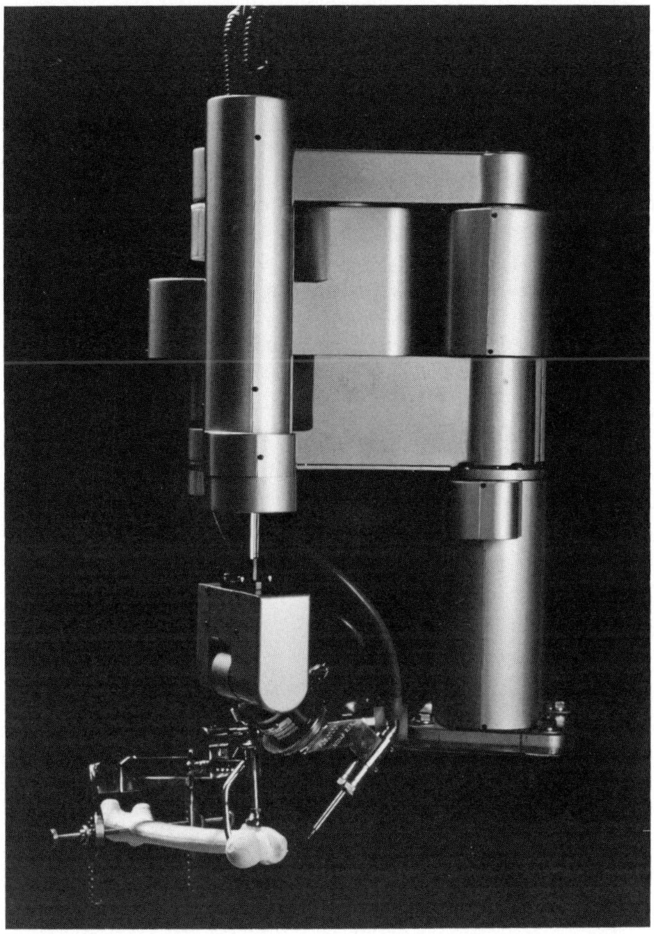

Figure 28–12. Macrorobotic surgery by computer-regulated, image-guided digital integration. (Courtesy of Integrated Surgical Systems, Sacramento, CA.)

REFERENCES

1. Moran, ME: Urologic laparoscopic surgery: Ethical and economic considerations. J Urol, submitted.
2. Wickham, JEA: The new surgery. Br Med J 295:1581, 1987.
3. Cuschieri, A; Terblanche, J: Laparoscopic cholecystectomy: Evolution, not revolution. Surg Endosc 4:125, 1990.
4. Gelet, A; Margonari, J; Chapelon, JY; et al: Treatment of Dunning R3327 prostatic adenocarcinoma in rats by ABLATHERM. The Society for Minimally Invasive Therapy, 3rd International Meeting, Boston, 1991, p. 85.
5. Rassweiler, J; Richter, GM; Kauffmann, GW; Alken, P: Capillary chemoembolization with ETHIBLOC pharmaceutical basis and results in a new model of renal rat tumors. The Society for Minimally Invasive Therapy, 3rd International Meeting, Boston, 1991, p. 68.
6. DerHaar, GR; Clarke, RL; Vaughan, MG; Hill, CR: Trackless surgery using focused ultrasound: Technique and case report. Min Invas Ther 1:13, 1991.
7. Wickham, JEA: Minimally Invasive Therapy. Min Invas Ther 1:1, 1991.
8. Wickham, JEA: From butcher to bioengineer. The John K. Lattimer Lecture, American Urological Association's 86th Annual Meeting, Washington, 1991.
9. Leadbetter, GW; Gillenwater, JY: Urology. JAMA 265:3175, 1991.
10. Winfield, HN; Donovan, JF; Wee, WA; et al: Urological laparoscopic surgery. J Urol 146:941, 1991.
11. Moran, ME: Integrated fluoroscopic/electronic video-imaging during complex endourologic surgery. J Endourol 6:135S, 1992.
12. Free, J: Digital holography. Pop Sci, January:84–87, 1991.
13. Fornari, F; Civardi, G; Cavanna, L; et al: Laparoscopic ultrasonography in the study of liver diseases. Preliminary results. Surg Endosc 3:33, 1989.
14. Briggs, TP; Parker, C; Smith, C; Miller, RA: Augmented hemostasis: A review of the pharmacology of hemostasis in endoscopic surgery. Min Invas Ther 1:7, 1991.
15. Szabo, Z; Bowyer, DW; Moran, ME: Operative laparoscopy in urology: Intracorporeal suturing of the lower urinary tract. J Urol 147:408A, 1992.
16. Avant, OL; Starr, GA: Vesicourethral reanastomosis by mechanical stapling and transurethral deep dorsal vein ligation: A new technique for radical retropubic prostatectomy (in press).
17. Rovsov, J: Fibrin glue: An effective hemostatic agent for nonsuturable intraoperative bleeding. Ann Thorac Surg 38:409, 1984.
18. Dapunt, O; Waclawiczek, HW: Prevention and treatment of lymphatic fistulae following lymph node dissections by means of fibrin sealing. In: Progress in Fibrin Sealing. Berlin, Springer-Verlag, 1991, p. 65.
19. Henderson, MR; Link, WJ; Incropera, FR; Glover, JL: Gas transport resulting from plasma-scalpel surgery. Med Biol Eng 12:208, 1974.
20. Bowyer, DW; Moran, ME; Szabo, Z: Laparoscopic hemostasis with an argon beam coagulator. J Endourol 6:165S, 1992.
21. Go, PMNYH; Bruhn, EW; Hunter, JG; et al: The erbium:YAG laser as a surgical tool. Lasers Surg Med 10(supplement 2):22, 1990.
22. Treat, MR; Oz, MC; Bass, LS: New technologies and future applications of surgical lasers. The right tool for the right job. Surg Clin North Am 72:705–742, 1993.
23. Greville, AC; Clements, EA; Erwin, DC; et al: Pulmonary air embolism during laparoscopic laser cholecystectomy. Anesthesia 46:113–114, 1991.
24. Bhatta, KM; Rattner, DW; Haw, T; et al: A new laser delivery device for laparoscopic procedures. Lasers Surg Med (in press).
25. Poppas, DP; Sutaria, P; Sosa, RE; et al: Re-establishing continuity of the ureter using laser tissue-welding techniques: Evaluation of new laser tissue-welding solders for laparoscopic surgery. J Urol 147:244A, 1992.
26. Schlossberg, SM; Poppas, DP: Tissue welding with lasers. Semin Urol 9:206, 1991.
27. Libutti, SK; Oz, MC; Forde, KA; et al: Canine colonic anastomoses reinforced with dye-enhanced fibrinogen and a diode laser. Surg Endosc 4:97, 1990.
28. Sauer, JS; Hinshaw, JR: A fiber optic exoscope for laser tissue welding. Lasers Surg Med 6:219, 1986.
29. Reed, WP; Taylor, LS: The microwave scalpel: Clinical use. Contemp Surg 36:22–25, 1990.
30. Sigel, B; Golub, RM; Loiacono, LA; et al: Technique of ultrasonic detection and mapping of abdominal wall adhesions. Surg Endosc 5:161–165, 1991.
31. Dagnini, G: New instruments. Fine needles for pneumoperitoneum. *In*: Laparoscopy and Imaging Techniques, Berlin, Springer-Verlag, 1990, pp. 9–11.
32. Moran, ME; Bowyer, DW; Szabo, Z: Laparoscopic visual access: Needle-scope techniques. J Endourol 6:165S, 1992.
33. Cuschieri, A: Minimal access surgery and the future of interventional laparoscopy. Am J Surg 161:404–407, 1991.
34. Ordorica, RC; Moran, ME: Celioscopic, intra-abdominal retraction: Comparison of two mechanical devices. Min Invas Ther 1:42, 1991.
35. Cuschieri, A: Variable curvature shape-memory spatula for laparoscopic surgery. Surg Endosc 5:179, 1991.
36. Clayman, RV; Kavoussi, LR; McDougall, EM; et al: Laparoscopic nephrectomy: A review of 16 cases. J Laparoendosc Surg (in press).

37. Sosa, ER; Weingram, J; Stein, B; et al: Hypercarbia in laparoscopic pelvic lymph node dissection. J Urol 147:246A, 1992.
38. Ferzli, G; Trapasso, J; Raboy, A; Albert, P: Extraperitoneal endoscopic pelvic lymph node dissection. J Laparoendosc Surg 2:39–44, 1992.
39. Gaur, DD: Retroperitoneoscopy. 10th World Congress on Endourology and Extracorporeal Shock Wave Lithotripsy, 8th Annual Research Symposium on Extracorporeal Shock Wave Lithotripsy, Singapore, September 6, 1992.
40. Brunt, LM; Molmenti, EP; Kerbl, K; et al: Retroperitoneal endoscopic adrenalectomy. J Endourol 6:158S, 1992.
41. Mancini, P; Cuttano, MG; Pistolesi, D; et al: Ileo-pelvic lymphadenectomy performed by extraperitoneal laparoscopy for staging of prostatic carcinoma. J Endourol 6:107S, 1992.
42. Chapple, CR; Osborne, JL: Laparoscopic colposuspension — a new procedure. J Urol 147:280A, 1992.
43. Coptcoat, MJ; Ison, KT; Wickham, JEA: Endoscopic tissue liquidization and surgical aspiration. J Endourol 2:321, 1988.
44. Clayman, RV; Kavoussi, LR; Soper, NJ; et al: Laparoscopic nephrectomy: Initial case report. J Urol 146:278, 1991.
45. Moran, ME: Robotic-assisted laparoscopic urologic pelvic surgery. J Laparoendosc Surg (in press).
46. Satava, RM: Ninetendo surgery. JAMA, 267:2331–2332, 1992.
47. Green, PE; Piantanida, TA; Hill, JW; et al: Telepresence: Dexterous procedures in a virtual operating field. Am Surg 57:192, 1991.
48. Flynn, AM: GNAT robots. Am Surg 57:192A, 1991.

CHAPTER 29

Virtual Reality, Robotics, and Surgery in the Twenty-first Century

Irwin B. Simon, MD

Most surgeons are well aware of the way in which their daily lives have been affected by computers. Computerized patient databases and electronic billing are common. The advent of computer networking, high-speed computers, and fiberoptic transmission of data will soon bring a paperless office a step closer.

Information gathered at a physician's office or hospital will be immediately available to any other physician or health care facility (on that particular network) who is a provider of health care services to a given patient. Patients will likely carry a credit card–sized medical and insurance record. Initially, networks will be local. Patients requiring health care at distant sites will be able to give their entire past medical history to the new facility, simply by passing the card through a magnetic or optical card-reader.

The education of current and future physicians, particularly those in the surgical specialties, may soon have a different format. Entire textbooks will be available on computer databases. Medical teaching files, including x-ray and video images of physical findings, will be digitized.

EDUCATION

The education and training of the surgical specialties has for years relied on the axiom "See one, do one, teach one." This is a relatively crude oversimplification of a complex and extended educational process. Nonetheless, there has always been a kernel of truth in it. The time has come for medical and surgical education to take action, following the lead of the military and industry in the use of computer simulation in training.

Consider military and commercial pilot training. The earliest attempts at flight simulation were the early Link Flight Simulators of the 1930s and 1940s. These simulator aircrafts were little more than blue soapboxes mounted on springs. Hand and foot levers manipulated a series of wires that tilted them. Despite their crude form, the simulators are credited with the rapid training of hundreds of pilots during World War II. Furthermore, they are credited with saving the lives of many pilots who would otherwise have died in training and in combat. Finally, they were extremely cost-effective in training these pilots.

The early Link Simulators have evolved into full-sized replicas of aircraft cockpits. Neither military nor civilian commercial pilots may fly a real aircraft until they have flown hundreds of hours in a computerized flight simulator. Sitting at the controls of a cockpit flight simulator, the individual is hard-pressed to tell whether the view out the cockpit window and the feel of the aircraft motion are real or simulated. Pilots are able to test their response to situations that they would not dare to encounter in a real aircraft. The sweating and racing heartbeats they experience are a testimonial to the perceived reality of the situation.

VIRTUAL REALITY

Modern aircraft simulators are perhaps the progenitors of the virtual reality surgical simulators of the near future. Virtual reality refers to a computer-generated world within which a human being may interact with other human beings and/or objects. He or she is "immersed" within this virtual world and experiences and interacts with objects in it through the senses, having the impression of truly being in this surreal, computer-generated world. The visual field is a stereoscopic video image of the world. This has been most often accomplished by the user's wearing a bulky headset consisting of two high-resolution video monitors directly in front of his or her eyes. The headset images are accompanied by stereo-audio input (Fig. 29–1). Within this world, objects can be manipulated by the computer user by simply moving some input device such as a joy stick. Early joy sticks are being replaced with input devices that mimic the human hand. One such mechanism is the DataGlove. Locomotion through the virtual world is accomplished by pointing a controlling finger from a DataGlove or similar input system, giving rise to the concept that users "fly" through virtual worlds. Objects touched or lifted can be "felt" by sophisticated computer simulation of tactile sensations, force feedback, and motion.

Other designations such as cyberspace and artificial reality are considered synonymous with the term *virtual reality* (VR). However, VR has been most commonly accepted.

In essence, modern flight simulators constitute a form of VR, since the simulators mimic actual cockpit experience. The thrust in the medical world is now to create a computer-simulated surgical world. It is anticipated that a surgeon or resident surgeon will be required to perform flawlessly an operation on a simulated surgical patient before being allowed to participate in an actual operation. Multiple computer-created scenarios of bleeding, adhesions, tumor ingrowth, and the like can be simulated to challenge the trainee. The trainee may thus cause bleeding from the iliac veins in a simulation of a laparoscopic pelvic lymph node dissection, yet no patient is harmed.

The concept of VR for surgical simulation has real impetus now for several reasons. The rapid evolution to more and more minimally invasive procedures has magnified the need for a training device that mimics a real patient and a real surgical theater. The simulation should be complete with video screens and the currently available array of minimally invasive instruments and techniques.

The computer world of VR can be used as an educational tool, allowing medical students and residents to view anatomy from viewpoints never before possible. The student can directly enter the globe of the eye, proceed down the optic nerve, across the optic chiasm, and eventually reach an intercellular synapse deep within the brain. Alternatively, it is possible to "fly" down the alimentary tract, turn into the common bile duct, and continue on through the biliary tree, visualizing biliary stones, choledochoceles, or an accessory duct of Luschke. This can eliminate or reduce the

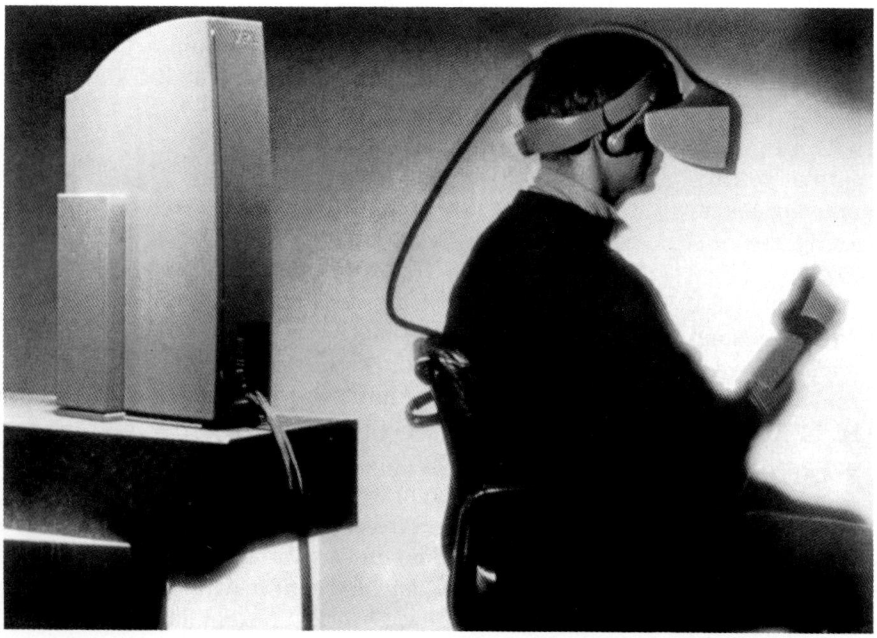

Figure 29–1. The head-mounted display and DataGlove used to view a virtual reality world. (From Satava, RM: High tech surgery: Speculation on future directions. In: Hunter, JG; Sackier, JM, eds: Minimally Invasive Surgery. New York, McGraw Hill, 1993, p. 343. Courtesy of VPL Research, Inc., Redwood City, CA.)

number of cadavers necessary in current training. Laboratory use of animals can be dramatically curtailed. All of this has significant financial and social implications.

It is beyond the scope of this chapter to detail any of the means currently under study to create computer-generated worlds. However, simply stated, they are created using sophisticated computer-assisted design (CAD) software packages. This software renders cartoon-quality images that are useful but are not at a level of realism considered adequate for surgical training. Additional software will allow moving, breathing, bleeding, deformability, and so forth necessary for a realistic appearing VR patient.

The goal is eventually to move from these cartoon images toward digitized video images that emulate realistic surgery. Such images require a level of computing power not currently available except in a few supercomputing centers around the world. When the next several generations of computers become available at a reasonable cost, real-time images of simulated surgical procedures should be usable by the typical resident in training as well as the practicing surgeon.

Practicing surgeons can use these training simulators to learn new procedures. For instance, had they been available, these devices would have been ideal for training the 33,000 general surgeons now practicing in the United States in the techniques of laparoscopic cholecystectomy. In addition, the computer will allow the surgeon to create an overlay of computed tomography (CT), magnetic resonance imaging (MRI), or any other imaging modality directly over the image of the patient. This will allow dry run-throughs of delicate operations before the actual procedures. Furthermore, heads-up display images may allow surgeons to visualize CT or MR images directly over the patient's real anatomy during the procedure, thus aiding in more complete removal of pathology yet sparing vital structures. Neurosurgical excision of intracranial tumors is an example of the use of such proposals.

Much of the early work in VR for surgical simulation has been carried out by Satava and co-workers in conjunction with VPL Research.*[1] At Dartmouth University, Rosen's laboratory is heavily involved in advanced VR projects. These projects have received significant attention from private sector medical manufacturers as well as from government agencies. Several commercial ventures are slated for availability in mid 1994.

Telepresence

Eventually, the computer workstation will allow more than a simulation of surgery. The very same workstation may be utilized as the control center for robotically assisted surgical procedures. The cornerstone of the surgical future may indeed be the linkage of VR and the science of telepresence.

The stage has been set for the introduction of telepresence surgery. Laparoscopic cholecystectomy is the paradigm and progenitor of innumerable minimally invasive procedures. Both medical and lay press constantly report new applications of laparoscopic technology. At present, most of these are minimally invasive adaptations of well-described and accepted open surgical procedures.

Urologic surgeons were among the first to take the great leap. They have been performing endoscopic surgery since the turn of the century when the first transurethral prostate resections were performed.

Gynecologic surgeons have been performing minimally invasive surgery since the early 1960s but were limited by the crude instruments and by the neck-craning required for one person to view through standard laparoscopes. The evolution of the charged coupled device (CCD) chip camera has brought the gynecologist, the urologist, and indeed all surgical disciplines into the 1990s world of videoscopic surgery.

From the 1800s through 1989, comparatively little change occurred in surgical technique. Now the surgical world has been dramatically changed forever by the application of techniques in minimal access surgery. These changes have evolved from the uniting of medicine and technology and are ubiquitous, crossing the boundaries into all surgical disciplines.

Currently, the art of surgery requires a true operating theater. Within this theater, the surgeon's instruments have been augmented with expensive, high technology props. These include the CCD chip camera, high-flow insufflators, high-resolution video monitors, argon-beam coagulators, and so forth. Most of these have been developed and initially used in the nonmedical world.

The latter part of this century has seen a resurgence of the surgical pioneering spirit. The names of those early surgical pioneers will be joined by such names as Dubois, Perrissat, and Reddick. In just three short years, laparoscopic cholecystectomy has been brought to the forefront as the currently accepted gold standard for removal of the diseased gallbladder.[2,3] The revolution that began with laparoscopic cholecystectomy has now advanced to the Laparoscopic Olympics of today[4] in which there is no intra-abdominal or intrathoracic procedure that cannot be performed by a laparoscopic surgeon with significant experience.

However, even the most adept surgeons are admittedly subject to the limitations of current technologies. Significant trade-offs are required in exchange for the privilege of these minimally invasive, or keyhole, techniques.

*Redwood City, CA.

The lack of depth perception is arguably the most critical limitation of current laparoscopic technology. This lack has been postulated as responsible for laparoscopic cholecystectomy having a higher rate of complications than its open counterpart. For this reason, stereoscopic videoscopy has become a high priority among major instrument producers today. The depth perception provided by one such product (3DSCOPE)* has been described in a review as "facilitating the performance of complex procedures."[5]

Despite the widespread acceptance and application of advanced laparoscopic procedures, the complaint of experienced surgeons has been that they could not perform such operations with the same facility as in open surgery. No real tactile, auditory, or olfactory signals reach the operator through the standard laparoscopic instruments and their two-dimensional images on a video monitor. In laparoscopy, the surgeon's dexterity is limited and worsened by the fulcrum effect of current laparoscopic instruments. The frustration is heightened whenever the two-dimensional camera angles (camera insertion port) are changed (Fig. 29–2).

Telepresence surgery is the name coined by Green and colleagues to describe the application of existing and developing robotic technologies as they are applied to minimally invasive surgical procedures.[6] The concept of robotic assistance in surgery is not altogether new. However, the concept of telepresence surgery is a refinement beyond robotics that is intended to give the future surgeon a realistic three-dimensional image with credible tactile feedback and dexterity as if he or she were actually present at the surgical site.

*American Surgical Technologies, Chelmsford, MA.

To understand telepresence surgery, some basic definitions must first be understood. The following stem from those of Sheridan.[7]

Robotics: The science and art of performing by means of an automatic apparatus or device functions normally ascribed to human beings.

Teleoperation: The extension of a person's manipulation capability to a remote location. It refers to direct and continuous human control (one to one) by the remote manipulator.

Telepresence: The concept of teleoperation with the added benefit of the system's sensing sufficient information about the remote manipulator and task environment and communicating this to the human operator so that the human feels as if he or she were physically present at the remote site.

Telerobotics: A form of teleoperation in which a human operator acts as supervisor. The telerobot executes the task based on information received from the human operator plus its own artificial sensing and intelligence.

Robotic technology is being utilized today in surgical procedures. Robodoc is the name given to a robotic arm placed at surgery that follows computer guidance from a preoperative CT scan. It is capable of extreme precision as a femur is drilled. The tolerances are fine enough to allow the surgeon to press-fit a hip prosthesis. Multiple animal trials have proved the utility of this computer-controlled robot. Early reports from human trials show tantalizing success.

In the United Kingdom, similar technology has been utilized by Timoney and Wickam. Their robotic surgery for transurethral resection of the prostate was the first totally robotic surgery in history.[8]

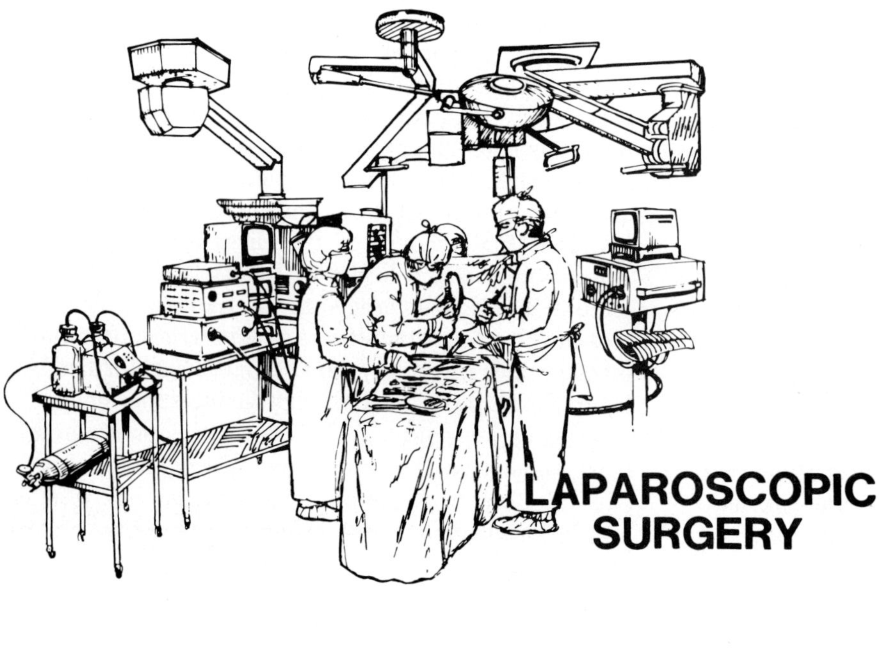

Figure 29–2. Laparoscopic surgery, as currently performed. (From Satava, RM: High tech surgery: Speculation on future directions. In: Hunter, JG; Sackier, JM, eds: Minimally Invasive Surgery. New York, McGraw Hill, 1993, p. 345.)

To date, surgical applications of robotic techniques have precluded any possibility of the human surgeon's interacting with the robot. Preprogrammed robotic movement is based on fixed spatial reference points. This type of technologic assistance would fail in the thoracic cavity or the abdomen, in which the organs are moving with respiration or physiologically with peristalsis, and in which there is great variability in size and location of the target of the operation.

Current state of the art in telepresence surgery is best exemplified by the Green Telepresence Surgery System. The surgeon performs the procedure while seated at a surgical computer workstation. The operative site may be any distance away—across the room or across the world, even above this world in a space station. Dual CCD cameras transmit stereoscopic images of the work site (Fig. 29–3). These images are received at the workstation. Simple polarizing lenses allow the alternating images to be viewed as a single three-dimensional image. This concept is known as field sequential vision.

The video monitor is situated in such a way that the surgeon looks down at it, much as a standing surgeon looks down into the operative field in conventional surgery. Articulations, designed in the remote manipulators, remove the awkward fulcrum effect of laparoscopic instruments. The surgeon's hands are placed below the three-dimensional video screen. In this fashion, a realistic illusion is created in which it seems that the surgeon's hands and instruments are actually within the patient's abdomen at the work site. The instruments respond deftly and in real time to the movements of surgeon's hands on controller actuators that actually are simple modifications of common operative instruments (Fig. 29–4).

Currently, early prototypes have been tested to demonstrate the realism of the visual effect and the versatility of force feedback. True tactile sensation and proprioception will eventually be added to the system as they become more feasible. Several engineering laboratories are working on mimicking human proprioception.

At this writing, there has been no human application of telepresence surgery. Laboratory experimentation has demonstrated the utility of early prototypes. Ex vivo application has demonstrated the system's ability to perform cholecystectomy and sutured bowel anastomoses. From a remote distance, the system is precise enough to allow the surgeon to deftly thread a 4.0 monofilament suture into the eye of a free needle.[9]

The system is easily scalable. Simple movements of the surgeon's hand can control gross motor movements such as those needed for intra-abdominal procedures. Alternatively, it is anticipated that scaling the movements down or up can allow gross hand movements of the surgeon to control microsurgical movements of the remote manipulators, such as for neurosurgical and microvascular surgical procedures. In fact, cellular surgery is not inconceivable.

Early human work will undoubtedly occur with the surgeon sitting only a few steps from the patient. However, once the system has been validated, the surgeon may operate from across the room, across the country, or around the world. In this fashion, telemedicine and telepresence surgery may be used to bring health care to underserved areas of the world.

Early candidates for telepresence surgery include placement of radioactive pellets for brachytherapy. Exposure of operating room personnel to the blood products of patients with communicable diseases such

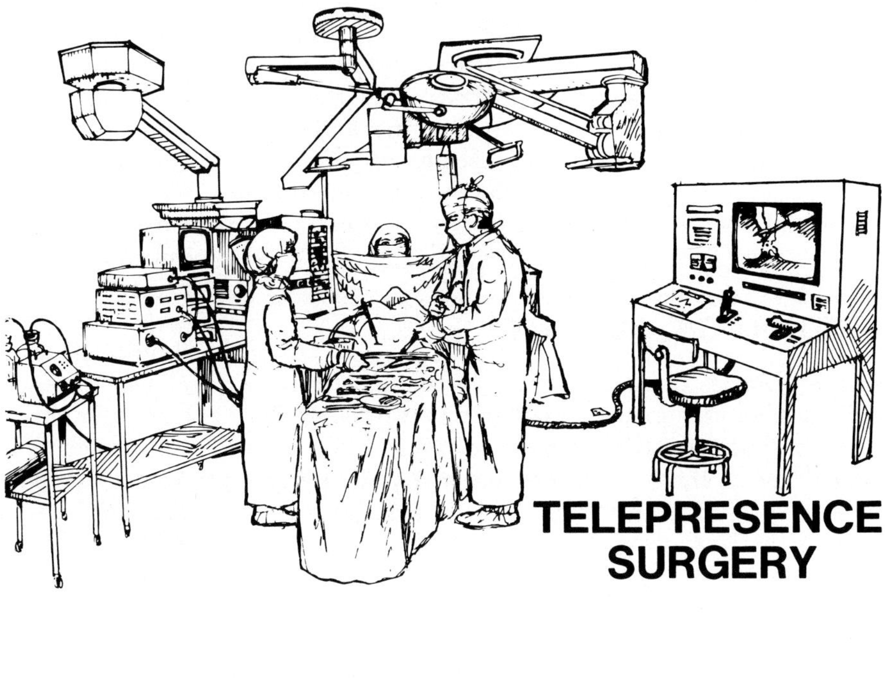

Figure 29–3. Telepresence surgery. Setting up the system identical to laparoscopic surgery but attaching the instruments and camera to robotic controls. (From Satava, RM: High tech surgery: Speculation on future directions. In: Hunter, JG; Sackier, JM, eds: Minimally Invasive Surgery. New York, McGraw Hill, 1993, p. 345.)

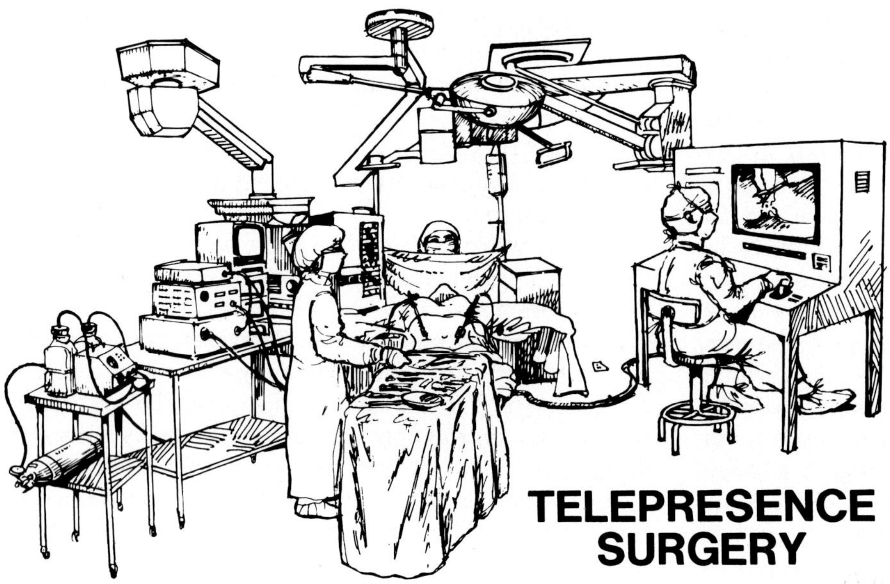

Figure 29–4. Telepresence surgery. Performing surgery remotely from the surgical workstations. (From Satava, RM: High tech surgery: Speculation on future directions. In: Hunter, JG; Sackier, JM, eds: Minimally Invasive Surgery. New York, McGraw Hill, 1993, p. 346.)

as AIDS and hepatitis can be minimized by application of telepresence principles.

Surgeons can assist each other from separate remote locations. The concept of computer networking will allow a surgeon in New York City to assist a local surgeon in rural America. This can occur by satellite transmission, fiberoptic networks, or some combination of the two. Earth-orbiting space stations and deep-space probes may become reality in the early twenty-first century. It is conceivable that with a trained technician on board the space station, the first surgery in space may be an appendectomy performed via telepresence by a surgeon at mission control.

The first commercially available telepresence surgery system will undoubtedly be followed closely by the introduction of specialty instruments manufactured by third parties. It is likely that every surgical specialty will have its own tool chest of specialized instruments to be used for telepresence in the performance of those procedures within the specialty. Adaptations for neurosurgery, vascular surgery, and urologic surgery will not lag behind the introduction of the initial telepresence technology.

TECHNOLOGIC ADVANCES

Entire libraries of medicine will be available to the individual physician along fiberoptic networks. Again, access will be through simple workstations. Efforts are under way to create hardware and software applications that will magnify the ability of the surgeon to perform surgical procedures with a precision never before attained. Three-dimensional images from ultrasound, computed tomographic (CT) scan, magnetic resonance imaging (MRI), and other evolving technologies may be transmitted to the visual field of the operating surgeon in the form of a heads-up, head-mounted display (HMD).

The HMD technology will allow the surgeon to perform a "dry run" of a technically demanding procedure on a VR "patient." Once satisfied, the surgeon can then flip a switch and the view changes to a real patient in the real world. This has application to training residents and to the practicing surgeon confronted with a difficult and demanding case.

CONCLUSIONS

This chapter has delineated some of the concepts of rapidly evolving technologies that have great potential to change the world. The urologic surgeon, along with surgeons in all disciplines, has become a laparoscopic-videoscopic surgeon and is more than ever dependent on advanced technologies. Such advances require a means to achieve education and training; this flow of information is most likely to arrive by the fiberoptic highways being constructed across the country and across the world. VR presents a way to create realistic simulation for training.

Telepresence surgery, teleradiology, and telemedicine offer the potential to alleviate some of the difficult problems facing health care in the modern world. Access to medical and surgical care can be simplified. The paperless office will come closer to reality as all medical access, transfers of information, and applications of therapeutic techniques are passed through the final common pathway, the computer workstation.

Through telepresence surgery, large-scale operations such as colon resections, Whipple procedures, and radical prostatectomies will become commonplace in a minimally invasive way. They will not be surgical curiosities rarely performed by a few aggressive and adept "Nintendo surgeons." Rather, they will become commonplace. Thus patient pain may be reduced, hospital stay may be shortened, and ultimately reduction of overall health care costs may benefit from this exciting new technology.

In Star Trek, Gene Roddenberry first described a "tricorder." This hand-held device was capable of diagnosis as well as therapeutic intervention. This chapter does not describe replacement of the surgeon by a small electronic box or a robot. Rather it portrays extension of the surgeon's abilities and accessibility to the patient.

REFERENCES

1. Satava, RM: Virtual reality surgical simulator: The first steps. Surg Endosc 7:203–205, 1993.
2. McSherry, CK: Cholecystectomy: The gold standard. Am J Surg 158:174–178, 1989.
3. Soper, NJ; Stockman, PT; Dunnegan, DL; Ashley, SW: Laparoscopic cholecystectomy: The new "gold standard"? Arch Surg 127:917–923, 1992.
4. Ponsky, JL: Presidential address of The Society of American Gastrointestinal Endoscopic Surgeons. Meeting, Washington, D.C., 1992.
5. MacFadyen, BV: Product review: Three-dimensional video system. Surg 2:3:273, 1992.
6. Green, P; Satava, R; Hill, J; Simon, I: Telepresence: Advanced teleoperator technology for minimally invasive surgery. (Abstract) Surg Endosc 6:62–67, 1992.
7. Sheridan, TB: Telerobotics. Automatica 25:487–507, 1989.
8. Timoney, AG; Ing, WF; Davis, BL; et al: The use of robots in surgery. The development of a frame for prostatectomy. J Endourol 5:165–168, 1991.
9. Simon, IB. Surgery 2001: Concepts of telepresence surgery. Surg Endosc 7:462, 1993.

Index

Note: Page numbers in *italics* refer to illustrations; page numbers followed by t refer to tables.

V

ISBN 0-7216-3766-3

90038

9 780721 637662